An Atlas of
FOOT AND ANKLE SURGERY

Second edition

An Atlas of
FOOT AND ANKLE SURGERY

Second edition

Edited by

Nikolaus Wülker
Orthopaedic Department
Tübingen University Hospital
Tübingen, Germany

Michael M. Stephens
Cappagh National Orthopaedic Hospital
Dublin, Ireland

Andrea Cracchiolo III
Orthopaedic Surgery
David Geffen School of Medicine at UCLA
Los Angeles, California, USA

With illustrations from

Andrea Rosenmeier
Cornelia Kaubisch
Léon Dorn
Karl-Horst Richardt

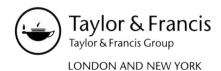

Taylor & Francis
Taylor & Francis Group

LONDON AND NEW YORK

© 2005 Taylor & Francis, an imprint of the Taylor & Francis Group

First published in the United Kingdom in 2005
by Taylor & Francis,
an imprint of the Taylor & Francis Group,
2 Park Square, Milton Park
Abingdon, Oxon OX14 4RN, UK

Tel.:   +44 (0) 20 7017 6000
Fax.:   +44 (0) 20 7017 6699
E.mail: info.medicine@tandf.co.uk
Website: www.tandf.co.uk/medicine

British Library Cataloguing in Publication Data

Data available on application

Library of Congress Cataloging-in-Publication Data

Data available on application

ISBN 1-84184-195-1

Distributed in North and South America by

Taylor & Francis
2000 NW Corporate Blvd
Boca Raton, FL 33431, USA

Within Continental USA
Tel.: 800 272 7737; Fax.: 800 374 3401
Outside Continental USA
Tel.: 561 994 0555; Fax.: 561 361 6018
E-mail: orders@crcpress.com

Distributed in the rest of the world by
Thomson Publishing Services
Cheriton House
North Way
Andover, Hampshire SP10 5BE, UK
Tel.: +44 (0) 1264 332424
E-mail: salesorder.tandf@thomsonpublishingservices.co.uk

Composition by C&M Digitals (P) Ltd., Chennai, India
Printed and bound by T.G. Hostench S.A., Spain

Contents

List of contributors

John Angel FRCS
26 The Grove
Radlett
Herts WD7 7NF
UK

Louis Samuel Barouk MD
Polyclinique de Bordeaux
151, rue du Tondu
33000 Bordeaux
France

Dr Martin Beck
Inselspital
3010 Bern
Switzerland

Wendy Benton-Weil DPM
Weil Foot and Ankle Institute
1455 Golf Road
Des Plaines, IL 60016
USA

Francesco Ceccarelli
Istituto Ortopedico Rizzoli
Via GC Pupilli 1
40136 Bologna
Italy

John Corrigan FRCSI FRCSI(Orth) MCh
Waterford Regional Hospital
Waterford
Ireland

Roderick Coull BA, FRCS(Orth)
Department of Orthopaedic Surgery
Watford General Hospital
Watford WD18 OHB
UK

Andrea Cracchiolo III MD
Orthopaedic Surgery
David Geffen School of Medicine at UCLA
PO Box 956902
10833 Le Conte Avenue
Los Angeles, CA 90095
USA

Alvin H. Crawford
Department of Orthopedics
Children's Hospital Medical Center
3333 Bennett Avenue
Cincinnati, OH 45229
USA

Georges Curvale
Service d'Orthopédie
Hôpital de la Conception
147 boulevard Baille
13005 Marseille
France

Greta Dereymaeker MD PhD
University Hospital Pellenberg
Catholic University of Leuven
Weligerveld 1
3212 Pellenberg
Belgium

Abubakar A. Durrani
Department of Orthopedics
Children's Hospital Medical Center
3333 Bennett Avenue
Cincinnati, OH 45229
USA

Dr Wolf Fröhlich
Unfallchirurgische Abteilung
AKH Linz
Krankenhausstrasse 1
4020 Linz
Austria

Renée-Andrea Fuhrmann MD PhD
Department of Orthopedic Surgery
University of Jena
Rudolf-Elle-Hospital
Klostelausnitzerstrasse 81
07607 Eisenberg
Germany

Johann Marian Gavlik MD
Klinik und Poliklinik für Unfall-
   und Wiederherstellungschirurgie
Universitätsklinikum Carl-Gustav Carus
Fetscherstrasse 74
01307 Dresden
Germany

Sandro Giannini MD
Istituto Ortopedico Rizzoli
Via GC Pupilli 1
40136 Bologna
Italy

David Grace FRCS
Chase Farm Hospitals NHS Trust
The Ridgeway
Enfield EN2 8JL
UK

Sigvard T. Hansen MD
Harborview Medical Center
University of Washington
325 Ninth Avenue
Seattle, WA 98104
USA

Nicholas J. Harris FRCS(Ed)
Leeds General Infirmary
Great George Street
Leeds LS1 3EX
UK

Beat Hintermann MD
Department of Orthopedic Surgery
University of Basel
Kantonsspital
4031 Basel
Switzerland

Suguru Inokuchi MD PhD
Department of Orthopedic Surgery
Keio University
35 Shinanomachi
Shinjuku-ku
Tokyo 160
Japan

Dr Kaj Klaue
Atos-Klinik
Bismarkstrasse 9–15
69115 Heidelberg
Germany

Patrick Laing FRCS(Ed)
Robert Jones and Agnes Hunt Orthopaedic Hospital
Oswestry
SY10 7AG
UK

Nilesh Makwana MS BS
   FRCS(Orth and Traum)
Robert Jones and Agnes Hunt
Orthopaedic Hospital
Oswestry SY10 7AG
UK

Prof Francesco Malerba
Istituto Ortopedico Galeazzi
Via R Galeazzi 4
Milano 20161
Italy

Roger A. Mann MD
3300 Webster Street, Suite 608
Oakland, CA 94609
USA

Alain C. Masquelet MD
Service d'Orthopédie et Traumatologie
Hôpital Avicenne
125 route de Stalingrad
93009 Bobigny
France

William C. McGarvey MD
Orthopedic Surgery
University of Texas Health Science Center
6500 Fannin, Suite 1006
Houston, TX 77030
USA

Thomas Mittlmeier MD
Chirurgische Klinik und Poliklinik der Universität
   Rostock
Unfall- und Wierderherstellungschirurgie
Schillingallee 35
18055 Rostock
Germany

Stephen Parsons FRCS FRCS(Ed)
Department of Orthopaedics
Royal Cornwall Hospital Treliske
Infirmary Hill
Truro TR1 3LJ
UK

Dr Jean Pfändler
Inselspital
3010 Bern
Switzerland

Stefan Rammelt MD
Klinik und Poliklinik für Unfall- und
Wiederherstellungschirurgie
Universitätsklinikum Carl-Gustav Carus
Fetscherstrasse 74
01307 Dresden
Germany

Prof Dr Rudolf Reschauer
Unfallchirurgische Abteilung
AKH Linz
Krankenhausstrasse 1
4020 Linz
Austria

Alexandre Rochwerger
Service d'Orthopédie
Hôpital de la Conception
147 boulevard Baille
13005 Marseille
France

Andreas Roth MD
Department of Orthopedic Surgery
University of Jena
Rudolf-Elle-Hospital
Klostelausnitzerstrasse 81
07607 Eisenberg
Germany

Thomas W.D. Smith FRCS(Ed) FRCS
Orthopaedic Department
Northern General Hospital
Herries Road
Sheffield S5 7AU
UK

Dr Mathias Speck
Inselspital
3010 Bern
Switzerland

Michael M. Stephens MSc FRCSI
Cappagh National Orthopaedic Hospital
Dublin 1
Ireland

Yoshinori Takakura MD
Department of Orthopedic Surgery
Nara Medical University Hospital
Kashihara
Nara 634-8522
Japan

Priv Doz Dr Hajo Thermann
Knie- und Fusschirurgie
ATOS-Klinik
D-69115 Heidelberg
Germany

Univ Doz Dr Hans-Jörg Trnka
Fusszentrum Wein
Mariannengasse 14/1/2
1090 Wien
Austria

Prof Dr Harald Tscherne
Unfallchirurgische Klinik
Medizinsche Hochschule Hannover
30006 Hannover
Germany

Victor Valderrabano MD
Clinic of Orthopedic Surgery
University of Basel
Kantonsspital
4031 Basel
Switzerland

Dr Bernard Valtin
72 Avenue Jack Gourevitch
94500 Champigny
France

Antonio Viladot Voegeli
Servicio de Cirurgia Ortopedica y
Traumatologica
Clinica Tres Torres
Barcelona 08017
Spain

Henry P.J. Walsh MCh(Orth) FRCS
Department of Orthopaedic Surgery
The Mater Hospital
Raymond Terrace
South Brisbane
Queensland 4101
Australia

Lowell Scott Weil Sr DPM FACFAS
Weil Foot and Ankle Institute
1455 Golf Road
Des Plaines, IL 60016
USA

Ian Winson FRCS
Avon Orthopaedic Surgery
Southmead Hospital
Bristol BS10 5NB
UK

Prof Dr Nikolaus Wülker
Orthopaedic Department
Tübingen University Hospital
Hoppe-Seyler-Strasse 3
72076 Tübingen
Germany

Hans Zollinger-Kies MD
Orthopedic Surgery
Bahnhofstrasse 56
8001 Zürich
Switzerland

Prof Dr Hans Zwipp
Klinik und Poliklinik für Unfall- und
Wiederherstellungschirurgie
Universitätsklinikum Carl-Gustav Carus
Fetscherstrasse 74
01307 Dresden
Germany

Preface

Foot and ankle surgery differs from other surgical specialities in a number of ways. Most importantly, foot and ankle surgery is very unforgiving. A little too much tension on the soft tissues or some over-correction of an osteotomy may cause considerable dissatisfaction of the patient. He or she will look at their feet every day and note that the result of surgery is not optimal. This is why surgical technique matters so much at the foot and ankle. It is the authors' hope that this second edition of *An Atlas of Foot and Ankle Surgery* will help surgeons understand the principles and the details of commonly used surgical procedures.

In addition, more surgical procedures have probably been described at the foot and ankle than anywhere else. Over 150 techniques exist for surgical correction of hallux valgus alone. This causes considerable confusion concerning the indications, technique and postoperative treatment of each procedure. This book is designed to assist surgeons in their choice of procedure for each individual patient.

Furthermore, technology, including implants and instruments, has only little influence on the outcome of foot and ankle procedures. It is mostly the surgeon's skills that decide the postoperative result. Therefore, surgeons may find the explanations in this book particularly helpful.

In the second edition of this Atlas, more than half of the material has been completely revised or rewritten. The reader will find more consistency between the chapters, as more procedures are described by the editors, who have particular expertise in a broad range of foot and ankle surgery. Some less important topics have been deleted, such as 'Subtalar arthrodesis', other important chapters have been added, such as 'The treatment of flat foot in children'. Again, a specific effort has been made to illustrate all important steps of the procedure with artful illustrations, and to present the corresponding detail in a comprehensive text. An important bibliography is listed at the end of each chapter.

The editors extend their gratitude to the great number of authors, who have spent much time on writing or rewriting their chapters and going through sometimes lengthy revision. Their efforts will be repaid by surgeons and patients who will all benefit from a high standard of surgical foot and ankle care. Ms Kaubisch is thanked for revising a number of the hand drawings that contribute much to the appearance of the book. Last, but not least, Robert Peden and the other editors from Taylor & Francis have always been helpful to this large and international group of editors and authors.

Nikolaus Wülker
Michael M. Stephens
Andrea Cracchiolo III

1

Hallux valgus: proximal phalangeal osteotomy

Louis Samuel Barouk

Introduction

Proximal phalangeal osteotomy in hallux valgus is most often performed in combination with other procedures [Akin 1925, Collof and Weitz 1967, Giannestras 1972, Silberman 1972, Seelenfreund and Fried 1973, Lavigne 1974, Magerl 1982, Bonnevialle et al. 1986, Goldberg et al. 1987, Barouk 1988, 1992, 1993a, Plattner and Van Manen 1990]. As a single procedure, it is generally insufficient to correct the deformity of the great toe [Gutzeit-Neidenburg 1914, Barouk 1993b]. Prior to proximal phalangeal osteotomy, congruity of the first metatarsophalangeal joint must be restored, sesamoid displacement must be corrected and metatarsus primus varus must be repaired [Groulier et al. 1988, Barouk 1994, 2000]. Therefore, lateral release of the first metatarsophalangeal joint and medial capsular tightening as well as correction of the intermetatarsal angle, generally by osteotomy of the metatarsal [Jarde et al. 1999], must be completed, if necessary, prior to osteotomy of the first phalanx. However, I now add the proximal phalangeal osteotomy in more than 80% of patients having an operation for hallux valgus.

Indication

The indication for proximal phalangeal osteotomy is determined using the load simulation test, once first metatarsophalangeal joint congruity, sesamoid position and first metatarsal alignment have been corrected, and after any necessary surgery of the lesser rays has been completed. This test reproduces the position of the great toe during standing. The surgeon pushes in a dorsal direction against the sole of the foot, under the metatarsal heads, using the palm of the hand. During this maneuver, the length of the great toe, in comparison with the second toe, and the varus–valgus alignment of the great toe are determined. If the great toe is correctly positioned, i.e. the metatarsophalangeal joint is in correct alignment and its length equals that of the second toe, there is no indication for first phalanx osteotomy. If correction of the hallux valgus deformity is insufficient even though metatarsophalangeal joint congruity has been restored, or if the great toe remains longer than the second toe, osteotomy of the proximal phalanx must be considered. This often occurs in advanced hallux valgus. In these cases, alignment of the great toe without proximal phalangeal osteotomy can be achieved only with slight overcorrection at the metatarsophalangeal joint.

There are two types of proximal phalanx (P1) osteotomy: the basal osteotomy and the shaft osteotomy each has separate indications and techniques (Figure 1).

Basal osteotomy

- It is indicated when the great toe is not too long (Greek or square type foot).

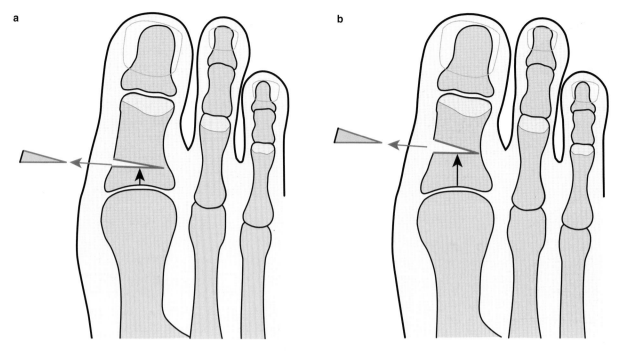

Figure 1

a. the basal osteotomy in the proximal metaphysis. The varization osteotomy removes a very thin wedge of medial cortex.
b. the shaft osteotomy can be used to shorten the hallux, as a derotation osteotomy or to correct interphalangeal valgus

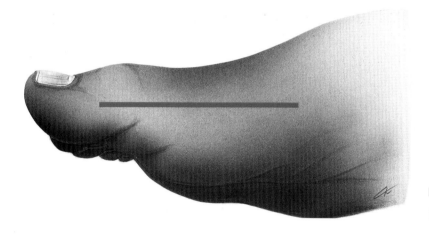

Figure 2

Incision for proximal phalangeal osteotomy

- It is performed in the proximal P1 metaphysis in cancellous bone and heals without problems.
- It preserves a lateral hinge located on the lateral cortex.
- Its fixation is easy thanks to a special small staple.

We distinguish two kinds of basal osteotomy:

1. Varization osteotomy (medial closing wedge) (Figure 1a). It is performed proximally to provide a large distal medial displacement despite removing a small medial wedge, because of the long distal lever arm.

2. Varization combined with derotation (Figure 1b). It is an oblique/plane osteotomy, described by P. Diebold (Nancy, France). This osteotomy is very useful for completing the hallux valgus correction, but the lateral hinge is more fragile. So, when large rotation is indicated we prefer to perform a shaft osteotomy.

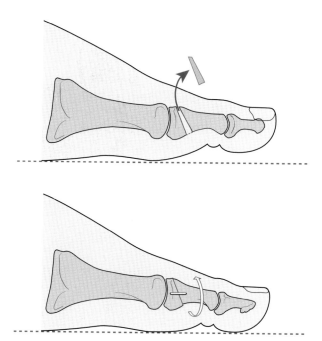

Figure 3

The basal osteotomy can be made obliquely, removing a plantar and medial wedge. A varus stress and derotation corrects mild rotation as well

Surgical technique

Basal osteotomy of the proximal phalanx

Proximal phalangeal osteotomy without shortening may be performed as a varus osteotomy and as a

derotation osteotomy. In many cases, a combination of both is necessary. The surgical approach is through a medial midline incision (Figure 2). The osteotomy is made proximally, generally within the proximal metaphysis of the phalanx. The cancellous bone in this location enhances bone healing. A proximal osteotomy also provides the greatest amount of medial correction of the great toe for a prescribed wedge size. It is important not to transect the lateral cortex, to provide maximum stability with minimum internal fixation. In the varus osteotomy, a smooth K-wire can be passed across the base of the phalanx parallel to the articular surface and just proximal to the osteotomy. The position of the K-wire can be checked using a fluoroscope to be certain it is not in the joint. A transverse cut is then made with a saw in the frontal plane, respecting the lateral cortex. The K-wire is removed and a second saw cut is made distal to the first and a medially based wedge is resected. However, only a very small wedge is generally required and it is preferable simply to widen the cut medially with the oscillating saw from inside the initial osteotomy. When varus stress is applied to the great toe, the two medial borders of the osteotomy come into contact. The lateral cortex at this location generally has sufficient elasticity to allow closure of the osteotomy without breaking. The varus osteotomy can also be performed in such a manner as to correct mild rotation, about 15°, of the hallux (Figure 3). The initial osteotomy is made obliquely, directed proximally and dorsally from the

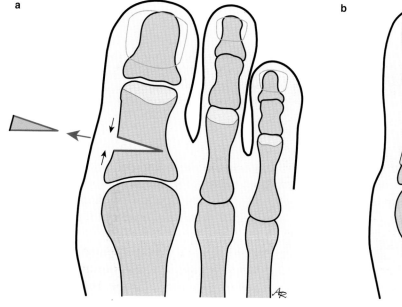
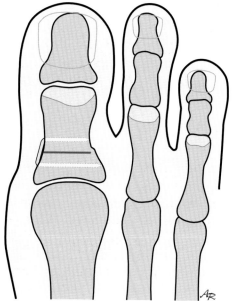

Figure 4

Varus osteotomy without shortening. a. before; b. after closure of the osteotomy and fixation with a specific oblique stainless steel staple

a

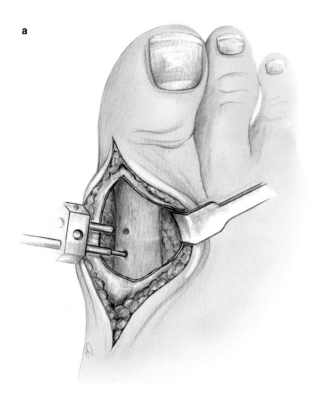

b

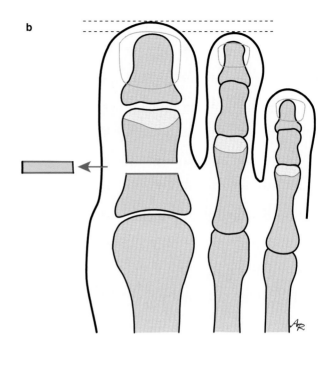

c

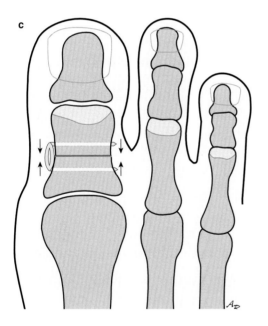

Figure 5

Osteotomy with shortening. a. intraoperative aspect: a guide is introduced around the Kirschner wire, which is inserted proximally into the medial aspect of the first phalanx. The proximal osteotomy is made at an equal distance between the proximal guide prong and the distal guide prong, which will later be used to drill the hole for the distal prong of the staple; b. osteotomy with shortening before closure of the osteotomy; c. osteotomy with shortening after closure; the staple provides bicortical medial and lateral compression

medial aspect of the proximal phalanx. A bone wedge with a medial and plantar base is removed. During closure of the osteotomy, a varus stress and derotation correct the deformity.

Fixation

A specific oblique staple may be used for fixation (Figure 4), while the varus position and the derotation of the great toe are maintained. This staple is shaped to conform to the obliquity of the medial proximal phalangeal surface. It thus avoids penetration of the proximal prong into the metatarsophalangeal joint, in spite of its proximal location. Prior to insertion of the staple, a hole is made distal to the osteotomy with a 1.0-mm Kirschner wire, which is the same diameter as the staple prong. The staple is directed laterally into the phalanx. Impaction of the staple is performed preferentially at its proximal prong. In the derotation osteotomy, instability of the fragments may require fixation with a cannulated threaded-head screw.

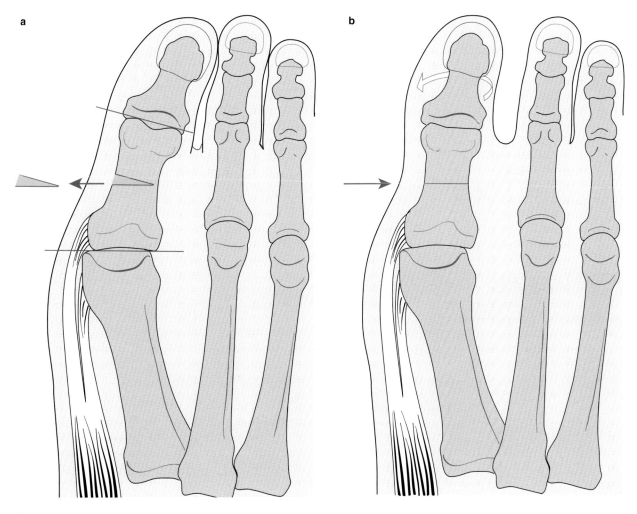

Figure 6

a–b. a shaft osteotomy, which is needed only to derotate the hallux in patients with moderate or severe rotational deformity

Shaft osteotomy

Osteotomy technique

- It is performed with a cut perpendicular to the shaft, so that it allows a large range of correction.
- It is less stable than the basal osteotomy, needing stronger fixation. We distinguish three kinds of shaft osteotomy: shortening, derotation and shaft varization.

Shortening osteotomy

This (Figure 5) is indicated when the great toe is too long (Egyptian type foot) compared to the second toe (more than 3 mm longer). The P1 shortening improves the correction by reducing the phalangeal arm (bowstring effect). It also reduces the dorsiflexion angle during the toe-off phase of gait, and reduces the longitudinal pressure provided by the shoe; the forefoot becomes square.

Derotation osteotomy

This (Figure 6) is indicated when moderate or large lateral rotation remains on the great toe (more than 20°) and also when there is need of only derotation, without varization.

Shaft varization osteotomy

This (Figure 1b) is indicated when there is interphalangeal valgus.

A cannulated threaded-head screw may be used for fixation (Figure 7). This screw has slightly different thread inclinations at its head and its core, in order to provide compression of the osteotomy. Prior to insertion of the screw, a Kirschner wire

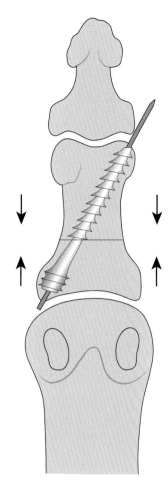

Figure 7

An alternative to the memory staple, a cannulated threaded-head screw can be used for fixation of a shaft osteotomy

(1 mm in diameter) is introduced obliquely into the proximal phalanx, from its proximal and medial corner to the lateral distal corner. The length of the screw can be measured from the guide wire or determined by intraoperative radiography. The screw must be accurately positioned in the lateral distal corner of the proximal phalanx, in order to obtain strong purchase of the screw thread. If the orientation of the screw is too oblique, fixation will not be sufficiently strong; if the screw is too much in line with the axis of the proximal phalanx, the screw may pass into the interphalangeal joint. The threaded proximal end of the screw must be positioned underneath the surface of the metaphyseal bone.

Alternatively, a specific metal staple can be used for fixation (Figure 5). When cooled and held in a forceps, this staple has parallel prongs and a slightly oval body. After removal of the forceps and warming of the staple to body temperature, the prongs converge to provide compression at the lateral side of the osteotomy, and the body of the staple takes a

more rounded shape for compression medially. This implant is also referred to as the memory staple (DePuy, Warsaw, Indiana). It is specifically shaped to the dimensions of the proximal phalanx and provides permanent bicortical compression both medially and laterally, even if bone resorption around the osteotomy should occur.

Following the osteotomy, temporary axial Kirschner wire fixation (1 mm in diameter) is recommended. This provides accurate control of the correction with regard to the valgus–varus alignment, and thereby yields a firm working plane during fixation of the osteotomy. The distal drill hole is then made with the use of the guide. The prongs have to be long enough to cross the lateral cortex, in order to provide strong fixation and to avoid penetration of the prongs into the osteotomy under compression. In most cases an equal length is necessary for the two prongs. However, the staple is also available with a length difference of 2 mm. A trial staple is inserted. If this does not pass into the drill holes with ease, the drill should be used in the holes one more time. After extraction of the trial staple, the memory staple is inserted into the proximal phalanx and impacted. Once the tourniquet is deflated, the memory staple warms and will provide compression at the lateral and at the medial cortex of the phalanx.

Postoperative care

For the osteotomy either with or without shortening, the described fixation is sufficiently strong to allow early functional postoperative treatment. For the first 15 days after surgery a heel support shoe is worn, followed by a flat postoperative shoe. Removal of the screws or staples is not necessary.

Complications

The flexor hallucis longus tendon must not be injured during the osteotomy. If, when doing the basal osteotomy, the integrity of the lateral cortex is not observed, loss of stability may require fixation with two staples or with the cannulated screw. When the varus osteotomy is combined with derotation, the preserved segment of the lateral cortex is small. If a large amount of derotation is necessary, it is preferable to perform the derotation in the shaft of the phalanx. In the shaft-shortening and derotation osteotomies, strong internal fixation with the threaded-head cannulated screw or with the memory staple is required. Excessive derotation can easily be avoided. Excessive varus alignment must be avoided, as this will result in painful contact with the shoe postoperatively. Staple expulsion or penetration of the prongs through the osteotomy cut should not occur, if details of the procedure are observed.

Conclusion

The great toe proximal phalanx osteotomies are very helpful, particularly as a complementary procedure to reduce hallux valgus deformity. The location, the technique and the indication have to be accurate to provide the required displacement and early functional recovery.

References

Akin O (1925) The treatment of hallux valgus: a new operative treatment and its results. Med Sentinel 33: 678

Barouk LS (1988) Indications et technique des osteotomies extra-articulaires du gros orteil. Med Chir Pied 4: 147–154

Barouk LS (1992) Osteotomies of the great toe. J Foot Surg 31 (4): 388–399

Barouk LS (1993a) Chirurgie de l'hallux valgus. Intérêt de l'ostéotomie de varisation-dérotation phalangienne. In: Benamou PH, Montagne J (eds) Actualités en médecine et chirurgie du pied. Paris, Masson, pp 93–105

Barouk LS (1993b) Le raccourcissement du gros orteil: intérêt de l'agrafe à mémoire spécifique. In: Benamou PH, Montagne J (eds) Actualites en médecine et chirurgie du pied. Paris, Masson, pp 93–105

Barouk LS (1994) Great toe osteotomies in the hallux valgus. Personal experience. Therapeutic proposition. Foot Diseases 1: 79–89

Barouk LS (2000) Scarf osteotomy for hallux valgus correction. Foot Ankle Clin 5 (3): 525–558

Bonnevialle P, Baudet B, Mansat M et al. (1986) Place de l'osteotomie phalangienne dans la cure chirurgicale de l'hallux valgus. In: Actualites en médecine et chirurgie du pied. Paris, Expansion Scientifique Francaise, pp 29–33

Colloff B, Weitz EM (1967) Proximal phalangeal osteotomy in hallux valgus. Clin Orthop 54: 105–113

Giannestras NJ (1972) Modified Akin procedure for the correction of hallux valgus. Am Acad Orthop Surg 21: 254–262

Goldberg I, Bahar A, Yosipovichz Z (1987) Late results after correction of hallux valgus deformity by basilar phalangeal osteotomy. J Bone Joint Surg 69A: 64–67

Groulier P, Curvale G, Prudent HP, Vedel F (1988) Resultats du traitement de l'hallux valgus selon la technique de Mac Bridge 'modifiée' avec ou sans osteotomie phalangienne ou metatarsienne complémentaire. Rev Chir Orthop 74: 539–548

Gutzeit-Neidenburg R (1914) Über Hallux valgus interphalangeus. Münchner Med Wschr 1: 1146

Jarde O, Tringquier JL, Gabrion A et al. (1999) Hallux valgus traité par une osteotomie de scarf du premier metatarsien et de la premiere phalange associée a une plastie de l'abducteur. Rev Chir Orthop 85: 374–380

Lavigne P (1974) L'osteotomie de la premiere phalange dans le traitement de l'hallux valgus. Ann Orthop Ouest 6: 11–16

Magerl F (1982) Stabile Osteotomien zur Behandlung des Hallux valgus. Orthopäde 11: 170–180

Plattner PF, Van Manen JW (1990) Results of Akin type proximal phalangeal osteotomy for correction of hallux valgus deformity. Orthopedics 13: 989–996

Seelenfreund M, Fried A (1973) Correction of hallux valgus deformity by basal phalanx osteotomy of the big toe. J Bone Joint Surg 55A: 1411–1415

Silberman F (1972) Proximal phalangeal osteotomy for the correction of hallux valgus. Rev Chir Orthop 85: 98–100

2

Hallux valgus: distal first metatarsal osteotomies

Nikolaus Wülker

Introduction

Lateral deviation of the great toe and a prominent bunion at the first metatarsal head are the obvious deformities in hallux valgus. However, the detailed pathology varies considerably between individuals and usually consists of a combination of the following factors:

- A soft tissue imbalance is present at the first metatarsophalangeal joint, with contracted soft tissues laterally (adductor tendon, joint capsule) and an insufficient capsule medially. This results in incongruence (subluxation) of the phalangeal joint surface on the metatarsal head surface, which is evident on the weightbearing dorsoplantar radiograph.
- The first metatarsal is deviated medially (metatarsus primus varus). The angle between the first and the second metatarsal (intermetatarsal angle) on the weightbearing dorsoplantar radiograph is often increased to more than 15°. The normal angle is less than 10°.
- The first metatarsal head articular surface is tilted laterally. The normal orientation is within 5–7° to the perpendicular to the diaphyseal axis of the first metatarsal (distal metatarsal articular angle; DMAA). In hallux valgus patients, deviation may be increased to more than 15°.
- The proximal phalanx of the hallux may be angulated in a lateral direction (hallux valgus interphalangeus).

Distal first metatarsal osteotomies correct the hallux valgus deformity by displacing the first metatarsal head into a more lateral position and rotating the articular surface medially. Metatarsal osteotomies do not correct the soft tissue balance at the metatarsophalangeal joint or hallux valgus interphalangeus. A number of different techniques have been used since the original description more than 100 years ago [Reverdin 1881]. The Hohmann osteotomy was most popular in Europe during the first half of the 20th century [Hohmann 1951]. The Mitchell osteotomy has mostly been used in North America [Mitchell et al. 1958]. Kramer modified the Hohmann osteotomy [Kramer 1990]. The Chevron osteotomy has rapidly gained popularity since its introduction in 1962 [Austin and Leventen 1981]. Other techniques of distal first metatarsal osteotomy have also been described [Gibson and Piggot 1962, Wilson 1963, Magerl 1982].

Indications for surgery

Increasing pain over the bunion, encroachment of the lesser toes, pain at the first metatarsophalangeal joint and transfer metatarsalgia are common indications for hallux valgus surgery. Reconstructive procedures at the great toe should not be performed for cosmetic reasons alone.

Distal first metatarsal osteotomies can correct the alignment of the articular surface by rotating the head fragment in a medial direction. Therefore, an increased DMAA is an indication. Metatarsus primus varus can be corrected by lateral displacement of the first metatarsal head. However, the head cannot be translated more than one-half the width of the distal first metatarsal, in order not to compromise stability. This limits correction of the intermetatarsal angle to approximately 5–7°.

Soft tissue imbalance at the first metatarsophalangeal joint is the predominant pathology in most advanced hallux valgus deformities. This cannot be corrected with the distal first metatarsal osteotomy alone. Also, malalignment at the proximal phalanx is not corrected.

In summary, the indication for distal first metatarsal osteotomy is mild to moderate hallux valgus (hallux valgus angle <35°) with no or only mild incongruence of the metatarsophalangeal joint and an intermetatarsal angle of less than 15°. More advanced hallux valgus with incongruence of the first metatarsophalangeal joint is corrected with the distal soft tissue procedure and proximal metatarsal osteotomy (see Chapter 3). If significant hallux valgus interphalangeus is present, this is corrected by additional osteotomy of the proximal phalanx (see Chapter 1).

Distal first metatarsal osteotomies are not indicated if significant degenerative changes have developed at the first metatarsophalangeal joint. As in all reconstructive hallux procedures, the prognosis for recovery of function of the hallux is significantly compromised if joint space narrowing is present on preoperative radiographs, if joint pain or a decreased range of motion are noted on clinical examination, or if degeneration of the articular surfaces is observed intraoperatively. These patients should rather undergo resection arthroplasty (if elderly, see Chapter 9) or arthrodesis of the metatarsophalangeal joint (if physically active, see Chapter 8).

Peripheral vascular disease with absent pedal pulses is the major contraindication to distal first metatarsal osteotomy. Delayed wound healing or necrosis may ensue if this is not observed.

Surgical technique

General considerations

- Biplanar osteotomies are inherently more stable than monoplanar osteotomies. This is particularly true for the Chevron osteotomy. Improved stability decreases postoperative swelling and the incidence of non-union and avascular necrosis. It also allows early postoperative weightbearing.

- Osteotomies within the first metatarsal head (e.g. the Chevron osteotomy) have larger bone surfaces than osteotomies proximal to the head (subcapital). This enhances bone healing and allows more lateral displacement of the head fragment. However, the risk of avascular necrosis of the head fragment is also increased.

- Most distal first metatarsal osteotomies include resection of a medially based bone wedge to reorient the first metatarsal head articular surface. A bone wedge can also be resected in biplanar osteotomies.

- Various methods of internal fixation are available for distal first metatarsal osteotomies. Some procedures have been used without internal stabilization. However, loss of reduction and nonunion may occur. Therefore, internal fixation with a screw or a wire has become the standard for all osteotomies.

- Simultaneous adductor tenotomy in distal first metatarsal osteotomies is controversial. This is generally performed through a separate incision in the first web space. It does not appear to increase the incidence of avascular head necrosis significantly, in spite of interruption of the blood supply lateral to the metatarsal head. Tenotomy may be indicated if significant contracture of the adductor tendon is present. However, hallux valgus patients with a significant soft tissue imbalance are better treated with a distal soft tissue procedure (see Chapter 3).

- Some surgeons perform distal first metatarsal osteotomies through a small stab incision. A high-speed burr is used to make the osteotomy, and fixation is usually with a Kirschner wire in the soft tissues. This technique requires little skill by the surgeon, but does not allow precise, anatomic realignment of the metatarsal head and joint.

Operative technique

The procedure is performed with the patient in the supine position. Regional, local or general anesthesia may be used. The foot is exsanguinated with a rubber (Esmarch) bandage.

Chevron osteotomy

A straight medial skin incision is made from the proximal phalanx to the proximal limit of the exostosis at the metatarsal head (Figure 1). Skin flaps are raised to expose the thick capsular tissue overlying

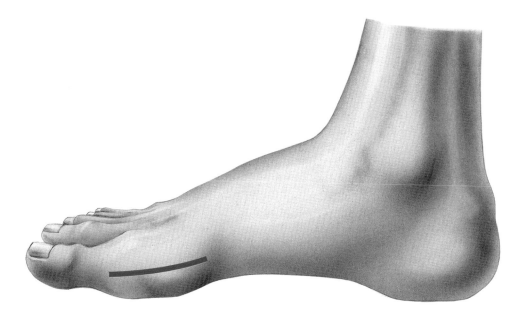

Figure 1

The skin incision for distal first metatarsal osteotomies reaches from the middle of the proximal phalanx to the middle of the first metatarsal

the exostosis. Flaps must be thick enough to secure postoperative perfusion and wound healing.

The capsule is divided parallel to the metatarsophalangeal joint line and immediately proximal to it. An L-shaped capsulotomy is created by extending the capsular incision at its dorsal end in a proximal direction. Alternatively, a longitudinal or V-shaped capsulotomy may be used. A bursa may be present over the exostosis. The thick capsular and bursal tissue is peeled off the exostosis, where it is usually quite adherent to bone. A pointed Hohmann retractor is inserted without further dissection at the plantar aspect just proximal to the first metatarsal head. A major portion of the blood supply to the head enters at this site and head perfusion must not be unduly disturbed. Dorsally, the periosteum immediately proximal to the capsular insertion is elevated and another Hohmann retractor is inserted.

Retraction of the hallux in a lateral direction exposes the articular surface of the first metatarsal head. A sagittal sulcus is usually found, separating the anatomic joint surface from the exostosis. Resection of the exostosis begins just medial to the bottom of this groove. Proximally, resection is in line with the medial border of the first metatarsal diaphysis. An oscillating saw is most convenient; alternatively, an osteotome may be used. Care must be taken to orient the resection in the sagittal plane, i.e. at a right angle to the sole of the foot. The resection edges are rounded with a rongeur.

A 2-mm drill hole is made medially to laterally through the center of the first metatarsal head (Figure 2a). This will serve as an exit point for the osteotomies and help to avoid fracture of the metatarsal head by excessive stresses at the apex of the saw cuts. The drill may be directed slightly in a plantar direction, which will move the head plantarward and improve loading of the first ray postoperatively. Some lengthening of the first metatarsal may also be desirable. However, distal displacement of the head fragment by distal orientation of the drill hole increases tension of the soft tissue and may prevent adequate lateral displacement of the head. Shortening of the first metatarsal should generally be avoided.

In the original description of the Chevron osteotomy two cuts were made at an angle of 60°, joined at the drill hole in the head center. A modified Chevron osteotomy is now commonly used, in which the plantar leg of the osteotomy is made in an almost horizontal orientation to exit the bone a few millimeters proximal to the resected surface of the medial exostosis (Figure 2b). The dorsal leg is almost vertical, exiting the bone just proximal to the insertion of the capsule. This modification provides several advantages: bone healing is promoted by larger osteotomy surfaces; the vascular supply at the plantar proximal aspect of the metatarsal head is better preserved; internal fixation is facilitated by a larger plantar fragment; and improved stability allows immediate postoperative weightbearing. The osteotomies must end precisely at the central drill hole in the head. Care is taken not to injure the lateral soft tissues with the saw. The head fragment is carefully mobilized with an osteotome. Fracture of the head fragment during this maneuver is a major complication and difficult to salvage.

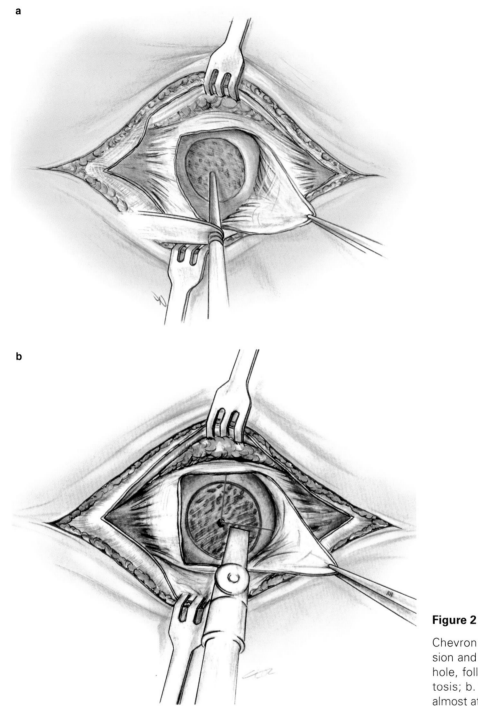

Figure 2

Chevron osteotomy. a. capsular incision and placement of the central drill hole, following resection of the exostosis; b. two osteotomies are placed almost at a right angle

In some hallux valgus patients, the articular surface of the first metatarsal head is significantly tilted in a lateral direction (increased DMAA). This is corrected by removing a small medially based bone wedge from the dorsal osteotomy cut, usually from the proximal fragment. The width of the wedge can be only roughly estimated and does not exceed 2–3 mm. Reorientation of the articular surface is observed when the head fragment is rotated medially by closing the osteotomy.

Lateral displacement of the head must be one-third to one-half of the first metatarsal diameter. This is usually achieved by a combination of tension and manipulation on the hallux, pressure on the head fragment in a lateral direction and manipulation of the osteotomy with an osteotome. In addition, the proximal fragment may have to be retracted medially with an elevator or a pointed clamp. Once sufficient displacement is attained, the surgeon must make sure that both the plantar and

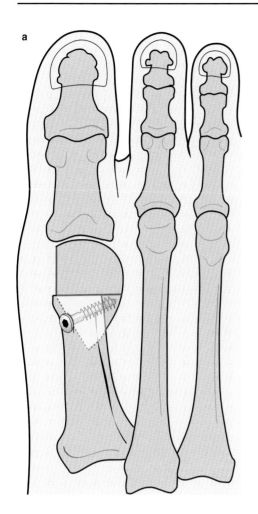

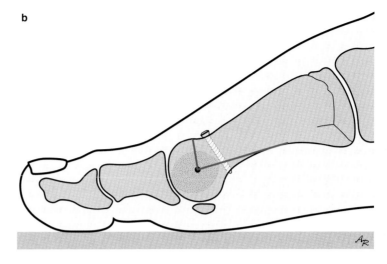

Figure 3

Stabilization of the laterally displaced first metatarsal head with a screw. The screw passes from dorsal medial through the osteotomy site and just out through the cortex plantar and lateral. a. dorsal aspect; b. medial aspect

the dorsal osteotomy surfaces are in immediate contact.

No internal fixation was used in the original description of the Chevron osteotomy. However, loss of reduction and non-union or malunion may occur. Internal stabilization with implants is now recommended. During fixation, the osteotomy is held reduced by axial pressure on the hallux by an assistant. Internal fixation may be with a 1.6-mm Kirschner wire inserted from the dorsomedial surface of the proximal fragment in a lateral and plantar direction, where it just penetrates the cortex. Care must be taken not to place the wire inside the joint. The upper end may be bent and left in the subcutaneous tissues, or the wire is left protruding through a stab incision in the skin, protected with a cap and pulled in the office 3 weeks postoperatively. A small fragment screw can also be used in the same orientation as the wire, preferably as a lag screw by overdrilling the dorsal cortex (Figure 3). The head must be sufficiently countersunk to avoid pressure under the skin. The screw is generally removed 1 year postoperatively. Depending on the skill and experience of the surgeon, intraoperative

fluoroscopy may be used to ascertain correct placement. Absorbable implants are now less frequently used, owing to their cost and because osteolysis around the implant may occur. Following fixation, prominent bone at the proximal fragment is removed with a saw or a rongeur.

The capsulotomy is closed with absorbable sutures. A vertical strip, 2–4 mm wide, may have to be resected prior to closure. It is imperative that the hallux be in anatomic alignment following closure of the capsule. The skin is closed in a routine fashion. Excess skin does not need to be excised as redundant skin reduces within 2 weeks after surgery. A soft dressing is applied and a protruding wire tip is protected. Following release of the tourniquet, skin perfusion at the hallux must be secured. If this does not return within a few minutes, the dressing must be removed.

Postoperatively, the patient is supplied with a firm shoe to prevent rolling over the operated toe. Full weightbearing is allowed immediately, but patients must largely limit their activities during the first 2 weeks to prevent swelling. Patients are instructed to apply the reduction bandage

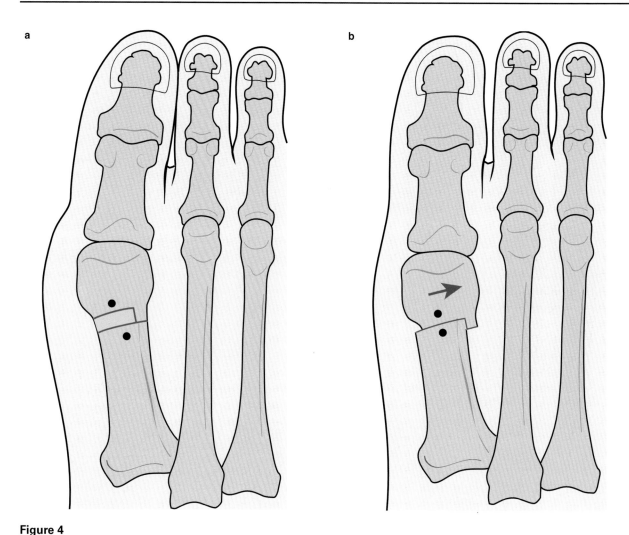

Figure 4

Mitchell osteotomy. a. area of bone resection; b. following lateral translation of the metatarsal head. Note the placement of drill holes for osteosutures

themselves daily. At 2 weeks, skin sutures are removed and gentle active and passive range of motion exercises are begun. At 3 weeks a Kirschner wire is pulled. Six weeks postoperatively, the postoperative shoe is discontinued and patients are instructed to use their great toe intentionally during walking.

Mitchell osteotomy

The joint capsule and the periosteum are opened with a distally opened Y-shaped incision, centered slightly proximal to the metatarsophalangeal joint. The exostosis is removed in line with the first metatarsal shaft. The level of the osteotomy cuts is determined through the neck of the first metatarsal. A first, complete osteotomy is made just proximal to the base of the neck of the first metatarsal (Figure 4). The second osteotomy is made parallel to the first osteotomy and 3 mm more distal. It does not go

through the lateral cortex, leaving a lateral spike. The distance between the osteotomies may be adjusted for the relative length of the first metatarsal. However, excessive shortening usually results if more than 3 mm is removed. The wedge may be made wider on the plantar than on the dorsal side to displace the head inferiorly. The head is shifted laterally, with the lateral cortex spike overlapping the shaft. The protruding portion of shaft at the medial side of the proximal fragment is removed.

Screw fixation with a small fragment cancellous screw is recommended, because the original suture fixation is quite unstable and requires non-weight-bearing postoperatively. The screw is placed in a proximal dorsomedial to distal plantar–lateral direction. The protruding fraction of shaft is removed with a saw. The capsule is tightened and closed in a Y–V fashion or with oblique capsular reefing. The skin is closed. Screw fixation is usually stable enough to allow early postoperative weightbearing.

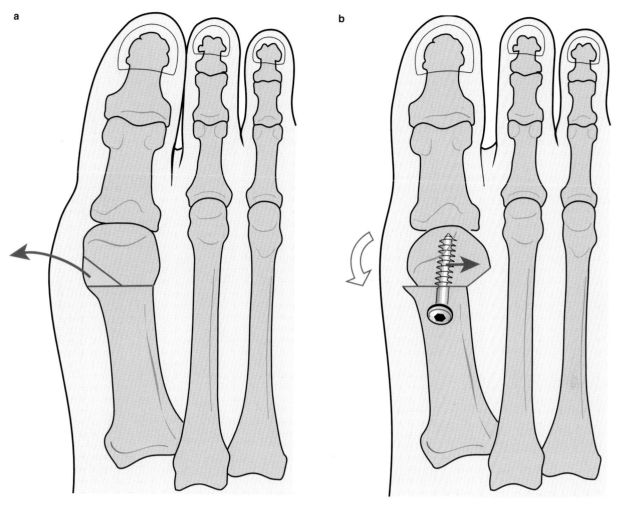

Figure 5

Hohmann osteotomy. a. area of bone resection; b. displacement of the metatarsal head and stabilization with a screw

Hohmann osteotomy

The skin incision must reach the first tarsometatarsal joint to allow dissection of the abductor hallucis tendon and muscle. The tendon is released to approximately mid-metatarsal level. The metatarsophalangeal joint is not generally opened. Retractors are placed behind the metatarsal neck. The first osteotomy is placed perpendicular to the metatarsal shaft at the juncture of the metatarsal head and neck, preferably with an oscillating saw (Figure 5). With the second osteotomy, a wedge-shaped section is removed from the head fragment, with a medial base. The width of the wedge corresponds to the desired angular correction of the hallux. The wedge may be shorter than the diameter of the first metatarsal, in order to avoid shortening of the first ray. A certain amount of plantar displacement of the first metatarsal head can be obtained by making the wedge wider on the plantar side. Following removal of the wedge, the distal fragment may be displaced laterally approximately one-third the diameter of the first metatarsal. It may also be moved in a plantar direction and rotated to decrease pronation of the toe. Excess bone at the medial side of the proximal fragment may have to be removed.

The Hohmann osteotomy was originally fixed with sutures through the joint capsule, with Kirschner wires in the soft tissues of the great toe or through the osteotomy fragments. Fixation with a small fragment cancellous screw is preferable because it allows immediate full weightbearing postoperatively. The capsule is reinforced medially with the abductor hallucis muscle. The distal end of its tendon is displaced distally and sutured to the insertion of the capsule at the proximal phalanx, then proximally and sutured to the attachment of the capsule at the metatarsal neck. This contributes to the correct alignment of the great toe and increases the stability

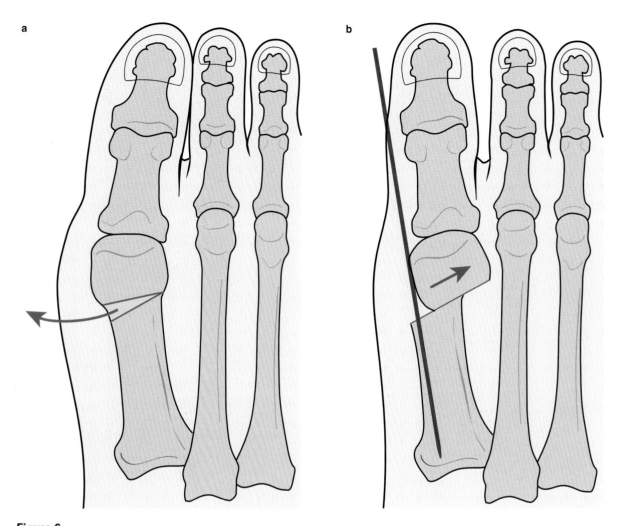

Figure 6

Kramer osteotomy. a. area of bone resection; b. displacement of the metatarsal head and stabilization with an axial Kirschner wire

of the osteotomy. Screw fixation is usually stable enough to allow early postoperative weightbearing.

Kramer osteotomy

Following the skin incision, the periosteum and the thickened bursa at the metatarsal head are incised longitudinally, without opening the joint. The metatarsal neck is exposed with retractors. A 2-mm Kirschner wire is placed medially through the soft tissues of the hallux, from distal to proximal. The first osteotomy is made with an oscillating saw, perpendicular to the metatarsal shaft, at the junction of the head and the neck (Figure 6). The more distal the osteotomy, the further the head can be displaced. However, the osteotomy should not be placed through the head itself because of the risk of avascular necrosis. With the second osteotomy, a medially based wedge is taken from the shaft, the

angle of the wedge corresponding to the desired correction. The head is mobilized laterally and plantarly with an osteotome. Lateral displacement should be half the diameter of the metatarsal shaft, but at least $0.5\,cm^2$ of bone contact must remain. A slight plantar displacement of the metatarsal head is recommended. The metatarsal is lengthened by shifting the head fragment laterally, compressing the osteotomy. Following displacement, the previously introduced Kirschner wire is directed around the medial side of the head fragment and into the shaft of the first metatarsal, to the subchondral bone at its base. An additional wire may be inserted for stability. Excessive bone at the medial side of the proximal fragment may have to be removed. Only the skin is closed. The toe is held in varus during the application of the dressing. Kirschner wire fixation requires the use of a heel support shoe for 6 weeks after surgery.

Complications

Avascular necrosis of the first metatarsal head is an uncommon complication that may occur with any type of distal first metatarsal osteotomy. Temporary disturbance of the circulation is quite common [Resch 1992] and this may manifest itself as focal osteolysis of the subchondral bone during the first postoperative weeks. It usually disappears with increased activity of the patient. Collapse of the articular surface is very rare. Gentle soft tissue dissection and stable internal fixation help to maintain the blood supply to the first metatarsal head.

Loss of reduction and non-union or malunion are observed occasionally, mostly because internal fixation was not sufficiently stable. With the Kramer osteotomy, complete radiographic union may take several months, because the axial Kirschner wire does not provide sufficient stability.

Delayed wound healing and postoperative infection occasionally occur but rarely require surgical revision. Prolonged swelling of the toe is observed if ambulation is allowed in spite of insufficiently stable fixation. Patients must be instructed to elevate the foot postoperatively and limit their activities to prevent swelling.

Neuromas may develop if the cutaneous nerves are transected with the skin incision. Sharp, local pain and tenderness usually resolve with local injections and rarely require surgical revision. Neuromas are most common with a dorsomedial skin incision, which may result in injury to the dorsomedial cutaneous nerve of the hallux.

Transfer metatarsalgia is improved in most patients compared to their situation preoperatively. Occasionally the hallux does not regain sufficient function postoperatively and the load under the foot is shifted to the lesser metatarsal heads. This is treated with vigorous active and passive range of motion exercises at the hallux and with insoles.

References

Austin DW, Leventen EO (1981) A new osteotomy for hallux valgus. Clin Orthop 157: 25–30

Das De S, Hamblen DL (1987) Distal metatarsal osteotomy for hallux valgus in the middle aged patient. Clin Orthop 218: 239–246

Gibson J, Piggot H (1962) Osteotomy of the neck of the foot metatarsal in the treatment of hallux valgus. J Bone Joint Surg 44B: 349–355

Hattrup S, Johnson K (1985) Chevron osteotomy: analysis of factors in patients' dissatisfaction. Foot Ankle 5: 327–332

Hohmann G (1951) Fuß und Bein, 5th edn. Munich, Bergmann, pp 145–180

Johnson K, Cofield R, Morrey B (1979) Chevron osteotomy for hallux valgus. Clin Orthop 142: 44–47

Kramer J (1990) Die Kramer-Osteotomie zur Behandlung des Hallux valgus und des Digitus quintus varus. Operat Orthop Traumatol 2: 14–38

Leventen E (1990) The Chevron procedure. Orthopedics 13: 973–978

Magerl F (1982) Stabile Osteotomien zur Behandlung des Hallux valgus. Orthopäde 11: 170–180

Meier PJ, Kenzora JE (1985) The risks and benefits of distal first metatarsal osteotomies. Foot Ankle 6: 7–17

Mitchell CLO, Fleming JL, Allen R (1958) Osteotomy-bunionectomy for hallux valgus. J Bone Joint Surg 40A: 41–58

Resch S, Stenström A, Gustafson T (1992) Circulatory disturbance of the first metatarsal head after chevron osteotomy as shown by bone scintimetry. Foot Ankle 13: 137–142

Resch S, Stenström A, Reynisson K et al. (1994) Chevron osteotomy for hallux valgus not improved by additional tenotomy. A prospective randomized study of 84 patients. Acta Orthop Scand 65: 541–544

Reverdin J (1881) De la déviation en dehors du gros orteil (hallux valgus, vulg. 'oignon', 'bunions', 'Ballen') et de son traitement chirurgical. Trans Int Med Congr 2: 408–412

Shereff MJ, Yang QM, Kummer F (1987) Extraosseous and intraosseous arterial supply to the first metatarsal and metatarsophalangeal joint. Foot Ankle 8: 81–93

Wilson JN (1963) Oblique displacement osteotomy for hallux valgus. J Bone Joint Surg 45B: 552–556

Wülker N (1997) Hallux valgus. Orthopäde 26: 654–664

3

Hallux valgus: soft-tissue procedure with proximal metatarsal osteotomy

Roger A. Mann

Introduction

The hallux valgus deformity usually occurs in adults as a result of chronic pressure against the hallux caused by wearing tight shoes. It is approximately ten times more common in women than men and is usually progressive with age. The changes that occur about the metatarsophalangeal joint as the proximal phalanx moves laterally on the metatarsal head consist of contracture of the lateral joint capsular structures, elongation of the medial joint capsular structures, the formation of a medial eminence of varying sizes, an increased intermetatarsal angle and uncovering of the sesamoids.

As a general rule, most patients complain of pain over the medial eminence, which is aggravated by activities and shoe wear. Usually barefoot walking is not a problem. As the deformity becomes more severe, there may be transfer metatarsalgia beneath the second metatarsal head. This often results in a diffuse callus beneath the second metatarsal. The transfer metatarsalgia is the result of decreased weightbearing due to lack of function of the windlass mechanism, which, during the last half of the stance phase, plantar flexes the first metatarsal

and transfers weight to the hallux. Without normal windlass function, weight is not transferred to the hallux in the last part of the stance phase and this results in increased pressure on the second metatarsal head. As a general rule, once the hallux valgus deformity is corrected, the transfer metatarsalgia resolves, or at least is significantly reduced [Mann et al. 1992]. It is for this reason that it is rarely necessary to perform any procedure on the second metatarsal, provided the metatarsophalangeal joint is not subluxed or dislocated when a hallux valgus repair is carried out.

Indications

The indication for the distal soft-tissue procedure and proximal metatarsal osteotomy is a hallux valgus deformity with a laterally subluxed or incongruent metatarsophalangeal joint [Mann et al. 1992, Sammarco et al. 1993, Borton and Stephens 1994]. If subluxation of the joint is not present, then the proximal phalanx cannot be rotated on the metatarsal head, which is an essential part of this surgical procedure.

Contraindications

The procedure is contraindicated when a congruent metatarsophalangeal joint is present [Mann and Coughlin 1981]. In this situation the proximal phalanx is not subluxed, and therefore the procedure should not be carried out because, if the proximal phalanx is rotated on the metatarsal head, an incongruent joint would be created. If there is more than mild to moderate arthrosis of the metatarsophalangeal joint, although satisfactory alignment can be achieved, the joint will often become stiff and painful. Arthrosis therefore represents a relative contraindication and is based upon the degree of arthrosis that is present [Mann and Pfeffinger 1991, Mann and Coughlin 1993].

Spasticity of any type, whether secondary to a stroke or head injury, is a contraindication. These patients unfortunately have a muscle imbalance which can be corrected, but an operation for hallux valgus will not result in a long-term correction, owing to the spasticity.

The presence of rheumatoid arthritis with more than minimal soft tissue involvement is a contraindication.

The circulatory status of the foot must be adequate in order to perform this procedure. If there is any doubt regarding the circulation to the foot, a Doppler arterial study should be carried out.

The age of the patient is not a significant factor – this procedure has been performed in children and in patients in their eighth decade – provided adequate circulation is present.

Radiographic evaluation

Weightbearing anteroposterior, lateral and oblique radiographs of the foot should be obtained prior to surgery, to look for the presence of arthrosis of the metatarsophalangeal joint, the degree of displacement of the sesamoids, the size of the medial eminence, the appearance of the metatarsocuneiform joint and the status of the lesser metatarsophalangeal joints (particularly evidence of subluxation or dislocation).

The following measurements should be obtained: hallux valgus angle (normal <15°), intermetatarsal angle (normal <9°) and the distal metatarsal articular angle (DMAA, normal <10° lateral deviation). The DMAA represents the relationship of the articular surface of the first metatarsal head to the long axis of the metatarsal [Coughlin 1996]. If more than 10–12° of lateral deviation is present, full correction of the deformity may not be possible without an osteotomy

of the base of the proximal phalanx. This is because if the DMAA is too large, despite the creation of a congruent joint, the hallux still tilts in a lateral direction. This may also occur in the presence of a hallux valgus interphalangeus and would require an osteotomy of the proximal phalanx to achieve full correction [Mann and Coughlin 1991] (see Chapter 1).

Treatment

Surgical technique

This procedure is usually carried out in an outpatient setting using an ankle block for anesthesia. An elastic tourniquet is applied in the supramalleolar area, wrapped over padding around the distal tibia and the underlying neurovascular structures. The first part of the procedure consists of three steps in order to prepare for the correction of the deformity:

1. Release of the adductor hallucis tendon, lateral joint capsule and transverse metatarsal ligament through a dorsal first web space incision.
2. Exposure of the medial aspect of the metatarsophalangeal joint, preparation of the joint capsule and excision of the medial eminence.
3. Exposure of the base of the first metatarsal and metatarsal osteotomy.

The second part of the procedure is the reconstruction of the metatarsophalangeal joint and consists of the following steps:

1. Placement of sutures in the first web space to re-attach the adductor hallucis tendon.
2. Correction of the intermetatarsal angle and fixation of the proximal metatarsal osteotomy.
3. Repair of the medial joint capsule.

The third part of the procedure is the application of the postoperative dressings.

Release of the lateral joint contracture

The initial skin incision is made in the first dorsal web space in the midline in order to avoid the superficial branches of the deep peroneal nerve which pass on either side of the web space (Figure 1). The incision is deepened to expose the adductor hallucis tendon, which crosses obliquely through the base of the wound, to insert into the plantar lateral aspect of the base of the proximal phalanx.

The knife blade is passed above the adductor hallucis tendon, into the space between the fibular

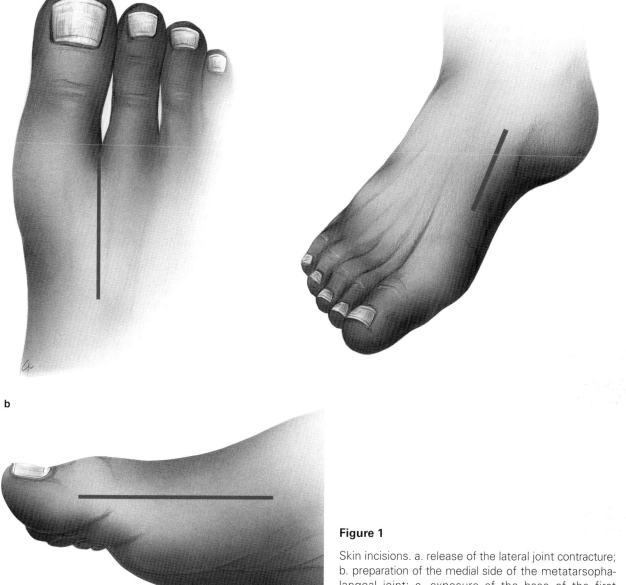

Figure 1

Skin incisions. a. release of the lateral joint contracture; b. preparation of the medial side of the metatarsophalangeal joint; c. exposure of the base of the first metatarsal and proximal metatarsal osteotomy

sesamoid and the metatarsal head at an angle of about 45°. Once in the interval, the capsule is cut distally until the knife blade strikes the base of the proximal phalanx; the blade is rotated laterally to release the insertion of the adductor hallucis from the base of the proximal phalanx (Figure 2).

The knife blade is then inserted into the initial capsular incision and brought proximally until the fleshy fibers of the flexor hallucis brevis and adductor hallucis are encountered. The adductor hallucis tendon is then carefully stripped from the lateral aspect of the sesamoid proximal to the level where the tendon ends and the muscle fibers of the adductor and flexor hallucis brevis begin.

A Weitlaner retractor is inserted between the first and second metatarsals, placing the transverse metatarsal ligament on stretch. The ligament is carefully released, with the tip of the knife (Figure 3). It should be kept in mind that the common digital nerve and vessels are beneath the ligament and should be avoided. The base of the wound should be carefully inspected to be sure that the entire transverse metatarsal ligament has been released.

The Weitlaner retractor is removed and the lateral joint capsule is detached from its proximal origin. This is achieved by placing the first metatarsophalangeal joint in mild valgus and carefully placing a knife blade between the lateral joint capsule and the metatarsal head. The knife is then brought proximally as the great toe is pulled in a medial direction. This places some tension on the capsule and makes its release easier. The hallux is pulled in a medial direction into about 25° of varus (Figure 4).

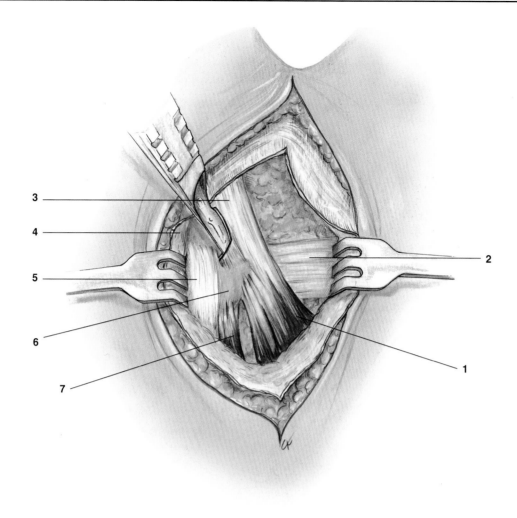

Figure 2

The adductor hallucis tendon is released from the base of the proximal phalanx with an incision that starts at the space between the fibular sesamoid and the metatarsal head

1 Adductor hallucis muscle
2 Deep transverse metatarsal ligament
3 Adductor hallucis tendon

4 Proximal phalanx
5 First metatarsophalangeal joint capsule
6 Fibular sesamoid
7 Flexor hallucis brevis muscle

Preparation of the medial side of the metatarsophalangeal joint

A medial midline incision is made extending for approximately 5 cm, centered over the metatarsophalangeal joint (see Figure 1). A full-thickness dorsal and plantar flap is created along the capsular plane. Care is taken to avoid the dorsal and plantar cutaneous nerves. A vertical incision is made 2–3 mm proximal to the base of the proximal phalanx, using a no. 11 blade.

A second incision is then made parallel to the first, anywhere from 3 mm to 8 mm more proximal, depending upon the size of the deformity (Figure 5). These two parallel cuts are connected by an inverted V on the dorsomedial aspect of the metatarsophalangeal joint and plantarward by a V-shaped incision through the abductor hallucis tendon [DuVries 1959]. When this plantar incision is made, it is imperative that the knife blade be kept inside the metatarsophalangeal joint so that the tip of the knife will strike the medial sesamoid bone and not inadvertently cut the plantar medial cutaneous nerve passing just below the abductor tendon.

An incision is made along the dorsomedial aspect of the capsule and the capsule is stripped off the medial eminence. After exposure of the medial eminence, it is removed in line with the medial aspect of the metatarsal shaft (Figure 6), starting

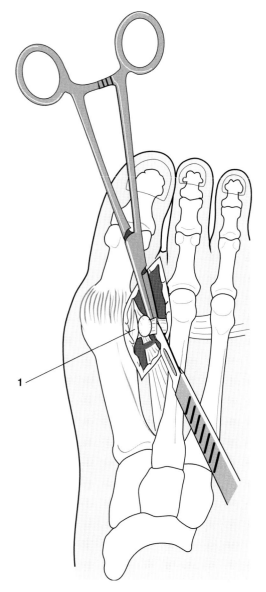

Figure 3

The transverse metatarsal ligament is released with a knife

1 Lateral capsule

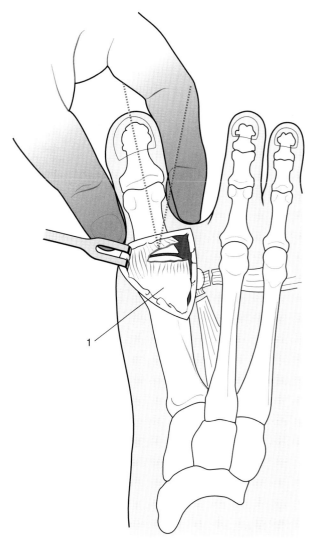

Figure 4

Following detachment of the adductor tendon, transection of the transverse metatarsal ligament and release of the lateral joint capsule from its proximal origin, all lateral contractures have been released and the great toe is forcefully brought into a varus position of 25°

1 Lateral capsule

2–3 mm medial to the sagittal sulcus. It is imperative that too much medial eminence is not removed, for fear of destabilizing the metatarsophalangeal joint. The edges of the bone are smoothed with a rongeur, particularly the dorsomedial aspect of the metatarsal head, where a sharp prominence is often present.

At this point in the operation, a decision must be made as to whether a metatarsal osteotomy is needed. For any deformity in which the intermetatarsal angle is greater than 12°, an osteotomy is almost always necessary. If the intermetatarsal angle is less than 12°, a clinical decision must be made at the time of surgery as to whether to perform an osteotomy. This is determined by pushing the metatarsal head in a lateral direction; if it tends to spring back towards the surgeon's finger, then an osteotomy should be carried out. In this situation the excursion of the metatarsocuneiform joint is insufficient to correct the intermetatarsal angle completely, if an osteotomy is not carried out.

Exposure of the base of the first metatarsal and proximal metatarsal osteotomy

An incision is made over the dorsal aspect of the base of the first metatarsal starting just proximal to the metatarsocuneiform joint and carried

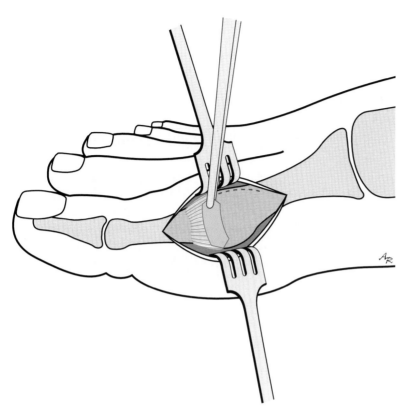

Figure 5

A vertical flap of capsular tissue measuring 3–8 mm is removed from the medial capsule, beginning 2–3 mm proximal to the base of the proximal phalanx. The capsular incision is then extended along the dorso-medial aspect (dashed line)

distally for a distance of approximately 3 cm (see Figure 1). The extensor tendon is retracted laterally. The metatarsocuneiform joint is identified and the site for the osteotomy is selected approximately 1 cm distal to the joint, slightly distal to the point where the metatarsal shaft widens, especially on the lateral side.

The author's preferred method is a crescentic osteotomy at the base of the first metatarsal. Other osteotomies, such as a basal chevron osteotomy [Sammarco et al. 1993, Borton and Stephens 1994], or a short oblique osteotomy, have also been described.

Approximately 1 cm distal to the site of the osteotomy a mark is made on the metatarsal shaft, which is where the fixation screw will be inserted. If a cannulated screw (4.0 mm) is to be used, the guide wire is inserted into the dorsal aspect of the metatarsal approximately 1 cm distal to the osteotomy site. It is placed at an angle of approximately 45° to the metatarsal and aimed in a proximal direction. It is important that it is not drilled in too far; if it is, it will cross the osteotomy site, preventing the blade from cutting the bone. If a 4.0-mm cancellous screw is to be used, then instead of placing the guide wire into the metatarsal 1 cm distal to the osteotomy, a glide hole is made using a 3.2-mm drill bit. As the glide hole is made it is imperative that it only be brought as far proximal as the anticipated osteotomy site or else it will

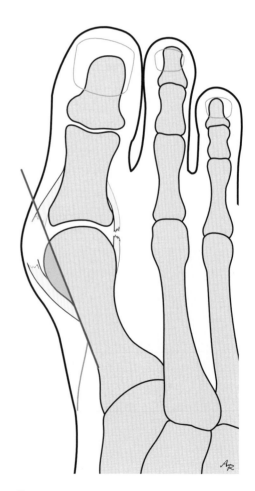

Figure 6

The medial eminence is removed in line with the medial aspect of the metatarsal shaft

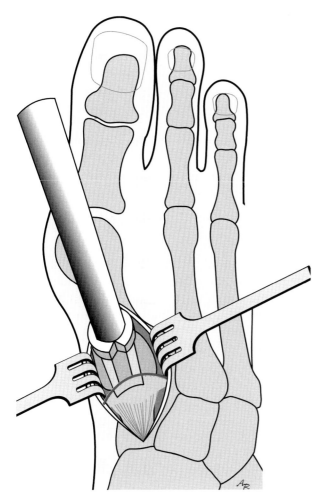

Figure 7

A crescentic osteotomy is made at the base of the first metatarsal, 1 cm distal to the metatarsocuneiform joint

interfere with the eventual correction of the osteotomy.

The osteotomy is made using a crescentic saw blade (Figure 7) and an oscillating saw. A short blade is used first. The osteotomy is started 1 cm distal to the metatarsocuneiform joint or just distal to the flare of the metatarsal. The angle of the saw blade is neither perpendicular to the metatarsal nor perpendicular to the bottom of the foot, but about halfway between. The concavity of the cut is directed towards the heel. As the saw blade is placed on the bone it is important that the blade penetrates the lateral aspect of the metatarsal shaft. If a small island of bone is left medially, it does not create a problem, because it is easily and safely osteotomized. If the osteotomy is not cut completely through on the lateral aspect, however, it is difficult to cut with an osteotome and the communicating artery may be damaged.

The oscillating saw is placed against the bone and a mark is made, following which the saw cut is produced by making a small arc with the blade in a medial–lateral direction. As this is carried out, the osteotomy is exactly cut. As the cut is deepened, the shoulder of the blade will strike the proximal portion of the metatarsal before the cut is complete and it is necessary to change to a longer blade in order to complete the cut. Once the cut has been made, if an island of bone is still present on the medial side, it is carefully cut using a small, sharp osteotome. The periosteum on the medial side is cut as well, so that the osteotomy site is freely moveable. If it is not freely moveable, it means that there is either a bony island still intact or the periosteum is not adequately stripped.

At this point in the procedure, each area of pathological anatomy has been adequately released and reconstruction of the deformity can be carried out.

Reconstruction of the first web space

A suture is placed into the adductor tendon and is left untied at this time. The purpose of this is to bring the adductor tendon along the lateral aspect of the metatarsophalangeal joint to re-form capsular tissue.

Correction of the osteotomy

The osteotomy site is corrected by placing a small elevator on the lateral aspect of the proximal fragment of the metatarsal. Pressure is then applied to the proximal fragment medially to rotate the metatarsocuneiform joint as far medially as possible (Figure 8). With the other hand, the metatarsal head is grasped and pushed in a lateral direction. This rotates the osteotomy site in such a way as to correct the intermetatarsal angle. The intermetatarsal angle is usually corrected when the lateral aspect of the first metatarsal touches the head of the second. It is imperative that the proximal fragment is stabilized as far medially as possible, or adequate correction of the deformity cannot be achieved.

If a cannulated screw system is used, the surgeon holds the osteotomy in the correct position while the cannulated guide pin is drilled across the osteotomy site. The dorsal cortex is then penetrated using the cannulated 4.0-mm drill bit, after which the hole is countersunk. As the hole is countersunk it is important that pressure be applied to the distal portion of the countersink cutter. The countersinking should be sufficient so that the rim of the head of the screw as it passes along the hole will not be cammed dorsally, thereby possibly cracking the osteotomy site.

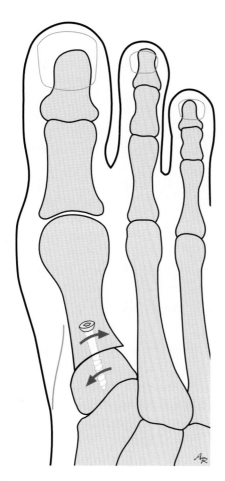

Figure 8

The osteotomy is reduced by pressure to the proximal fragment medially and to the metatarsal head laterally. A small screw is used for fixation

Usually a 26-mm cannulated screw with long threads is inserted in order to stabilize the osteotomy site. In large patients sometimes a longer screw is necessary. As a general rule, a 26-mm screw stops just short of the metatarsocuneiform joint. If the metatarsocuneiform joint is penetrated, it usually does not cause the patient any significant problem, although occasionally the screw may break. If a cannulated screw system is not used, once the osteotomy site has been stabilized by the surgeon, a drill sleeve is placed into the glide hole and it is drilled with a 2.7-mm drill bit. The hole is tapped and countersunk as described above and a fully threaded 4.0-mm screw inserted.

As the screw is tightened, care must be taken not to crack the bone island, which is somewhat fragile, although with proper countersinking fracture of the island is uncommon. If fracture were to occur and the fixation was felt to be unstable, then several Kirschner wires could be added to produce stability.

Repair of the medial joint capsule

The hallux is held in corrected alignment. This consists of placing the toe in line with the long axis of the metatarsal, bringing the toe into approximately 5° of varus and then rotating it to correct any pronation that is present. The latter maneuver brings the sesamoids back underneath the metatarsal head. With the great toe held in correct alignment, the capsule is then carefully inspected to see whether or not more capsular tissue needs to be removed to create a side-to-side repair.

Four or five sutures are placed into the medial joint capsule, starting at the plantar aspect which places the suture through the abductor hallucis tendon. The plantar two-thirds of the capsule is the strongest, and adequate sutures in this area are imperative for a good repair. Dorsally at times the tissue becomes flimsy and is not capable of supporting the sutures.

At this point adequate alignment of the hallux should be present. Intraoperative radiographs may be useful, but are not a necessary part of the procedure. The suture that is in the adductor tendon is placed through the lateral joint capsule, which is attached to the base of the proximal phalanx. If the hallux has a tendency to drift a little into varus, more tension is placed on this suture and, if the alignment is tending to drift a little into valgus, no tension is placed on this suture. The wounds are closed in a routine manner. A compression dressing is applied to squeeze the metatarsal heads together and hold the great toe in correct alignment.

Postoperative care

The patient is seen approximately 24–48 h following surgery, after which the compression dressing is removed and a spica dressing consisting of a 4-cm gauze bandage and 1-cm adhesive tape is applied. The postoperative dressing is changed on a weekly basis for 8 weeks. The patient is permitted to walk in a postoperative shoe.

The postoperative dressing is a critical part of this procedure [DuVries 1959]. The principle of the dressing is to bind the metatarsal heads together, which helps support the osteotomy site and holds the hallux in correct alignment, which is about 0–5° of valgus, correction of all pronation and in line with the first metatarsal. Avoid dressing the toe into too much varus or valgus, or allowing it to dorsiflex. With this in mind, dress the right foot (when viewing the patient from the foot of the bed) by wrapping the bandage in a counterclockwise direction, in order to keep the sesamoids beneath the metatarsal head, and dress the left foot by wrapping the bandage and adhesive tape in a clockwise direction.

Radiographs are obtained usually 1 week after surgery, at which time the alignment of the metatarsophalangeal joint is assessed. Based on this radiograph one can decide exactly how the dressings should be applied and whether a slight varus or valgus force should be applied to the great toe to achieve an optimal result.

Complications

Hallux varus may occur in up to 8% of patients, and this may be related to excessive excision of the medial eminence or overcorrection of the intermetatarsal angle. Varus angulation is usually between 5° and 8° [Mann et al. 1992]. In most patients this does not cause symptoms and almost never requires further surgery. Recurrence of the deformity may be due to an inadequate postoperative dressing, insufficient plication of the medial joint capsule, inadequate release of the lateral joint contracture, insufficient medial capsular tissues secondary to degenerative changes or cyst formation, and failure to treat a metatarsus primus varus. Persistent stiffness of the metatarsophalangeal joint may be caused by unrecognized arthrosis or postoperative infection. Occasionally the dorsal or plantar cutaneous nerve to the great toe is injured or entrapped. This complication is avoided by using a straight medial incision.

Pseudarthrosis of the proximal metatarsal osteotomy rarely occurs. The average shortening of the first metatarsal is 2 mm. Some first metatarsal dorsiflexion may be observed on lateral radiographs, but this rarely causes transfer metatarsalgia [Mann et al. 1992].

References

Borton DC, Stephens MM (1994) Basal metatarsal osteotomy for hallux valgus. J Bone Joint Surg 76B: 204–209

Coughlin MJ (1996) Hallux valgus. J Bone Joint Surg 78A: 932–966

DuVries HL (1959) Surgery of the Foot. St Louis, Mosby, pp 381–440

Mann RA, Coughlin MJ (1981) Hallux valgus: etiology, anatomy, treatment and surgical considerations. Clin Orthop 157: 31–41

Mann RA, Coughlin MJ (1991) Video Textbook of Foot and Ankle Surgery. St Louis, Medical Video Productions, pp 146–184

Mann RA, Coughlin MJ (1993) Adult hallux valgus. In: Mann RA, Coughlin MJ (eds) Surgery of the Foot and Ankle, 6th edn. St Louis, Mosby-Yearbook, pp 167–296

Mann RA, Pfeffinger L (1991) Hallux valgus repair: DuVries modified McBride procedure. Clin Orthop 272: 213–218

Mann RA, Rudicel S, Graves SC (1992) Repair of hallux valgus with distal soft tissue procedure and proximal metatarsal osteotomy. A long term followup. J Bone Joint Surg 74A: 124–139

Sammarco GJ, Brainard B, Sammarco VJ (1993) Bunion correction using proximal Chevron osteotomy. Foot Ankle 14: 8–14

Veri JP, Pirani SP, Claridge R (2001) Crescentic proximal metatarsal osteotomy for moderate to severe hallux valgus: a mean 12.2 year follow-up study. Foot Ankle Int 22: 817–822

4

Hallux valgus: scarf bunionectomy

Louis Samuel Barouk
Lowell Scott Weil Sr

Introduction

The surgical treatment of hallux valgus deformity is patient dependent. Although the great majority of these deformities can be accommodated with a wide toe-box shoe, secondary deformities such as painful hammer digit syndrome and metatarsalgia, coupled with patient demand, often drive the need for operative intervention. In addition, some individuals are averse to wearing any type of special shoe and wish to have the deformity corrected rather than accommodated.

When an operation is indicated in the opinion of the surgeon and in concert with the patient's wishes, the goals for the ideal hallux valgus operation are as follows:

- Joint congruity, pain free, full range of motion postoperatively
- Improved cosmesis and ability to wear varied shoe styles
- Wide range of indications
- Long-term predictability
- Minimum postoperative disability and interference with the activities of daily living
- Minimal and salvageable complications
- Ability to be performed bilaterally.

The scarf bunionectomy can significantly improve hallux valgus correction. It is versatile, is structurally sound, has a wide range of indications and applications, and allows for an early, functional recovery.

The scarf bunionectomy is not purely an osteotomy, but a combination of techniques involving a fibular sesamoid release, scarf osteotomy, a unique form of rigid internal fixation, capsule–tendon balancing and a rigorous postoperative rehabilitation. Every component of this bunionectomy contributes to its success.

History

The authors' collective experience of 70 years of performing hallux valgus surgery has taken them through procedures such as the McBride, Keller, chevron, crescentic and Lapidus. Although each of these procedures was successful for the perfect indication, the versatility and predictability for success were not optimal. Since 1990, the authors have used the scarf bunionectomy as their primary hallux valgus procedure.

Scarf osteotomy history

In 1976, J. M. Burutaran presented a preliminary report of four cases using a combination of the Keller operation with a 'Z' osteotomy of the first metatarsal to correct hallux valgus deformity.

Gudas and Zygmund began using a full-length horizontal 'Z' cut in the first metatarsal and shared their early observations (with LSW) in 1984, as did LSW with LSB in 1990. The authors promptly embraced the procedure, while developing modifications and increased indications, and popularized the 'scarf bunionectomy' worldwide.

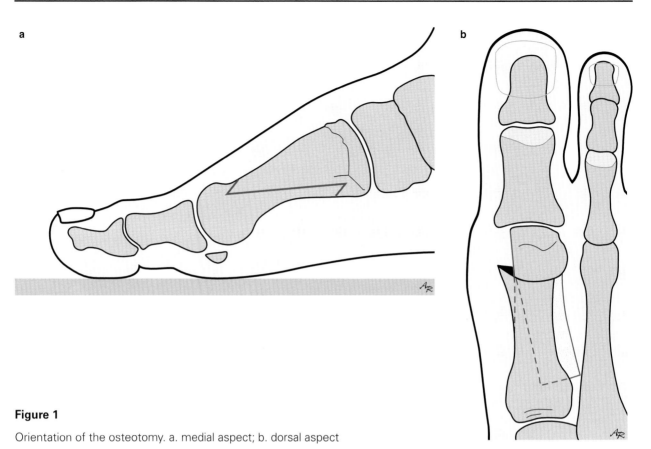

Figure 1

Orientation of the osteotomy. a. medial aspect; b. dorsal aspect

The term 'scarf' is an architectural and carpentry term defined as 'a joint made by notching, grooving, or otherwise cutting the ends of two pieces and fastening them together so that they lap over and join firmly into one continuous piece' (Figure 1).

The scarf osteotomy has great versatility by allowing:

- Lateralization of the head-shaft fragment to reduce the intermetatarsal angle. Unlike the crescentic or proximal chevron, this lateral displacement does not increase the distal metatarsal articular angle (DMAA), also called the proximal articular set angle (PASA), thereby maintaining joint congruity and avoiding the long-term complication of arthrosis;
- Medialization of the capital fragment (in cases of hallux varus);
- Plantar displacement to increase the first ray load;
- Dorsal displacement to decrease the ray or tibial sesamoid load;
- Elongation in cases of a short first metatarsal;
- Shortening in cases of a long first metatarsal or severe deformity;
- Transverse plane rotation up to 15° to correct an increased DMAA;
- Axial rotation (supination) in cases of first metatarsal pronation.

Local vascular anatomy as applied to the scarf

LSB performed anatomic vascular studies, injecting five cadaveric feet to study the effects of the scarf bunionectomy on local blood supply to this region.

The dorsal blood supply

The first dorsal metatarsal artery first gives rise to the nutrient artery, which penetrates the metatarsal shaft in the distal one-third of the plantar border (deep to the scarf horizontal cut). Distal branches penetrate the head through the dorsal–lateral capsule. However, the main blood supply comes from the plantar side.

The plantar blood supply

The plantar medial artery is located dorsal to the abductor hallucis and flexor hallucis muscles. At the distal metaphyseal level, it divides into a branch for the sesamoids and metaphyseal capital branches. The lateral plantar artery divides into a lateral sesamoid artery and capital branches to the metaphysis, where an anastamosis occurs forming an important vascular arch under the metatarsal neck.

The scarf cut does not jeopardize this blood supply. Special care is taken during the lateral release, whether it is performed from the lateral incision, intermetatarsal approach or through the intra-articular approach.

Indications

The indications for the scarf osteotomy are:

- Hallux valgus deformity with an intermetatarsal angle of 12–28° (the length of the horizontal cut is increased as the intermetatarsal angle becomes greater);
- Increased PASA–DMAA;
- Range of motion of the first metatarsophalangeal joint of greater than 40° without severe joint arthrosis.

Surgical technique

The authors are generally in agreement with regard to the technique. However, small differences, based on personal preference, will be noted.

The scarf osteotomy is only one of the three components of the scarf bunionectomy. The three steps are: (1) release of the metatarsophalangeal–lateral sesamoidal complex (lateral release); (2) scarf osteotomy of the first metatarsal with supportive and rigid fixation; (3) medial capsulorrhaphy and capsuloplasty.

The addition of a phalangeal osteotomy (Akin or shortening) is commonly performed with the scarf bunionectomy (see Chapter 1).

The procedure may be performed under a general anesthetic or under a combination of intravenous sedation and local anesthesia. A Mayo block, utilizing 10–12 ml of 0.5% bupivacaine, is administered just prior to inflation of an ankle tourniquet to 250 mmHg.

A medial incision approach is used and is made where the skin of the plantar surface meets the skin of the dorsum (Figure 2). The length of the incision varies depending on the intended horizontal length of the osteotomy (the larger the intermetatarsal angle, the longer the osteotomy (although LSB prefers a long osteotomy in all cases); the neurovascular structures are identified and preserved and the wound edges are retracted using four flexible skin hooks, which then encircle the foot and are clamped laterally.

A lenticular capsular incision is made, removing a small ellipse of capsule adjacent to the dorsoplantar midline of the metatarsal head. The capsule and periosteum are then reflected dorsally along the medial side of the metatarsal head and shaft and distally to the base of the proximal phalanx, preserving the dorsal capsule. The plantar reflection is made to expose the joint but preserve the vascular network just proximal to the sesamoids, and is then deepened more proximally by blunt dissection. A self-retaining retractor is placed between the plantar capsule and the metatarsal head to allow for exposure and release of the suspensory ligament of the fibular sesamoid (Figure 3). Following release, the self-retainer is removed and a limited lateral release is performed through the joint, making certain to preserve the lateral joint capsule. If additional lateral release is desired, a careful release of the anterior fibular sesamoid ligament is made, thus releasing the contracture in advanced deformities. The fibular sesamoid is removed only in cases of severe arthrosis to the undersurface of the first metatarsal head.

LSB prefers to perform the lateral release through a small dorsal incision, just lateral to the first metatarsal head. The fibular sesamoid suspensory ligament is divided, allowing the sesamoid to move plantarward. The phalangeal insertional band is also divided, to release the joint contracture. The authors have used both of these approaches successfully.

The scarf osteotomy may be performed with or without an osteotomy guide. The osteotomy is designed to separate a proximally based dorsal fragment and a plantar fragment, which comprises the plantar surface and the metatarsal head. The longitudinal or horizontal cut is then followed by two transverse cuts.

An osteotomy guide may be used to facilitate the bone cuts (Figure 4). First, a 1.1-mm K-wire is inserted 3–4 mm below the dorsal medial surface of the metatarsal head and directed at a lateral and plantar declination of about 25–30° (aiming just plantar to the fifth metatarsal head).

The proper direction of this guide pin is essential, since it will formulate the displacement of the metatarsal head-shaft. If the pin is directed lateral and plantar, the metatarsal head will be displaced laterally and plantarward; if directed slightly proximal, it will cause a small shortening of the metatarsal as well. In the great majority of cases, plantar displacement of 2–3 mm is desirable to offset the elevation of the first metatarsal and thereby decrease the load under the second metatarsal.

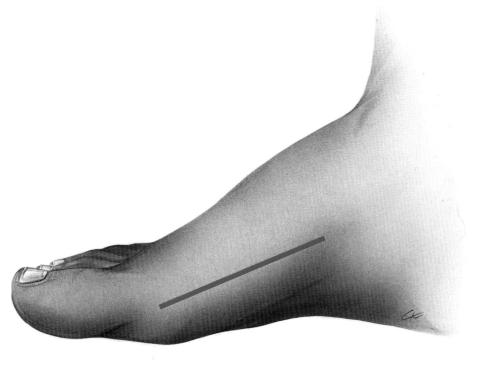

Figure 2

A direct medial approach is used for the osteotomy

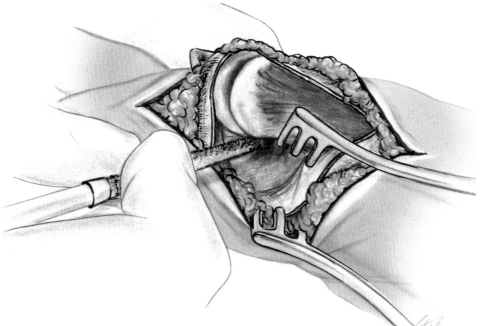

Figure 3

Intra-articular release of lateral sesamoid suspensory ligament allowing for reduction of the hallux valgus contracture. Note preservation of proximal sesamoid vascular supply. (LSW)

The osteotomy guide is then placed over the pin and a 12-mm wide sagittal saw blade is used to create the dorsal cut. This cut is made about 5 mm proximal to the margin of the dorsal cartilage and is made at a 60–70° angle. (It is mandatory to keep this distal cut in the cancellous bone of the metatarsal head to avoid troughing and channeling during the lateral displacement). The osteotomy guide is then rotated toward the long axis of the metatarsal shaft and directed toward the inferior and proximal portion of the metatarsal, extending to about 2 cm distal to the metatarsal cuneiform articulation. The osteotomy should end about 3–4 mm above the plantar cortex (Figure 5). (Making this cut at the plantar portion of the metatarsal is essential to avoid stress risers leading to stress fractures.) A 20-mm wide sagittal saw is used to make the long cut. The length of this osteotomy is increased by up to 10 mm in cases of large intermetatarsal angles in order to transpose a greater volume of bone and thus

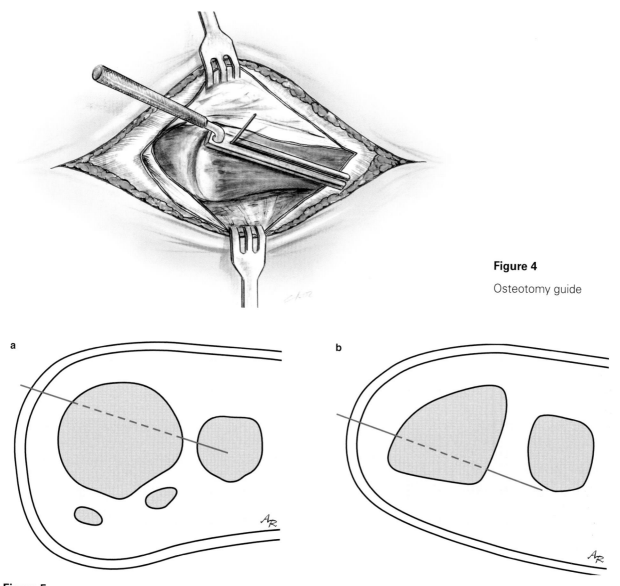

Figure 4

Osteotomy guide

Figure 5

a. Transverse section at metatarsal neck level; b. transverse section at proximal metatarsal level

prevent recurrence due to reverse buckling of the intermetatarsal angle. The typical length of the osteotomy is about 40 mm, but it can be as long as the entire length of the metatarsal shaft to the cancellous bone in the base of the metatarsal. (This is the preference of LSB in every case.)

As the cut is made through the shaft in a lateral direction, careful attention is paid to avoid burying the saw blade in the intermetatarsal space, thus preserving the vital structures in this area. The osteotomy guide is then removed distally and the vertical and horizontal cuts are connected using the side of the saw blade as a cutting tool. Finally, the plantar cut is completed, connecting the long cut of the shaft at a 60° angle to form a locking mechanism once the bones are displaced and compressed.

Traction of the hallux during this final cut will facilitate its completion. (LSB prefers to complete the proximal cut first and the distal cut last.) The head-shaft is now mobile and, while an assistant places a small clamp on the intact shaft and pulls medially, the free-floating head-shaft is displaced laterally until resistance is encountered (this is called the pull–push maneuver).

The hallux is then held firmly with pressure in a proximal direction while the specially designed scarf bone clamp is applied. Alterations of the distal cut can be made to correct the PASA up to 15°.

The osteotomy is then fixed with the two threaded-head screws (Figure 6). The distal screw is placed obliquely into the metatarsal head to add additional, longitudinal, compressive support to the

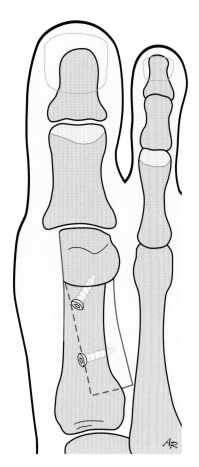

Figure 6

Following displacement of the fragments, the osteotomy is stabilized with two screws and excess bone at the dorsal fragment is resected

plantar fragment and to avoid any possible irritation of the sesamoid apparatus by a penetrating screw. Typically, we use threaded-head screws that will be flush with the dorsal cortex and avoid the minor complication of a prominent screw head. Following fixation, the great toe is aligned congruent to the first metatarsal head and a decision is made whether to perform a phalangeal osteotomy (Akin) or shortening to correct a hallux abductus interphalangeus deformity or a congenitally long proximal phalanx.

Finally the redundant bone on the medial side of the head and shaft is removed, preserving the plantar articulation of the tibial sesamoid. A rotary burr is used to smooth the dorsimedial aspect of the metatarsal head, which is the most likely site of prominence postoperatively.

Capsuloplasty is accomplished with 2–0 absorbable sutures, with the suture being placed immediately medial to the tibial sesamoid and connected to the dorsal portion of the capsule. The tensioning of the repair is important to correct the deformity but not cause a postoperative hallux varus.

The wound is closed with a subcuticular 5–0 absorbable suture and augmented with half-inch (12-mm) Steri-strips. The great toe is bandaged without any additional attempts at correction through the use of the bandage. A 6-inch (15-cm) elastic bandage is applied with mild tension from the toes to the mid-calf.

Typically, the operation consumes 30 min of operating time once the learning curve is mastered. Bilateral hallux valgus is corrected at the same operative encounter.

Postoperative care

An LSB type I or typical surgical shoe is used postoperatively and the patient is permitted to bear weight without crutches or cane. LSW returns patients home the same day as surgery and LSB's patients remain in the hospital for 1–2 days.

Non-steroidal anti-inflammatory medication is used for 10 days and augmented when necessary by moderate analgesic drugs. Most patients experience little to almost no postoperative pain, probably as a result of the long duration of local anesthesia.

Patients are instructed to limit weightbearing to the essentials: bathroom and getting something to eat. The elastic bandage is removed and re-applied daily, during which the subtalar joint and ankle are rotated for several minutes to prevent splinting of the musculature.

Patients are called the first postoperative day and further instructed to contact the office in the event of severe pain, swelling, throbbing or other possible signs of infection.

One week following surgery, all bandages are removed and radiographs taken to confirm maintenance of fixation. The patient is evaluated by a physical therapist who provides a comprehensive program in home physical therapy. A 3-foot (1-m) long, 2-inch (5-cm) wide piece of an Esmarch bandage is used to exercise the great toe in plantar flexion. With the foot held at a right angle to the leg, the strip is placed around the patient's great toe and the patient holds the strip as if holding the reins on a horse. Initially, the strips will provide little resistance as they flex the toe plantarward, but with time and confidence they increase the tension for a dynamic exercise of the great toe flexors. The flexion exercise is performed in three sets of 25 each for a total of 75 times, twice daily.

There are no sutures to remove and therefore the patient may resume bathing immediately and leave the Steri-strips in place until they come off with wear. Patients are further instructed to return to a roomy athletic shoe or an LSB type II shoe (LSW patients prefer to use their old stretched-out athletic shoes; LSB patients prefer something a bit more esthetic) immediately and avoid wearing the surgical shoe. We have found that the surgical shoes are non-supportive, do not control swelling and are not comfortable to wear. The power of this procedure allows us to have confidence that the correction will be maintained. LSB prefers to keep patients in the type I shoe for 15 days before allowing a closed shoe.

Patients, of course, supinate for several weeks postoperatively until the strength and comfort of the great toe is sufficient to off-load the medial side of the foot.

The patient is again cautioned to avoid extended periods of weightbearing or any type of physical exercise in a weightbearing mode for an additional 5–6 weeks. They may drive a car when they have the confidence and comfort to step on the brake in an emergency situation. Most patients are able to accomplish this in 1–2 weeks following surgery.

At 7 weeks postoperatively, a final radiograph is taken and usually the bone has healed enough to allow the patient full activity to their tolerance. Range of motion and strengthening exercises are to be continued for a total of 8 weeks, but realistically most patients probably quit after 3–4 weeks.

In our collective experience of more than 10 000 bunionectomies, we have found that it takes 3–5 months for complete reduction of swelling, full range of motion and maximum improvement. Some patients say it can be as long as 1 year.

Complications

As with any surgical procedure, the scarf osteotomy is not without complications.

Stress fracture

Prior to our modification of plantarizing the proximal portion of the cut that preserves the lateral face of the first metatarsal shaft, stress fracture through the dorsal cortex at the proximal metatarsal was observed. However, even when this did occur, the dorsal migration of the metatarsal was minimal and not nearly as devastating as noted in base osteotomies. In the past 5 years, stress fracture has been rare.

Prominent hardware

Since we have switched exclusively to threaded-head screws, there have been only three cases of screw removal.

Osteonecrosis

There has been less than 0.2% of osteonecrosis in our entire series. Five patients developed painful arthritis and their treatments were revised with arthrodesis. The remaining cases did not have sufficient symptoms to warrant intervention. Poor patient selection, such as those with advanced joint arthrosis and loss of fixation, were the predisposing factors.

Overcorrection

The scarf osteotomy is a very powerful procedure to correct hallux valgus deformity. In the first 5 years of our series, postoperative hallux varus occurred in 8% of the operated feet. Although revision was not necessary in every case, it is our belief that any postoperative hallux varus is unacceptable. Since then, the incidence of hallux varus has remained at 3% for LSW and less than 1% for LSB. All cases of hallux varus were attributed to surgeon error of extensive lateral release, exaggerated lateral shift of the metatarsal, excessive exostosis resection, or overzealous medial capsulorrhaphy.

Undercorrection or recurrence of hallux valgus requiring revision

This is a rare complication in our collective series. Untreated hallux abductus interphalangeus often accounts for this complication. In fact, LSB believes that the phalangeal osteotomy improves the correction even when an interphalangeus deformity is minimal or does not exist.

Postoperative joint stiffness

This occurs much less frequently than any prior bunion operation that we have performed. We attribute this to a small shortening that we apply to all cases of limited range of motion, rigid internal fixation, early mobilization and the dynamic exercise program that the patients perform postoperatively.

Summary

The scarf bunionectomy has been shown to be a versatile and powerful procedure to correct various degrees of hallux valgus deformity. Through modifications of bone cut lengths and in combination with a phalangeal osteotomy, most hallux valgus deformities can be corrected. In cases of extreme ligamentous laxity of the first ray or arthrosis of the first metatarsocuneiform joint, the Lapidus operation may be more appropriate.

The comprehensive approach to the total forefoot imbalance is a point of discussion between the authors. LSB prefers to consider the most affected segment as the keystone of forefoot imbalance, around which the entire forefoot should be corrected, whereas LSW prefers to deal with the most affected segment independently and the correction of the remainder of the forefoot subject to the symptoms expressed by the patient.

The results of the scarf bunionectomy compare favorably with the results reported for other popular bunion surgeries, but in the whole realm of choice one must consider the following: which operation allows the patient to ambulate postoperatively without a cast or the use of crutches? Which allows a return to bathing and a closed athletic shoe in 1–2 weeks? Which allows the performance of bilateral surgery, maintaining cost effectiveness as well as returning the patient to their desired lifestyle more quickly? The scarf bunionectomy clearly excels in these areas.

It has been said that surgery is both a science and an art. The authors believe that bunion surgery is as much art as science, hence the success of so many procedures in one surgeon's hands and the failure in another's hands. The scarf osteotomy is a technically demanding procedure that has a large learning curve. However, once mastered, the scarf can provide a highly predictable and satisfying outcome for both patient and foot surgeon.

Bibliography

Barouk LS (2000) Scarf osteotomy for hallux valgus correction: local anatomy, surgical techniques and combination with other forefoot procedures. Foot Ankle Clin 5: 525–558

Dereymaeker G (2000) Scarf osteotomy for correction of hallux valgus: surgical technique and results compared to distal chevron osteotomy. Foot Ankle Clin 5: 513–524

Jarde O, Trinquier Lautard JL, Garbrion A et al. (1999) Hallux valgus treated by scarf osteotomy of the first metatarsus and the first phalanx associated with an adductor plasty. Apropos of 50 cases with a 2-year follow up. Revue de chirurgie orthopédique et réparatrice de l'appareil moteur 85: 374–380

Schoen NS, Zygmunt K, Gudas C (1996) Z-Bunionectomy: retrospective long-term study. J Foot Ankle Surg 35: 312–317

Weil LS (2000) Scarf osteotomy for correction of hallux valfus: historical perspective, surgical technique and results. Foot Ankle Clin 5: 559–580

5

Metatarso-cuneiform fusion for hallux valgus

Sigvard T. Hansen Jr

Introduction

In 1935, Dudley Morton published a study of the human foot in which he identified gastrocnemius contracture and excessive mobility of the first ray as major causes of foot pathology [Morton 1935]. Since then, first ray hypermobility has been the subject of debate and confusion in foot and ankle surgery. Often regarded as increased translation of the first tarsometatarsal (metatarsocuneiform) joint, first ray hypermobility is better defined as elevation of the first metatarsal head relative to the lesser metatarsals, resulting in inadequate weight-bearing by the first metatarsal. Pathological mobility can be seen on clinical examination when the first metatarsal head is elevated approximately 5–8 mm above the lesser heads with simulated weightbearing. Even stronger evidence of pathology is greater callosity under the second and third metatarsal heads than under the first. The second or second and third metatarsophalangeal (MTP) joints are frequently tender, usually a sign of synovitis. Lesser MTP joint dislocation is a later and more troublesome finding.

Pathological mobility of the first ray is frequently a major component of hallux valgus. Hallux valgus has traditionally been described as a deformity in a single transverse plane, but 'bunion' surgery based on this premise has been fraught with problems. In a significant number of cases, the scope of deformity includes both the transverse and the sagittal planes, allowing metatarsal mobility in both dorsal and medial directions. Weight that is normally borne by the first ray is thus transferred laterally to

the second metatarsal head, resulting in 'transfer metatarsalgia' and skin callosity.

Around the same time that Morton described first ray hypermobility, Paul Lapidus described an operation for hallux valgus consisting of first metatarsal–cuneiform fusion and MTP joint soft tissue realignment [Lapidus 1934]. Lapidus shared Morton's opinion that the pathology of hallux valgus originated in the midfoot. However, the procedure he originally described was largely unsuccessful, owing to lack of adequate internal fixation (he used suture to hold the position of the re-aligned first metatarsal). With the advent of modern fixation techniques, malunion and non-union rates have fallen well below 10%. The modified Lapidus procedure can be a powerful tool for correction of hallux valgus [Sangeorzan and Hansen 1989].

The loss of motion that results from fusion of the first tarsometatarsal joint is not a functional problem, as motion in the normal first tarsometatarsal joint is negligible. Lack of motion here is certainly preferable to hypermobility. The medial midfoot joints, including the navicular, the cuneiforms and the medial three metatarsals, are all normally very stable. The posterior tibial tendon inserts broadly on all these bones, and the three medial metatarsals act as an anterior extension of the rigid midfoot block.

By definition, hallux valgus includes abnormalities in the soft tissues around the first MTP joint. As the head of the metatarsal moves medially away from the lesser metatarsals, the medial side of the MTP joint capsule stretches both longitudinally and transversely. The metatarsal head is first subluxated and, eventually, dislocated from the sesamoids, which are held in place by the intermetatarsal ligaments. During this process, the flexor and extensor tendons come to lie lateral to the head and become valgus-producing forces at the MTP joint. Since soft-tissue pathology is associated with bony malalignment, correction of metatarsal instability must also address secondary soft-tissue problems at the MTP joint at the time of tarsometatarsal fusion.

Excessive sagittal mobility of the first ray is usually associated with gastrocnemius contracture. A tight gastrocnemius manifests symptoms through the foot by driving the metatarsal heads into the ground during the stance phase of gait, thus aggravating the symptoms of metatarsalgia. Because a tight gastrocnemius is seen in most cases of hallux valgus, reconstruction of an unstable first ray must be accompanied by gastrocnemius recession whenever this muscle is tight. Other deformities, such as clawing of the lesser toes from extensor recruitment, should be addressed at the same time. In late stages, particularly in rheumatoid patients with synovitis or diabetic patients with intrinsic musculature denervation, the lesser MTP joints may be already dislocated. In these cases, reconstruction (not resection), including MTP reduction and flexor and extensor intrinsic-plasty, is necessary.

Technique

The original procedure described by Lapidus included fusion of the first tarsometatarsal joint and fusion between the first and second metatarsal bases. The resulting rate of malunion was unacceptable because, lacking rigid fixation, he used catgut for fixation. Advances in internal fixation made popular in trauma surgery allowed Lapidus' basic concepts to be applied more effectively. There are several key principles to be followed:

1. The first metatarsal must be anatomically aligned in the transverse and sagittal planes. In other words, the first metatarsal head must be parallel to the second for even weightbearing.
2. The MTP capsule and plantar adhesions must be released to allow the metatarsal head to be centered over the sesamoids and flexor tendons.
3. The length of the first metatarsal must be maintained.
4. The metatarsocuneiform joint must be adequately prepared for fusion.
5. The fusion must be stabilized with adequate internal fixation using two or three screws. These screws must be placed with appropriate

technique to maximize their leverage on the fusion (long screws are better than short ones).
6. Shear strain-relieved bone graft must be added to encourage union.

A dorsal skin incision is made over the first ray to expose the tarsometatarsal joint without jeopardizing the anterior tibial tendon. The long extensor is held medial and the extensor brevis is kept lateral during dorsal exposure of the proximal first metatarsal. The incision can be extended proximally for fusion of the medial intercuneiform joint (needed in approximately 10% of cases) and is routinely extended distally for soft-tissue procedures at the lateral first MTP joint. After the joint has been opened, cartilage is denuded with small curettes or osteotomes, leaving bare subchondral bone on both sides of the joint (Figure 1). The bone is then drilled in multiple locations with a 2.0-mm drill to facilitate bony union. The joint is manually held reduced while the surgeon makes sure that the elevation of the first metatarsal head is at the same level as the lesser heads for uniform weightbearing.

This technique maintains the length of the first ray and is an excellent tool for correction of excessive dorsal mobility, but it may not be as effective in dealing with severe deformity. Cases in which the first tarsometatarsal joint faces medially, so that the cuneiform is wedge-shaped rather than rectangular, require a different technique. An oscillating saw with a blade 3.0 cm long and 1.0 cm wide is used to resect bony surfaces. Just enough bone is removed to correct the angulation. Most of the bone is resected from the lateral side of the first cuneiform and very little is taken from the medial side. Similarly, minimal bone is resected dorsally, whereas a small wedge may be removed from the plantar side to keep the metatarsal down in its proper position. The cuts must be precise, since multiple cuts will result in shortening of the first ray and may damage the insertions of the anterior tibial and long peroneal tendons.

Following joint preparation, it is essential that the first metatarsal head lies in an appropriate position next to the second. Excessive elevation will result in transfer metatarsalgia under the second metatarsal, and excessive plantar flexion will lead to pain under the first metatarsal head with weightbearing. After the joint has been properly positioned, internal fixation is carried out with lag screws. The first screw (3.5 or 4.0 mm cortical) is placed through a trough made in the dorsal shaft of the first metatarsal 2.0 cm distal to the tarsometatarsal joint (Figure 2a). The trough prevents the head of the

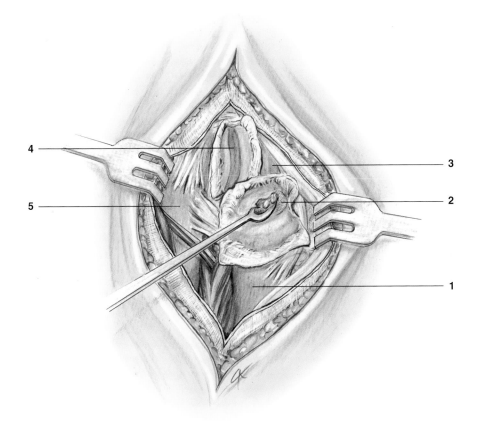

Figure 1

Cartilage is removed with a curette or an osteotome for arthrodesis of the first tarsometatarsal joint

1 First metatarsal
2 First tarsometatarsal joint
3 First cuneiform
4 First–second intercuneiform joint
5 Second metatarsal

screw from riding up on the dorsal cortex and splitting the base of the metatarsal. The screw should be placed parallel to the medial border of the foot with approximately 2.0 cm of length in the metatarsal and another 2.0 cm in the cuneiform. The length of this screw provides excellent leverage for fixation. The second screw may then be placed starting dorsally from the medial cuneiform and going into the first metatarsal. This screw is usually 36–40 mm long and is aimed plantar and parallel to the medial border of the foot (Figure 2b).

When the first metatarsal has a significant varus deformity, fixation calls for three screws. The third screw is placed in lag fashion from the medial side of the proximal first metatarsal into the base of the second metatarsal (Figure 3). Since the diameter of the second diaphysis is small and its cortex is hard, the screw should be directed somewhat proximally, where larger bone and thinner cortex are easier to penetrate. Two or three 6–8-mm burrholes are

drilled across the reduced joint to act as a 'trough' for later placement of shear strain-relieved bone graft. Bone graft for this purpose may be harvested from Gerdy's tubercle in the proximal lateral tibial metaphysis. The graft bridges the fusion site for healing and, together with good fixation, will reduce the risk of non-union.

Occasionally, the first ray is truly shorter than all the lesser rays. In this case, the joint is excised and an interpositional bone graft is placed in the fusion to restore length (Figure 4). Following debridement, the joint is opened more dorsal than plantar with a lamina spreader until the first metatarsal head is appropriately aligned with the second. A bone block may be harvested from the iliac crest, but it is often easier to take a small block from the calcaneal tuberosity. Prior to placement of internal fixation, the surgeon must make sure that the first MTP joint is not too stiff. Excessive lengthening tightens up soft tissues and, if excessive tightness is

a

Trough

Gliding hole

Tap hole

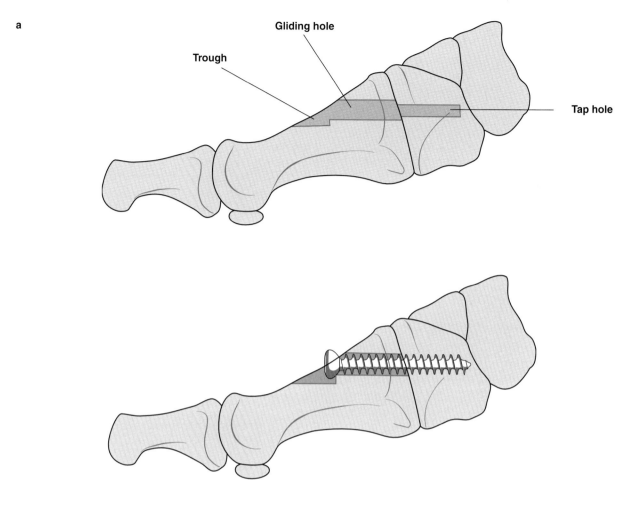

b

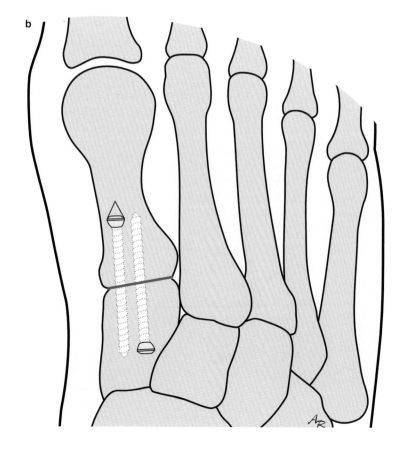

Figure 2

a. a trough made on the proximal dorsal side of the first metatarsal and the gliding hole.
b. screw in place with the head of the screw in the trough to prevent fracture of the metatarsal

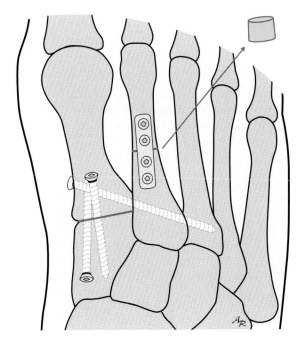

Figure 3

Screw placement when correcting a significant varus deformity of the first metatarsal. An overly long second metatarsal may be shortened in addition to the arthrodesis to eliminate excessive weightbearing

noted, the first ray should be lengthened a smaller amount. If that is the case, the lesser metatarsals may have to be shortened (see below).

A dorsal buttress plate, a quarter-tubular plate with 2.7-mm screws molded across the dorsal aspect of the fusion, holds the block in place and maintains alignment. Additional screws may be placed across the second ray, and the addition of a shear strain-relieved bone graft may be beneficial.

When the second metatarsal is quite long compared to the first and third, it may be shortened to prevent metatarsalgia postoperatively (Figure 3). Shortening is done after the first ray has been stabilized. Although the Weil sliding osteotomy has become quite popular, we have more extensive experience with diaphyseal osteotomies. A small segment of shaft is removed with an oscillating saw, making sure that the ends of the segment are parallel so that the metatarsal head is not accidentally plantarflexed. The metatarsal is shortened and held reduced by a quarter-tubular plate and 2.7-mm screws. A small amount of bone graft is added. Using this technique, the second metatarsal head stays exactly where it was placed.

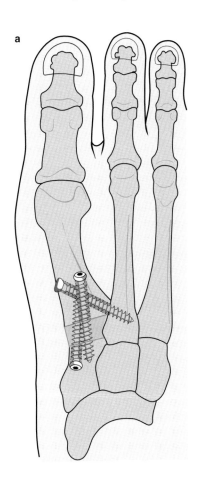
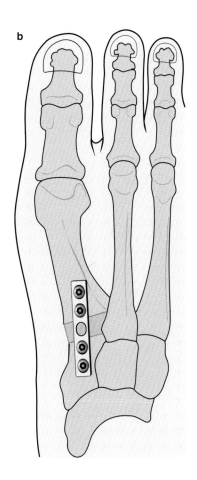

Figure 4

Interpositional bone graft from the iliac crest placed to lengthen an already shortened first metatarsal. Fixation can be achieved with 3.5-mm lag screws (a) or by utilizing a dorsal plate (b)

Distal soft tissue re-alignment

The surgical treatment of hallux valgus must include soft-tissue re-alignment around the first MTP joint. This technique is discussed in greater detail in other chapters, but it is important enough to be briefly described here. The dorsal incision is brought over the first interspace at the level of the MTP joints. The lateral first MTP capsule is incised longitudinally, but the adductor tendon is usually not transected. A small second incision is made over the medial MTP joint, carefully avoiding the sensory nerves. The medial capsule is also opened longitudinally and, after adhesions under the head and neck are released, it is reefed to tighten medially. The sesamoids should now be in their reduced positions under the metatarsal head. A medial eminence of osteophyte is removed only rarely, for the simple reason that it rarely exists. It is possible to overreduce the MTP joint by releasing the adductor tendon and removing the medial head of the metatarsal, thus leading to hallux varus.

Opening wedge osteotomy of the first cuneiform

This type of opening wedge osteotomy is useful to treat hallux valgus in adolescents, usually boys with an open physis who have several years of growth remaining. A medial cuneiform osteotomy re-aligns the first metatarsal by re-positioning the first metatarsocuneiform joint. As with fusion, soft-tissue balancing is also necessary to restore the alignment of the MTP joint. A dorsal incision is made, and the anterior tibial tendon crossing the medial surface of the first cuneiform on its way to the medial plantar surface of the first metatarsal is carefully avoided. A long, narrow oscillating saw is used to cut vertically across the middle of the medial cuneiform, leaving the lateral cortex intact. A distal capsulorrhaphy should be done prior to opening the osteotomy so that the metatarsal head can be pushed laterally while the sesamoid complex is held medially with a clamp. An osteotomy is then carried out to lever open the cuneiform medially and sometimes dorsally as well. It is essential to get the first metatarsal head level with the second. A block of iliac crest allograft bone may be shaped to fill the open wedge. The block is held in place with a small quarter-tubular 2.7-mm plate, which also buttresses the osteotomy.

Postoperative care

The foot is immobilized in a cast, and weightbearing is limited to a minimal amount needed for balance during ambulation. The sutures are removed at 2.5 weeks, and the foot is placed into a cast or a cast boot. If radiographs taken at 8 weeks show bony union, weightbearing is increased as tolerated, and the foot is gently phased into a normal shoe. Walking in a pool is an excellent form of early rehabilitation.

Occasionally, the intermetatarsal screw is prominent and symptomatic. This screw may be removed in the office after 3–6 months using a local anesthetic.

Complications

If the principles of the procedure are followed rigorously, few complications will occur. The most troublesome problems occur when the first metatarsal is not reduced level with the second. This results in metatarsalgia under the prominent head. Although mild cases can be treated with an orthotic to reduce pressure under the symptomatic head, revision surgery may be needed to restore proper alignment. In general, revisions are quite simple.

The use of suture or wires for internal fixation leads to unacceptably high rates of malunion and non-union. Adequate joint preparation and internal fixation with two or three screws plus a shear strain-relieved bone graft help to avoid this problem.

Finally, the surgeon should avoid performing bilateral fusions. Patients are unable to protect both feet postoperatively, making malunion more likely to occur.

References

Hansen ST (2000) Functional Reconstruction of the Foot and Ankle. Philadelphia, Lippincott Williams & Wilkins

Lapidus PW (1934) Operative correction of the metatarsus varus primus in hallux valgus. Surg Gynecol Obstet 58: 183–191

Morton DJ (1935) The Human Foot: Its Evolution, Physiology and Functional Disorders. Morningside Heights, Columbia University Press

Sangeorzan BJ, Hansen ST Jr (1989) Modified Lapidus procedure for hallux valgus. Foot Ankle 9: 262–266

6

Hallux varus: split extensor hallucis longus transfer

Roger A. Mann

Introduction

Hallux varus is medial deviation of the proximal phalanx on the first metatarsal head. Although it may be congenital or caused by trauma, it is usually a complication following hallux valgus surgery. The presence of a hallux varus deformity per se does not necessarily mean that the patient is symptomatic or needs surgical correction of the deformity. Following hallux valgus surgery, a varus deformity of up to 8–10° is compatible with almost normal foot function. Dorsiflexion of the metatarsophalangeal joint associated with the varus is the main factor that makes a hallux varus deformity symptomatic. If it is a single-plane deformity with the great toe deviated only medially, instead of a biplane deformity in which the great toe deviates both medially and dorsally, a moderate degree of varus is often tolerated.

The hallux varus deformity may be of several types, depending upon the etiology. Most commonly it is a single-plane deformity in which the great toe is deviated in a medial direction with no dorsiflexion component to it. Generally speaking, this is the easiest type of deformity to correct. A biplane deformity is a more severe deformity, in which there is almost always an associated flexion deformity of the interphalangeal joint of the hallux, which may be either flexible or fixed.

The etiology of hallux varus can be the result of a soft tissue imbalance or secondary to a malalignment of the metatarsal. The soft tissue causes include overplication of the medial joint capsule and inadequate re-formation of the lateral joint capsule. The lateral joint capsule includes not only the collateral ligament, but also the insertion of the adductor hallucis tendon into the base of the proximal phalanx.

The bony causes for hallux varus include the deformities resulting from excision of the fibular sesamoid (which in essence is a disruption of the lateral joint capsule), from medial subluxation of the tibial sesamoid, from excessive excision of the medial eminence, or from excessive lateral translation of the metatarsal head following either a proximal or a distal metatarsal osteotomy. Finally, the cause may be iatrogenic, from improper postoperative management in which the dressing or cast holds the toe in excessive varus following a hallux valgus repair.

Clinical findings

When considering a patient for reconstruction of the hallux varus deformity, a careful physical examination is very important. It must be determined what type of deformity is present, e.g. single plane or biplane. The patient is asked to stand, and it should be noted that in a single-plane deformity the great toe moves medially only in the transverse plane, whereas in the biplane deformity the great toe will deviate both medially and into dorsiflexion. In the biplane deformity, a flexion deformity of the interphalangeal joint of the hallux is always present, whereas it is seldom present in the single-plane deformity. The degree of tightness of the deformity should also be determined, although this is somewhat subjective; when a deformity is very rigid it is more difficult to correct than when it is flexible. The range of motion of the first metatarsophalangeal joint and the interphalangeal joint is also determined. If there is a rigid flexion deformity of the interphalangeal joint of more than about 35–40°, an interphalangeal joint arthrodesis will probably be necessary. If the deformity is fairly flexible, however, then an arthrodesis may not be necessary if the deformity can be passively straightened to approximately 25°. If the range of motion of the first metatarsophalangeal joint is reduced to less than 40–50% of that of the opposite side, then rather than attempting a soft-tissue reconstruction of the hallux varus deformity an arthrodesis of the metatarsophalangeal joint would be preferable. When checking range of motion, it is important to establish whether or not it is painful; pain may indicate the presence of arthrosis, which also precludes a soft tissue reconstruction. The placement of the surgical scars and the condition of the skin must also be taken into account: if marked adhesions and soft-tissue contractures are present, a skin slough may result from an attempted soft-tissue reconstruction.

Radiographic findings

The weightbearing radiographic analysis of the foot includes observation of the metatarsophalangeal joint, looking for the presence of a significant degree of arthrosis, assessing whether or not too much medial eminence has been excised, and the location of the sesamoids. If there is insufficient width of the metatarsal head or if there is significant arthrosis, a soft-tissue procedure will fail and an arthrodesis should be considered. A displaced sesamoid bone can usually be excised or freed up and re-aligned in the course of a soft-tissue repair. The intermetatarsal angle is observed to see whether or not following a proximal metatarsal osteotomy excessive lateral deviation of the first metatarsal has occurred. Pressure of the proximal phalanx on the medial side of the metatarsal head will produce a narrowing of the intermetatarsal angle, and this has to be differentiated from excessive lateral displacement of the metatarsal caused by an osteotomy. The distal portion of the metatarsal also has to be evaluated, since following a chevron or other distal metatarsal osteotomy, lateral deviation of the head may occur, which can also result in a varus alignment of the hallux.

If a hallux varus deformity is present and the metatarsophalangeal joint is satisfactory, then a soft-tissue re-alignment procedure utilizing the split extensor hallucis longus transfer can be expected to produce an acceptable result in approximately 80% of cases. If, however, there is significant arthrosis of the metatarsophalangeal joint or an excessive amount of medial eminence has been excised, then an arthrodesis is indicated.

If the varus deformity is due to malalignment of the first metatarsal, caused by either excessive lateral deviation following a proximal metatarsal osteotomy or abnormal rotation of the metatarsal head following a distal metatarsal osteotomy, it is necessary to determine whether a bony correction should accompany the soft-tissue correction.

Treatment

Surgical technique

The procedure is divided into three parts: the first is the harvesting of the lateral two-thirds of the extensor hallucis longus tendon and the preparation of the lateral aspect of the base of the proximal phalanx; the second is a medial approach in which the contracted capsular tissues are released; and the third is the reconstructive phase in which the tendon is passed beneath the transverse metatarsal ligament and inserted into the base of the proximal phalanx.

The results of this procedure have been satisfactory. If the tendon transfer is not tightened sufficiently, or if the soft tissue contracture is not completely released, full correction cannot be achieved. Approximately 50% of normal dorsiflexion and plantar flexion at the metatarsophalangeal joint is achieved following the procedure. If the procedure fails and the patient is dissatisfied, a fusion of the metatarsophalangeal joint can be carried out.

Obtaining the extensor hallucis longus tendon graft and preparation of the base of the proximal phalanx

The skin incision starts distally just lateral to the extensor hallucis longus tendon, is carried in a lateral direction towards the first web space, and then gently swings back medially towards the extensor hallucis longus tendon to the level of the metatarsocuneiform joint (Figure 1a). The skin flap is dissected full thickness to avoid a slough, exposing the extensor hallucis longus tendon throughout

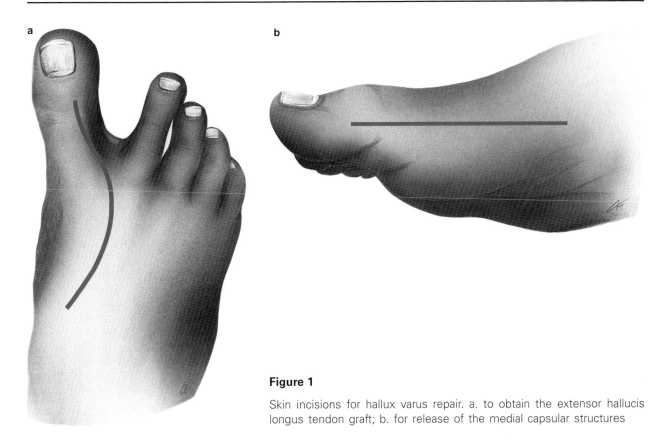

Figure 1

Skin incisions for hallux varus repair. a. to obtain the extensor hallucis longus tendon graft; b. for release of the medial capsular structures

the entire length of the wound. The lateral two-thirds of the extensor hallucis longus tendon is harvested by removing its insertion from the distal phalanx and then carefully teasing it proximally to the level of about the metatarsocuneiform joint (Figure 2). The lateral aspect of the base of the proximal phalanx is exposed by sharp and blunt dissection approximately 5 mm distal to the level of the metatarsophalangeal joint.

Release of the medial capsular structures

Through a separate medial longitudinal incision (Figure 1b), starting at the level of the interphalangeal joint, an incision is brought proximally to the level of the midportion of the metatarsal. It is deepened through the skin down to the capsule and a full-thickness dorsal and plantar flap is created (Figure 3). At times this dissection is hampered by scar tissue from previous surgery. Care is taken to avoid the dorsal and plantar medial cutaneous nerves during this portion of the dissection. The joint capsule is removed from its origin along the dorsomedial aspect of the metatarsal head in such a way that it can be slid distally as one sheet of tissue (Figure 3). At times it is impressive how thick this tissue layer can be. The abductor hallucis tendon is identified and an incision is made along its dorsal

aspect, separating it from the medial joint capsule. If the tibial sesamoid is subluxed medially, it is dissected free of the abductor hallucis tendon, so that it can be re-aligned if possible underneath the first metatarsal head. If the sesamoid bone, when restored underneath the metatarsal head, is too prominent on the sole of the foot, it can be excised. This is necessary in about one-third of cases. The abductor hallucis tendon is then cut obliquely, completing the release of the medial structures of the metatarsophalangeal joint. At this point, when the hallux is lightly pushed into a lateral position it should have a tendency to remain there. If, however, there is resistance to lateral deviation of the hallux, it means there still is some soft-tissue contracture present medially, which needs to be released. Keep in mind that a tendon transfer will not be successful in the presence of any fixed soft-tissue contracture. Occasionally the dorsal capsule needs to be released if there is a dorsiflexion contracture at the metatarsophalangeal joint. The metatarsal head is carefully inspected for evidence of arthrosis.

Reconstruction

A drill hole of adequate size is made across the base of the proximal phalanx distal to the articular

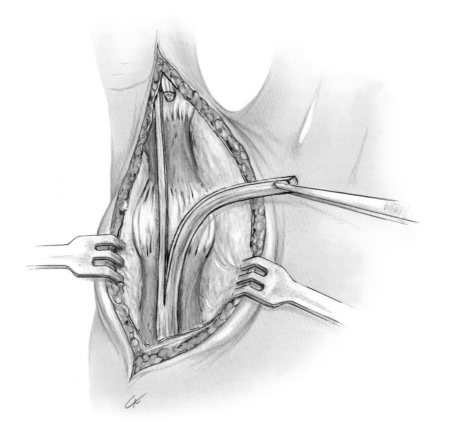

Figure 2

The lateral two-thirds of the extensor hallucis longus tendon is detached

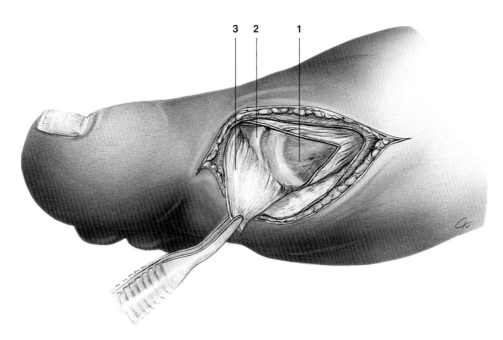

Figure 3

The medial joint capsule is released through the medial incision

1 First metatarsal head
2 Proximal phalanx
3 Joint capsule

surface of the joint from medial to lateral. This should be made in the midline (Figure 4). A ligature carrier or large right-angle clamp is passed deep or plantar to the transverse metatarsal ligament from distal to proximal leaving a piece of suture behind (Figure 5). Two sutures are placed into the stump of the extensor hallucis longus tendon. It is attached to the suture, which is beneath the transverse metatarsal ligament and brought out distally into the first web space.

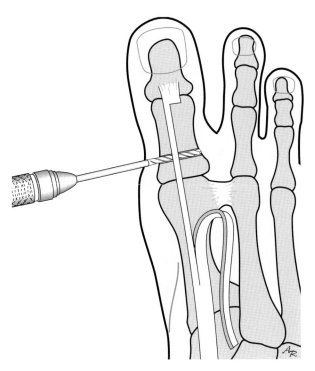

Figure 4

A horizontal drill hole is made from medial to lateral at the base of the proximal phalanx

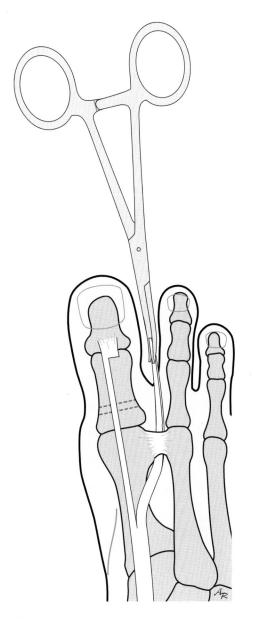

Figure 5

A clamp is passed underneath the transverse metatarsal ligament and the tendon graft is pulled through

The sutures in the extensor hallucis longus tendon are now passed through the drill hole in the base of the proximal phalanx from lateral to medial. The extensor hallucis longus tendon is pulled through the base of the proximal phalanx (Figure 6) as the phalanx is brought into lateral deviation and the ankle joint into dorsiflexion in order to relieve the tension on the extensor hallucis longus tendon. Usually 5–7 mm of tendon can be pulled through to the medial side of the phalanx, placing the hallux in about 25° of valgus. The tendon is anchored into the soft tissues along the medial side of the base of the proximal phalanx. The hallux should now stay in a valgus position when the ankle joint is brought from dorsiflexion to a neutral position. If the tendon is not under sufficient tension, it will need to be tightened further. If the position of the hallux is satisfactory, the medial third of the extensor hallucis longus tendon is loose and needs to be tightened in order for the patient to resume active extension of the metatarsophalangeal joint. A 4–0 nylon suture with a needle at each end is woven through the medial third of the extensor hallucis longus tendon over a distance of approximately 2.5 cm. Once this has been achieved, the suture is gently tightened, which brings the remaining extensor hallucis longus tendon into multiple folds. The tension is increased until the interphalangeal joint of the hallux is brought into full extension with the ankle in neutral position. With the hallux in the desired valgus position, the abductor hallucis tendon is sutured in its lengthened position. The medial joint capsule is left covering the bone over the medial aspect of the metatarsal.

Postoperative care

The wounds are closed with interrupted sutures and a snug compression dressing is applied, holding the great toe in approximately 25° of valgus. The

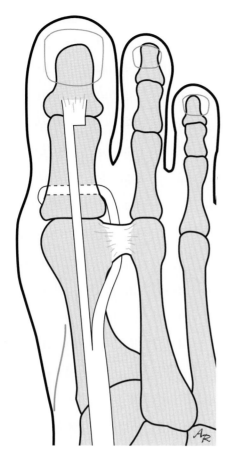

Figure 6

The tendon graft is passed through the drill hole and sutured to the medial aspect of the joint capsule, with the hallux in the desired position

postoperative dressing is changed after approximately 24–36 h and a new dressing maintaining the valgus alignment of the hallux is applied. The patient is permitted to walk in a postoperative shoe. The dressings are changed every 7–10 days for a total of 8 weeks.

Further reading

Hawkins FB (1971) Acquired hallux varus: cause, prevention and correction. Clin Orthop 76: 169–176

Jahss MH (1983) Spontaneous hallux varus: relation to poliomyelitis and congenital absence of the fibular sesamoid. Foot Ankle 3: 224–226

Johnson KA, Spiegl PV (1984) Extensor hallucis longus transfer for hallux varus deformity. J Bone Joint Surg 66A: 681–686

Joseph B, Chacko V, Abraham T, Jacob M (1987) Pathomechanics of congenital and acquired hallux varus: a clinical and anatomical study. Foot Ankle 8: 137–143

Mann RA, Coughlin MJ (1993) Adult hallux valgus. In: Mann RA, Coughlin MJ (eds) Surgery of the Foot and Ankle, 6th edn. St Louis, Mosby-Yearbook, pp 167–296

Miller JW (1975) Acquired hallux varus: a preventable and correctable disorder. J Bone Joint Surg 57A: 183–188

Mills JA, Menelaus MB (1989) Hallux varus. J Bone Joint Surg 71B: 437–440

Skalley TC, Myerson MS (1994) The operative treatment of acquired hallux varus. Clin Orthop 306: 183–191

Tourne Y, Saragaglia D, Picard F, De Sousa B, Montbarbon E, Charbel A (1995) Iatrogenic hallux varus surgical procedure: a study of 14 cases. Foot Ankle Int 16: 457

Turner RS (1986) Dynamic post-surgical hallux varus after lateral sesamoidectomy: treatment and prevention. Orthopedics 9: 963–969

7

Hallux rigidus: cheilectomy and osteotomies around the first metatarso-phalangeal joint

Andrea Cracchiolo III
Francesco Malerba

Introduction

Hallux rigidus is a condition of the hallux metatarsophalangeal joint characterized by pain and limitation of motion. This entity has been known for 100 years and is probably second only to hallux valgus as a cause of hallux symptoms. The condition has a rich orthopedic history and its original description was probably by Nicoladoni [1881] and by Davies-Colley [1887], who used the term 'hallux flexus'. Many other names have been used to characterize the pathology, such as hallux dolorosa, dorsal bunion, hallux limitus, hallux arthriticus and hallux equinus. However, the name proposed by Cotterill [1887] – hallux rigidus – is today the most accepted and refers to degenerative arthrosis involving the hallux metatarsophalangeal joint. The condition begins as a flexible, functional sagittal-plane deformity, frequently called 'hallux limitus', and then becomes rigid. No matter what the grade or stage, the hallux usually remains well aligned. However, a few patients may also show a valgus deformity, hence the term 'hallux valgus rigidus'.

The symptoms of pain and restriction of motion in the hallux metatarsophalangeal joint are usually of gradual onset, and the patient may give a completely negative history for any possible etiology. One characteristic of pain in hallux rigidus is that it is usually present with walking, whereas patients with hallux valgus complain of pain mostly when walking in shoes [Moberg 1979]. The motion initially most severely restricted is dorsiflexion. Plantar flexion may be unaffected, especially early in the disease. However, patients may also present with some restriction of almost all motion. Various degrees of inflammation can be seen within the joint. However, the foot often appears completely normal, with no detectable swelling or erythema and with only some degree of spasm of the extensor hallucis longus. There is usually considerable tenderness when the joint is palpated, and one can usually feel a dorsal bone spur. Any forceful movement, especially dorsiflexion, causes pain. Patients with hallux rigidus have a particularly difficult time finding shoes that will allow more comfortable walking. Whenever a shoe with any significant elevation of the heel is worn, pain increases and walking is more limited. Patients with this condition usually show no sign of arthrosis in any other joints.

Hallux rigidus is found in both men and women, being somewhat more common in women [McMaster 1978, Mann et al. 1979]. However, since restriction of dorsiflexion is more disabling in women, they may more often seek care. The condition may be present in any age group from adolescence onwards. Unilateral cases are the most common.

Etiology

Many factors have been implicated as possibly causing or contributing to the development of hallux rigidus:

- Abnormalities of anatomy, such as a long, narrow foot, a pronated foot, a long first metatarsal, abnormalities of the hallux metatarsophalangeal joint and elevation of the first ray, called metatarsus primus elevatus [Jack, 1940];
- Unsuitable shoes, especially those causing hyperextension of the great toe;
- Abnormality of gait;
- Osteochondritis dissecans;
- Miscellaneous factors such as obesity and occupation;
- Trauma to the joint – patients occasionally report a specific history of injury that seems consistent with the degree of pathology seen clinically and radiographically, and at the time of surgical exploration of the joint;
- Chip fractures of the dorsal lip of the proximal phalanx, as well as small subchondral defects in the metatarsal head [McMaster 1978].

Pathology, clinical and radiographic findings

Patients are usually seen initially with advanced changes that resemble the pathology of degenerative joint disease. Extensive osteophytes are present, usually on the dorsum of the metatarsal head and the base of the proximal phalanx and along the tibial and fibular borders of the head, which makes the metatarsal head seem radiographically flattened. The joint space is greatly narrowed and almost obliterated at times. Subchondral sclerosis is seen, and cysts may be present in the head and may also occur in the phalanx. However, patients seen early in their disease may have minimal radiographic changes showing only some narrowing of the joint and slight flattening of the head. A loose body has been described within the joint, as well as a traumatic flap of cartilage found between the apex of the dome of the head and its dorsal border [McMaster 1978]. Therefore, it appears that direct trauma or indirect trauma such as stubbing of the hallux can produce lesions that result in hallux rigidus. Elevation of the first ray, called metatarsus

primus elevatus, was also thought to play a role in the pathogenesis of hallux rigidus. However, the same degree of metatarsus primus elevatus (8 mm average) has been found in normal subjects as is found in patients with hallux rigidus.

Treatment

Patients with considerable pain, especially those who are active, usually cannot find sufficient relief with non-operative measures and require surgery. A variety of operations have been performed to correct painful hallux rigidus.

Cheilectomy is a debridement of the joint with special emphasis on removing the osteophytes about the metatarsal head. A dorsal closing wedge of the base of the proximal phalanx has been used as the sole treatment for this condition [Kessel and Bonney 1958, Moberg 1979]. This is also an excellent adjunct procedure to a cheilectomy. The osteotomy positions the hallux in some degree of dorsiflexion during heel lift. If there is 20–30° of plantar flexion remaining in the joint then the hallux remains plantigrade during stance.

The enclavement procedure was originally described by Regnauld [1986] and has been used by surgeons in Europe for the treatment of both hallux rigidus and hallux valgus. Many variations of the procedure exist, but basically it is an osteotomy of the proximal third of the proximal phalanx, which is excised, remodeled and re-inserted as an osteocartilaginous graft.

Other treatment options are an excisional arthroplasty of the joint, an arthrodesis of the hallux metatarsophalangeal joint, and implant arthroplasty using a double-stem silicone implant.

Indications

Choosing the correct procedure depends on several factors: the severity of the disease, the patient's age and sex, and postoperative activity expectations.

Severity of disease

Hallux rigidus has been divided into various grades or stages, depending on the degree of arthrosis present within the joint [Hattrup and Johnson 1988]. Grade I disease shows little or no radiographic abnormality, with the patient presenting because of limited dorsiflexion of the hallux. Grade II hallux rigidus is characterized by markedly decreased and painful dorsiflexion, with dorsal joint space narrowing or osteophyte formation on radiographs. Grade III represents end-stage arthritic changes of the joint, with complete obliteration of the joint space radiographically. Feltham et al. [2001] utilized the grading system proposed by Regnauld [1986], which is somewhat different and more complicated than that proposed by Hattrup and Johnson [1988]. Moreover, Feltham et al. divided their patients into two groups when deciding which operation to advise. The division was based on whether or not the patient had predominantly extra-articular symptoms, for which they advised cheilectomy. Those having intra-articular pain (pain at rest, prior to activity or at night) were advised to have an arthrodesis. (See Malerba classification pp. 56–57.)

Age, sex and activity level

It would indeed be a rare patient who required an operation prior to completion of skeletal growth. Patients with chip fractures or osteochondritis would be best treated by removal of the fragments. A young active patient could be a candidate for cheilectomy, especially where there is less severe joint space narrowing [Graves 1993]. Middle-aged active patients may consider a cheilectomy if it appears that some viable joint surfaces remain with only mild to moderate osteophytes and a good joint space [Hattrup and Johnson 1988]. However, cheilectomy may not result in an absolutely painless, moveable joint; the patients are better but not 'normal'. In such patients cheilectomy can be combined with a dorsal closing wedge of the base of the proximal phalanx. This is a good option if the joint has a relatively normal amount of plantar flexion. In patients with more advanced degenerative joint changes, an arthrodesis should be advised. However, some patients resist this recommendation and prefer cheilectomy. Such patients must be told that, should cheilectomy fail, an arthrodesis will be required. Women usually prefer to regain dorsiflexion motion, and if they are inactive may be considered as suitable for an excisional or capsular interpositional arthroplasty or a silicone implant. Elderly patients are candidates for implants or arthrodesis. Implant arthroplasty may be preferable in an older patient with low activity expectations, because the postoperative course is much shorter than for an arthrodesis.

Contraindications

Apart from the absolute contraindications for surgery, such as poor general health, peripheral vascular disease, poor skin coverage and local infection, each of the following procedures has specific drawbacks.

- Cheilectomy of a severely arthritic joint was not advocated if significant motion and function were the goals. While these joints may show some increase in motion in the face of cartilage deterioration [Mann and Clanton 1988], long-term improvements in function were not reported. Pain relief was not achieved in 30–40% of these patients with more advanced degenerative changes [Hattrup and Johnson 1988]. However, Feltham et al. [2001] and Easly et al. [1999] both reported good results when cheilectomy was performed on any patient with extra-articular pain, regardless of the radiographic features or the patient's age. However, 7% failed [Feltham et al. 2001] and required subsequent arthrodesis.
- Excisional arthroplasty frequently results in a loss of hallux function. In addition, malalignment of the hallux may develop.
- Arthrodesis will certainly relieve pain if successful. However, interphalangeal motion should be normal preoperatively and must not be damaged by the procedure. Should the interphalangeal joint deteriorate later, the patient's gait may be further impaired. The technique of arthrodesis must be

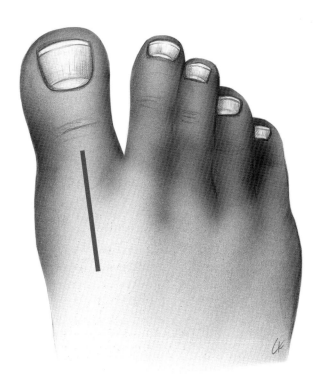

Figure 1

A dorsal longitudinal incision just medial to the extensor hallucis longus is usually the most efficient incision to give adequate exposure

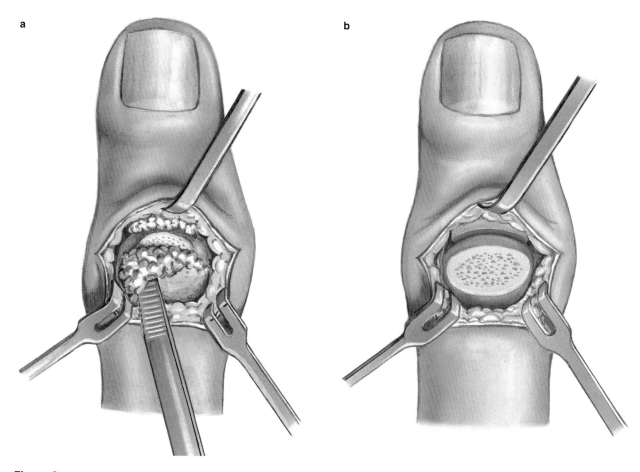

Figure 2

An osteotome or a thin oscillating saw can be used for resection of the osteophyte. a. prior to removal of osteophyte; b. following removal of the dorsal 25–35% of the head with the osteophyte, and of the osteophyte at the base of the proximal phalanx

precise, and the angle of arthrodesis is critical. Time required for fusion as well as immobilization may be lengthy and may produce difficulties, especially for the older patient. Lastly, fusion may not occur.

- The single-stem silicone implant arthroplasty, although giving good relief of pain and restoring functional motion, does deteriorate with time. Radiographs show fragmentation of the implant requiring its removal [Shankar 1995] and the procedure is no longer recommended. A double-stem silicone implant protected by titanium grommets may still be used [Sebold and Cracchiolo 1996]. However, even this implant should not be used in young or highly active patients, such as those wanting to continue with sports requiring running or jumping. Any implant can fail or become infected, requiring its removal.

Operative techniques

Several steps are common to all operations involving the hallux metatarsophalangeal joint in patients with hallux rigidus. Most surgeons prefer to use a tourniquet so that the procedure is performed in a bloodless field. The incisions are almost always longitudinal and may be dorsomedial, or a direct dorsal longitudinal incision may be preferable.

Cheilectomy

Cheilectomy is performed on an outpatient basis and can be done under regional ankle block anesthesia. The hallux metatarsophalangeal joint is exposed through a dorsal longitudinal incision (Figure 1). The capsule is incised in a similar longitudinal line. The capsule and the extensor hallucis longus are retracted laterally, exposing the dorsal bone spurs and any lateral osteophytes. Bony spurs can be removed using rongeurs and the metatarsal head further trimmed using either a sharp osteotome or a power oscillating saw (Figure 2).

Approximately 25–35% of the dorsal portion of the metatarsal head should be obliquely excised (Figure 3), with the cut beginning distally and being made in a proximal and dorsal direction. This also

a

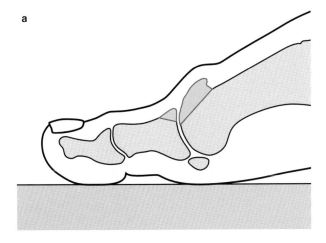

b

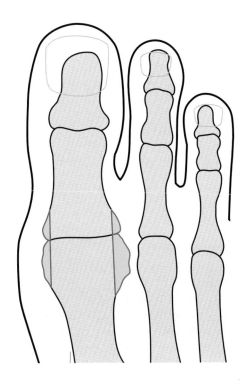

Figure 3

The dorsal 25–35% of the metatarsal head and remaining osteophytes at the lateral and medial aspects of the metatarsal head are excised. At the base of the proximal phalanx a wedge of bone is removed, which usually contains the dorsal osteophyte and some eburnated joint surface. a. medial aspect; b. dorsal aspect

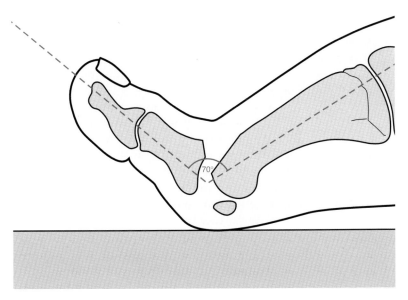

Figure 4

Between 70 and 90° of passive extension should be obtained at the conclusion of the cheilectomy

avoids fracture of the head if an osteotome is used. A small amount of bone wax can be used to decrease the postoperative bleeding. The medial and lateral osteophytes should be removed in a similar fashion. Any significant osteophytes on the dorsum of the base of the proximal phalanx should also be removed, together with some eburnated joint surface. It may be necessary to excise the same amount of the dorsum of the proximal phalanx as was removed from the metatarsal head, in order to regain the desired amount of dorsiflexion. At this point, at least 70–90° of passive dorsiflexion must be obtained (Figure 4).

Approximately half that motion will be lost post-operatively. If achieving this degree of dorsiflexion proves difficult, insufficient bone may have been removed, or there may be adhesions between the sesamoids and the metatarsal head on the plantar surface. This area should be routinely inspected, which can be easily done by plantarflexing the hallux. The area can be probed with a smooth elevator. Blunt dissection is usually sufficient to clear these restrictive adhesions (Figure 5). If the sesamoids are ankylosed to the plantar condyle of the metatarsal head, this usually indicates advanced degenerative arthrosis, and a cheilectomy may fail in such a patient. The dorsal capsule is closed loosely with an absorbable suture and the skin is closed in a routine manner. A sterile compression dressing is placed which should hold the hallux in a normal alignment.

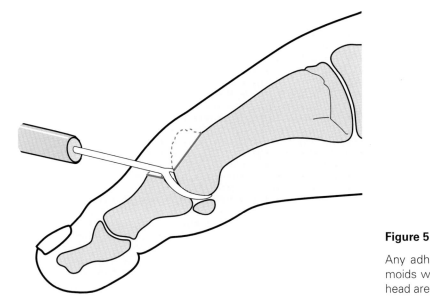

Figure 5

Any adhesions at the articulation of the sesamoids with the plantar surface of the metatarsal head are divided

Postoperatively, the patients are allowed to walk on the first day after surgery using a hard-soled postoperative shoe. An oversize, inexpensive, flexible athletic shoe, to accommodate postoperative swelling, should be worn once the bulky postoperative dressing has been removed, about 5–7 days postoperatively. The sutures remain in place for 10–14 days. Passive and active exercises are initiated during the first few postoperative days, with an emphasis on dorsiflexion of the hallux.

Phalangeal osteotomy

A dorsal closing wedge osteotomy can be performed at the junction between the metaphysis and diaphysis of the base of the proximal phalanx. This osteotomy has been described for the treatment of hallux rigidus in adolescents [Kessel and Bonney 1958] and adults [Moberg 1979] (Figure 6). It is most frequently used as an adjunct procedure, if sufficient passive extension cannot be achieved during cheilectomy. However, the patient should have about 20° of flexion at the hallux metatarsopharyngeal joint preoperatively. This motion will allow sufficient flexion postoperatively so the hallux should touch the floor. This osteotomy should not be used if there is no flexion, as the toe may be in extension postoperatively. The proximal part of the phalanx can be easily exposed via the distal limit of the skin incision. The periosteum should be carefully elevated both medially and laterally, but not circumferentially. Small right-angled retractors are used to protect the medial and lateral soft tissues. An oscillating saw with a thin, narrow blade is used to remove a dorsal wedge of bone about 2–3 mm thick. The blade should not cut through the plantar cortex. This avoids the risk of damage to the flexor hallucis longus. Producing a

greenstick-type fracture of the plantar cortex closes the dorsal side of the wedge and provides good stability to the hallux. Internal fixation can be used to secure the osteotomy and may be necessary if the osteotomy is unstable. This can be done using a thin wire as a suture, a small staple, an absorbable pin, or preferably a 2.7-mm screw for postoperative stability. If possible, the soft tissues over the osteotomy should be closed with a few interrupted 4–0 absorbable sutures.

Postoperatively, the patients can walk using crutches and should use a wooden-soled shoe for about 10 days. However, active and passive motion of the hallux should be instituted as soon as possible, usually at about 5 days postoperatively. Patients can leave off their wooden shoe and walk either barefoot or in sandals. The postoperative dressing is changed again at about the 10th day; the sutures can be removed if wound healing is satisfactory. A smaller dressing is placed to hold the hallux in a corrected position, permitting more potential motion. Pain and swelling usually subside after 2–3 months, and best results are usually seen by 6 months. It must be stressed that the patients must actively participate in a vigorous rehabilitation program if they are to regain motion, and that success is not achieved immediately.

Excisional arthroplasty

In the past, the Keller resection arthroplasty was used to treat hallux rigidus. The results were unpredictable, and frequently the hallux would drift into valgus or varus. However, if good soft-tissue repair is added after the base of the proximal phalanx has been resected, it may be possible to achieve a good result with excisional arthroplasty. Hamilton and

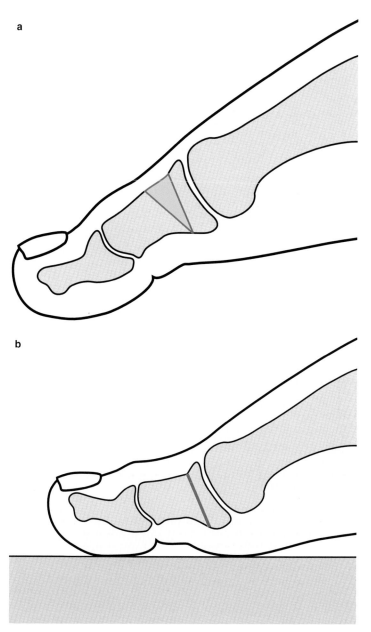

Figure 6

A dorsal closing wedge osteotomy has been used to provide a relative increase in extension of the hallux in patients with hallux rigidus. a. prior to removal of the bone wedge; b. following closure of the osteotomy

Hubbard [2000] reported good to excellent results using a capsular interposition arthroplasty in patients with severe (grade III) hallux rigidus. This procedure utilizes the thickened dorsal capsule as an interposition into the space created by excision of the base of the proximal phalanx (Figure 7). It is sutured to the stumps of the flexor hallucis brevi just distal to the sesamoids. Soft-tissue balance must be preserved, and unless the extensor hallucis longus is lengthened, a Kirschner wire is not used.

Complications

Superficial wound infection and delayed healing are rare complications of these operations. Unsatisfactory results are usually due to progression of the degenerative process, with recurrent or continued pain on dorsiflexion of the hallux. In this case, a

further procedure such as arthrodesis, resection arthroplasty or implant arthroplasty may become necessary.

Hallux rigidus: role of distal first metatarsal osteotomies

Francesco Mallerba

Hallux rigidus is a pathology of the first metatarsophalangeal (MP1) joint clinically characterized by a restriction of motion, whatever the cause. Abnormal biomechanics at the MP1 joint as a possible cause of hallux rigidus is of great interest: in the propulsive phase of gait the subtalar joint should be supinated

a

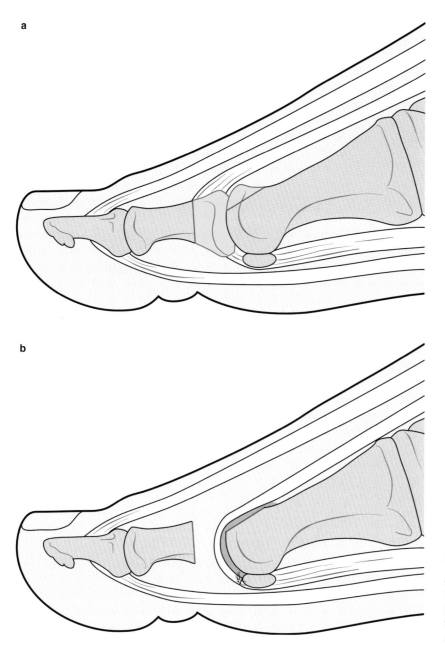

b

Figure 7

a. Excision of the base of the proximal phalanx and the dorsal osteophytes on the metatarsal head. b. the dorsal capsule is sutured to the stumps of the flexor hallucis brevis

to transform the forefoot into a rigid lever suitable for effective propulsion. Any condition that forces the subtalar joint to remain pronated in the propulsive phase of gait results in an instability of the first ray. The metatarsal is not able to counteract the ground reaction forces, and the first metatarsal elevates. As the hallux, at that moment, is firmly fixed on the ground, a dorsal subluxation at the MP1 joint may occur with a dorsal impingement of the joint, especially when a forefoot rectus morphotype is present. In the initial phases the elevation of the first ray is evident only when weightbearing (functional limitus). With time the inflammatory processes caused by impingement at the MP1 joint may result in the development of dorsal osteophytes of the first metatarsal and in a contracture of the plantar soft structures, and finally the elevatus of the first

metatarsal is present also when non-weightbearing (structured hallux limitus).

The frequency of a biomechanical progressive failure of the MP1 joint causing hallux rigidus is unknown and this is not a universally accepted phenomenon. In any case an elevated position of the first metatarsal is often observed in the radiological and clinical findings of hallux rigidus, and this condition should be considered when planning treatment. Hallux rigidus in the past was also called 'hallux flexus' and 'first metatarsal elevatus' to identify the important anatomical pathological condition of the deformity. This hallux rigidus classification recognizes four stages based on the degree of MP1 arthritis:

1. Functional limitus is characterized by the clinical observation of an elevated position of the

first metatarsal in the propulsive phase of the gait, causing pain and synovitis at the MP1 joint without any radiographic changes.

2. Hallux rigidus first degree: the pathology is characterized by clinical and radiographic evidence of MP1 joint adaptation to the impingement and increased pressure acting on the joint. The head of the first metatarsal flattens, osteochondral pathology may be seen, small dorsal exostoses are observed and a limitation of the range of motion of the MP1 joint is evident.

3. Hallux rigidus second degree: MP1 joint arthrosis is observed with severe flattening of the head of the first metatarsal, joint space narrowing and cartilage erosions, and the dorsal exostosis becomes larger. Motion is limited and painful.

4. Hallux rigidus third degree, the stage of ankylosis: the head of the first metatarsal is severely flattened and the joint space obliterated. There is extensive erosion of the cartilage and exuberant exostosis of the head of the first metatarsal. Minimal motion or ankylosis of the MP1 joint is observed.

The classification is important for prognosis and the selection of treatment, but there can be many variations in each stage.

Conservative treatment is limited to the functional limitus stage of hallux rigidus (orthotics to control pronation at the subtalar joint) or in patients with general or local contraindications to undergoing a surgical procedure (special shoes, pads, insoles).

Surgical treatment depends on the etiology and the severity of the deformity. Surgical procedures are grouped as reconstructive joint techniques (MP1 would be preserved via distal osteotomies of the first metatarsal) and destructive joint techniques (arthrodesis, arthroplasty, joint replacement).

The purpose of osteotomies in hallux rigidus is to re-align the joint when an elevatus of the first metatarsal is present and/or to decompress the joint as a narrowing of the articular space occurs associated with extensive stiffness of the soft tissues around the joint. Viable articular cartilage is an absolute prerequisite for these procedures in hallux rigidus of the first degree and selected cases of the second degree.

Re-alignment of the joint occurs by means of a distal osteotomy of the first metatarsal designed to plantar displace the metatarsal head, restoring the normal relationships between the first metatarsal and the hallux, and to decompress the joint. Decompression of the joint occurs by moving the first metatarsal head more proximally to restore the joint space and relax the contracted soft tissues. By

starting active and passive joint motion immediately, the soft tissues begin to remodel, allowing more joint motion. Removal of dorsal osteophytes also aids in restoring motion.

The aims of distal osteotomies of the first metatarsal are to reduce symptoms, improve function, correct pathology and delay more aggressive procedures. The following treatment can be considered for two stages of hallux rigidus: first-degree hallux rigidus with mild elevatus; and first- or second-degree hallux rigidus with any elevatus of the first metatarsal.

Hallux rigidus of the first degree with mild elevatus of the first metatarsal

The author (FM) has extensive experience using an osteotomy proposed by Youngswick. It consists of a V-shaped distal osteotomy of the first metatarsal directed proximally (Figure 8a). The apex of the osteotomy is at the dorsal two-thirds of the metatarsal head, and is variously angled (from 60 to 90°) depending on the elevatus (the greater the elevatus the greater the angle). The plantar cut is always proximal to the plantar blood supply for the metatarsal head, to avoid avascular necrosis. A dorsal wedge is removed from the dorsal aspect of the osteotomy, which decompresses the joint. The osteotomy design can be facilitated by using an osteotomy guide to achieve more precise and congruous cuts. When a dorsal exostectomy is not required, the osteotomy is performed without detaching the dorsal capsule and synovial recess of the joint, minimizing the risks of iatrogenic arthrofibrosis. Rigid internal fixation is mandatory, to avoid postoperative loss of correction, to allow immediate passive and active motion and to provide rapid healing of the osteotomy. The use of screws completely embedded into the bone avoids the need for a second operation to remove screws that cause discomfort (Figure 8b).

The procedure may be considered a modification of the chevron osteotomy proposed by Austin for hallux valgus. The metatarsal head can be moved laterally when there is an abnormal intermetatarsal angle.

The postoperative management includes nonweightbearing for 3 weeks, with the support of special shoes and immediate motion of the joint.

In 31 cases with an average follow-up of 6 years, 26 patients had an excellent result (the score considered motion, pain and radiographic changes

a

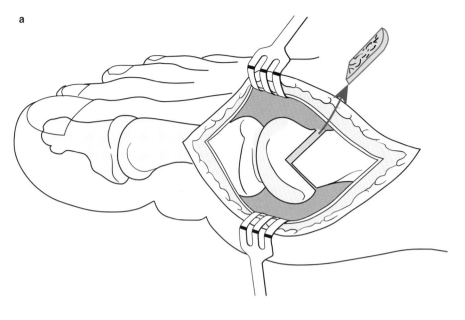

b

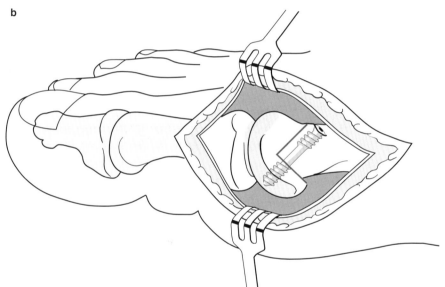

Figure 8

a. Removing the dorsal wedge allows decompression of the metatarsophalangeal joint; b. solid internal fixation is obtained using a threaded-head screw which is completely embedded in the bone

at the MP1 joint), five patients had a poor result with increased pain and rigidity of the joint, and four of these underwent further surgery. Of the patients with excellent results at 6 years' average follow-up, 51% showed progressive arthrosis radiographically. The complications observed were the same as those seen after any distal osteotomy of the first metatarsal, and may require further surgery. Arthrodesis was successful in the four patients with a poor result. The risk of avascular necrosis is extremely limited, as the main blood supply to the metatarsal head is preserved.

Moderate to severe elevatus of the first metatarsal is a contraindication for this procedure.

Hallux rigidus of the first degree with moderate to severe elevatus of the first metatarsal, or second degree with any elevatus and good cartilage at the first metatarsophalangeal joint

The author (FM) in 1995 presented a personal technique called 'oblique distal osteotomy of the first metatarsal' which can be performed with any degree of elevatus [Malerba and De Marchi 1995]. This procedure also decompresses the MP1 joint.

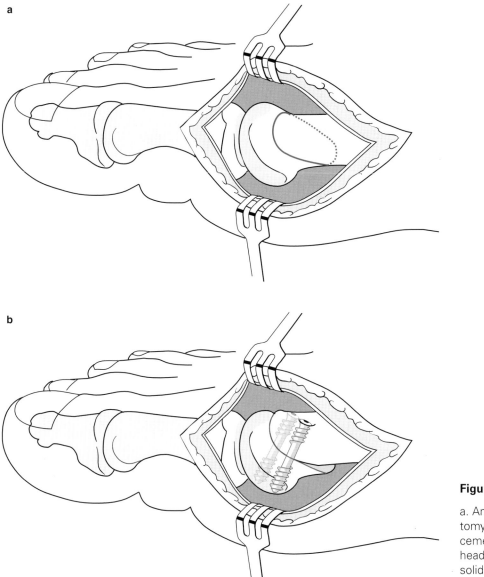

a

b

Figure 9

a. An oblique shortening osteo-tomy with proximal displa-cement of the first metatarsal head; b. a lateral view showing solid internal fixation with two threaded-head screws

Surgical technique

The osteotomy is a linear one that starts dorsally at the articular cartilage of the first metatarsal and goes proximally and plantarly to exit the metatarsal proximal to the plantar vessels which provide blood supply to the metatarsal head. As the osteotomy is completed the lateral soft tissues, which are still intact and tight, draw the metatarsal head proximally and plantarly, spontaneously restoring normal alignment and decreasing the intra-articular pressure at the MP1 joint. The plantar–proximal position may be guided by the surgeon to achieve a better relationship of the first metatarsal to the proximal phalanx of the hallux and an acceptable decompression of the joint. It is not possible to give in millimeters the amount of displacement that is required of the osteotomy;

however, the learning curve is short and the procedure is not demanding. As a proximal displace-ment occurs the metatarsal shortens but transfer metatarsalgia is avoided, as plantar displacement of the first metatarsal head always occurs, owing to the direction of the osteotomy. Thus, the shortening of the first metatarsal is balanced by the associated plan-tar displacement of the metatarsal head. In cases when the elevatus of the first metatarsal is the domi-nant deformity, the direction of the osteotomy should be more vertical (Figure 9a).

The osteotomy is intrinsically unstable and rigid internal fixation is required. This is provided by using two screws or two threaded pins to control any rotatory forces (Figure 9b). Rigid fixation allows immediate motion of the joint, which is particularly important in this procedure.

a

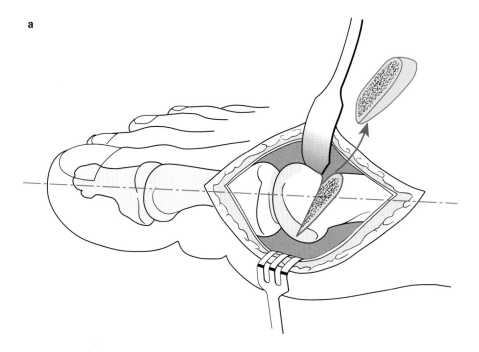

b

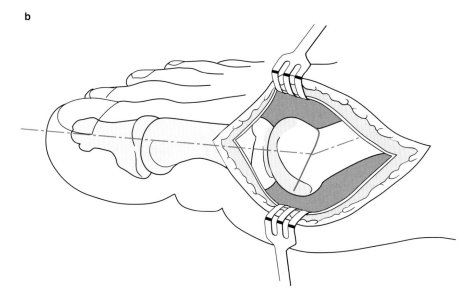

Figure 10

a. The osteotomy of LS Weil. A dorsal wedge of bone is excised from the metatarsal head, with the apex of the osteotomy being plantar and distal; b. a threaded-head screw is used for internal fixation

It is important to smooth the dorsal aspect of the osteotomy after the displacement, to avoid impingement of the joint during motion. The base of the proximal phalanx should glide smoothly on the head of the metatarsal, to allow free motion of the joint.

The metatarsal head may also be moved in the transverse plane in case of an associated abnormal intermetatarsal angle, and even rotated in case of an abnormal proximal set angle (PASA; or distal metatarsal articular angle, DMAA). The healing time is short as the osteotomy is performed in cancellous bone. In 78 cases with an average follow-up of 5 years, 42 patients were rated excellent (the evaluation considered motion, pain and radiological changes at the MP1 joint), 14 patients were rated poor, as they had more pain than preoperatively, and

six of these underwent a further procedure (four MP1 joint arthrodeses). In two of these cases the failure was due to a technical error, as the dorsal aspect of the osteotomy was not resected, causing an impingement at the MP1 joint. As we are dealing with a progressive degenerative pathology, 53% excellent results demonstrates the effectiveness of the procedure at a medium follow-up.

Avascular necrosis of the metatarsal head was observed in two cases; in both, the bone necrosis was marginal and lateral and the patients were pain free with improved motion and function.

Good articular cartilage is an absolute prerequisite for distal reconstructive osteotomies in hallux rigidus. However, in some cases of hallux rigidus of the second degree, there are extensive erosions of

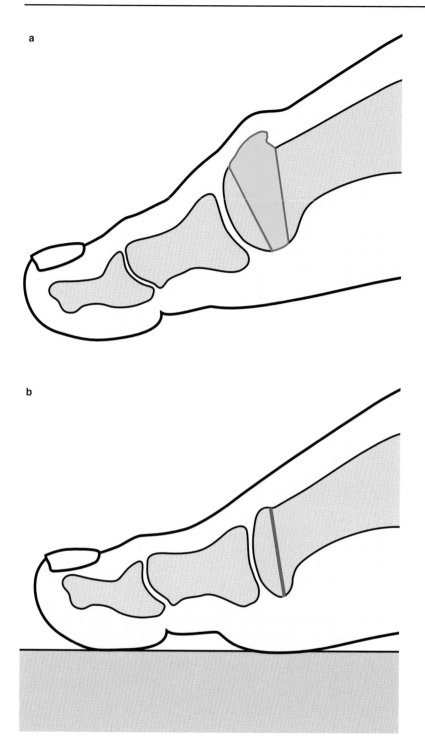

Figure 11

The articular surface of the metatarsal head may be redirected with an osteotomy of the neck of the metatarsal. a. prior to removal of bone wedge; b. following closure of the osteotomy

the cartilage in the dorsal and frontal area of the metatarsal head, making the joint unsuitable for motion. In these patients a distal osteotomy of the first metatarsal proposed by L.S. Weil in 1989 [personal communication] has been a valid alternative procedure. The operation consists of the removal of a dorsal bone wedge from the metatarsal head (Figure 10). The apex of the osteotomy is plantar and distal and terminates as close as possible to the subchondral bone. The wedge is removed and the osteotomy closed by forcing the hallux into

dorsiflexion. Rigid internal fixation is mandatory and the use of a screw that is completely embedded into the bone is necessary, as the screw should enter the bone from distal to proximal through the cartilage. The use of an osteotomy guide is helpful to excise a precise and congruous wedge of bone.

As the osteotomy is incomplete with the apex at the subchondral bone close to the cartilage, the gap created by the removal of the dorsal bone wedge is easily closed, owing to the elasticity of the cartilage. Waterman [1927] (Figure 11) had described a cuneiform dorsal osteotomy of the distal end of the first metatarsal. However, this procedure was used primarily to decompress the joint. Internal fixation was probably not used and long-term results have not been reported.

The postoperative management allows immediate weightbearing and early motion.

In a continuous series of 17 patients with an average follow-up of 4 years, eight were rated excellent (motion, pain and radiological changes were considered in the score) and five had a poor result as they had much more pain and less function than preoperatively (three underwent further surgery). At medium-term follow-up the procedure maintains encouraging results and appears to be a valid alternative to arthrodesis or to arthroplasties.

Avascular necrosis was not detected in this series, despite the distal fragment being almost completely detached from its blood supply. However, the distal fragment is very thin and could be easily integrated by the viable proximal cancellous bone.

Distal osteotomies of the first metatarsal, with proper indications, are recommended as effective procedures taking into account the pathology and the available alternatives. Long-term results are uncertain, but in any case revision procedures can be easily performed.

References

Cotterill JM (1887) Condition of great toe in adolescence. Edinburgh Med J 33: 459

Davies-Colley JNC (1887) Contraction of the metatarsophalangeal joint of the great toe. Br Med J 1: 728

Easley ME, Davis WH, Anderson RB (1999) Intermediate to long-term follow-up of medial-approach dorsal cheilectomy for hallux rigidus. Foot Ankle Int 20: 147–152

Feltham GT, Hanks SE, Marcus RE (2001) Age-based outcomes of cheilectomy for the treatment of hallux rigidus. Foot Ankle Int 22 (3): 192–197

Graves SC (1993) Hallux rigidus: treatment by cheilectomy. In: Myerson M (ed) Current Surgical Therapy in Foot and Ankle Surgery. St Louis, Mosby Yearbook, pp 74–76

Hamilton WG, Hubbard CE (2000) Hallux rigidus excisional arthroplasty. Foot Ankle Clin 5 (3): 663–671

Hattrup SJ, Johnson KA (1988) Subjective results of hallux rigidus following treatment with cheilectomy. Clin Orthop 226: 182–191

Jack EA (1940) The aetiology of hallux rigidus. Br J Surg 27: 492

Kessel L, Bonney G (1958) Hallux rigidus in the adolescent. J Bone Joint Surg 40B: 668

Malerba F, De Marchi F (1995) Hallux limitus rigidus: surgical strategy. Foot Dis 2: 97–104

Mann RA, Clanton TO (1988) Hallux rigidus: treatment by cheilectomy. J Bone Joint Surg 70A: 400–406

Mann, RA, Coughlin MJ, DuVries HL (1979) Hallux rigidus. Clin Orthop 142: 57

McMaster MJ (1978) The pathogenesis of hallux rigidus. J Bone Joint Surg 60B: 82

Moberg E (1979) A simple operation for hallux rigidus. Clin Orthop 142: 55

Nicoladoni C (1881) Uber Zehenkontrakturen. Wien Klin Wochenschr 51: 1418–1419

Regnauld B (1986) Hallux rigidus. In: The Foot. Berlin, Springer, 335–350

Sebold EJ, Cracchiolo A (1996) Use of titanium grommets on silicone implant arthroplasty of the hallux metatarsophalangeal joint. Foot Ankle 17 (3): 145–151

Shankar NS (1995) Silastic single-stem implants in the treatment of hallux rigidus. Foot Ankle Int 15: 487–491

Vanore JV, O'Keefe RG, Bidny MA et al. (1992) Hallux rigidus. In: Marcinko DE (ed) Medical and Surgical Therapeutics of the Foot and Ankle. Baltimore, Williams & Wilkins, 209–241

Waterman H (1927) Die arthritis deformans des grobetazehengrundgelenkes als selbst ndiges krankheitsbild. Z Orthotop chir 48: 346–355

Bibliography

Austin DW, Leventen EO (1981) A new osteotomy for hallux valgus. Clin Orthop 57: 25–30

Blyth MJ, Mackay DC, Kinninmouth AW (1998) Dorsal wedge osteotomy in the treatment of hallux rigidus. J Foot Ankle Surg 37: 8–10

Drago JJ, Oloff L, Jacobs AM (1984) A comprehensive review of hallux limitus. J Foot Surg 23: 213–220

Duke HF, Kaplan EM (1984) A modification of the Austin bunionectomy for shortening and plantarflexion. J Am Podiatr Assoc 74: 209–215

Klosok JK, Pring DJ, Jessop JH, Maffulli N (1993) Chevron and Wilson metatarsal osteotomy for hallux valgus. J Bone Joint Surg 75B: 825–829

Lambrinudi C (1938) Metatarsus primus elevatus. Proc Roy Soc Med 31: 1273

Lundeen RO, Rose JM (2000) Sliding oblique osteotomy for the treatment of hallux abducto valgus associated with functional hallux limitus. J Foot Ankle Surg 39: 161–167

Regnauld B (1986) The Foot. Berlin, Springer-Verlag, pp 271–280

Ronconi P, Monachino P, Baleanu PM, Favilli G (2000) Distal oblique osteotomy of the first metatarsal for the correction of hallux limitus and rigidus deformity. J Foot Ankle Surg 39: 154–160

Root ML, Orien WP, Weed JH (1977) Normal and Abnormal Function of the Foot, vol. 2. Los Angeles, Clinical Biomechanics, pp 218–363

Youngswick F (1982) Modification of the Austin bunionectomy for treatment of metatarsus primus equinus associated with hallux limitus. J Foot Surg 21: 114–116

8

Arthrodesis of the hallux metatarso-phalangeal joint and inter-phalangeal joint

Andrea Cracchiolo III
Hans-Jörg Trnka

Metatarsophalangeal joint arthrodesis

Introduction

Arthrodesis of the hallux metatarsophalangeal joint is almost always performed in painful and arthritic joints. The arthrodesis can be performed as a primary procedure, as in a patient with advanced hallux rigidus, for joint destruction due to rheumatoid arthritis, or in a patient with hallux valgus and secondary degenerative arthrosis. Arthrodesis is usually one of the best salvage procedures in treating a patient with a painful arthritic joint who has already had an unsuccessful operation. Although it is possible to fuse a joint after removing a failed implant, this usually requires a bone graft, and the time to union is much longer than if two stable surfaces with satisfactory bone are present. For this reason, implant removal and a distraction-type excisional arthroplasty may be preferred. In the rare case of an infected joint, this should be debrided and treated with antibiotics. If a delayed arthrodesis is needed, it can be performed after the infection has been eradicated if the patient still complains of pain or significant malalignment.

Treatment

Surgical technique

It is important to position the hallux correctly when performing an arthrodesis. The hallux should be parallel to the floor or in slight dorsiflexion, with the foot plantigrade. It should be in 20–30° dorsiflexion in relation to the first metatarsal (Figure 1). This angle must therefore be adjusted in cases of pes planus or pes cavus. The hallux should also be in some degree of valgus, but not impinging on the adjacent second toe. In a patient with hallux rigidus this may be only 5° of valgus, while in a patient with rheumatoid arthritis or a failed bunion surgery the valgus may be 15–20°. Rotation of the hallux is usually neutral, i.e. the toenail should be dorsal. Positioning may be facilitated by using a phalangeal guiding device. The base plate for the phalangeal guide is fixed on the dorsal aspect of the first metatarsal after preparation of the bone surfaces. Attached to the base plate is a kind of goniometer to set extension and flexion as well as varus and valgus.

Before the correct position for the arthrodesis is obtained, the joint surfaces must be properly prepared. This requires resection of the articular surface. A minimal amount of the joint should be

a

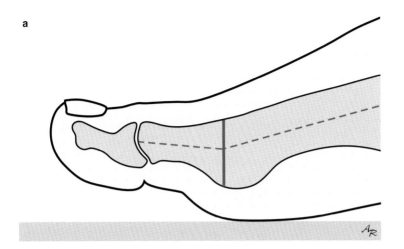

b

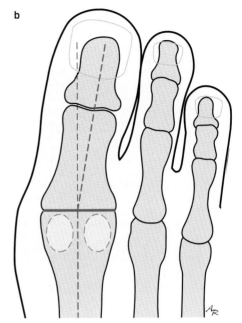

Figure 1

The position of the great toe should be in slight dorsiflexion or parallel to the floor, and in some valgus. a. medial aspect; b. dorsal aspect

excised, consistent with having good-quality bone surfaces that will fuse and avoiding excessive shortening of the first ray. Only in patients with rheumatoid arthritis may it be necessary to shorten the first ray, if the other rays have had a resection of the arthritic metatarsal head. In such a patient the hallux ray should not be too long in relation to the lateral metatarsals, especially rays two and three. The articular surface of the metatarsal head is best resected with a thin, solid oscillating saw. The articular surface of the base of the proximal phalanx is similarly resected, removing only the concave surface and resecting as little bone as possible. The short flexor tendon attachments are retained. The sesamoid articulations are not disturbed unless they are grossly abnormal.

Several methods for preparing the articular surfaces of the metatarsal head and the base of the proximal phalanx have been described. These include flat surfaces, 'tongue and trough' technique for conical surfaces prepared manually with a burr, or a reamer system. Flat surfaces can be achieved by using an oscillating saw. A disadvantage of this method is that one must achieve the optimum position of the cuts at the first attempt. Re-positioning requires further bone cuts and may lead to more bone loss. Other options are to shape the head and base of the proximal phalanx into a congruent cone–cup surface or into spherical surfaces.

There are several sets of instruments commercially available which shape the head into a cone

that fits into a concave, cup-shaped surface in the base of the proximal phalanx [Marin 1968, Alexander 1993, Coughlin and Abdo 1994]. This may also be achieved by using a burr, although it is not possible to achieve as much congruency of the two articular surfaces as if performed with instruments. However, two flat surfaces may give more stability to the arthrodesis site, and no special instrumentation is required.

Incision

A dorsal longitudinal incision is made just medial to the extensor hallucis longus tendon (Figure 2). This incision should extend from the neck of the proximal phalanx across the joint and across the neck and distal diaphysis of the first metatarsal. Good exposure is critical in performing a successful arthrodesis. The extensor tendon is usually retracted laterally. The dissection is carried through the capsule, exposing the entire metatarsal head and the proximal third of the base of the proximal phalanx. A lateral soft-tissue release may be necessary to correct a valgus deformity of 20° or greater. The sesamoids should be located under the metatarsal head by soft-tissue dissection, if necessary. Occasionally it may be necessary to excise a single grossly deformed sesamoid, especially if it caused significant preoperative pain. If a large medial eminence is present it can be excised with an oscillating saw.

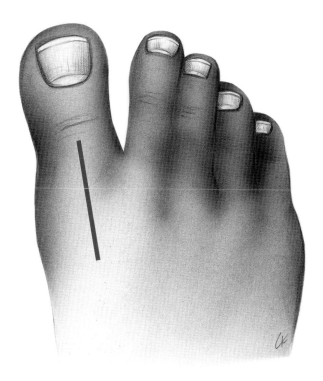

Figure 2

A dorsal longitudinal incision is used to expose the hallux metarsophalangeal joint

Joint resection

Flat surfaces

The base of the proximal phalanx is exposed and held by an assistant while the surgeon resects a thin wafer of what remains of the articular surface, using the oscillating saw. This cut is made at a right angle to the shaft of the phalanx. It is important not to resect too much bone, especially at the medial shoulder of the metaphysis of the phalanx, as this may be needed for internal fixation. However, satisfactory cancellous bone must be exposed to promote the arthrodesis. The first ray should not be excessively shortened in most patients who require an arthrodesis. Occasionally, in a patient with rheumatoid arthritis who is undergoing excision of the lateral metatarsal heads or metatarsophalangeal joints, it may be necessary to shorten the first ray more than is usual in a non-rheumatoid patient. The final position is determined by resecting the surface of the metatarsal head. By draping the involved lower extremity above the knee joint, the knee can be flexed and (using a few towels or a metal tray) the foot can be placed in the plantigrade position. An assistant holds the hallux in the desired position, and the surgeon resects the surface of the metatarsal

head parallel to the cut made across the base of the proximal phalanx, again resecting as little bone as possible. The final position is then carefully checked and small adjustments can be made using a rasp or the power saw. The sagittal position of the hallux in relationship to the metatarsal is most important in performing a successful arthrodesis. The usual angle is approximately 20–30° as measured between the line drawn along the metatarsal and one drawn along the proximal phalanx. It is helpful to do this on a weightbearing radiograph, and also to position the foot in a weightbearing posture during the operation when the joint is exposed. The tip of the toe should be just raised off a flat surface.

Cup and cone preparation by reamers

Using a phalangeal guide, a guide wire is placed in the center of the base of the proximal phalanx parallel to the axis of the toe. The cylindrical reamer is then advanced over the wire until the reamer stop sits flush to the phalangeal base. The phalangeal truncated reamer then replaces the cylindrical reamer until the rim of the base of the cone is even, sharp and devoid of articular surface. The guide wire for the metatarsal reamer is inserted with the help of a metatarsal guide that allows the surgeon to set the valgus angle from 0° to 20° and dorsiflexion from 0° to 50°. The reamer is now used until the cancellous truncated cone completely fills the window in the side of the reamer head. The male and female cones are apposed and longitudinal pressure is applied. The arthrodesis is secured with screw fixation.

Spherical articular surfaces

The base of the proximal phalanx is exposed by inserting a small Hohmann retractor medially and laterally, and placing the great toe in maximal plantarflexion. Using a burr, the residual cartilage or the sclerotic surfaces are removed until good bleeding cancellous bone is visible, and a concave surface is obtained. Following this the metatarsal head is also exposed using the Hohmann retractors. The remnant cartilage or sclerosis is removed with the burr in a convex fashion leaving a peripheral rim (Figure 3).

The two surfaces are then apposed, and the final position is checked clinically as described previously.

Internal fixation

Depending on the size of the hallux and the metatarsal and the quality of the bone, one of the

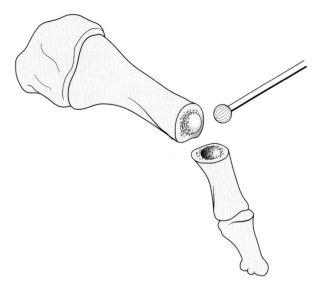

Figure 3

Freehand shaping of surfaces with power burr

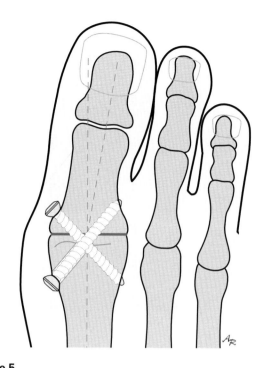

Figure 5

Alternatively, both screws can be placed in a crossed fashion from medial to lateral

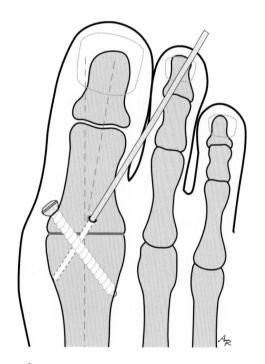

Figure 4

Fixation of the arthrodesis. Following temporary fixation with guide wires, the first screw can be placed from distal–medial to proximal–lateral. It may be inserted as a compression screw by overdrilling the distal hole or by using a lag screw. The second screw is placed over the second guide wire. Cannulated 3.5-mm screws facilitate screw fixation

following methods may be used to secure the resected joint surface.

With small fragment cancellous bone screws, two screws provide good internal fixation. The orientation of the screws may be either crossed (Figure 4) or parallel. Screw placement is usually determined by the size and quality of the bone adjacent to the arthrodesis site. Screws are placed only in large bony fragments, otherwise there is not enough room for them to be placed. The advantage of parallel screw placement is that no secondary incisions for screw insertion are necessary. For crossed screw placement one additional incision may be necessary.

Self-reaming, self-tapping cannulated screws, 3.0 mm or 3.5 mm, which can be placed over a guide wire, are optimal as internal fixation for this small joint. For crossed screw placement, the surfaces may first be temporarily fixed with a single 1.5-mm Kirschner wire. Subsequently, the first screw is placed across the joint from proximal in the medial side of the metatarsal, to distal lateral on the proximal phalanx (Figure 5). If the bone is not too sclerotic, by using self-reaming, self-tapping cannulated screws, drilling is usually not necessary [Cracchiolo 1993]. It is usually possible to exit the opposite cortex, so the screw will have good purchase. A second screw should be placed from medial–distal to proximal–lateral, particularly if the patient is large with good-quality bone. Crossed screws provide excellent fixation for arthrodesis of the hallux metatarsophalangeal joint if there is sufficient bone. This method is also well accepted by patients, as nothing protrudes from the skin

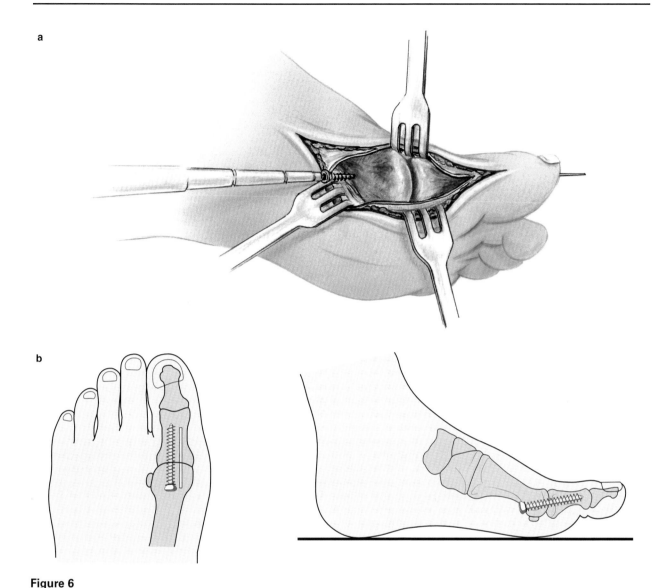

Figure 6

a. skin incision on the plantar side of the midline. b. fixation with screw and K-wire

and the screws usually produce no discomfort postoperatively.

Internal fixation can also be placed across the plantar portion of the metatarsal neck distally into the proximal phalanx [Hansen 2000, Castro and Klaue 2001]. This can be done only when there has been no loss of bone at the metatarsophalangeal joint. The anatomy of the head and neck of the metatarsal allows for a buttressing of the head of a compression screw and gives solid internal fixation. The skin incision proximally must be on the plantar side of the midline and the digital nerve must be protected (Figure 6a). The incision continues distally in the midline or can curve to the dorsal medial side of the joint. The surfaces are prepared and the proper position is secured with a 1.5-mm Kirschner wire placed as laterally as possible. A 3.5-mm cortical or 4.0-mm cancellous screw, preferably cannulated,

is placed in a lag fashion to secure the joint. The K-wire is removed and the screw tightened. The K-wire is re-inserted more medially parallel to the screw to provide rotational stability [Castro and Klaue 2001] (Figure 6b). Hansen [2000] prefers to use a single 6.5-mm lag screw and a K-wire if the bone is large or if there is osteoporosis. Alternatively, in a small bone, or if the bone is hard, he utilizes two 3.5-mm cortical screws placed as lag screws (Figures 7a and b).

Dorsal plate technique with or without a single screw fixation

Using a plate may be appropriate when two screws cannot be placed because the bones are small, or when the bone quality is poor. In such conditions,

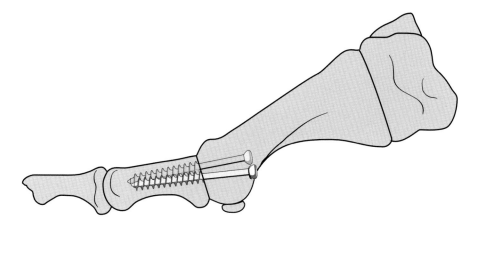

Figure 7

Hansen's alternative approach

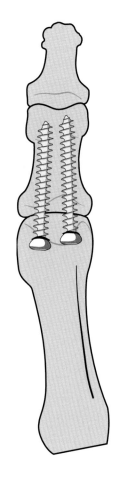

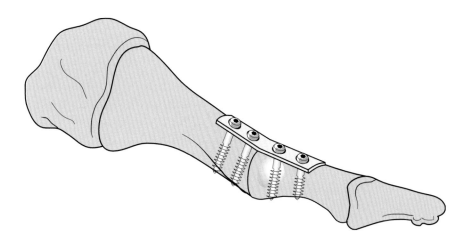

Figure 8

Dorsal plate for internal fixations

the plate probably gives a more stable construct for internal fixation (Figure 8). A high rate of fusion has been reported, even though the plate is placed on the compression surface rather than on the tension surface. A three- to five-hole one-third tubular plate is bent and secured dorsally with the distal screw holes over the proximal phalanx and the proximal screw holes over the first metatarsal [Holmes 1992]. An additional screw can be placed from distal–medial to proximal–lateral across the joint.

Alternatively, a six-hole Vitallium mandibular plate may be used [Coughlin and Abdo 1994, Coughlin 2000]. The plates may be prominent, requiring removal postoperatively.

Fixation with one staple and one cortical screw

After positioning of the arthrodesis and temporary fixation with a K-wire, a drill guide for the staple system is placed at the dorsal aspect of the metatarsal head and the proximal phalanx. Using the drill guide, two parallel holes are drilled, each at one side of the arthrodesis measuring of the length. The staple is placed and brought under tension. For rotational stability, either a second staple or a crossed screw is placed.

Threaded Steinmann pin fixation

Threaded Steinmann pin fixation [Mann and Thompson 1984] is an excellent method of securing the joint for an arthrodesis, especially if the bone is of poor quality [Cracchiolo 1993]. It results in a solid arthrodesis whenever used, but it has two disadvantages: (1) the pins protrude through the tip of the hallux and must be removed after radiographs indicate that fusion is present; and (2) the pins must traverse the interphalangeal joint, which may produce some postoperative stiffness in that joint.

Two pins are placed in a retrograde fashion. It is important that they have trocar points at both ends. The diameter of pins selected may be 3.6 mm, 3.2 mm, 2.7 mm or 2.4 mm. Pin selection depends on the size of the bone remaining in the hallux. Any combination of pins is acceptable. The pins are first passed through the proximal phalanx, exiting the tip of the toe just below the nail. An assistant must then hold the phalanx tightly to the metatarsal while the pins are drilled across the arthrodesis site into the metatarsal. This must be done using a large power drill. The pins are cut long enough distally to permit subsequent removal. Well-fitting caps should be placed over the cut end of the pins to keep them from impinging on the patient's dressings, socks or bed covers. Despite early evidence of fusion, which may occur as early as 8 weeks, the average time to fusion is about 12 weeks postoperatively. Therefore, pins should not be removed prematurely.

Bone graft salvage of short first ray

A bone graft is usually not required for the standard arthrodesis of the hallux metatarsophalangeal joint. However, there may be three exceptions: a first ray that has been shortened as a result of trauma or extensive osteonecrosis of the metatarsal head; in the salvage of a failed implant, where pain persists after the implant has been removed; and in the salvage of a painful joint after an earlier excisional arthroplasty. Grafts are difficult to use successfully for several reasons: the recipient site is usually

scarred with poor-quality soft tissue, the bone ends are eburnated, most of the intramedullary cancellous bone is either missing or of poor quality, and the blood supply to the bone may have been damaged by previous trauma, sepsis or surgery.

Salvage of first metatarsophalangeal arthrodesis with iliac crest bone graft

Patients with a painful first metatarsophalangeal joint, a short first ray and a loss of bone may require an arthrodesis. Lengthening is achieved using an autogenous tricortical iliac crest graft [Brodsky et al. 2000, Myerson et al. 2000] or unicortical or bicortical allograft from a femoral head [Myerson et al. 2000]. The average increase in length of the first ray has been reported to be 7.5–13 mm. A dorsal or dorsomedial incision is preferred. Skin flaps are required and meticulous soft-tissue and bone preparation is essential. The intramedullary canals are packed with cancellous bone. The interposition graft is provisionally fixed with a smooth K-wire, and a dorsal plate is the most commonly used internal fixation (Figure 9). Screws and K-wires are used as supplemental fixation. Arthrodesis has been reported an average of 12–13 weeks postoperatively. Non-union and complications occur in these difficult cases.

Postoperative care

Immobilization is provided by a below-knee cast or by a compression dressing and a wooden-soled shoe. This is determined by the bone quality and the degree of secure internal fixation. Depending on the type of fixation, it may be difficult to determine when arthrodesis has been achieved. Despite early evidence of fusion, the internal fixation device should not be removed prematurely. In many cases, internal fixation screws or a plate do not need to be removed unless they cause irritation.

If a bone graft is used or if the bone quality is poor or the fixation marginal, a short leg cast is usually helpful to protect the patient and emphasizes the need for caution and protected weight-bearing. If there is some evidence of fusion clinically and radiographically at about 6 weeks postoperatively, the cast may be changed to a removable boot or hard-soled postoperative shoe. It may take 10–12 weeks before an arthrodesis can be achieved. The patient having such an operation must understand the time involved and the difficulty of obtaining a fusion, and be able to co-operate with the treatment plan.

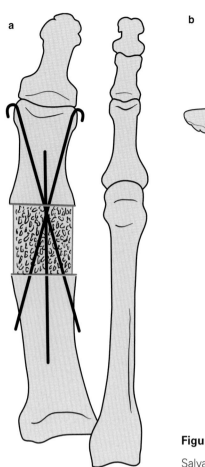

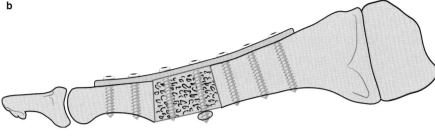

Figure 9

Salvage arthrodesis using an interpositional bone graft

Complications

The incidence of postoperative non-union has been indicated to be between 0 and 13%, and may vary with the fixation method used. A non-union rate of 3–5% must be expected, even if stable internal fixation can be achieved. The incidence is higher if bone graft interposition is used. A pseudarthrosis may remain asymptomatic and not require revision. Delayed wound healing may be a problem. Again, this is more frequent with bone graft interposition. It may also be related to the bulk of the internal fixation. Secondary degenerative changes at the interphalangeal joint have been observed in approximately 10% of patients on long-term follow-up, but most cause only minor symptoms or are asymptomatic.

Interphalangeal joint arthrodesis

Historically, arthrodesis of the hallux interphalangeal joint has been performed as part of the extensor hallucis longus tendon transfer operation. The joint was fused to prevent a flexion deformity occurring as a result of the unopposed pull of the long flexor tendon. Arthrodesis was also recommended when there was irreparable damage to the flexor hallucis longus or following a neglected or unrecognized laceration of the tendon. Thus the arthrodesis was performed on a normal or near-normal joint. Arthrodesis is also indicated if there is degeneration of the joint. This is usually due to a crush injury of the hallux, intra-articular fracture, or an arthrosis. Arthrodesis of the joint is well tolerated, especially if there is a normal metatarsophalangeal joint. Therefore, fusion of this joint in a patient who has rheumatoid arthritis may not be indicated, since the metatarsophalangeal joint is frequently involved in the arthritic deformity of the forefoot. In such a patient it is preferable to do a soft-tissue release to re-align the joint if necessary and remove the fibrous debris from within the joint. A threaded Kirschner wire is passed across the joint to hold the surfaces distracted. The wire is removed about 3–4 weeks postoperatively.

Treatment

Exposure is through a curved dorsal incision (Figure 10). The transverse portion of the incision is

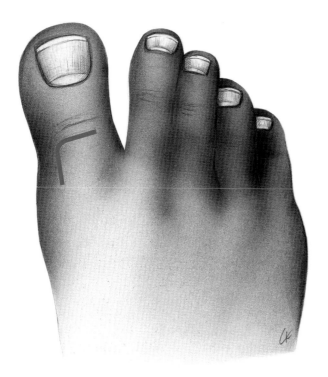

Figure 10

A curved skin incision is used for arthrodesis of the interphalangeal joint

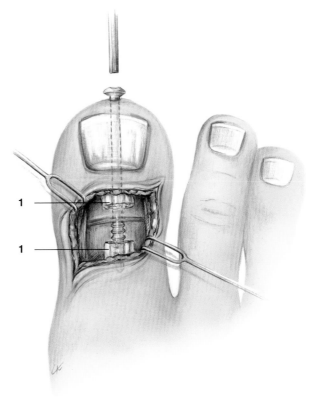

Figure 11

A cannulated cancellous bone screw can be passed over a guide wire

1 Extensor tendon, divided

made directly over the interphalangeal joint. The extensor tendon is divided transversely to expose the joint. The articular surfaces are removed using either a small oscillating saw blade or a sharp curette. Very little bone should be resected. After the joint surfaces have been resected, the surfaces should be held together manually to check the alignment of the hallux. The joint should be aligned in neutral orientation, any excessive interphalangeal valgus should be corrected and the toenail should point dorsally.

Internal fixation

A guide wire or drill is passed in a retrograde fashion through the distal phalanx, exiting the skin just below the toenail. The wire is then directed back into the distal phalanx with the joint surfaces well approximated and passed into the proximal phalanx, stopping at the junction of the diaphysis and the proximal metaphysis. It should not enter the metatarsophalangeal joint. A 4.0-mm or 3.5-mm cannulated cancellous bone screw is used for fixation [Shives and Johnson 1980], making certain that the threads are all in the proximal phalanx (Figure 11). Newer screws that are self-reaming and

self-tapping and are also cannulated make this screw placement relatively easy. A supplemental 1-mm Kirschner wire may also be passed obliquely across the joint to control rotation [Alexander 1993]. This is always helpful if the bone is osteoporotic (Figure 12). Both the screw and the wire are removed about 3 months later, if the fusion is radiographically solid.

Alternative fixation

In some patients, the bones are small or of poor quality so that screw fixation is not possible. In such circumstances, two 1.5-mm Kirschner wires with trocar tips on each end are passed in a retrograde direction through the distal phalanx and out through the tip of the toe. A large-bore needle is then drilled from medial to lateral across the base of the distal phalanx plantar to the Kirschner wire. A strand of 24-gauge wire is then passed through the needle. Using the same technique, the same strand of wire is then passed from lateral to medial

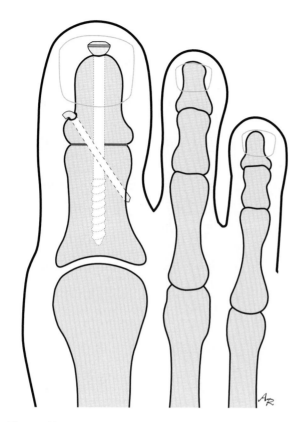

Figure 12

An additional Kirschner wire may be passed obliquely across the joint to control rotation

transversely across the metaphysis of the proximal phalanx. The resected surfaces of the joint are then manually compressed and the Kirschner wires are drilled into the proximal phalanx. The ends of what is now the cerclage 24-gauge wire are then twisted to compress the resected joint further. The Kirschner wires are cut and their ends covered with rubber protectors. The wires are removed postoperatively when there is some radiographic evidence of an arthrodesis. The cerclage wire can be removed later if it is causing symptoms.

Postoperative care

In most patients a compression dressing and postoperative wooden-soled shoe are sufficient if only an interphalangeal fusion has been done. It will require 6–8 weeks for fusion to be sufficient so that a closed shoe can be used, and this requires radiographic evidence of fusion. If percutaneous K-wires have been placed, they should not be removed until there is radiographic evidence of a solid fusion.

References

Alexander IJ (1993) Arthrodesis of the metatarsophalangeal and interphalangeal joints of the hallux. In: Myerson M (ed) Current Therapy in Foot and Ankle Surgery. St Louis, Mosby-Year Book, pp 81–90

Brodsky JW, Ptaszek AJ, Morris SG (2000) Salvage of first MTP arthrodesis utilizing ICBG: clinical evaluation and outcome. Foot Ankle Int 21 (4): 290–296

Castro MD, Klaue K (2001) Revisiting an alternative method of fixation for first MTP joint arthrodesis. Foot Ankle Int 22 (8): 687–688

Coughlin MJ, Abdo RV (1994) Arthrodesis of the first metatarsophalangeal joint with Vitallium plate fixation. Foot Ankle 15 (1): 18–28

Coughlin MJ (2000) Rheumatoid forefoot reconstruction. J Bone Joint Surg 82A: 322–341

Cracchiolo A (1993) The rheumatoid foot and ankle: pathology and treatment. Foot 3 (3): 126–134

Hansen ST (2000) Functional Reconstruction of the Foot and Ankle. Philadelphia, Lippincott Williams & Wilkins, pp 343–347

Holmes GB (1992) Arthrodesis of the first metatarsophalangeal joint using interfragmentary screw and plate. Foot Ankle 13 (6): 333–335

Mann RA, Thompson FM (1984) Arthrodesis of the first metatarsophalangeal joint for hallux valgus in rheumatoid arthritis. J Bone Joint Surg 66A: 687–692

Marin GA (1968) Arthrodesis of the first metatarsophalangeal joint of hallux valgus and hallux rigidus. Int Surg 50: 174–178

Myerson MS, Schen LC, McGuigan FX, Ozmir A (2000) Results of arthrodesis of the hallux metatarsophalangeal joint using bone graft for restoration of length. Foot Ankle Int 21 (4): 297–306

Shives TC, Johnson KA (1980) Arthrodesis of the interphalangeal joint of the great toe: an improved technique. Foot Ankle 1: 26–29

9

Resection arthroplasty of the great toe

Nikolaus Wülker

Introduction

Resection arthroplasty has been used for more than 100 years for the treatment of hallux valgus and hallux rigidus. Generally, the phalangeal articular surface is removed, including up to one-half of the proximal phalanx. Metatarsal head resections have been used in the past [Hueter 1871] but are now largely abandoned because they severely compromise the load-bearing capacity of the first ray.

Resection arthroplasty is a relatively easy and forgiving technique and less demanding than reconstructive procedures, which better preserve the anatomy and the function of the great toe. Resection arthroplasty must not be used indiscriminately, because it destroys the metatarsophalangeal joint of the hallux and significantly impairs forceful motion of the great toe. Decreased plantarflexion power during toe-off is of particular relevance. Resection arthroplasty shifts the load from the first ray to the lesser rays. Transfer metatarsalgia under the lesser metatarsal heads is a common late sequela of resection arthroplasty. It may occur a few months to a number of years after the procedure, in particular in physically active or athletic individuals.

In consequence, resection arthroplasty is the technique for the physically less demanding and elderly patient. The indication depends more on the level of physical activity than on chronological age. Patients over 60 years are usually good candidates for the procedure, and resection arthroplasty is the preferred technique in patients over 70 years of age. It is also used in younger patients who are permanently handicapped for other health problems.

Hallux valgus is the most common indication for resection arthroplasty. However, the soft-tissue imbalance that causes the deformity is not corrected by resection of the articular surface alone. Recurrent late postoperative deformity is a common problem – in particular valgus and dorsiflexion malalignment – owing to loss of short flexor muscle power. Temporary postoperative wire fixation may help, but is not able to maintain alignment in all patients. In addition, hallux valgus is often associated with medial deviation of the first metatarsal (metatarsus primus varus). This may have to be corrected with an additional proximal first metatarsal osteotomy.

Hallux rigidus is another indication for resection arthroplasty. However, patients are usually younger and physically more active, which is a contraindication to resection arthroplasty. In addition, hallux rigidus patients have usually become accustomed to diminished metatarsophalangeal motion at the hallux and benefit more from an arthrodesis (see Chapter 8), which maintains the weightbearing capacity of the hallux better than resection arthroplasty. Endoprosthetic replacement is another alternative in these patients (see Chapter 10).

The major contraindication to resection arthroplasty is peripheral vascular disease, which is particularly common and often undiagnosed in elderly patients. If the dorsalis pedis or tibialis posterior pulses are not palpable, Doppler studies and possibly angiography must be performed.

Anatomically, the short flexor and extensor tendons of the hallux insert at the base of the proximal phalanx. Their insertions will be lost following

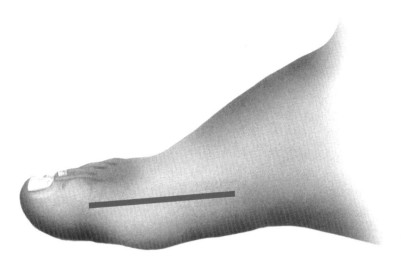

Figure 1

A straight medial skin incision is used for resection arthroplasty

resection arthroplasty. The sesamoid bones, which are embedded into the short flexor tendons, usually displace proximally following the resection. The long flexor tendon is located between the two short flexor tendons and must not be injured during the procedure.

Surgical technique

The procedure is performed with the patient in the supine position. Regional, local or general anesthesia may be used. The foot is exsanguinated with a rubber (Esmarch) bandage.

A straight medial skin incision is made from the interphalangeal joint of the hallux to the proximal limit of the exostosis at the first metatarsal head (Figure 1). Skin flaps are raised to expose the periosteum at the proximal phalanx and the thick capsular tissue overlying the exostosis. Skin flaps must be thick enough to secure postoperative perfusion and wound healing.

Interposition of capsular tissue into the resection space is recommended to avoid painful contact between the resection surface at the proximal phalanx and the metatarsal head articular surface postoperatively. The thick capsular tissue overlying the exostosis is best suited for this purpose. A U-shaped incision of capsule and periosteum is used to raise a distally based flap approximately 1 cm wide (Figure 2). At the metatarsal head, the capsule is usually quite adherent to bone and sharp dissection with a knife must be used. At the proximal phalanx, the periosteum is thin and is carefully

raised with a periosteal elevator. Distal attachment of the flap is not crucial for perfusion but should be maintained for mechanical anchorage.

The bone surface medially at the metatarsal head is fully exposed with sharp Hohmann retractors. The capsular incision may have to be extended proximally for this purpose. The hallux is held laterally by an assistant. At the articular surface of the metatarsal head a sagittal sulcus is usually found, separating the joint from the exostosis. The bottom of this groove is the distal landmark for resection of the exostosis. Proximally, resection is in line with the medial border of the first metatarsal diaphysis. Resection is most conveniently carried out with an oscillating saw. Alternatively, an osteotome may be used. Care must be taken to orient the resection in the sagittal plane, i.e. at a right angle to the sole of the foot. The resection edges are rounded with a rongeur.

The dorsal and plantar periosteum at the base of the proximal phalanx are elevated and round Hohmann retractors are inserted. The long flexor and extensor tendons must clearly be outside the retractors to avoid injury with the saw. The capsular flap is retracted distally away from the oscillating saw. Resection should comprise approximately one-third of the proximal phalanx, equivalent to 1 cm in the average patient. The osteotomy must be placed at a right angle to the longitudinal axis of the hallux (Figure 3). If it is directed too far distally, recurrent valgus deformity may ensue. An orientation too far proximally may result in postoperative hallux varus.

The base fragment of the proximal phalanx is grasped with a pointed clamp and retracted medially. An osteotome may be inserted into the

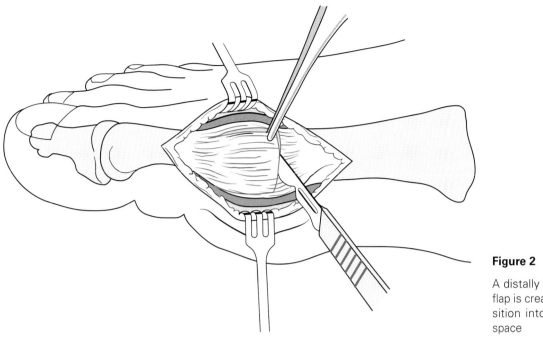

Figure 2

A distally based capsular flap is created for interposition into the resection space

osteotomy to lever the base fragment out of the resection space. The firm attachments of the short flexor and extensor tendons must be divided with a scalpel, carefully avoiding injury to the long tendons. Once the base fragment is removed, the surgeon's little finger should fit snugly into the resection space. Excessive resection will result in a floppy, powerless great toe and in cosmetically unacceptable shortening. Inadequate resection will lead to contact between the resection surface and the metatarsal head, which may impair postoperative motion and be painful in spite of soft-tissue interposition.

An assessment must now be made about the position of the first metatarsal bone. Metatarsus primus varus, i.e. medial angulation, may be soft and easily correctable by pressure on the first metatarsal head in a lateral direction. In this case, the sesamoid bones under the metatarsal head are carefully mobilized with a periosteal elevator and the position of the first metatarsal is corrected by a tight capsular closure at the end of the procedure. Closure following resection of the flap will push the first metatarsal head laterally. This is also referred to as the 'cerclage fibreux'.

If there is rigid resistance against lateral displacement of the first metatarsal, a proximal first metatarsal osteotomy is carried out. The skin incision is extended proximally to the level of the first tarsometatarsal joint. Round Hohmann retractors are inserted following elevation of the periosteum at the base of the first metatarsal. The osteotomy

is made approximately 1 cm distal to the joint and oriented slightly in a lateral–distal direction. A small wedge of bone with a lateral base of 2–3 mm is removed. The wedge fragment is removed and the osteotomy is closed by manual correction of the first metatarsal alignment. Fixation with a longitudinal Kirschner wire is usually adequate (see below).

The capsular flap is tagged with absorbable sutures and attached to the remaining capsule at the lateral aspect of the resection space. Temporary fixation with a longitudinal 1.8-mm Kirschner wire is recommended to avoid postoperative malalignment (Figure 4). The wire is first inserted into the bone resection surface at the proximal phalanx and advanced into the tip of the hallux in a retrograde direction. Subsequently, the wire is driven proximally into the first metatarsal head while the hallux is maintained in neutral alignment. The capsular flap is secured in the resection space by an assistant to prevent twisting. The wire is advanced until it exits the first metatarsal at the plantar aspect of its diaphysis. If a proximal first metatarsal osteotomy was performed in addition to the resection arthroplasty, the hallux is held in slight plantarflexion so that the wire enters the metatarsal diaphysis and crosses the osteotomy and the first tarsometatarsal joint. This is usually adequate for fixation of the osteotomy.

The capsule is closed longitudinally with absorbable, interrupted sutures (Figure 5). Closure should be tight enough to push the metatarsal head in a lateral direction, especially if metatarsus primus varus was present preoperatively. If this is not

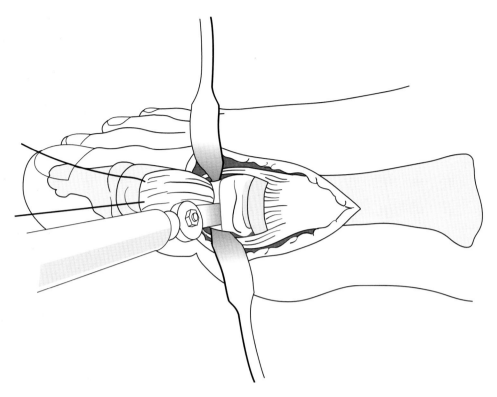

Figure 3

The base of the proximal phalanx is resected with an oscillating saw

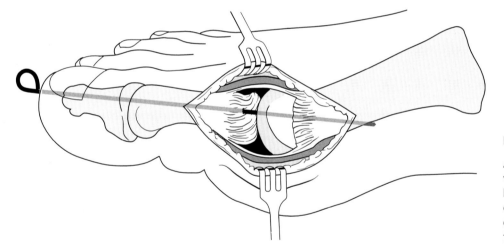

Figure 4

A longitudinal Kirschner wire is advanced into the bone resection surface, drilled distally and then drilled proximally into the first metatarsal

achieved with the previous resection of the capsular flap, an additional horizontal strip of capsular tissue of adequate width must be excised.

The skin is closed in a routine fashion. No skin is excised because skin redundancy at the medial aspect of the first metatarsal head will reduce within 2 weeks after surgery. A soft dressing is applied and the wire tip is protected. Following release of the tourniquet, skin perfusion at the hallux must carefully be assessed. If this does not return to normal within a few minutes, the dressing should be removed and the wire may have to be drawn.

Postoperatively, full weightbearing is allowed in a postoperative shoe, which mainly features a firm sole to avoid rolling over the operated toe. The wire is removed in the office at 2 weeks after surgery, together with the skin sutures. Subsequently, motion and ambulation exercises are performed. Usually, normal ambulation is regained after 6 weeks.

Complications

Delayed wound healing is the most common immediate postoperative complication and this may progress to necrosis of the entire hallux if preoperative circulation was not adequate.

Shortening and some loss of power of the hallux always follow resection arthroplasty, but they are usually tolerable to the elderly and less physically

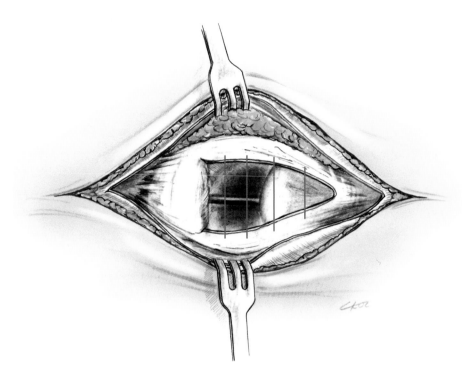

Figure 5

The capsule is closed with interrupted absorbable sutures

active patient. Younger patients frequently develop transfer metatarsalgia, which is difficult to salvage.

Postoperative malalignment of the great toe is particularly common in hallux valgus patients. It is due to uncorrected soft tissue balance and to loss of the short flexor muscles. Malalignment is also common if deviation of the first metatarsal is not corrected.

Neuromas may develop if the cutaneous nerves are transected with the skin incision. Sharp, local pain and tenderness usually resolve with local injections and rarely require surgical revision. Neuromas are most common with a dorsomedial skin incision, which may result in injury to the dorsomedial cutaneous nerve of the hallux.

Bibliography

Brandes M (1929) Zur operativen Therapie des Hallux valgus. Zentralbl Chir 56: 2434

Hueter K (1871) Klinik der Gelenkkrankheiten. Leipzig

Jordan HH, Brodsky AE (1951) Keller operation for hallux valgus and hallux rigidus. An end result study. Arch Surg 62: 586–596

Keller WL (1904) The surgical treatment of bunions and hallux valgus. NY Med J 80: 741

Viladot A (1979) Pathologie de l'avant-pied. Paris, Expansion Scientifique

Wülker N (1997) Hallux valgus. Orthopäde 26: 654–664

10

Endoprosthetic first metatarso-phalangeal joint

Alexandre Rochwerger
Georges Curvale

Introduction

A stable, pain-free and mobile great toe is essential for normal foot function and gait. In the case of degenerative changes on a stiff and painful metatarsophalangeal joint, endoprosthetic replacement seems to be a logical method of treatment. That so many procedures are described and no single one is universally accepted suggests that there is as yet no ideal solution.

The general aim of implant surgery should be to relieve metatarsophalangeal joint pain and to provide for better joint motion, stability, function and cosmesis. Different types of prosthesis have been described over the past 50 years.

Interposition hemi-arthroplasties are designed to seat in the proximal phalanx. They act as a 'spacer' which could improve the results of the Keller–Brandes procedure. These implants are made from silicone or metal.

Total replacement prostheses are divided into constrained and non-constrained systems. The well-known Swanson hinged toe implant is a silicone constrained prosthesis the results of which have been widely published in the international medical literature. Non-constrained implants include two components. The metatarsal component is metallic, usually chrome/cobalt with a titanium-coated intramedullary stem if non-cemented. The phalangeal component is composed of ultra-high-molecular-weight polyethylene with or without a metal back. More recently, non-constrained ceramic implants have been introduced on to the market.

Review of the literature

Silicone implants

The forces that act for instance on the knee and the first metatarsophalangeal joint during walking are different. The implant on the metatarsophalangeal joint must withstand more shearing stresses than compression stresses. These biomechanic constraints expose the implant to many complications, which have been regularly reported in the past 20 years. About 20% of the papers are devoted to complications in the silicone implants. The attempt to retain length of the great toe by using silicone may lead to recurrence of the deformity, silicone synovitis and breakage of the implant [Cracchiolo et al. 1981, 1992, Kampner 1984, Weil et al. 1984, Lauf et al. 1985, Verhaar et al. 1989, Swanson et al. 1991, Papagelopoulos et al. 1994, Shankar 1995, Sebold and Cracchiolo 1996, Neumann et Reisch 1996, Bonet et al. 1998, Hanyu et al. 2001]. The breakage of the implant will produce a soft-tissue reaction around the metatarsophalangeal joint, destroying the bony architecture [Verhaar et al. 1989]. Recurrence of pain and stiffness will then appear. This phenomenon may occur in all kinds of silicone implants. For instance, hemiarthroplasties [Kampner 1984, Shankar 1995] have good immediate postoperative results, but with a longer follow-up the rate of failure increases to 35%.

Double-stem implants also give disappointing results with time. The use of grommets [Sebold and Cracchiolo 1996] decreases the rate of implant breakage and ectopic bone formation. Nevertheless, passive range of motion decreases and few patients have a functional weightbearing great toe joint.

Metallic hemi-arthroplasty

Very little has been published about these implants [Chen and Wertheimer 1991, Leavitt et al. 1991, Townley and Taranow 1994]. According to the authors in the largest series, the results remained satisfactory at a follow-up beyond 10 years, with no wearing of the implant or significant alteration of the metatarsal head.

Total replacement arthroplasty

Few well-documented series are available in the literature comparing the different types of implant [Johnson and Buck 1981, Merkle and Sculco 1989, Blair and Brown 1993, Koenig 1994, Gerbert and Chang 1995, Koenig and Horwitz 1996, Olms and Dietze 1999]. The main indication in the literature is hallux rigidus, and most of the authors opt for other procedures in chronic deformities of the forefoot. Although long-term results have not been noted to date (ranging from 12 to 48 months), results are encouraging, with a passive dorsiflexion ranging from 20 to 40° on average. Eighty per cent of the patients are pain free at the time of follow-up.

In order to avoid jeopardizing the final outcome, some principles should be respected: the patient should have a good bone stock, a normal alignment of the first metatarsal and a normal to short first metatarsal. The complications, which are not uncommon, are attributed to the negligence of these points. The stiffness of the first metatarsophalangeal joint is related to insufficient joint capsule release, a first metatarsal left unshortened, and an uncorrected pronation of the phalanx. Loosening of the implant is attributed to severe biomechanical constraints on an insufficient bone stock.

There are still some unsolved concerns about the implant itself:

- In how far should the implant be anatomic?
- Should the concept take into account the proximal articular set angle (PASA)/distal metatarsal articular angle (DMAA)?
- How many sizes should be available?
- Are various angulations between the stem and the metatarsal head necessary?
- Which is the best fixation: cement or cementless?

If there is a good indication for such an implant, the choice nevertheless remains difficult. It is clear that silicone implants have fallen into disfavor and have been totally abandoned in most countries. Despite so many reservations with respect to the two-component arthroplasty this still seems an interesting area of research, but also a challenge. The indications should remain very restricted. Patients should be informed that joint preservation procedures (osteotomies, cheilectomy) and other joint destructive procedures (arthrodesis) are available and reliable [Curvale and Rochwerger 1997], and that a failure after a total joint replacement usually requires demanding salvage arthrodesis [Coughlin and Mann 1987, Hecht et al. 1998, Brodsky et al. 2000, Myerson et al. 2000, Rochwerger et al. 2002].

Treatment

Indications

The main indication is hallux rigidus, usually at a stage compatible with a joint-destructive procedure such as arthrodesis. In order to allow for the best long-term result, the following points should be considered:

- Good bone stock
- Normal alignment of the first metatarsophalangeal joint in both planes
- Normal to short first metatarsal
- Absence of a metabolic arthritic process
- Low-demand users
- Patients aged above 55 years.

Once the implant is inserted, if structural malalignment of the first metatarsal is left uncorrected, complications and abnormal stresses on the prosthesis will occur. A long first metatarsal, if not shortened, will limit the range of motion on the prosthetic joint. Similarly, residual pronation in the phalanx will have the same effect.

Surgical technique

The operation is carried out under general or regional anesthesia. Additional peripheral nerve block is used for postoperative pain. The patient is positioned supine. A thigh tourniquet is used. Routine skin preparation and draping of the whole foot, including the ankle, is performed.

A dorsomedial incision (Figure 1) is employed to expose the capsule, which is medially incised longitudinally. This places the skin and capsular incisions at different levels. A sharp dissection elevates capsular structures from around the metatarsal

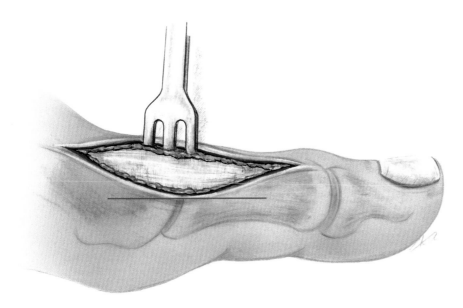

Figure 1

Dorsomedial incision. Skin and capsular incisions are at different levels

head and proximal phalanx base. The head of the first metatarsal is exposed, the medial eminence removed, and dorsal, lateral and plantar osteophytes are excised.

Soft-tissue procedures are used when a valgus deformity is present. A lateral capsular release, adductor tendon release and abductor tendon repositioning are performed. In some cases extensor tendon lengthening is necessary. Special care is taken in releasing the tendon of the flexor hallucis brevis from the plantar base portion of the first phalanx in order to prevent extension deformity at the metatarsophalangeal joint postoperatively. It is performed very close to the bone–periosteum interface.

The periosteum is elevated from the neck of the metatarsal to allow placement of two bone levers to expose the metatarsal head (Figure 2). The resection is made just proximal to the articular margin. An appropriate amount of bone is removed. More should be resected from the proximal phalanx than from the metatarsal head in order to prevent further shortening of the first ray, which may be a cause of postoperative metatarsalgia. Some types of implant offer the help of a jig for resecting the metatarsal and phalangeal end. Usually a total of 10–15 mm of bone needs to be resected.

Resection through the proximal phalanx is made perpendicular to its long axis. The metatarsal head is sized and central holes are then bored into the shaft (Figure 4). The metatarsal implant is inserted first (Figure 5) with an adapted holder (cementless press-fit fixation). A spacer is selected and the joint is taken through its range of motion. Laxity or restriction of motion is adjusted by changing the spacer. The definitive (Figure 6) component should

not be inserted too tightly and dorsiflexion of at least 70° should be obtained intraoperatively.

When the fixation requires the use of cement, the implants are removed, the bone surfaces cleaned and dried, and a grouting of cement is applied to the components. They are pressed firmly into place and held until the cement has hardened.

An increased intermetatarsal angle (over 12°), or an elevated position of the first ray must be corrected by proximal metatarsal osteotomy prior to implantation.

The joint is irrigated and the tourniquet let down, and the bleeding points are coagulated. The wound can then be closed. A small hole (1.5 mm) is drilled in the metatarsal neck which will allow anchorage of the plantar capsule to the bone with a nylon suture. The capsule is closed under tension, making sure that passive range of motion remains complete. The skin is re-approximated over a drain as preferred, and a bulky dressing is applied.

The leg is kept elevated for 4 days and the drain is removed. The patient is discharged on the 5th postoperative day and allowed to walk in special postoperative shoes with weightbearing on the heel, in order to avoid all weightbearing on the forefoot for 3 weeks. After wound healing, normal mobility and activity are encouraged.

Complications

Deep infection must be taken seriously, as with other joint replacements. Specific complications are more frequently described. Lack of hallux toe purchase occurs in half of the cases, owing to the

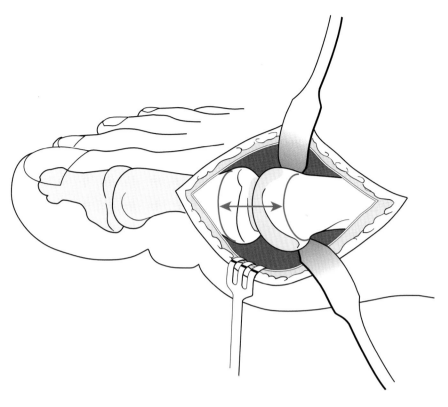

Figure 2

Placement of two bone levers to expose the head

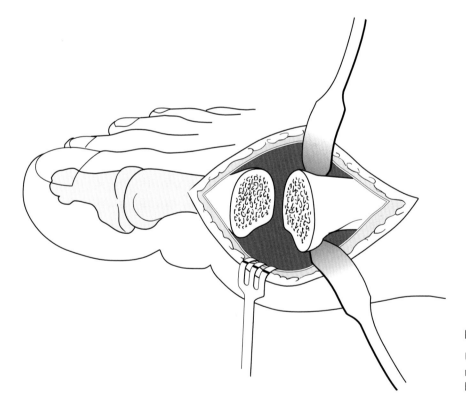

Figure 3

Usually a jig helps the surgeon to resect an appropriate amount of bone

relative inefficiency of both the flexor hallucis brevis and the flexor hallucis longus. This may require suture of the flexor hallucis longus tendon to the base of the phalanx.

Postoperatively some patients may complain about residual metatarsalgia. Usually this is successfully treated with orthotics. In some cases it is related to a metatarsus primus elevatus, which should have been treated with plantarflexor osteotomy.

Residual pain and limited range of motion may demand removal of the implant, leaving the patient with a resectional arthroplasty or an arthrodesis.

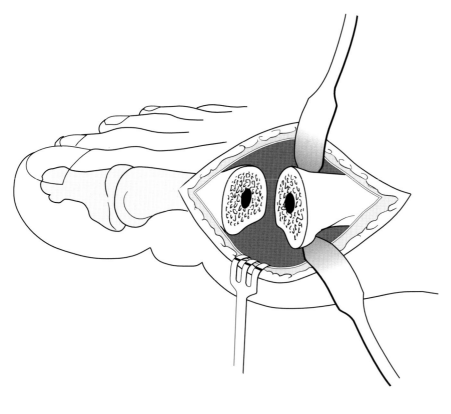

Figure 4

Central holes are bored using an adapted template

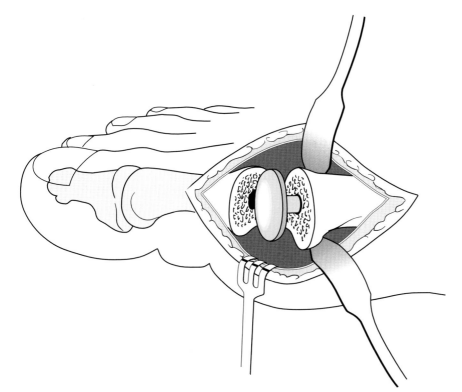

Figure 5

The metatarsal implant is inserted first with a special holder (cement-less press-fit fixation)

The causes of this complication are various. Impingement of the sesamoids on the metatarsal head may lead to a removal of the involved sesamoid, or of both if they are too arthritic. This latter procedure has its own complications and requires an interphalangeal joint fusion. (This leaves very few 'salvage procedures' in case of implant failure.) Limited range of motion is in some cases attributed to the tightness of the plantar fascia. Intraoperatively this point should be checked and, if necessary, the fascia released through a different incision on the metatarsal shaft.

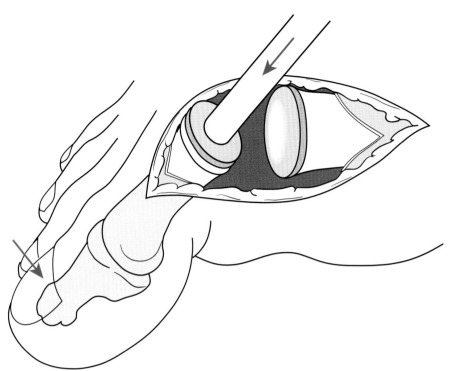

Figure 6

The polyethylene component and its metal back is inserted after testing the mobility in dorsiflexion with a spacer

Fractures of the phalanx and radiolucency have also been described as complications in the first 2 years after surgery. The result of an arthroplasty needs to be reassessed yearly. These complications prove that the results of implants are never definitive.

References

Blair MP, Brown LA (1993) Hallux limitus/rigidus deformity: a new great toe implant. Foot Ankle Surg 32 (3): 257–262

Bonet J, Taylor DT, Lam AT et al. (1998) Retrospective analysis of Silastic implant arthroplasty of the first metatarsophalangeal joint. J Foot Ankle Surg 37 (2): 128–134

Brodsky J, Ptaszek A, Morris S (2000) Salvage first MTP arthrodesis utilizing ICBG: clinical evaluation. Foot Ankle 21: 290–296

Chen DS, Wertheimer S (1991) The Keller arthroplasty with use of the Dow Corning titanium hemi-implant. J Foot Surg 30 (4): 414–418

Coughlin MJ, Mann RA (1987) Arthrodesis of the metatarsophalangeal joint as salvage for the failed Keller procedure. J Bone Joint Surg 69A: 68–75

Cracchiolo A 3rd, Swanson A, Swanson GD (1981) The arthritic great toe metatarsophalangeal joint: a review of flexible silicone implant arthroplasty from two medical centers. Clin Orthop 157: 64–69

Cracchiolo A 3rd, Weltmer JB Jr, Lian G et al. (1992) Arthroplasty of the first metatarsophalangeal joint with a double stem silicone implant. J Bone Joint Surg 74A (4): 552–563

Curvale G, Rochwerger A (1997) Surgical treatment of hallux rigidus. Rev Chir Orthop 83 (Suppl III): 35–38

Gerbert J, Chang TJ (1995) Clinical experience with two-component first metatarsal phalangeal joint implants. Clin Podiatr Med Surg 12 (3): 403–413

Hanyu T, Yamazaki H, Ishikawa H et al. (2001) Flexible hinge toe implant arthroplasty for rheumatoid arthritis of the first metatarsophalangeal joint: long-term results. J Orthop Sci 6 (2): 141–147

Hecht PJ, Gibbons MJ, Wapner KL et al. (1998) Arthrodesis of the first metatarsophalangeal joint to salvage failed silicone implant arthroplasty. Foot Ankle Int 19: 59–60

Johnson KA, Buck PG (1981) Total replacement arthroplasty of the first metatarsophalangeal joint. Foot Ankle 1 (6): 307–314

Kampner SL (1984) Total joint prosthetic arthroplasty of the great toe – a 12-year experience. Foot Ankle 4 (5): 249–261

Koenig RD (1994) Revision arthroplasty utilizing the Biomet Total Toe System for failed silicone elastomer implants. J Foot Ankle Surg 33 (3): 222–227

Koenig RD, Horwitz LR (1996) The Biomet Total Toe System utilizing the Koenig score: a five-year review. Foot Ankle Surg 35 (1): 23–26

Lauf E, McLaughlin B, McLaughlin E (1985) Swanson great toe flexible hinge endoprosthesis. Design, flexibility, and function. J Am Podiatr Med Assoc 75 (8): 393–400

Leavitt KM, Nirenberg MS, Wood B, Yong RM (1991) Titanium hemi-great toe implant: a preliminary study of its efficacy. J Foot Surg 30 (3): 289–293

Merkle PF, Sculco TP (1989) Prosthetic replacement of the first metatarsophalangeal joint. Foot Ankle 9 (6): 267–271

Myerson M, Schon L, McGuigan F, Oznur A (2000) Results of arthrodesis of the hallux metatarsophalangeal joint using bone graft for restoration of length. Foot Ankle 21: 297–306

Neumann R, Reisch P (1996) Silastic arthroplasty of the great toe metatarsal joint. Orthopäde 25 (4): 332–337

Olms K, Dietze A (1999) Replacement arthroplasty for hallux rigidus. 21 patients with a 2-year follow-up. Int Orthop 23 (4): 240–243

Papagelopoulos PJ, Kitaoka HB, Ilstrup DM (1994) Survivorship analysis of implant arthroplasty for the first metatarsophalangeal joint. Clin Orthop 302: 164–172

Rochwerger A, Lecoq C, Curvale G, Groulier P (2002) Reconstruction arthrodesis of the first metatarsophalangeal joint iatrogenic bone defects. Rev Chir Orthop Reparatrice Appar Mot 88: 501–507

Sebold EJ, Cracchiolo A 3rd (1996) Use of titanium grommets in silicone implant arthroplasty of the hallux metatarsophalangeal joint. Foot Ankle Int 17 (3): 145–151

Shankar NS. Silastic single-stem implants in the treatment of hallux rigidus. Foot Ankle Int 16 (8): 487–491

Swanson AB, de Groot Swanson G, Maupin BK et al. (1991) The use of a grommet bone liner for flexible hinge implant arthroplasty of the great toe. Foot Ankle 12 (3): 149–155

Townley CO, Taranow WS (1994) A metallic hemiarthroplasty resurfacing prosthesis for the hallux metatarsophalangeal joint. Foot Ankle Int 15 (11): 575–580

Verhaar J, Bulstra S, Walenkamp G (1989) Silicone arthroplasty for hallux rigidus. Implant wear and osteolysis. Acta Orthop Scand 60 (1): 30–33

Weil LS, Pollak RA, Goller WL (1984) Total first joint replacement in hallux valgus and hallux rigidus. Long-term results in 484 cases. Clin Podiatry 1 (1): 103–129

11

Hammer toes: condylectomy and arthrodesis of the inter-phalangeal joints

Reneé-Andrea Fuhrmann
Andreas Roth

Introduction

The rigid hammer toe occurs primarily in the sagittal plane and is described as a fixed plantarflexion deformity at the proximal interphalangeal joint. It may also involve the distal interphalangeal joint, where the deformity may include either hyperextension or hyperflexion. If there is additional dorsal subluxation or dislocation at the metatarsophalangeal joint, this is mostly referred to as a claw toe, which requires additional surgical procedures.

The mallet toe is an isolated flexion deformity at the distal interphalangeal joint [Grace 1993]. It is less common as an isolated deformity but may occur with hammer toe deformities.

Etiology and pathogenesis

The etiology of hammer toes and mallet toes is multifactorial. They may develop as a congenital or an acquired deformity. Hammer toes most frequently involve the second and third toes. Lesser toe deformities are often associated with hallux valgus. Owing to the lateral deviation and subduction of the great toe the first interspace is narrowed, which may force the second toe to dorsal subluxation at the metatarsophalangeal joint. Depending on the insufficiency of the great toe with hallux valgus deformity, lesser toes

are strained to plantarflexion in order to rebalance the forefoot during weightbearing. This mechanism may lead to flexion contracture at the proximal interphalangeal joint. After a period of time insufficiency of the intrinsic apparatus and elongation of the plantar plate is followed by a dorsiflexion at the metatarsophalangeal joint. Long flexor muscle activity then endeavors to correct this deformity, which further increases the plantarflexion of the proximal and distal interphalangeal joints. Long extensor activity, which occurs to counterbalance flexor activity, then leads to increasing dorsiflexion at the metatarsophalangeal joint, resulting in the classic claw-toe deformity [Myerson 1992]. A similar pathomechanism may occur as a consequence of inflammatory changes at the metatarsophalangeal joint, leading to an insufficiency of the plantar plate.

Other predisposing factors resulting in hammer toes or mallet toes may be an excessive length of the second toe, i.e. a Greek foot, or a significantly longer second and third metatarsal relative to the first metatarsal. Owing to the resulting increased pressure of the shoe, lesser toe deformity may develop [Scheck 1977, Thompson 1995].

Sometimes hammer toes and claw toes occur in association with severe hindfoot deformities because of neuromuscular disease, e.g. Charcot–Marie–Tooth disease, Friedreich ataxia, cerebral palsy or multiple sclerosis.

Valgus deformity of the hindfoot associated with a pronation causes instability of the tarsal joints and may result in a relative instability of the entire forefoot. This leads to an increased extrinsic muscle activity, which weakens the interosseous muscles and enhances the development of hammer toes [McGlamry 1992]. Additional relative weakness of the tibialis posterior and peroneus longus muscles, which act as a sling to elevate the longitudinal arch of the foot, may also contribute to toe deformity. The other extrinsic flexors attempt to compensate this mechanism by forced contraction, which compels the lesser toes to migrate into flexion. This patho-mechanism also occurs in rheumatoid forefoot deformities [Coughlin and Mann 1993].

Cavus foot deformity leading to greater tension of the extrinsic extensor muscles is followed by relative weakness of the toe-stabilizing lumbrical muscles. During plantarflexion at the beginning of the swing phase, the proximal phalanges remain in forced dorsiflexion and the plantar plate becomes stretched [Myerson and Shereff 1989]. Forced dorsi-flexion of the metatarsophalangeal joints leads the intrinsic flexors to enhanced activity [Coughlin and Mann 1993, McGlamry 1992]. In consequence, the extrinsic extensor tendon loses its tenodesis effect at the interphalangeal joints, resulting in flexion deformity.

Taking this mechanism into account, it should be clearly stated that the isolated flexion contracture of the proximal interphalangeal joint is a rare entity. In most cases hammer toes develop according to a subluxation or dislocation of the metatarso-phalangeal joint. This treatment influences the algorithm.

Clinical and radiographic findings

Clinical examination of the entire foot is essential to determine the surgical procedure. Concomitant hindfoot deformities have to be taken into account to obtain suitable results. This has to be accom-plished with and without weightbearing.

Hyperkeratotic lesions at the proximal or distal interphalangeal joints indicate a chronic skin irrita-tion within the shoe. In a mallet toe with plantar-flexion deformity at the distal interphalangeal joint, painful calluses may develop at the tip of the toe. This is often associated with toenail deformities. Plantar callosities beneath the metatarsal head indicate a pathologically elevated loading in that region, which can be a symptom of deranged fore-foot biomechanics.

Assessing the forefoot itself should include the 'push-up' test. Manual pressure proximal to the metatarsal heads demonstrates whether the defor-mity at the proximal interphalangeal joint is still flexible or whether it is a rigid contracture. If the toe straightens during this maneuver, the deformity is still flexible and does not require any osseous procedures. A flexor-to-extensor transfer may be sufficient to re-align the toe. During the push-up test it is recommended to observe the adjacent lesser toes, to see whether there is additional short-ening of the long flexor tendons.

Dorsal hyperextension at the metatarsophalangeal joint can be easily detected during weightbearing. Again the additional push-up test is a suitable tool to distinguish flexible from rigid deformities. A drawer test, also known as a Lachman test, is appropriate to assess the stability of the plantar plate.

The radiographic examination includes a dorso-plantar and a lateral radiograph of the weight-bearing foot. Subluxation or dislocation at the metatarsophalangeal joint can be visualized for evaluating the joint space, which is narrowed. Owing to the flexion at the interphalangeal joints, radiological assessment is not worthwhile.

Treatment

Indications for operative treatment

A mild lesser toe deformity can often be treated conservatively. If the patient's complaints do not respond well to orthotic devices, a flexor-to-extensor tendon transfer may be chosen for flexible hammer toes [Coughlin and Mann 1993]. However, this will not succeed in a rigid flexion contracture.

Prior to choosing the appropriate procedure, assessment of the metatarsophalangeal joint posi-tion is crucial. If the metatarsophalangeal joint is well aligned, condylectomy of the proximal phalanx or arthrodesis of the proximal interphalangeal joint is indicated [Alvine and Garvin 1980, McGlamry 1992]. If even a mild dorsal dislocation at the metatarsophalangeal joint is not taken into consid-eration, the toe will develop a recurrent deformity.

A mild hyperextension at the metatarsopha-langeal joint may be sufficiently corrected by releas-ing the dorsal capsule and reefing the plantar plate. In cases of severe or longstanding dorsal disloca-tions, metatarsal shortening may be necessary to achieve joint congruency.

In isolated mallet toe deformities, arthrodesis of the distal interphalangeal joint is recommended.

This procedure will lead to a stable and well-aligned distal toe, whereas resectional arthroplasty may cause painful instability.

A concomitant hallux valgus deformity must always be corrected at the same time to achieve adequate space for the re-aligned lesser toes.

Alternative treatment

Non-operative treatment includes metatarsal padding, which supports the transverse arch and reduces pressure against the metatarsal heads. Soft padding of the dorsal hyperkeratoses may also relieve pressure symptoms. Ready-made foam rubber bolsters or custom-made silicone cushions can be used for this purpose. Well-fitting shoes with a sufficiently wide toe box are the most important prerequisites for successful non-operative treatment [Thompson 1995].

Apart from condylectomy and arthrodesis, hammer toes can be corrected by diaphyseal shortening of the proximal phalanx, combined with manual reduction of the rigid proximal interphalangeal joint [Uhthoff 1990, Kuwada 1992]. This may be indicated in patients with a long second toe. Shortening can be achieved either by the resection of a small diaphyseal part of the proximal phalanx or by a Z-shaped osteotomy, which is technically demanding.

Shortening of a lesser metatarsal together with manual reduction of the rigid flexion contracture at the proximal interphalangeal joint has also been suggested to treat hammer deformities associated with a dorsal dislocation at the metatarsophalangeal joint. This procedure requires precise metatarsal length adjustment relative to the adjacent metatarsals to avoid overloading symptoms. Shortening of the metatarsal is supposed to result in a relaxation of the soft tissues, allowing restoration of the joint congruency at the metatarsophalangeal joint. Additional manual reduction of the hammer toe deformity is thought to correct the distal deformity sufficiently [Jaworek 1973, Reikeras 1983, McGlamry 1992]. During recent decades the shortening osteotomy predominantly involved the second to fourth metatarsals and was performed over a short distance from proximal–dorsal to distal–plantar [Helal 1975]. Upward sliding of the metatarsal heads depended on immediate postoperative weight-bearing. This technique was often followed by large callus formations, malalignment and pseudarthrosis. Shortening the metatarsal over a long diaphyseal distance from distal–dorsal to proximal–plantar [Barouk 1994], however, allows precise restoration of the metatarsal length and stable screw fixation.

Plantar condylectomy [Mann and Coughlin 1993] as an additional procedure is suggested in patients with marked metatarsalgia.

Tenotomy of the short extensor tendon, together with a Z-shaped lengthening of the long extensor tendon, may be helpful in reducing a mild dorsal dislocation at the metatarsophalangeal joint.

Resection of the base of the proximal phalanx should not be performed routinely, as this leads to an irreversible instability of the metatarsophalangeal joint.

Surgical technique

The operation can be performed under local, regional or general anesthesia. A tourniquet should be used, which may be applied above the ankle or at the thigh. The patient is in the supine position, with the foot slightly elevated.

Skin incision

Condylectomy of the proximal phalanx/arthrodesis of the proximal interphalangeal joint

The type of skin incision depends on the deformity. If any additional procedure around the metatarsophalangeal joint cannot be ruled out, an S-shaped or an angular skin incision is recommended (Figure 1). The incision should not be perpendicular to the transverse skin folds, because of the risk of postoperative contracture. S-shaped and angular incisions allow extension in both directions. This may be essential if other procedures, such as exploration of the metatarsophalangeal joint, lengthening of the extensor tendon or metatarsal shortening, have to be added. The disadvantage of these incisions is that callosities at the extensor side of the proximal interphalangeal joint can only partly be removed.

The transverse incision courses exactly parallel to the skin fissure lines over the proximal interphalangeal joint and is therefore cosmetically more favorable. It is suggested if a condylectomy or an arthrodesis is sufficient to correct the deformity. Elliptical excision of the dorsal callosities results in a dermodesis effect, which additionally contributes to the correction of the deformity [Kuwada 1992, McGlamry 1992]. In case of a condylectomy, this incision is placed approximately 3 mm proximal to the palpable joint line to address the distal part of the proximal phalanx. The incision extends to the

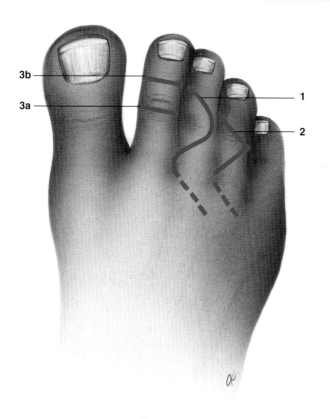

Figure 1

The skin incision may be S-shaped (1), angular (2), or transverse (3). 3a. incision for condylectomy of the proximal phalanx; 3b. incision for condylectomy of the middle phalanx. S-shaped and angular incisions may be extended proximally to expose the metatarsophalangeal joint (dashed lines)

end of the skin folds at the dorsal toe. Deep lateral incisions should be avoided in order to protect the adjacent neurovascular bundles.

Arthrodesis of the distal interphalangeal joint

To perform an arthrodesis of the distal interphalangeal joint, a transverse incision corresponding to the course of the skin fissure lines proximal to the distal interphalangeal joint is most useful. A more extensive exposure can be obtained with an S-shaped or angular incision. In this case, the nail root must be preserved to avoid growth disturbances of the nail.

Soft-tissue dissection

In a hammer toe deformity, bursa-like tissue may be found beneath the hyperkeratotic lesions,

which have to be excised. Following a transverse incision, the skin is retracted with two small sharp retractors. In an angular or S-shaped incision, the skin should be retracted with sutures, to avoid injury to the skin flaps. The extensor hood is now exposed (Figure 2a). Following a transverse skin incision, it may be incised in the same direction (Figure 2b). To facilitate wound closure in layers at the end of the procedure, it is useful to release the extensor hood from the underlying capsule. With a modified longitudinal skin incision the extensor tendon may be divided longitudinally, so that subsequent elongation with a Z-plasty will be possible. Depending on the metatarsophalangeal joint position, the short extensor tendon, running laterally to the long extensor tendon, can be cut sharply and allowed to retract. The underlying capsule is then incised transversely (Figure 2c). Exposition of the proximal interphalangeal joint is facilitated by maximum flexion of the distal toe. The lateral parts of the capsule, together with the collateral ligaments, are transected close to the bone with a small blade under direct vision (Figure 2d). Subsequently, the joint can be dislocated and the condyles exposed dorsally. Care must be taken not to damage the neurovascular bundle and the flexor tendons.

Condylectomy at the proximal interphalangeal joint

The distal part of the proximal phalanx must be exposed subperiosteally with an elevator. Two round retractors at the distal end of the phalanx are helpful to protect the flexor tendons. The extent of the resection depends on the severity of the deformity (Figure 3). As a rule, the resection must be proximal to the condyles but not comprise more than one-third of the proximal phalanx [Richardson 1987, Johnson 1989]. Insufficient resection may result in a painful pseudarthrosis, whereas excessive resection will lead to a floppy toe. The plane of resection should be exactly vertical to the axis of the shaft. Following oblique resection, lateral or medial deviation of the toe may ensue [Coughlin and Mann 1993]. An oscillating saw is strictly recommended for the osteotomy. A rongeur should not be used as it may splinter the phalanx, especially if the bone is osteoporotic. Following resection, the integrity of the flexor tendons must be assured. The edges of the bone are smoothed with a rongeur, if necessary.

Subsequently, the transverse arch of the foot is manually elevated (push-up test) to examine

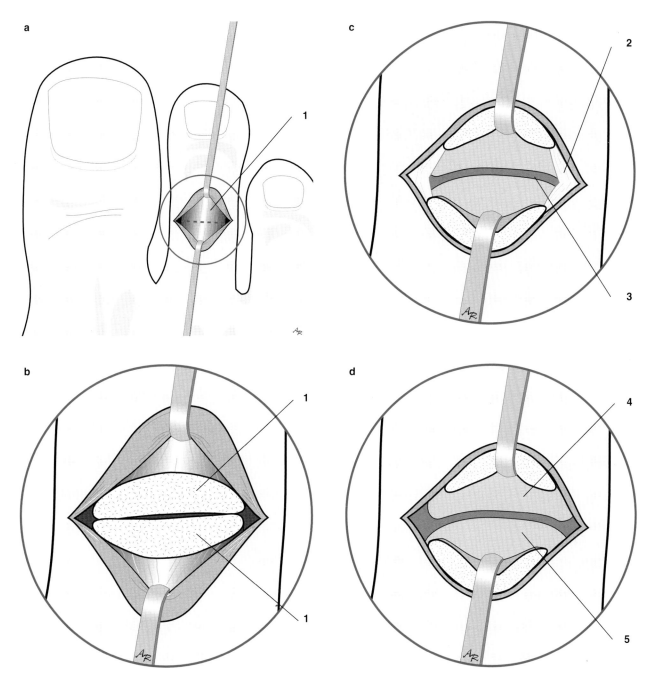

Figure 2

Surgical approach for condylectomy of the proximal phalanx. a. the extrinsic extensor tendon and its hood are exposed; b. the extrinsic extensor tendon and its hood are incised; c. following transverse incision of the capsule, the joint is exposed; d. the lateral parts of the capsule and the lateral ligaments are transected to enlarge the exposure of the joint

1 Extensor tendon
2 Joint capsule (incised)
3 Proximal interphalangeal joint
4 Base of middle phalanx
5 Condyle of proximal phalanx

whether the toe alignment and the extent of the resection are adequate [Coughlin and Mann 1993]. Axial traction on the distal toe should result in a distance of approximately 5 mm. The flexion deformity must be completely corrected. If this is not the case, additional procedures must be carried out.

To maintain the alignment it may be helpful to stabilize the proximal interphalangeal joint. A 1.0-mm Kirschner wire is drilled from proximal to

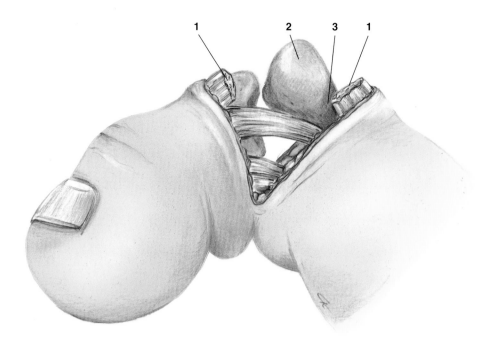

Figure 3

The resection of the phalanx is proximal to the condyles

1 Extensor tendon (divided)
2 Condyle of the proximal phalanx
3 Resection

distal through the middle phalanx, exiting at the tip of the toe. The wire is then drilled back proximally through the remainder of the proximal phalanx. In case of additional soft-tissue procedures at the metatarsophalangeal joint, the wire can be driven into the metatarsal bone [Richardson 1987].

Arthrodesis at the proximal interphalangeal joint/arthrodesis at the distal interphalangeal joint

The technical procedure concerning an arthrodesis of the interphalangeal joints does not differ significantly from the condylectomy. After exposure of the proximal condyles, limited resection of the cartilage is performed using an oscillating saw. It is very important to achieve a resection plane that is perpendicular to the long axis of the proximal phalanx. A slight plantar flexion of 5° may be advantageous at the proximal interphalangeal joint to facilitate ground contact, while the distal interphalangeal joint should be aligned in a straight position. The cartilage at the base of the middle phalanx can be removed with a rongeur. Trial reduction should result in the desired toe alignment. Prior to the stabilization it is further recommended to assess the toe length according to the adjacent toes in order to avoid any malalignment.

As an alternative to perpendicular bone resection, the articular cartilage may be removed with conical reamers, leading to a cup-and-cone fit [Lehman and Smith 1995, Weil 1999].

Stabilization of the arthrodesis at the proximal interphalangeal joint is mostly performed by using a Kirschner wire. The insertion technique does not differ from the method that is described for the condylectomy. Nevertheless, this fixation will neither control rotational forces nor lead to any compression. An additional wire cerclage may therefore be recommended to provide sufficient stability. Arthrodesis at the distal interphalangeal joint can be stabilized by a cannulated screw (2.0 mm) to achieve sufficient compression.

Additional procedures

If a slight flexion deformity at both the proximal and the distal interphalangeal joint remains after adequate condylectomy, tenotomy of the long flexor tendon may be indicated [Ross and Menelaus 1984, Lehman and Smith 1995]. This can be done by a stab incision at the distal flexion crease. This tenotomy can also be a successful procedure for an isolated flexion contracture at the distal interphalangeal joint.

A persistant dorsal position of the concerned toe during the push-up test after condylectomy or arthrodesis of the proximal interphalangeal joint points to an unsolved problem at the metatarsophalangeal joint. It is then suggested to follow a stepwise algorithm. At first the short extensor tendon should be detached at its insertion at the base of the middle phalanx. The long extensor tendon is then separated from its hood and is transected with a Z-shaped incision. This 'Z' should include at least 1.5 cm. Stay sutures are attached to the two ends of the tendon. In cases of a very mild tendency to dorsal dislocation these tendon procedures may be sufficient to correct the deformity.

The position of the metatarsophalangeal joint is again examined, with manual plantar pressure (push-up test) under the metatarsal head region. Even slight dorsal subluxation of the metatarsophalangeal joint should be thoroughly corrected to prevent a dorsiflexion deformity of the toe. To release the metatarsophalangeal joint the dorsal capsule is opened obliquely. Even if this procedure does not lead to an adequate toe position, the capsule is released circumferentially, including the collateral ligaments. The neurovascular bundles must be protected. Subsequently, the plantar plate is inspected. Any distal avulsion or elongation should be repaired after meticulous release [Mann and Coghlin 1991], although this is a very demanding procedure even after manual distension of the joint.

In case of a dorsal dislocation at the metatarsophalangeal joint, shortening of the metatarsal should be precisely planned preoperatively. Although this procedure is highly effective [Barouk 1996], it may offer many problems concerning the metatarsophalangeal joint, the transverse arch and the metatarsal alignment.

The wound closure has to include periosteal re-fixation of the collateral ligaments. Sutures of the dorsal capsule should be performed only if this can be achieved without tension. The extensor hood, including the lengthened long extensor tendon, requires a precise reconstruction [Sarrafian 1995] in order to create a dorsal tenodesis effect.

Closure

The tourniquet should be released and hemostasis performed. This is of special interest in recurrent deformities, where perfusion may be impaired. Both the capsule of the interphalangeal joints and the long extensor tendon should be closed with single sutures, using monofilament absorbable suture. This should also be done if the tendon was incised longitudinally, following an S-shaped or angular skin incision. If the extensor tendon was lengthened with a Z-plasty, the ends of the tendon have to be sutured side to side. The skin is closed with interrupted sutures after partial or complete resection of the hyperkeratotic lesions.

Bandaging technique

After cleansing and disinfecting the wound, a small gauze dressing is applied. Following condylectomy, long wound dressing sponges should be placed around the operated toe following a figure-of-eight pattern, pulling the proximal phalanx in a plantar direction and the middle phalanx in a dorsal direction. This is not necessary if the toe was fixed with a Kirschner wire. Small dressing sponges are also placed between all toes to keep the interdigital spaces dry. A narrow elastic bandage is applied and provides compression of the forefoot. A cushion may be placed under the metatarsal head region to elevate the transverse arch of the forefoot. If a Kirschner wire was used, its tip should be turned back and protected.

Postoperative care

If only a condylectomy at the proximal interphalangeal joint or an arthrodesis at the distal interphalangeal joint was performed, immediate plantigrade weightbearing can be permitted. Arthrodesis at the proximal interphalangeal joint may require partial weightbearing in an appropriate postoperative shoe. This corresponds to procedures where a Kirschner wire was used for stabilization of the metatarsophalangeal joint. Otherwise, the Kirschner wire may break or loosen [Coughlin and Mann 1993]. Longer periods of resting with the foot in an elevated position are advised for 3–5 days to prevent postoperative edema. Simultaneous systemic administration of nonsteroidal anti-inflammatory medication is optional.

Following simple condylectomy of the proximal interphalangeal joint, the Kirschner wire can be removed after 2 weeks, because it only serves to maintain the toe alignment and to preserve the distance after resection arthroplasty. If a capsular release and a reduction at the metatarsophalangeal joint were performed in addition, the Kirschner wire should remain for at least 4 weeks [Mann and Coghlin 1991].

Apart from that, the position of the operated toe has to be maintained for approximately 12 weeks. This is achieved by forced passive plantarflexion exercises of the metatarsophalangeal joint, which have to be performed regularly by the patient. Active foot exercises, such as grasping with the toes, may also accelerate rehabilitation. In cases of severe postoperative edema, lymphatic drainage may be advantageous.

The position of the toe should be maintained with a tape bandage for at least 6–12 weeks, depending on the severity of the deformity.

Complications

Swelling of the operated toe may persist for up to 6 months. This can be treated with elevation, lymphatic drainage and anti-inflammatory medication. Pain at the proximal interphalangeal joint after condylectomy and restriction of motion may be caused by insufficient bone resection and the development of a pseudarthrosis [Kuwada 1992]. This can be relieved by further resection or by an arthrodesis. With resection arthroplasty or arthrodesis at the proximal interphalangeal joint, restriction of active toe motion must be expected. Lateral deviation of the toe occurs if the resection plane is not perpendicular to the shaft. Interdigital corns at the adjacent toes may require re-operation.

Shortening of the toe changes the configuration of the forefoot, but this usually does not impair the cosmetic appearance or worsen forefoot function. 'Floppy toes' may result from an excessive resection of bone during condylectomy. Although this is usually not painful, it may be responsible for a loss of active movement and lack of ground contact. Recurrence of the deformity is rare if the indication and the operative technique were correct. Recurrent deformities almost always result if subluxation or dislocation of the metatarsophalangeal joint was not adequately treated.

Arthrodesis at both interphalangeal joints can result in a fibrous pseudarthrosis, which normally does not lead to any functional impairment or complaints. Comparing the possible complications of condylectomy and arthrodesis at the proximal interphalangeal joint, arthrodesis seems to be the more reliable and safer procedure.

References

Alvine FG, Garvin KL (1980) Peg and dowel fusion of the proximal interphalangeal joint. Foot Ankle 1: 90–94

Barouk LS (1994) L'ostéotomie cervico-capitale de Weil dans les métatarsalgies médianes. Méd Chir du Pied 10: 1–11

Barouk LS (1996) Die Metatarsalosteotomie nach Weil zur Behandlung der Metatarsalgie. Orthopäde 25: 338–344

Coughlin MJ, Mann RA (1993) Lesser toe deformities. In: Mann RA, Coughlin MJ (eds) Surgery of the Foot and Ankle, 6th edn. St Louis, Mosby, pp 341–411

Grace DL (1993) Surgery of the lesser rays. Foot 3: 51–57

Helal B (1975) Metatarsal osteotomy for metatarsalgia. J Bone Joint Surg 57B: 187–188

Jaworek T (1973) Diaphyseal resection: a modified approach to contracted digits. J Foot Surg 12: 118–119

Johnson KA (1989) Problems of the lesser toes. In: Surgery of the Foot and Ankle. New York, Raven Press, pp 101–150

Kuwada GT (1992) Surgery of the lesser digits. In: Butterworth R, Dockery GL (eds) A Colour Atlas and Text of Forefoot Surgery. London, Wolfe, pp 137–158

Lehman DE, Smith RE (1995) Treatment of symptomatic hammer toes with a proximal interphalangeal joint arthrodesis. Foot Ankle Int 16: 535–541

Mann RA, Coughlin MJ (1991) Lesser toe deformities. In: Jahss M (ed) Disorders of the Foot and Ankle. Philadelphia, WB Saunders, pp 1205–1228

Mann RA, Coughlin MJ (1993) Keratotic disorders of the plantar skin. In: Mann RA, Coughlin MJ (eds) Surgery of the Foot and Ankle, 6th edn. St Louis, Mosby, pp 413–465

McGlamry ED (1992) Lesser ray deformities. In: McGlamry ED, Banks AS, Downey MS (eds) Comprehensive Textbook of Foot Surgery, 2nd edn, vol 1. Baltimore, Williams & Wilkins, pp 321–378

Myerson MS, Shereff NJ (1989) The pathological anatomy of claw and hammer toes. J Bone Joint Surg 71A: 45–49

Myerson MS (1992) Arthroplasty of the second toe. Semin Arthroplasty 3: 31–38

Reikeras O (1983) Metatarsal osteotomy for relief of metatarsalgia. Arch Orthop Traumatol Surg 101: 177–178

Richardson EG (1987) The foot in adolescents and adults. In: Crenshaw AH (ed) Campbell's Operative Orthopedics, 7th edn. St Louis, Mosby, pp 2729–2755

Ross ERS, Menelaus NB (1984) Open flexor tenotomy for hammer toes and curly toes in childhood. J Bone Joint Surg 66B: 770–771

Sarrafian SK (1995) Correction of fixed hammertoe deformity with resection of the head of the proximal phalanx and extensor tendon tenodesis. Foot Ankle Int 16: 449–451

Scheck M (1977) Etiology of acquired hammer toe deformity. Clin Orthop 123: 63–69

Thompson GH (1995) Bunions and deformities of the toes in children and adolescents. J Bone Joint Surg 77A: 1924–1936

Uhthoff HK (1990) Operative Behandlung der nicht kontrakten Hammerzehe. Operat Orthop Traumatol 2: 46–50

Weil LS (1999) Hammertoe arthrodesis using conical reamers and internal pin fixation. J Foot Ankle Surg 38: 370–371

12

Hammer toes: flexor tendon transfer and metatarsophalangeal soft-tissue release

Henry P. J. Walsh

Introduction

Toe deformities such as hammer, claw and mallet toe commonly affect the lesser toes of the foot. The accepted definition of 'hammer toe' deformity is that the middle and distal phalanges are flexed on the proximal phalanx, with the main deformity being at the proximal interphalangeal joint, there being little or no hyperextension of the metatarsophalangeal joint [Mann and Coughlin 1993].

The etiology of the condition has a definite link with ill-fitting shoes, especially those with a small toe box, which restricts normal movement and impedes intrinsic activity as well as causing buckling of the toes. These problems are exacerbated by the wearing of high heels. Certain conditions can predispose the foot to secondary development of hammer toe deformities. These include neurological conditions such as cerebral palsy, spinal dysraphism and multiple sclerosis, inflammatory disorders such as rheumatoid disease, generalized disorders such as diabetes mellitus with associated neuropathy and post-traumatic compartment syndromes after lower leg or foot trauma.

To understand the basis for treatment for hammer toe deformity, it is important to study the anatomy and biomechanics of the toe [Coughlin 1989]. The flexor digitorum longus inserts into the distal phalanx and contraction flexes the distal interphalangeal joint. The flexor digitorum brevis flexes the proximal interphalangeal joint as it is inserted into the base of the middle phalanx (Figure 1). Over the proximal phalanx, the flexor digitorum longus is deep to the flexor digitorum brevis. Neither flexor tendon has a significant influence in metatarsophalangeal joint flexion. This is largely controlled by the intrinsic muscles, i.e. the interosseous and lumbrical muscles. The lumbrical muscles pass deep to the transverse metatarsal ligament to be inserted into the extensor hood. They thus act as flexors of the metatarsophalangeal joints and as extensors of the proximal and distal interphalangeal joints. The interosseous muscles have a similar influence on joint motion to the lumbrical muscles, with an additional abduction/adduction effect. The plantar aspect of the metatarsophalangeal joint is stabilized by the plantar aponeurosis and capsular condensation. These structures are referred to as the 'plantar plate'.

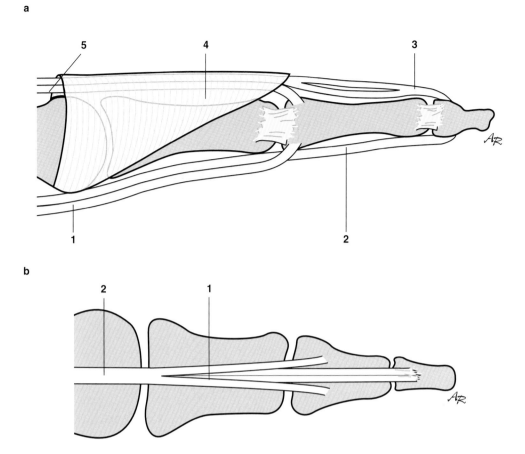

Figure 1

Anatomy of the lesser toe tendons. The flexor digitorum longus is deep to the flexor digitorum brevis and is inserted into the base of the distal phalanx. The flexor digitorum brevis is inserted into the base of the middle phalanx by two slips. The flexor digitorum brevis can be separated surgically over the proximal phalanx to expose the flexor digitorum longus, which has a central raphe over this area. a. lateral aspect; b. plantar aspect

a
1 Short flexor tendon
2 Long flexor tendon
3 Long extensor tendon
4 Extensor hood
5 Short extensor tendon

b
1 Long flexor tendon
2 Short flexor tendon

If the toes are held in hyperextension at the metatarsophalangeal joint over extended periods, several things occur. First, the plantar plate stretches and the metatarsophalangeal joint begins to subluxate. This, combined with a small toe box, will encourage the metatarsophalangeal joint extension to increase. Proximal interphalangeal joint flexion will arise as the toe buckles. In this position the intrinsic muscles are significantly disadvantaged and their actions of metatarsophalangeal joint flexion and proximal and distal interphalangeal joint extension are compromised. The hammer toe position is adopted. At first the toe deformity is correctable, but it will ultimately become fixed as the contractures develop principally in the proximal interphalangeal joint. Hyperextension forces across the metatarsophalangeal joint will also ultimately cause instability, with dorsal subluxation of the proximal phalanx.

Clinical assessment

The patients may be asymptomatic, but ultimately they can present with pain due to the callosities on the dorsal aspect of the proximal interphalangeal joint or over the plantar aspect of the metatarsal head, as the metatarsophalangeal joint begins to hyperextend. The second toe, which is frequently longer than the first, can develop a callosity over the tip due to local pressure within the shoe. The circulation and neurological status require careful assessment, not only to exclude a primary underlying condition, but also bearing in mind that any surgery to the toe can be extensive and compromise an already critical circulation still further.

It is important to distinguish between correctable and fixed hammer toe deformity. The flexible type will be apparent only on weightbearing. When the patient lies down with the foot held in equinus, the toe straightens at the proximal interphalangeal joint and metatarsophalangeal joint. The deformity of the toes is then reproducible by dorsiflexion of the ankle. The deformity can also be corrected by local pressure on the toe itself, thus confirming the flexibility of the joints. In addition, while the patient is in the standing position the other toes are examined to make sure there is room between them for the corrected toe, as it may be compromised by other deviated adjacent toes, particularly with the hallux valgus. Tightness of the flexor digitorum longus in the other toes is also assessed, as some individuals have naturally shortened flexor digitorum longus muscles, which emphasizes that the flexor digitorum longus in the symptomatic toe requires release at the time of surgery. Finally, the position of the metatarsophalangeal joint is examined. If there is a tendency to early hyperextension deformity, metatarsophalangeal joint surgery may be necessary in addition to distal surgery, to correct the deformity totally [Thompson and Hamilton 1987].

Treatment

Conservative treatment includes advice about shoes: patients should purchase shoes with high and wide toe boxes, with soft uppers and soft soles to avoid callosities. Foam toecaps can also bring symptoms under control. For more extensive problems, extra-depth shoes with appropriate metatarsal bars can give adequate relief. However, if these methods fail, surgical intervention can be considered. It is important to classify the type of deformity present, as this dictates which procedure is most suitable. While the deformity remains correctable, a flexor tendon transfer to the extensor aspect is the treatment of choice, as it is aimed at re-establishing the normal anatomy and biomechanics of the proximal interphalangeal and metatarsophalangeal joints. One would hope to re-establish intrinsic activity within the toes.

Surgical options are as follows:

- For flexible hammer toe deformity with normal metatarsophalangeal joints, a flexor tendon transfer should be used.
- Flexible hammer toe deformity with a tendency to metatarsophalangeal joint hyperextension or

subluxation is corrected with a flexor tendon transfer and soft-tissue release of the metatarsophalangeal joint [Parrish 1973].
- In fixed hammer toe deformity with normal metatarsophalangeal joints, condylectomy of the proximal phalanx and soft-tissue repair [Johnson 1989], such as extensor tendon tenodesis [Sarrafian 1995] or proximal interphalangeal joint fusion, are indicated (see Chapter 11).
- Fixed hammer toe deformity with metatarsophalangeal joint subluxation or hyperextension is treated with condylectomy of the proximal phalanx, arthrodesis of the proximal interphalangeal joint and soft-tissue release of the metatarsophalangeal joint, which must be adequate to correct any hyperextension at this joint. This is checked by dorsiflexion of the ankle through pressure on the plantar aspect of the metatarsal head of the joint that is being corrected.

Flexor tendon transfer

Girdlestone is credited with developing the procedure to transfer the long flexor tendon of the toe to the dorsal expansion of the extensor tendon to substitute for lack of intrinsic activity at the metatarsophalangeal and proximal interphalangeal joints [Taylor 1951]. Others have used the flexor digitorum brevis for this purpose, but the transfer was weaker and more difficult to execute [Parrish 1973]. Several toes can be corrected at one time, but it is critical to check the circulation carefully preoperatively, as the toe or toes are approached from both the plantar and the dorsal aspects and the surgery is carried out over such a large area that neurovascular compromise can be a problem.

Local blocks can be used by infiltrating a mixture of 0.5% plain lignocaine and 0.25% plain bupivacaine into the intermetatarsal spaces in the midfoot to allow blockage in the metatarsophalangeal joints and the toes. Further local infiltration of the skin is also usually necessary, as the superficial layers are rarely adequately anesthetized by standard blocks. For these reasons it may be preferable to perform the surgery under general anesthesia, as this does not compromise the operative field. Local blocks can be inserted after induction of anesthesia to aid with postoperative analgesia.

An ankle or a thigh pneumatic tourniquet can be used, according to the surgeon's preference. The usual pressure can be double systolic for the thigh and 50 mmHg above systolic for the ankle. Esmarch

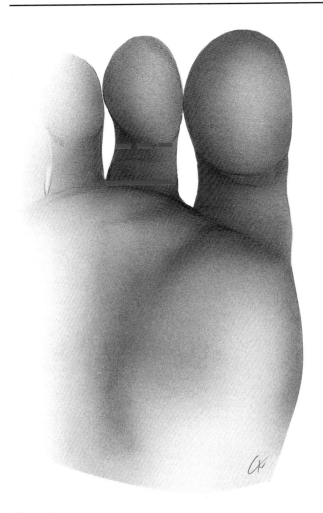

Figure 2

Initial incision at the level of the proximal flexor crease of the second toe. A more distal incision will be used to detach the flexor digitorum longus tendon (dashed line)

exsanguination for the thigh tourniquet, or a compression tube if available and elevation for 5 min for the ankle tourniquets should be used.

The procedure is carried out with the patient in the supine position and with the surgeon seated.

The preoperative assessment is repeated to confirm that the proximal interphalangeal joint deformity is fully correctable. Metatarsophalangeal joint stability is tested for [Thompson and Hamilton 1987].

Surgical technique

The first incision is made horizontally in the plantar skin at the level of the proximal flexor crease of the affected toe. It is 5–6 mm long and goes down to the level of the flexor tendons (Figure 2). A Z-incision can also be used [Johnson 1989]. The soft tissues are separated off the flexor tendon sheath, which is then opened longitudinally. Note that there are three tendons within the sheath (Figure 3a). The central deep one is the flexor digitorum longus. The flexor digitorum brevis tendon can be separated at this level into two lateral strands. The flexor digitorum longus is mobilized by blunt dissection with a mosquito forceps and by gentle flexion of the toe (Figure 3b). With a second small incision, which is made over the distal flexor crease, the flexor digitorum longus is tenotomized as distally as possible (Figure 3b). The flexor digitorum longus is then pulled into the original wound and the central raphe is divided longitudinally, so that two equal strips of tendon are held within a mosquito forceps (Figure 3c). The surgeon's attention then turns to the dorsum of the foot, and through a longitudinal incision over the proximal phalanx and over the metatarsophalangeal joint, the extensor expansion is exposed (Figure 4). The two strands of the flexor digitorum longus are then passed dorsally toward the extensor expansion on the medial and lateral aspects of the proximal phalanx, deep to the neurovascular bundle (Figure 5). They are then sutured to the extensor digitorum longus tendon at about the middle portion of the proximal phalanx, with the toe held in 20° of plantar flexion at the metatarsophalangeal joint and tensioned to obtain slight overcorrection when the ankle is in neutral position.

Alternatively, the flexor digitorum longus tendon can be passed wholly through a drill hole made in the base of the proximal phalanx from plantar to dorsal [Kuwada and Dockery 1980]. The hole is approximately 2–3 mm in diameter and the flexor tendon is sutured to the extensor expansion. This technique is useful when there is demonstrated instability of the metatarsophalangeal joint.

A Kirschner wire can be used as reinforcement of the transfer. The wire is driven into the base of the proximal phalanx, through a small dorsal transverse incision at the metatarsophalangeal joint, and passed retrogradely across the metatarsophalangeal joint into the metatarsal head. However, the wire must not be used to correct any suggestion of hyperextension deformity at the metatarsophalangeal joint or to hold the toe down to compensate for lack of correction by the transfer. In this case, a soft-tissue correction of the metatarsophalangeal joint is necessary (see below).

Closure and postoperative care

The wounds are sutured with interrupted absorbable material. The toe is then bandaged with sterile wool and crêpe dressings over a non-adhesive dressing. The tourniquet is released and the return of

a

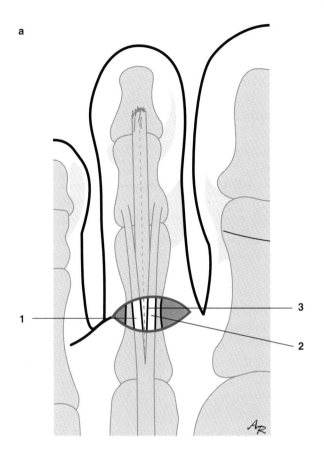

b

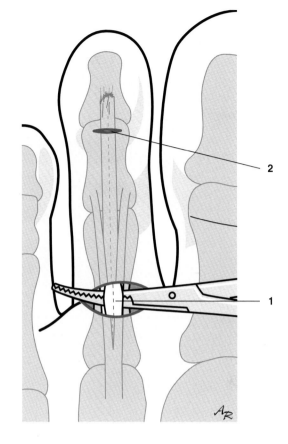

c

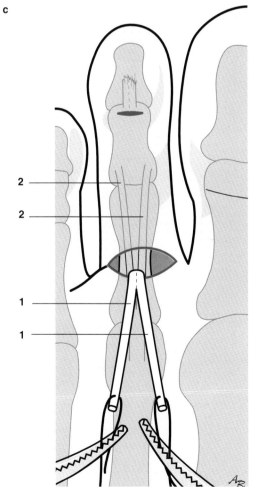

Figure 3

Dissection of the flexor digitorum longus tendon (plantar aspect). a. the flexor digitorum longus tendon is exposed behind the split flexor digitorum brevis; b. it is pulled out of the wound beneath a small clamp and detached from its insertion through the small distal incision; c. the tendon is divided along its central raphe

a
1   Short flexor tendon
2   Short flexor tendon
3   Long flexor tendon

b
1   Long flexor tendon
2   Distal incision

c
1   Long flexor tendon (divided)
2   Short flexor tendons

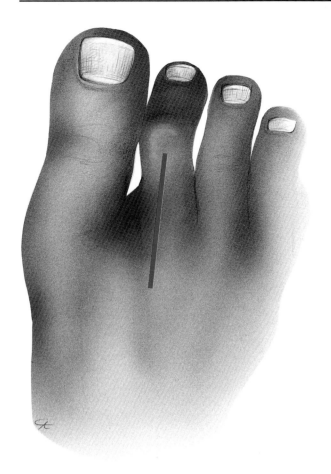

Figure 4

The extensor tendon with the metatarsophalangeal joint underneath is exposed through a dorsal incision

removal may occasionally be necessary to allow quicker return of the blood supply. Postoperatively, the patient is mobilized in a wooden-soled shoe for essentials only in the first 2 weeks, keeping the foot elevated for the remainder of the time. The sutures are removed at 2 weeks. If a Kirschner wire has not been used, the toe is strapped in a crossover fashion from that time for a further 4 weeks. Patients are then instructed in this strapping technique so that they can change the splintage themselves as necessary. If a Kirschner wire has been used, this is removed at 4 weeks postoperatively and the strapping is then commenced for a further 2 weeks as above.

Metatarsophalangeal joint soft-tissue correction

On transfer of the flexor digitorum longus tendons to the dorsum of the toe, it may become apparent in some instances that the flexor tendon transfer will not correct the toe fully at the metatarsophalangeal joint. Under normal circumstances, the flexor tendon transfer should be such that under tension it holds the metatarsophalangeal joint in 20° of plantar flexion. If this is not so, then there is residual deformity at the metatarsophalangeal joint which requires a soft-tissue release of this joint.

circulation to the toe is checked. If there is delay in revascularization, then loosening the bandages allows the return of the circulation in the vast majority of cases. If a Kirschner wire is used, its early

Surgical technique

Through the dorsal incision the extensor digitorum longus tendon is divided horizontally at the level of

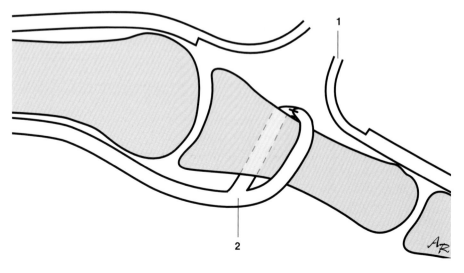

Figure 5

Lateral aspect. The extensor expansion is split longitudinally at about the mid-portion of the proximal phalanx, and the split portions of the flexor tendons are sutured to one another and to the extensor tendon, with the toe held at 20° of plantar flexion at the metatarsal phalangeal joint. Tension of the transfer is important to obtain slight overcorrection, with the ankle held at 90°

1　Extensor tendon (divided)
2　Long flexor tendon transfer

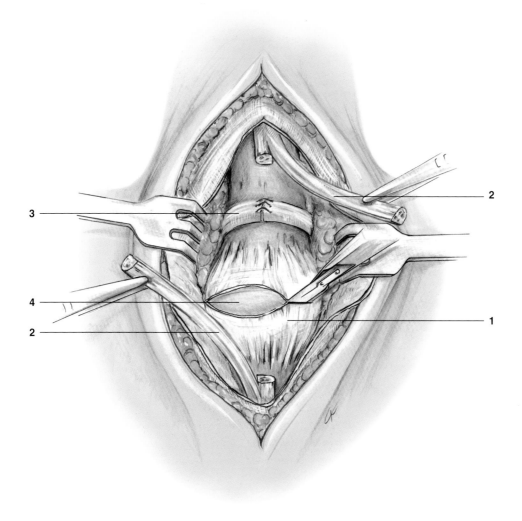

Figure 6

Dorsal aspect following suture of the transferred flexor digitorum longus tendon. In order to allow correct tension with the transfer, the extensor digitorum longus and dorsal capsule of the metatarsophalangeal joint sometimes have to be divided. Further soft-tissue releases medially and laterally in a dorsoplantar direction of the joint may also be necessary

1   Metatarsophalangeal joint capsule (incised)
2   Extensor tendon (Z-lengthened)
3   Transferred flexor tendon
4   Metatarsophalangeal joint

the metatarsophalangeal joint in a Z-fashion to allow subsequent lengthening. The capsule of this joint is also divided dorsally (Figure 6).

In flexible hammer toes this can be sufficient to correct the metatarsophalangeal joint deformity, but occasionally rebalancing the joint will be necessary, owing to some associated deviation to the medial or lateral side. This is carried out through appropriate release of the collateral ligaments in a dorsal to plantar direction as necessary.

A Kirschner wire is then introduced as described in the flexor tendon transfer, and the closure and postoperative care are as above.

Complications

The results of this procedure for primary flexible hammer toe deformity are usually satisfactory. However, in the presence of secondary disease the outcome is less predictable.

Kirschner wire fixation with protrusion through the tip of the toe can be associated with superficial infection [Johnson 1989]. In addition, the pin may fracture as it crosses the joint. If a broken wire protrudes into the middle phalanx, then surgical removal may be necessary. However, if it is buried within bone, then it is unlikely to cause any long-term problems. Persistent swelling around the toe may be a problem and the use of Kirschner wires with associated superficial infection may prolong this process. However, this subsides with time.

Vascular compromise is a rare complication. If the circulation is checked thoroughly prior to surgery and gentle mobilization of the soft tissue is carried out, with attention to the neurovascular bundles, it is not likely to cause significant problems. If it occurs in the immediate postoperative period, then loosening of the dressings or even total removal of the bandages may be necessary and this almost inevitably allows return of the circulation. If a Kirschner wire has been inserted, its removal may also be necessary to help return of the blood supply. For these reasons, it is important for the surgeon to make sure that the deformity has been appropriately corrected before the Kirschner wire is inserted. The wire should be acting as only a reinforcement rather than a fundamental part of the procedure.

Because of the transfer of the tendon from the plantar to the dorsal aspect, occasionally numbness of the toe develops; this is usually transient.

Recurrent metatarsophalangeal joint extension can be due to scarring in the soft tissues. This soft-tissue problem may be corrected by Z-plasty, with good short-term to medium-term results [Myerson et al. 1994]. However, the surgeon must also be aware of the possibility that inadequate soft-tissue correction of the metatarsophalangeal joint was performed at the time of the flexor tendon transfer surgery; a more extensive soft-tissue release of the metatarsophalangeal joint may be necessary.

References

Coughlin MJ (1989) Subluxation and dislocations of the second metatarsophalangeal joint. Orthop Clin North Am 20 (4): 535–551

Johnson KA (1989) Surgery of the Foot and Ankle. New York, Raven Press

Kuwada GT, Dockery GL (1980) Modification of the flexor tendon transfer procedure for the correction of flexible hammertoes. J Foot Surg 19: 38–40

Mann RA, Coughlin MJ (1993) Surgery of the Foot and Ankle. St Louis, Mosby–Year Book

Myerson MS, Fortin P, Gurard P (1994) Use of skin Z-plasty for management of extension contracture in recurrent claw and hammer toe deformity. Foot Ankle Int 15 (4): 209–212

Parrish TF (1973) Dynamic correction of claw toes. Orthop Clin North Am 4 (1): 97–102

Sarrafian SK (1995) Correction of fixed hammer toe deformity with resection of the head of the proximal phalanx and extensor tendon tenodesis. Foot Ankle Int 16: 449–451

Taylor RG (1951) The treatment of claw toes by multiple transfers of flexor into extensor tendons. J Bone Joint Surg 33B: 539–542

Thompson FM, Hamilton WG (1987) Problems of the second metatarsophalangeal joint. Orthopedics 10 (1): 83–89

13

Bunionette deformity: osteotomies of the fifth metatarsal bone

Nikolaus Wülker

Introduction

Bunionette deformity (tailor's bunion) is a prominence or enlargement of the fifth metatarsal head, causing pressure symptoms particularly when wearing a shoe. It is comparable to a bunion at the first ray but, unlike hallux valgus, toe deformity is usually absent and symptoms are isolated to the metatarsal head. Medial deviation of the fifth toe is usually congenital and treated with various soft-tissue corrections (see Chapter 14).

Bunionette is most often treated in young adults, mostly women. The etiology is unknown. It some-times occurs in conjunction with hallux valgus and is then often related to splaying of the midfoot, i.e. an increased angle between the metatarsal bones.

Various deformities at the fifth metatarsal bone may cause bunionette. The fifth metatarsal head may be enlarged (in approximately 25% of patients). The fifth metatarsal may also have an increased lateral curvature (25%), or the angle between the fourth and the fifth metatarsal may be increased (50%).

Symptoms are closely related to footwear. Fashion shoes with a narrow toe box and with high heels may cause bunionette symptoms even without a notable deformity. Pain may be present not only laterally but also underneath the fifth metatarsal head. Other causes of metatarsalgia must be excluded, e.g.

cavus foot. Physical examination usually reveals an area of inflamed skin or a callus with local tenderness at the prominent fifth metatarsal head.

Standing dorsoplantar radiographs are required. An enlarged fifth metatarsal head has an increased width (normal < 13 mm) and is often larger than the heads of the fourth and third metatarsals. Normally, the fifth metatarsal bone is straight. An angle between the proximal and the distal segments (lateral deviation angle, normal < 8°), i.e. lateral bowing of the fifth metatarsal, causes prominence of the head and bunionette symptoms. The inter-metatarsal angle between the fourth and the fifth metatarsal is usually 10° or less. If increased, this may also lead to bunionette symptoms.

Treatment

Inadequate footwear must be corrected before any treatment is begun. Non-operative treatment such as cushions, local anti-inflammatory treatment and callus debridement usually provide only temporary relief. If symptoms are sufficiently severe, surgery is indicated.

Treatment must be individualized to the defor-mity. Bunionette is always a bone deformity and soft-tissue procedures are not adequate. Malalignment

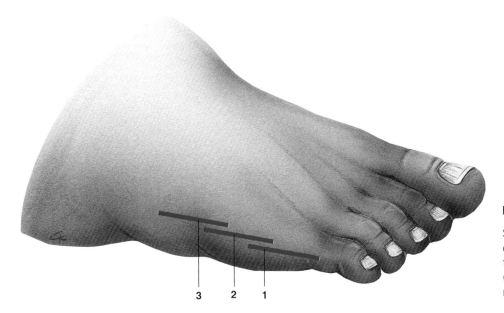

Figure 1

Skin incisions for the distal chevron osteotomy (1), for the diaphyseal osteotomy (2) and for the proximal fifth metatarsal osteotomy (3)

must be corrected where it occurs. Enlargement of the fifth metatarsal head with lateral prominence is best treated with a distal fifth metatarsal osteotomy. Various techniques may be used. The chevron osteotomy is relatively stable and has few complications. Other distal osteotomies provide less predictable results. Lateral bowing of the fifth metatarsal requires a diaphyseal osteotomy, which is usually oblique. Bunionette due to an increased intermetatarsal angle to the fourth ray is treated with a proximal fifth metatarsal osteotomy.

Significant varus deviation of the fifth toe, whether isolated or in conjunction with bunionette deformity, must be corrected with soft-tissue procedures (see Chapter 14), and osteotomy alone is not adequate.

Resections of the fifth metatarsal head have been used in the past. However, they invariably lead to transfer metatarsalgia under the fourth and third metatarsal heads and should therefore be avoided.

Peripheral vascular disease with absent pedal pulses is the major contraindication to fifth metatarsal osteotomy. Delayed wound healing or necrosis may ensue if this is not observed.

Surgical technique

The procedure is performed with the patient in the supine position. Regional, local or general anesthesia may be used. The foot is exsanguinated with a rubber (Esmarch) bandage.

Chevron osteotomy

A straight lateral skin incision is made from the proximal phalanx to the proximal limit of the exostosis at the metatarsal head (Figure 1). Skin flaps are raised to expose the thick capsular tissue overlying the head. Flaps must be thick enough to secure postoperative perfusion and wound healing.

The capsule is divided longitudinally. A bursa may be present over the exostosis. The thick capsular and bursal tissue is peeled off the head, where it is usually quite adherent to bone. Pointed Hohmann retractors are inserted.

The lateral projection of the fifth metatarsal head is resected in line with the lateral border of the fifth metatarsal diaphysis. An oscillating saw is most convenient; alternatively, an osteotome may be used. Care must be taken to orient the resection in the sagittal plane, i.e. at a right angle to the sole of the foot. The resection edges are rounded with a rongeur.

A 2-mm drill hole is made lateral to medial through the center of the fifth metatarsal head (Figure 2a). This will serve as the exit point for the osteotomies and help to avoid fracture of the metatarsal head by excessive stresses at the apex of the saw cuts. The drill may be directed slightly in a dorsal direction, which will move the head dorsally and relieve pressure underneath the metatarsal head if this caused symptoms preoperatively. Shortening of the fifth metatarsal should generally be avoided.

The two cuts are made at an angle of 60°, joined at the drill hole in the head center. The osteotomies must end precisely at the central drill hole in the head. Care is taken not to injure the medial soft tissues with the saw. The head fragment is carefully mobilized with an osteotome. Fracture of the head fragment during this maneuver is a major complication and difficult to salvage.

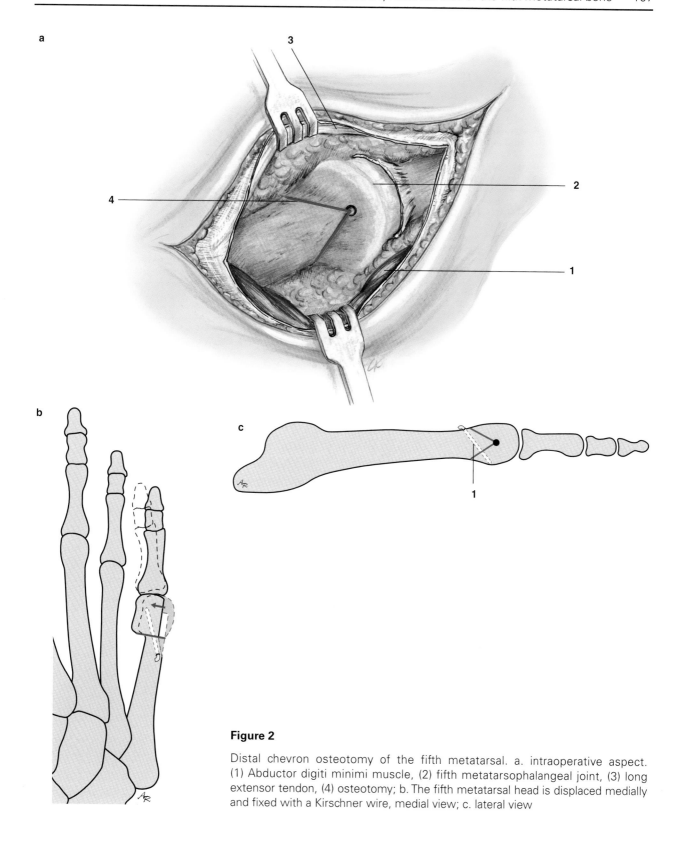

Figure 2

Distal chevron osteotomy of the fifth metatarsal. a. intraoperative aspect. (1) Abductor digiti minimi muscle, (2) fifth metatarsophalangeal joint, (3) long extensor tendon, (4) osteotomy; b. The fifth metatarsal head is displaced medially and fixed with a Kirschner wire, medial view; c. lateral view

Medial displacement of the head must be one-third to one-half of the fifth metatarsal diameter (Figure 2b). This is usually achieved by a combination of tension and manipulation on the hallux, pressure on the head fragment in a medial direction and manipulation of the osteotomy with an osteotome. In addition, the proximal fragment may have to be retracted laterally with an elevator or a pointed clamp. Once sufficient displacement is attained, the surgeon must make sure that both the plantar and the dorsal osteotomy surfaces are in immediate contact.

Internal stabilization with a Kirschner wire is recommended (Figure 2c). During fixation, the

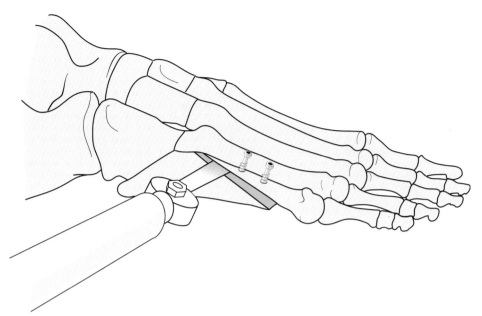

Figure 3

Oblique diaphyseal osteo-
tomy and fixation with two
mini-fragment screws

osteotomy is held reduced by axial pressure on the
hallux by an assistant. Internal fixation may be with
a 1.2-mm Kirschner wire inserted from the dorsolateral surface of the proximal fragment in a medial,
distal and plantar direction. The wire should not
penetrate the articular surface and care must
be taken not to place the wire inside the joint.
The upper end may be bent and left in the subcutaneous tissues, or the wire is left protruding
through a stab incision in the skin, protected with
a cap and pulled in the office 3 weeks postoperatively. Depending on the skill and experience of
the surgeon, intraoperative fluoroscopy may be
used to ascertain correct placement. Following fixation, prominent bone at the proximal fragment is
removed with a saw or a rongeur.

The capsulotomy is closed with absorbable
sutures. The skin is closed in a routine fashion.
Excess skin does not need to be excised, as skin
redundancy reduces within 2 weeks after surgery. A
soft dressing is applied and a protruding wire tip is
protected. Following release of the tourniquet, skin
perfusion at the fifth toe must be secured. If this
does not return within a few minutes, the dressing
must be removed.

Postoperatively, the patient is supplied with a firm
postoperative shoe to prevent rolling over the operated toe. Full weightbearing is allowed immediately,
but patients must largely limit their activities during
the first 2 weeks to prevent swelling. At 2 weeks, skin
sutures are removed. At 3 weeks, the Kirschner wire
is pulled if it was left outside the skin. Six weeks
postoperatively, the postoperative shoe is discontinued and patients are instructed to use their forefoot
intentionally during walking.

Oblique, diaphyseal osteotomy

A straight lateral skin incision is made from the
head to the base of the fifth metatarsal (Figure 1).
The incision is carried straight on to the bone
and unnecessary soft-tissue dissection is avoided.
The periosteum at the fifth metatarsal diaphysis is
elevated and round Hohmann retractors are
inserted.

An oblique osteotomy is used for correction. This
extends through most of the metatarsal diaphysis
(Figure 3). The preferred orientation is from dorsal
and proximal to plantar and distal. If pressure symptoms were present not only laterally but also underneath the fifth metatarsal head, the saw cut is
oriented slightly upwards, so that the distal fragment will be elevated with medial displacement.
The saw should just penetrate the cortical bone but
not reach into the intermetatarsal soft tissues. The
periosteum is loosened with an osteotome, which is
used as a lever to open the osteotomy.

The distal fragment is rotated medially. The amount
of rotation can be estimated at the osteotomy. The
fifth metatarsal head must no longer be prominent
following the correction. The osteotomy is temporarily fixed with a pointed reduction clamp, which is
applied with caution in order not to break the relatively fragile fragments.

Screws are preferred for fixation. According
to the diameter of the fifth metatarsal diaphysis,
mini-fragment screws with an internal diameter of
1.5 mm are most suitable. They should be inserted
as lag screws by overdrilling the dorsal hole to the
outer diameter of the screw. The head must be
sufficiently countersunk to avoid pressure under

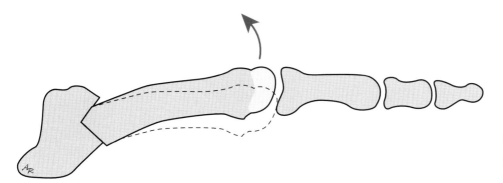

Figure 4

Proximal fifth metatarsal osteotomy

the skin. Again, care must be taken not to fracture the fifth metatarsal during tightening of the screw.

The reduction clamp is removed and stability as well as correct alignment of the osteotomy is ascertained. Following irrigation of the wound, only the skin is closed with interrupted sutures. A soft compression dressing is applied. Following release of the tourniquet, skin perfusion at the fifth toe must be secured. If this does not return within a few minutes, the dressing must be removed.

Postoperative treatment is identical to that following chevron osteotomy. The screws are generally not removed unless they cause symptoms.

Proximal fifth metatarsal osteotomy

A longitudinal, dorsolateral skin incision is made over the base of the fifth metatarsal (Figure 1). The incision is carried straight on to the bone and unnecessary soft-tissue dissection is avoided. The periosteum is elevated and pointed Hohmann retractors are inserted. The capsule of the fifth tarsometatarsal joint should be exposed at the proximal end of the incision but does not need to be opened.

A proximal chevron-type osteotomy provides most stability, because it is in two planes (Figure 4). The dorsal cut is made with an oscillating saw approximately 5 mm distal to the joint and in a vertical orientation, half way through the metatarsal base. The plantar cut is then made at an angle of approximately 45° so that it exits the plantar cortex of the metatarsal approximately 1 cm distal to the dorsal cut. A small bone wedge is removed from the dorsal osteotomy, with a medial base of 2–3 mm at the proximal fragment. Following removal of the wedge and closure of the osteotomy, alignment of the fifth metatarsal must be corrected.

Internal fixation is preferably with a small-fragment screw, inserted dorsally in a plantar and medial direction to enter the plantar spike of the proximal fragment. The head must be sufficiently countersunk to avoid pressure under the skin. Alternatively, a Kirschner wire can be used. It may be left protruding through the skin and removed in the office 3 weeks postoperatively.

Following irrigation of the wound, only the skin is closed with interrupted sutures. A soft compression dressing is applied. Following release of the tourniquet, skin perfusion at the fifth toe must be secured. If this does not return within a few minutes, the dressing must be removed.

Postoperative treatment is identical to that following chevron osteotomy. The screws are generally not removed unless they cause symptoms.

Bibliography

Coughlin MJ (1991) Treatment of bunionette deformity with longitudinal diaphyseal osteotomy with distal soft tissue repair. Foot Ankle 11: 195–203

Diebold PF, Bejjani FJ (1987) Basal osteotomy of the fifth metatarsal with intermetatarsal pinning: a new approach to tailor's bunion. Foot Ankle 8: 40–45

Karasick D (1995) Preoperative assessment of symptomatic bunionette deformity: radiographic findings. Am J Roentgenol 164: 147–149

Kasparek M, Knahr K (1996) Operative Behandlung der Bunionette. Z Orthop Ihre Grenzgeb 134: 520–523

Kitaoka HB, Holiday AD (1992) Lateral condylar resection for bunionette. Clin Orthop 278: 183–192

Kitaoka HB, Leventen EO (1989) Medial displacement metatarsal osteotomy for the treatment of painful bunionette. Clin Orthop 243: 172–179

Moran MM, Claridge RJ (1994) Chevron osteotomy for bunionette. Foot Ankle Int 15: 684–688

Yancey HA (1969) Congenital lateral bowing of the fifth metatarsal. Report of 2 cases and operative treatment. Clin Orthop 62: 203–205

14

Overriding fifth and curly toe

Thomas W. D. Smith
Nicholas J. Harris

Overriding fifth toe

The overriding fifth toe usually presents in children and adolescents. The toe adopts an extended, adducted and supinated position at the metatarsophalangeal joint with a typical 'cock-up' appearance over the fourth toe. Pain and callosity formation are indications for surgery, although some patients request surgery for cosmetic reasons.

The deformity is associated with a tight extensor tendon and contracture of the dorsal metatarsophalangeal joint capsule.

Treatment

The V–Y elongation is a useful technique for mild overlapping deformity of the fifth toe [Wilson 1953]. For more severe deformity the Butler procedure was reported to give good results in 90% of cases up to 10 years after surgery and is especially useful in children [Cockin 1968, Hassan et al. 2004]. Transfer of the extensor digitorum longus tendon around the proximal phalanx has also been used to treat overriding of the fifth toe [Lapidus 1942].

Surgical technique

V–Y plasty for the overlapping fifth toe

The V incision is performed with two limbs, the apex proximally extending over the dorsum of the fourth interspace and over the dorsal surface of the fifth toe (Figure 1). The fifth metatarsophalangeal joint is then released after an extensor tenotomy is performed; the capsule of the joint requires radical release on the medial and dorsal aspects (Figure 2). The toe is then pulled down into a flexed position and the ensuing Y-shaped skin flap is closed with interrupted nylon sutures.

Butler procedure

The Butler procedure is best performed under general anesthesia with the patient in the supine position using tourniquet control.

A standard circumferential 'racket' incision is used, with a 'handle' on the plantar aspect of the foot (Figure 1). The neurovascular bundles are identified early in the dissection and protected. The tight extensor tendon is divided, revealing the contracted dorsal capsule of the metatarsophalangeal joint. This is also released. It should then be possible to swing the toe laterally and plantarwards into the corrected position, rather like changing gear in a car (Figure 2). Occasionally there may be difficulty in correcting longstanding deformities owing to adherent capsule on the plantar aspect of the metatarsal head. This should also be released using blunt dissection. With the toe held in the corrected position, the skin around it can be closed without tension using interrupted nylon sutures. No splintage is required and the patient is able to heel weightbear the same day.

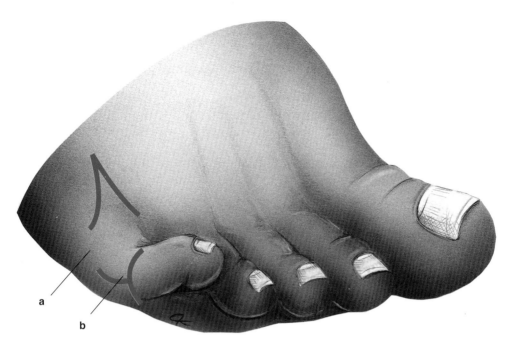

Figure 1

(a) Incisions for the V–Y plasty; (b) a circumferential racket incision is used for the Butler procedure

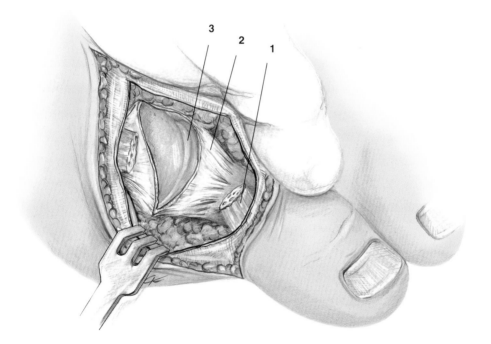

Figure 2

The position of the fifth toe can be corrected following division of the tight extensor tendon and the dorsal metatarsophalangeal joint capsule

1 Extensor tendon
2 Metatarsophalangeal joint capsule
3 Metatarsal head

Complications

Neurovascular complications are rare in childhood, provided the neurovascular bundles are identified and protected, although transient vascular spasm is common. Recurrence of the deformity may be treated by proximal phalangectomy or even by amputation through the metatarsophalangeal joint.

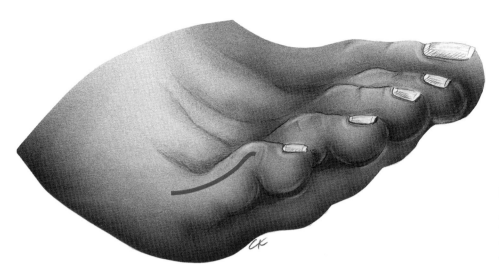

Figure 3

A lateral incision is used for flexor tenotomy and for flexor to extensor tendon transfer

Curly toes

The etiology of curly toes remains unclear. It may be the result of intrinsic muscle imbalance [Duchenne 1883], although some investigators could find no evidence of this [Taylor 1951, Mann and Inman 1964]. In cases with increasing deformity, an underlying cause such as spinal dysraphism should be suspected. The condition is most commonly found in children and young adults and often involves several toes in both feet. The principal deformity consists of flexion at the interphalangeal joints with some adduction and supination of the toe. There is no fixed deformity in curly toes, but more severe cases may develop pain and callosity formation on the dorsal surface of the flexed interphalangeal joints. The major deforming force in the development of curly toes appears to be the flexor digitorum longus, because of either weaker toe extensors or increased pull of the flexor itself. There may also be some incompetence of the fibular collateral ligament at the metatarsophalangeal joint, allowing the toe to drift into a more adducted position.

Treatment

In the newborn child, treatment with strapping is often advised. Improvement of the deformity may occur with or without such treatment, and early surgery is not indicated in the absence of pain or callosity formation. There is no evidence to suggest that curly toes, if left untreated, will progress to more serious deformity.

Several soft-tissue procedures have been described in the treatment of curly toes, such as the Girdlestone flexor to extensor transfer [Taylor 1951] and the simple flexor tenotomy [Ross and Menelaus 1984]. Simple flexor tenotomy and flexor to extensor transfer gave equally good results in children at 4 years' follow-up [Hamer et al. 1993].

Modifications of the flexor digitorum longus transfer have been described to give a more direct flexion force to the proximal phalanx [Coughlin 1993, Kuwada 1988]. These techniques appear more effective than the original Girdlestone transfer and are especially useful when there is subluxation of the metatarsophalangeal joint in association with a claw toe.

Surgical technique

Flexor tenotomy

Flexor tenotomy is best performed with the patient in a supine position under general anesthesia using a tourniquet control. A short transverse plantar incision may be used, but in cases where there is significant varus of the toe, the lateral scar contracture produced by a lateral incision may help to correct the toe. This incision commences at the metatarsophalangeal joint and extends just distal to the proximal interphalangeal joint (Figure 3). The lateral neurovascular bundle is identified and retracted in the plantar skin flap. The lateral aspect of the flexor sheath is then identified and incised. The opening in the sheath is enlarged and the flexor tendons identified. A

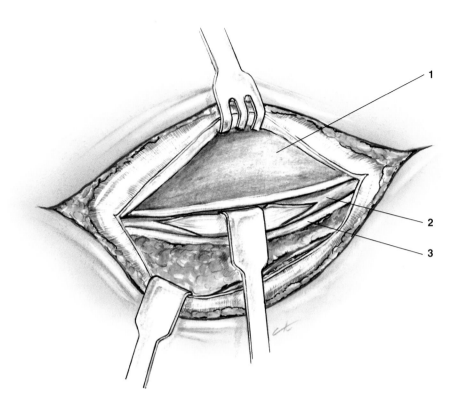

Figure 4

The long flexor tendon is retrieved with a small retractor and divided

1 Proximal phalanx
2 Flexor tendon sheath
3 Plantar neurovascular bundle

small, blunt hook is used to retrieve the long flexor tendon from the sheath, and the tendon is then divided (Figure 4). This is facilitated if the toe is hyperflexed.

The skin is closed using an absorbable subcuticular suture.

The traditional Girdlestone procedure [Taylor 1951] is now less frequently performed. It seems to have no advantage over the less invasive flexor tenotomy, but although it was originally described for severe claw toe in children with poliomyelitis, it may still have a place in the older patient with severe mobile clawing of the toe.

There is no need to transfer both flexor tendons in mild or moderate curly toe deformity.

In more severe cases, the procedure is performed by the same incision as for flexor tenotomy. The long flexor tendon is divided as distally as possible and then transferred around the lateral aspect of the proximal phalanx of the toe. It is then passed through a midline split in the extensor tendon at this level and sutured into place under moderate tension.

Closure and postoperative management are identical to those of flexor tenotomy. A Lambrinudi splint, as originally recommended for the Girdlestone procedure, should not be used, as it is dangerous to the circulation of the toe.

Postoperative care

The patient is able to heel weightbear and is discharged the same day. Correction may not be immediate and the child's parents need to be reassured that in time the pull of the transferred tendon will correct residual deformity.

Complications

Care must be taken to avoid damage to the neurovascular bundle. Despite this, some patients may experience transient vascular spasm following surgery. Failure to correct the deformity and recurrence of the deformity may require subsequent bony correction.

References

Cockin J (1968) Butler's operation for an over-riding 5th toe. J Bone Joint Surg 50B: 78–81

Coughlin MJ (1993) Second metatarsophalangeal joint instability in the athlete. Foot Ankle 14: 309–319

Duchenne GBA (1883) Selection of Clinical Works of Duchenne (translated by GV Poore). London, New Sydenham Society

Hamer AJ, Stanley D, Smith TWD (1993) Surgery for curly toe deformity: a double blind, randomised, prospective trial. J Bone Joint Surg 75B: 662–663

Hassan FO, Shannak A, Stephens M (2002) V–Y arthroplasty for congenital overriding fifth toe. Foot Ankle Surg 8: 49–52

Kuwada G (1988) A retrospective analysis of modification of the flexor tendon transfer for correction of hammer toe. J Foot Surg 27: 57–59

Lapidus PW (1942) Transplantation of the extensor tendon for correction of the overlapping of the fifth toe. J Bone Joint Surg 24: 555–559

Mann R, Inman VT (1964) Phasic activity of the intrinsic muscles of the foot. J Bone Joint Surg 46A: 469

Ross ERS, Menelaus MB (1984) Open flexor tenotomy for hammer toes and curly toes in childhood. J Bone Joint Surg 66B: 770–771

Taylor RG (1951) The treatment of claw toes by multiple transfers of flexor into extensor tendon. J Bone Joint Surg 33B: 539

Wilson JN (1953) V–Y correction for varus deformity of the fifth toe. Br J Surg 41: 133–135

15

Rheumatoid arthritis: excisional arthroplasty of the metatarsophalangeal joints

Andrea Cracchiolo III

Introduction

Rheumatoid arthritis is a systemic disease which frequently involves the foot. Since there are many synovia-lined joints within the foot, active rheumatoid disease can produce widespread foot pain.

The classic findings of rheumatoid arthritis in the forefoot include hallux valgus with intra-articular degeneration of the metatarsophalangeal joints [Cracchiolo et al. 1996]. The toes usually drift laterally with dorsal subluxation or dislocation. As this occurs, the metatarsal heads are directed more plantarwards, the toes develop a claw toe deformity, and the weightbearing plantar fat pad is drawn further forward, losing its normal location underneath the metatarsal heads. Large bursae with overlying calluses are frequent under the middle metatarsal heads and, at times, under the hallux. Web space pathology, usually an intermetatarsal bursa, gives neuroma-like symptoms as early evidence of forefoot involvement, and may be an early sign of rheumatoid arthritis.

Pathology of the hindfoot frequently affects the forefoot, is more subtle and can progress rapidly. Synovitis of the hindfoot joints and subsequent loss of articular cartilage and erosion of the talonavicular

and subtalar joints lead to a persistent valgus deformity of the hindfoot. The talonavicular joint becomes unstable, with the head of the talus drifting medially and plantarwards. The remainder of the midfoot and forefoot drifts into abduction. The calcaneus may also abut against the distal fibula producing pain at the lateral malleolus. The posterior tibial tendon may rupture [Michelson et al. 1995], or if intact may not function effectively as the medial stabilizer of the hindfoot owing to the altered hindfoot mechanics. A standard set of radiographs should be obtained when evaluating any rheumatoid patient with significant involvement of the foot. These should include a weightbearing anteroposterior (A-P) and lateral view of the foot. Also, a weightbearing A-P view of the ankle is important, especially if there is any ankle or hindfoot pathology.

The most important aspect of non-operative care is proper footwear. Usually a shoe must be selected or modified to fit the patient's deformity. Shoes do not correct deformities, rather they accommodate the deformities and thus reduce pain. Since the forefoot is the most common area of symptoms and pathology, a shoe with a wide, deep toe box is important in patients with rheumatoid arthritis. The most common shoe modification is a metatarsal pad, which should be placed with the apex of the pad just proximal to the area of maximum tenderness or callus formation, usually the second and third metatarsal heads.

Treatment

Effect of medication on the surgical procedures

One of the most important preoperative considerations should be the type of medication that the patients are taking for their arthritis. Patients taking doses of prednisone over 10 mg are at higher risk for failure of primary wound healing and for developing subsequent sepsis. Methotrexate also delays wound healing and if possible should be discontinued about 1 week before the surgery and for about 2 weeks postoperatively.

Surgical procedures to correct rheumatoid deformities of the forefoot

Over the years, many operative procedures have been described to correct rheumatoid forefoot deformities. Fowler [1959] used a dorsal approach to resect the joints and a plantar incision to reposition the fat pad. Lipscomb et al. [1972] described a plantar condylectomy and excision of the proximal third of the proximal phalanx through a dorsal incision.

Clayton [1982] popularized excision of both the metatarsal head and the base of the proximal phalanx. The sesamoids were excised only if they were fused to the bottom of the first metatarsal head or if they were grossly deformed. Clayton's observations after extensive clinical experience indicated that, if one or two joints were relatively spared by the disease, they should also be excised so that in general all metatarsophalangeal joints should be included in the forefoot operation. He also emphasized that the postoperative results of these procedures on the rheumatoid forefoot, if the patient was followed long enough, would gradually deteriorate. Rheumatoid disease is frequently progressive in most patients and if deformities increase in the remaining joints of the foot, particularly the hindfoot joints, then forefoot deformities may recur. Coughlin [2000], however, has followed his rheumatoid patients for an average of 74 months and reports a continued high success rate following arthrodesis of the hallux metatarsophalangeal joint and excisional arthroplasty of the lateral four joints. One should avoid the indiscriminate resection of bone as the only method of correcting the forefoot deformity. It is as important to re-align the soft-tissue structures as it is to resect the bone. More recently, Clayton [1992] described resection of the metatarsophalangeal joints with interposition of the plantar plate.

The operation advocated by Stainsby [1992] resected the proximal two-thirds of the proximal phalanx and sutured the extensor tendon to the flexor tendon. Most series report satisfactory results in up to 85% of patients, and failures in less than 10% [McGarvey and Johnson 1988]. Factors associated with unfavorable results [Barton 1973] include:

- Inadequate bony resection
- Recurrent hallux valgus
- Wound problems
- Disease progression
- Neurovascular problems.

Surgical technique

Usually it is best to perform forefoot surgery in rheumatoid patients under thigh-high tourniquet control. There are often gross deformities of the toes and a tourniquet applied above the ankle tends to bind the tendons, interfering with the soft-tissue correction of deformities. Contraindications for use of a tourniquet are evidence of vasculitis or peripheral vascular disease.

Exposure is facilitated by operating on the four lateral metatarsophalangeal joints before operating on the hallux. It is frequently difficult to gain full correction of the hallux metatarsophalangeal joint first, when there is severe deformity of the other four joints. Dorsal longitudinal incisions provide an excellent exposure to the metatarsophalangeal joints and usually heal well [Cracchiolo et al. 1996]. Three incisions are usually required (Figure 1). The first two incisions are made in the second web space and in the fourth web space to expose the lateral four metatarsophalangeal joints. If possible, the hallux incision and correction of the hallux follow the correction of the lateral four joints. In severe hallux valgus deformity, the incision over the hallux metatarsophalangeal joint will be necessary to free the hallux and allow it to be brought away from the lateral toes so that their operative procedures can be accomplished. A dorsal medial incision is made to expose the hallux metatarsophalangeal joint (Figure 1). A plantar approach to the metatarsophalangeal joints also gives a good exposure and is the

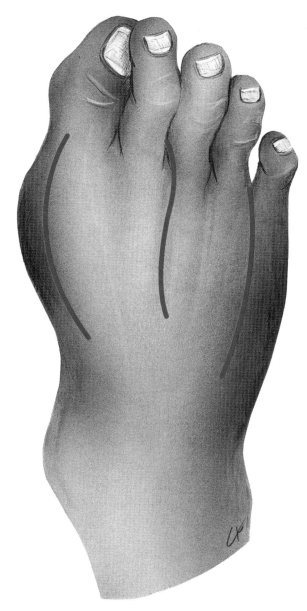

Figure 1

Three dorsal longitudinal incisions are used for the exposure of the deformed metatarsophalangeal joints in a patient with rheumatoid arthritis

easiest approach to the dislocated metatarsal heads [Kates et al. 1967] (see Figure 5). The incision is transverse and is placed at the level of the metatarsal necks, to the heel side of the dislocated metatarsophalangeal heads.

Surgical correction of the lateral four metatarsophalangeal joints

The metatarsal head is most frequently resected because it is usually grossly destroyed and pushed plantarwards by the dorsally dislocated toes. A decision must be made whether to resect the base

of the proximal phalanx. This is seldom necessary, and excision of the proximal third usually results in loss of control of the toe. If not surgically syndactylized, the toe may become floppy. Where it is necessary to excise a significant amount of the proximal phalanx, syndactylization of the adjacent toes should therefore be performed [McGarvey and Johnson 1988, Daly and Johnson 1992]. It is a most useful procedure to correct severely deformed toes or when revision forefoot operations are performed. There are two basic surgical techniques for correcting the rheumatoid deformities in the lateral four metatarsophalangeal joints.

Plantar plate arthroplasty

Plantar plate arthroplasty [Clayton 1992] appears to be a distinct improvement in the technique of excisional arthroplasty. The lateral four metatarsophalangeal joints are approached in sequence [Cracchiolo 1988]. It is best to perform both dorsal incisions and to release the extensor tendons, ligaments and capsules of all four joints before attempting to expose the metatarsal heads. It is important to excise the metatarsal head in an oblique direction (Figure 2), removing more bone from the plantar aspect of the distal metatarsal, as some plantar bone may regrow, causing a painful callus. Sufficient bone should be excised and soft tissues released to allow a 1.5-cm space between the resected end of the metatarsal and the proximal phalanx. After resection of the metatarsal heads the metatarsal lengths should be in a smooth arc, with the third metatarsal being 2–3 mm shorter than the second, and the fourth and fifth being progressively shorter (Figure 3). The plantar plate (Figure 4) is carefully dissected from the base of the proximal phalanx, using a scalpel with a no. 11 blade. Care is taken not to cut the flexor tendon. If necessary, the articular surface can also be removed, or what remains of the surface of the base of the proximal phalanx. Excision of a third to half of the proximal phalanx will require other soft-tissue procedures to stabilize the toe. Resection of the base of the proximal phalanx frees the plantar plate, and it can be placed over the resected end of the metatarsal and transfixed with a 1.8-mm Kirschner wire passed in a retrograde direction through the toe to exit the pulp just underneath the toenail, and then across the plate and into the metatarsal shaft (Figure 4). Alternatively, the plantar plate can be sutured to any portion of the extensor tendon or the capsule that remains. The plantar plate simply holds the flexor tendon aligned under the ray. If a flexor tendon

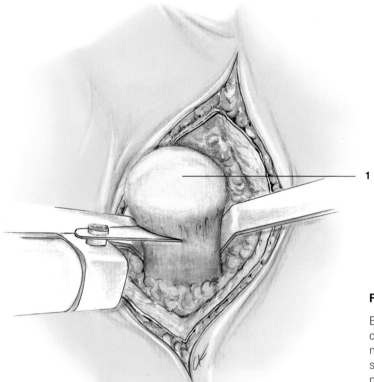

Figure 2

Excision of the metatarsal head through a dorsal approach. Any bursal tissue and the metatarsal head are carefully exposed. Care should be taken to avoid injury to the plantar fat pad, the digital nerves and the flexor tendons

1 Metatarsal head

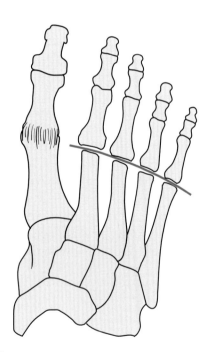

Figure 3

Following excision of the lateral metatarsal heads the relative lengths of the metatarsals should form a smooth arc

remains dislocated, then there is a much greater chance of recurrent deformity in the direction of the dislocated tendon postoperatively. Prior to drilling the Kirschner wire, any toe deformities

at the interphalangeal joints must be corrected. Usually these are hammer toe deformities involving the proximal interphalangeal joint, and they can usually be manipulated to straighten the toe. Occasionally, in a severe fixed deformity, e.g. a claw toe, it is necessary to excise the head of the proximal phalanx, and this is done through a short dorsal incision, either transverse or longitudinal. Securing the plantar plate is important as it helps centralize the flexor tendon under the involved ray. One can also determine that the tendon is intact, which is usually the case. It is best not to advance the Kirschner wire across the base of the metatarsal, as this then 'skewers' the toe, leaving it immobile and perhaps jeopardizing its vascular supply. The Kirschner wire should be passed 2–3 cm into the intramedullary canal of the metatarsal, so that it stabilizes the alignment of the ray. All deformities must be completely corrected before placement of the Kirschner wire. The wire simply holds the correction, as soft postoperative dressings are inadequate to control all five operated toes. The Kirschner wire must *not* produce any of the correction, as the deformity will recur after the wire is removed. Some patients have a 'stiff' type of rheumatoid disease, and the wires can be removed at about 2–3 weeks. Patients with a 'loose' type should have the wires in place for about 4–5 weeks. Operative correction

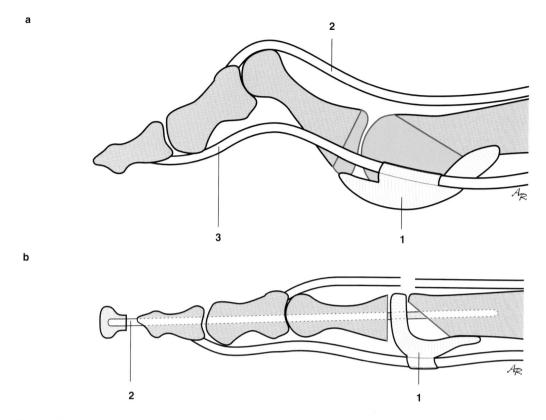

Figure 4

Plantar plate arthroplasty. The deformed metatarsal head is resected in an oblique direction, removing more bone from the plantar side than the dorsal side. If a plantar plate is present then either it can be skewered onto the Kirschner wire, or it can be sutured to any portion of the extensor tendon or capsule that remains. a. preoperatively; b. following arthroplasty

a
1   Plantar plate
2   Long extensor tendon
3   Long flexor tendon

b
1   Plantar plate
2   Kirschner wire

of the hallux metatarsophalangeal joint is then performed (see below). A sterile compression dressing is placed and then the thigh-high tourniquet is deflated. The combination of good wound closure and the dressing ensures minimal wound hematoma.

Stainsby developed an alternative method for correcting claw toe deformities in rheumatoid arthritis. The procedure is based on the concept that flexion of the toes at the metatarsophalangeal joint is provided by the action of the plantar aponeurosis. Clawing of the toes with extension indicates a failure of this mechanism. His procedure emphasizes freeing of the plantar plate without dividing its attachments to the deep transverse metatarsal ligament and plantar anpeneurosis, repositioning it underneath the metatarsal head. This removes the downward force on the metatarsal head exerted by tension

in the plantar aponeurosis and deep transverse metatarsal ligaments through the displaced plantar plate. The plantar plate and forefoot fat pad are restored to their normal functional position and can be maintained there only if the metatarsal length is preserved. Thus, Stainsby resects most of the proximal phalanx and retains the metatarsal heads even if they are severely eroded, removing only spicules of bone from their plantar surface; likewise, the metatarsals are not shortened (Figure 5). A Keller-type excisional arthroplasty is performed to the hallux along with lengthening of the extensor hallucis longus, release of the extensor hallucis brevis, and reefing of the medial capsule to reposition the sesamoids under the metatarsal head. Briggs and Stainsby [2001] reported a good or excellent result in 38/41 feet (93%) at a mean follow-up of 5 years.

a

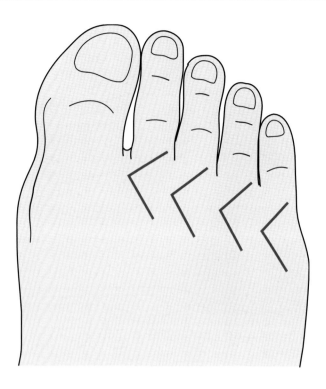

b

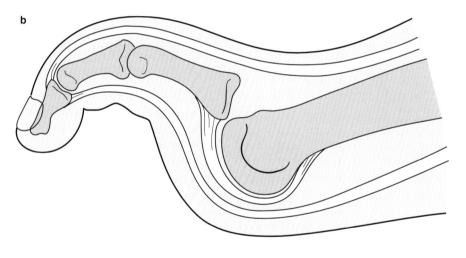

c

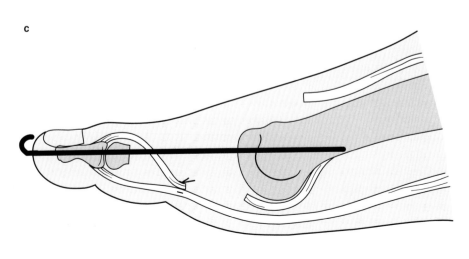

Figure 5

a. Dorsal angled skin incisions are used to expose the lateral metatarsophalangeal joints; b. the proximal phalanx is usually dislocated dorsally on the metatarsal head; c. the extensor is divided proximally and reflected distally, exposing the proximal phalanx. The proximal phalanx is divided at the neck and excised; the plantar plate is freed under the metatarsal head and the toe brought plantarward, freeing the fat pad. The toe is stabilized with a K-wire into the metatarsal head and the extensor tendon sutured into the flexor to avoid reconnection of the extensor mechanism

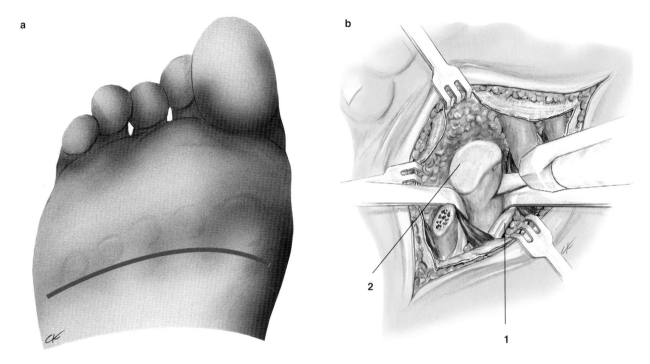

Figure 6

a. Skin incision for the plantar approach at the level of the necks of the dislocated metatarsal heads; b. Following plantar exposure, the metatarsal head is resected with an oscillating saw

1   Long flexor tendon
2   Metatarsal head

Excisional arthroplasty through a plantar approach

A plantar approach (Figure 6) to the dislocated metatarsophalangeal joints has been described with only the metatarsal heads being resected [Kates et al. 1967]. Excision of some of the redundant skin, as much as 2 cm from the proximal side of the incision, helps to keep the fat pad properly re-positioned. This incision should be used when the dorsal skin is poor, or when the patient has had previous operations with inappropriately placed dorsal scars. A combination of both dorsal and plantar approaches to the rheumatoid forefoot has also been used [Fowler 1959]. In this technique most of the bony surgery is performed through a dorsal incision and then the plantar incision is used to excise an ellipse of skin and to draw the toes into more plantar flexion.

Tillmann [Tillmann 1979, Cracchiolo et al. 1996] has modified the plantar approach to resect the lateral metatarsal heads (Figure 6a). A plantar transverse skin excision across the distal forefoot is used, excising all callosities and removing an ellipse of skin. The metatarsal head is exposed by dividing the flexor tendon sheath and what remains of the plantar plate longitudinally. Care should be taken to avoid cutting the flexor tendon. The metatarsal head is excised at the metatarsal neck (Figure 6b). This is done with a narrow oscillating saw and the soft tissues are protected using two narrow Hohmann retractors. The metatarsal resection surfaces are rounded and smoothed. A tenolysis is performed and a reconstruction of the flexor tendon is attempted, if the tendon is found to be ruptured. Whatever remains of the plantar plate is sutured on the tibial side of the second, third and fourth metatarsophalangeal joints. This suture is placed to maintain a neutral alignment of the toe. For the fifth toe a purse-string suture is placed around the fibular structures of the capsule and what remains of the plate to hold the toe in a corrected position. The toes should be held distracted about 6–8 mm from the resected metatarsal. Use of Kirschner wires is seldom necessary. When sutured closed, the elliptical skin incision produces a dermodesis.

Surgical treatment of the hallux metatarsophalangeal joint

Rarely, the hallux metatarsophalangeal joint may be spared. However, if there is significant synovitis,

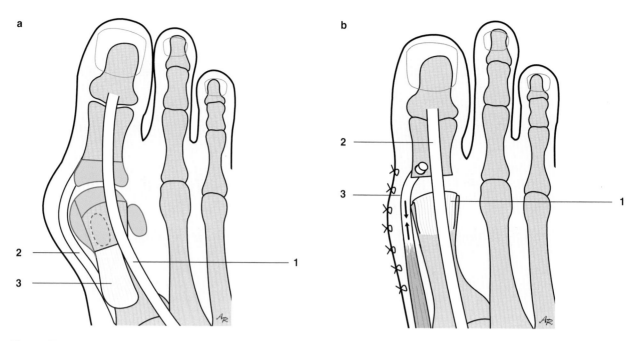

Figure 7

At the great toe, the metatarsal head and the base of the proximal phalanx should be excised. The reshaped and short-ened metatarsal head is covered by a proximal-based capsular flap. The abductor tendon is repositioned to the medial side of the joint and may be shortened by weaving a suture through its substance (arrows). The excised joint space should be distracted about 8 mm. a. prior to resection; b. following resection

a

1 Long extensor tendon
2 Abductor tendon
3 Capsular flap

b

1 Capsular flap
2 Long extensor tendon
3 Abductor tendon

an arthrotomy should be performed through a longitudinal incision, and a synovectomy carried out. If there is significant hallux valgus deformity with a good joint space, this must be corrected to accommodate the more normal realignment of the lateral four toes. Such joints, however, may deterio-rate, although it may be many years before they require operative treatment [Graham 1994]. However, in most cases there is significant destruc-tion of this joint with a severe valgus deformity. Two operations are used by the author for treating the hallux metatarsophalangeal joint: an arthrode-sis [Mann and Thompson 1984] (see Chapter 8) or a double-stem silicone implant arthroplasty [Cracchiolo et al. 1992, Moeckel et al. 1992, Sebold and Cracchiolo 1996]. Either is performed after cor-rection of the lateral four metatarsophalangeal joints. Excisional arthroplasty has been used as an alternative.

Excisional arthroplasty of the hallux metatarsophalangeal joint

A modification of the first metatarsal head resection of Hueter and Mayo has been developed by Tillmann, who advocates its use in most patients with rheumatoid arthritis [Tillmann 1979, Cracchiolo et al. 1996] (Figure 7). The hallux metatarsopha-langeal joint is exposed through a dorsomedial incision. A proximally based flap of the medial and dorsal portions of the joint capsule and extensor hood is fashioned, which also exposes the metatarsal head. A portion of the head is excised, much as recommended in the Hueter–Mayo arthroplasty (Figure 7). Excessive bone should not be removed: merely enough to correct the hallux deformity. The tibial sesamoid is usually excised, if it is destroyed, and the fibular sesamoid can also be excised if necessary. The gap in the short flexor tendon is

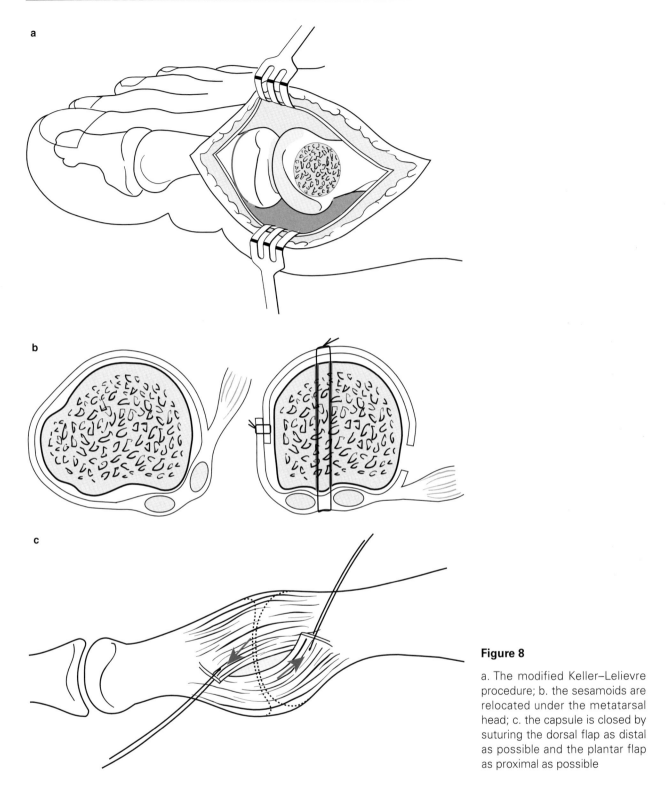

Figure 8

a. The modified Keller–Lelievre procedure; b. the sesamoids are relocated under the metatarsal head; c. the capsule is closed by suturing the dorsal flap as distal as possible and the plantar flap as proximal as possible

closed with sutures to prevent hyperextension of the hallux and subsequent interphalangeal joint flexion deformity. The adductor tendon and fibular collateral ligament are also released. Crucial to the arthroplasty is the fashioning of the proximal-based flap, which is then sutured over the resected metatarsal head. The abductor tendon is reinforced and shortened using a non-absorbable suture woven through the tendon from distal to proximal (Figure 7). This will add to the soft-tissue re-alignment of the hallux. The excised joint space should be distracted about 8 mm and adjusted to that width by the soft-tissue closure. This position is held using a soft-tissue dressing; no internal fixation is used. In severe deformities, i.e. in more than 60° of valgus, it may be necessary to resect the base of the proximal phalanx to avoid excessive shortening of the first metatarsal. Alternatively, such patients may be better candidates for an arthrodesis. Dereymaeker et al. (1997) prefer using the Keller–Leliévre procedure to correct the rheumatoid hallux deformity in patients over age 55. The hallux metatarsophalangeal joint is approached through a longitudinal dorsomedial incision. The capsule is similarly divided, and the medial eminence is excised. The base of the proximal phalanx is excised and the capsular attachment to the lateral sesamoid is released. The sesamoids are mobilized and centered under the metatarsal heads. The drill holes from dorsal to plantar are then made in the head and a suture is passed to secure the position of the sesamoids and is tied dorsally over the head. The medial capsule is closed by suturing the dorsal flap as distal and plantar as possible, and the plantar flap is sutured as proximal and dorsal as possible (Figure 8). In younger patients the authors prefer to perform an arthrodesis. The lateral metatarsals are corrected by an excisional arthroplasty.

Recently there has been renewed interest in using a shortening osteotomy to correct metatarsalgia. This can be considered if the joint is only mildly involved and the metatarsal head not severely destroyed. However, long-term results have not been reported and other osteotomies attempted in the past have been largely discarded.

Complications

Patients with rheumatoid arthritis have a systemic disease which varies in severity with time. They also must take a wide variety of medications on a daily basis. Therefore, these patients probably experience more complications than other patients. Interestingly the most common cited complication in patients with rheumatoid arthritis following forefoot operations was the development of arthrosis in the interphalangeal joint of the hallux [Nassar and Cracchiolo, 2001]. Plantar callosities were the next most frequent postoperative complaint, followed by hammer-toe deformities, delayed wound healing, wound infection and pin tract infection. A reoperation rate of between 11 and 30% is also reported.

References

Barton NJ (1973) Arthroplasty of the forefoot in rheumatoid arthritis. J Bone Joint Surg 52B: 126

Briggs PJ, Stainsby GD (2001) Metatarsal head preservation in forefoot arthroplasty and the correction of severe claw toe deformity. Foot Ankle Surg 7: 93–101

Clayton ML (1982) Evolution of surgery of the forefoot in rheumatoid arthritis. J Bone Joint Surg 64B: 640

Clayton ML (1992) Management of the rheumatoid foot. In: Clayton ML, Smyth CJ (eds) Surgery for Rheumatoid Arthritis. New York, Churchill Livingstone, pp 307–344

Coughlin MJ (2000) Rheumatoid forefoot reconstruction. J Bone Joint Surg 82A: 322–341

Cracchiolo A (1988) Rheumatoid arthritis of the foot and ankle. In: Gould J (ed) The Foot Book. Baltimore, Williams & Wilkins, pp 239–267

Cracchiolo A, DeStoop N, Tillmann K (1996) The rheumatoid foot and ankle. In: Helal B, Rowley DI, Cracchiolo A, Myerson M (eds) Surgery of Disorders of the Foot and Ankle. London, Martin Dunitz, pp 443–476

Cracchiolo A, Weltmer JB, Lian G et al. (1992) Arthroplasty of the first metatarsophalangeal joint with a double stem silicone implant: results in patients who have degenerative joint disease, failures of previous operation in rheumatoid arthritis. J Bone Joint Surg 74A: 552–563

Daly PJ, Johnson KA (1992) Treatment of painful subluxation or dislocation at the second and third metatarsophalangeal joints by partial proximal phalanx excision and subtotal webbing. Clin Orthop 278: 164–170

Dereymaeker G, Mulier T, Stuer P et al. (1997) Pedodynographic measurements after forefoot reconstruction in rheumatoid arthritis patients. Foot Ankle 18 (5): 270–276

Fowler AW (1959) The method of forefoot reconstruction. J Bone Joint Surg 41B: 507

Graham CE (1994) Rheumatoid forefoot metatarsal head resection without first metatarsophalangeal arthrodesis. Foot Ankle Int 15 (12): 689–690

Kates A, Kessel L, Kay A (1967) Arthroplasty of the forefoot. J Bone Joint Surg 49B: 552

Lipscomb PR, Benson GM, Sones DA (1972) Resection of proximal phalanges and metatarsal condyles for deformities of the forefoot due to rheumatoid arthritis. Clin Orthop 82: 24–31

Mann RA, Thompson FM (1984) Arthrodesis of the first metatarsophalangeal joint for hallux valgus in rheumatoid arthritis. J Bone Joint Surg 66A: 687

McGarvey WC, Johnson KA (1988) Keller arthroplasty in combination with resection arthroplasty of the lesser metatarsophalangeal joints in rheumatoid arthritis. Foot Ankle 9 (2): 75–80

Michelson J, Easley M, Wigley FM, Hellmann D (1995) Posterior tibial tendon dysfunction in rheumatoid arthritis. Foot Ankle 16 (3): 156–161

Moeckel BJ, Sculco TP, Alexiades MM et al. (1992) The double-stem silicone-rubber implant for rheumatoid arthritis of the first metatarsophalangeal joint: long term results. J Bone Joint Surg 74A: 564–570

Nassar J, Cracchiolo A (2001) Complications in surgery of the foot and ankle in patients with rheumatoid arthritis. Clin Orthop 391: 140–152

Sebold EJ, Cracchiolo A (1996) Use of titanium grommets in silicone implant arthroplasty of the hallux metatarsophalangeal joint. Foot Ankle 17 (3): 145–151

Stainsby GD (1992) A modified Keller's procedure for the lateral four toes. Annual Meeting of the British Orthopaedic Foot Surgery Society, Stanmore, 20 November

Tillmann K (1979) The Rheumatoid Foot. Stuttgart, Thieme

16

Metatarsalgia: metatarsal osteotomies

Andrea Cracchiolo III
Bernard Valtin

Introduction

Metatarsalgia, or generalized pain under the forefoot in the area of the metatarsal heads, is one of the most common symptoms of the adult forefoot. Although patients can present with this symptom alone, they frequently have associated disorders such as a splay foot, hallux valgus or bunionette deformities, or failed previous operations either to the hallux or to one of the other metatarsals. Other pathologies which may lead to metatarsalgia, either localized or generalized, are: hammer toes, sesamoid pathology, interdigital nerve compression, osteochondritis of the metatarsal head and a cavus foot. Metatarsophalangeal joint, synovitis, subluxation, dislocation and crossover toe deformities can also be involved. Lastly, in the author's experience, patients with osteoporosis can present with metatarsalgia. Such patients have no detectable mechanical pathology; they have a thin plantar fat pad, and may have evidence of a metatarsal stress fracture. These patients may have an abnormal bone density scan. At times it is difficult to appreciate the etiology of the pain. Frequently patients will have a callus which is centered under either the second or the third metatarsal head. When painful, this is commonly called an 'intractable plantar keratosis'. Rarely does it extend across the entire forefoot. There are a number of predisposing causes which may produce increased plantar pressure and the resulting intractable plantar keratosis. Imbalance of the intrinsic muscles of the foot may be a factor. This imbalance may be due in part to wearing unsuitable shoes, particularly the continuous use of high-heeled shoes with a pointed toe box. As a result there may be dorsal subluxation of the proximal phalanx and increased plantar pressure under a metatarsal head. Other etiologies may be mechanical or anatomical abnormalities; these usually follow trauma to the forefoot or a failed prior operation.

Metatarsalgia is a symptom, not a diagnosis. The term 'pressure metatarsalgia' has been used specifically to define pain under the metatarsophalangeal joints or the metatarsal heads during weightbearing [Helal 1975]. Additionally, there is displacement of the anterior fat pad forward with the subluxating or dislocated toes, so that it no longer functions in its normal anatomical position. Mobility of the metatarsal heads depends upon the status of the tarsometatarsal joints and the adherence of the soft tissue around the metatarsal heads. If the metatarsal heads are mobile, and this mobility is within normal limits, then the hindfoot should be examined for a fixed pronation or even a supination deformity which can lead to abnormally high pressures under the forefoot.

Many different types of operation have been performed to treat patients with metatarsalgia, including claw toe corrections, flexor-to-extensor transfers and plantar fascia release, even with Dwyer's osteotomy of the calcaneus. Therefore, the treatment for metatarsalgia can include correction of all forefoot deformities. This chapter will specifically cover the use of metatarsal osteotomies in the treatment of metatarsalgia.

Clinical and radiographic appearance

Tenderness is usually present directly underneath the involved metatarsal head, but not in the intermetatarsal space. There may be marked atrophy of the plantar fat pad in the involved area. Callus is usually present underneath the involved metatarsal heads, but may not always be seen, especially if the patient has reduced the amount of walking.

It is difficult to examine the foot while the patient is weightbearing, but standing or walking is what usually produces the symptoms. However, the forefoot can be examined to determine the status of the metatarsophalangeal joints, whether they are unstable, swollen, subluxated or (in some cases) dislocated. The relative length of the metatarsals can be assessed, particularly the second and third metatarsals compared with the first, as well as the flexibility of the tarsometatarsal articulations. In patients who do not have arthritis and who have pressure metatarsalgia the second metatarsal is usually the longest, even longer than the first. This is also the case when the first metatarsal has been shortened or the first metatarsal head has been elevated by a fracture or a failed operation for a bunion deformity. The presence of other abnormalities such as hallux valgus or a toe deformity should be noted. If there is an associated hallux valgus deformity with displacement of the sesamoids, then even greater pressures are placed under the second and sometimes the third metatarsal heads.

Many of the above features can be better evaluated using weightbearing radiographs, particularly the length of the metatarsals, the status of the metatarsophalangeal joints and the presence of other pathological conditions or previous operative procedures on the forefoot. A shortened first metatarsal or dorsal displacement of the metatarsal head from a previous operation on the first ray will explain the presence of pain or a callus under the head of a longer second and possibly third metatarsal. This is the classic transfer lesion. When excessive pressure has been transferred to the second metatarsal, its medial cortex will be thickened and the cortices of the first metatarsal are thinned.

Indications for surgery

The forefoot must be carefully evaluated to determine the pathology that is causing the metatarsalgia. Occasionally, this may be a single abnormality, such as synovitis of a metatarsophalangeal joint. More frequently, there are multiple causes: hallux valgus, long second metatarsal, subluxation usually of the second metatarsophalangeal joint, and hammer-toe deformity. An operation on the metatarsals, whether it be at the base, along the diaphysis or at the neck distally, is determined mostly by clinical judgment

and experience. A pedobarograph can measure pressures beneath the forefoot. However, it has not been effective in selecting patients who might benefit from an operation to decrease the pressure under the metatarsal head to eliminate symptoms of metatarsalgia [Dreeben et al. 1989]. Operations on the metatarsals are designed either to shorten the metatarsal and elevate the metatarsal head, or only to elevate the metatarsal head in the hope of relieving the pressure causing the pain.

Since evaluation methods are imprecise at best, patients with an intractable plantar keratosis should be considered for treatment with non-operative measures to see whether pain can be improved or alleviated. When such measures have failed, or it appears that they are only a futile attempt at treatment, then an operation can be considered. Some patients seem to have plantar skin that is prone to callus formation. Thus, if there are numerous areas of callus, especially involving the heel or the toes, in the absence of an obvious mechanical abnormality, an operation may be contraindicated. Such patients should be referred for dermatological consultation.

Surgical correction of metatarsalgia must address the correction of all of the deformities thought to be producing the forefoot pain. This may involve a number of procedures, which are covered in Chapters 1–5, 11–14 and 16–18. Osteotomies of the metatarsals (usually second, third and occasionally fourth) have been described by many different authors in the past 25 years. They can be divided into those performed proximally at the base of the metatarsal, within the diaphysis of the metatarsal, and at the metatarsal neck. Historically, there has initially been great optimism after the description of a new osteotomy. However, the favorable results frequently initially reported have worsened over time and at times cannot be reproduced by others. Two philosophies have developed regarding fixation of these osteotomies. Initially, internal fixation was not recommended. It was thought that the osteotomy should allow the metatarsal head to find its optimal final location by having the patient bear weight, and hopefully the osteotomy would heal solidly. In defense of that philosophy was the fact that power equipment and internal fixation had not developed sufficiently to allow the type of surgical techniques available in recent years. The second philosophy, prevalent in all recently described osteotomies, is precision osteotomy with solid internal fixation.

Some authors emphasize that an osteotomy to elevate a depressed metatarsal head must be considered only when there is an absence of any toe deformity [Thomas 1974]. Such feet are uncommon.

Proximal metatarsal osteotomies

A narrow 2-mm dorsal closing wedge osteotomy at the base of the involved metatarsal may be used [Thomas 1974, Mann 1986], which allows the metatarsal head to drift slightly dorsally. Osteotomy of only one metatarsal at a time has been recommended [Mann 1986]. However, the second and third metatarsals are frequently both longer than the first metatarsal, and an osteotomy of the second and third may be considered.

A dorsal wedge V-osteotomy at the base of the metatarsal has also been recommended to correct a plantar callus brought about by a prominent metatarsal head that does not lie at the same level as the other metatarsal heads [Sclamberg and Lorenz 1983]. This is not designed to shorten the metatarsal, and patients who have a plantar callus under an overly long metatarsal head are not candidates for this operation. The osteotomy is said to be relatively stable. L.S. Barouk, P. Ripstein and E. Troullec [personal communication 2001] have recently described an oblique proximal osteotomy, which they use only to elevate the metatarsal head in patients with localized metatarsalgia and no other pathology of the involved ray.

A diaphyseal osteotomy is advocated by Hansen [2000] when one wishes to shorten a metatarsal. This procedure removes a segment of the diaphysis and requires fixation with a plate.

Distal metatarsal osteotomies

These have been the most popular over time. A number have been described and until recently none were fixed internally [Helal 1975]. Helal suggested that an osteotomy is indicated in the presence of a painful callosity which is under the metatarsal head and when the metatarsal does not move dorsally when pressure is applied to its plantar surface. The operation shortens the metatarsal, producing significant soft-tissue laxity, which aids in re-aligning the toe deformity. Results have been variable, and good or excellent results have been reported in a wide range (47–85%) of patients [Helal and Greiss 1984, Pedowitz 1988, Winson et al. 1988, Trnka et al. 1996]. Fifteen per cent of patients were found to have radiographic evidence of non-union. The following factors were associated with patients having a poor result: age greater than 65 years; first and fifth metatarsal osteotomies; postoperative plaster immobilization; and poor toe function at the time of review [Winson et al. 1988].

Dorsal closing wedge osteotomy at the neck of the metatarsal has also been used [Wolf 1973, Leventen and Pearson 1990]. The protocol to determine which metatarsal to osteotomize was based on the location of the intractable plantar keratosis [Leventen and Pearson 1990]. Thus, a patient with an intractable plantar keratosis under the second metatarsal head required an osteotomy on both the second and third metatarsals, to lessen the chance of a transfer lesion. An intractable plantar keratosis under the fourth metatarsal head was treated by osteotomy of the third and fourth metatarsals. If the symptomatic intractable plantar keratosis was under the third metatarsal head, an osteotomy of all three middle metatarsals was performed. Recently, Weil has described a distal metatarsal osteotomy, which at the time of this chapter's preparation is currently the most popular of the distal osteotomies.

Treatment

Surgical technique

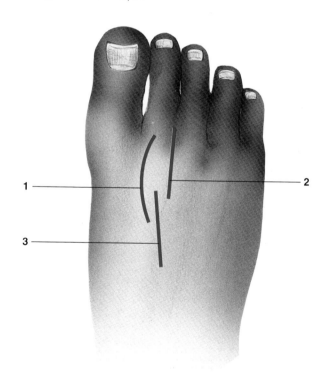

Figure 1

A curved dorsal incision is used to approach the metatarsophalangeal joint (1). A longitudinal incision in the web space is a good alternative, particularly if exposure of the adjacent metatarsal bone is required (2). Thus, to expose metatarsals II and III, a longitudinal incision would be made in the second web space. The length of the incision can vary, depending on the portion of the metatarsal that requires exposure. For an osteotomy at the base of the metatarsal, a longitudinal incision approximately 4 cm long is made (3)

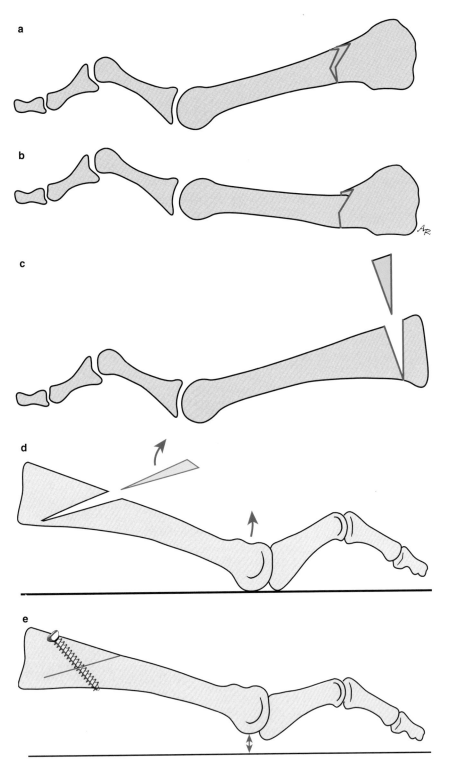

Figure 2

A V-type osteotomy at the base of the metatarsal. a. removal of a bone wedge; b. following closure. c. osteotomy at the base of the metatarsal [Thomas 1974, Mann 1986]; d. osteotomy of Barouk, Ripstein and Troullec. A thin dorsal wedge is removed and the plantar cortex should be preserved; e. fixation with a single 2.7 mm cannulated screw

Osteotomy at the base of the metatarsal

Osteotomy at the base of the metatarsal was described by Sclamberg and Lorenz [1983]. A longitudinal incision approximately 4 cm long is made over the base of the involved metatarsal (Figure 1). If two metatarsals are to be sectioned then the

incision is made in the intermetatarsal space. The extensor tendons are retracted and the periosteum is elevated about the proximal metatarsal base. A marking pen is used to outline an inverted V with the apex pointing towards the metatarsal base (Figures 2a–b). The angle of the V should be approximately 60° with the metatarsal shaft. An oscillating saw with a thin blade is used for the osteotomy. The saw cut does not extend through the plantar cortex. A second inverted V-osteotomy is made approximately 3–4 mm distal to the first one (Figure 2c). The two osteotomies should converge at the same point on the inferior cortex, allowing removal of a dorsal V-shape wedge of bone. It is important to remember that the metatarsal head can be displaced dorsally a significant distance by removing only a small wedge of bone from the base of the metatarsal. Therefore, it is critical not to remove too much bone using any type of osteotomy at the base. Pressure is exerted plantarwards over the dorsal aspect of the metatarsal head until the inferior cortex fractures. The distal metatarsal is then pushed upwards and manipulated until the osteotomy becomes mobile, hinging on the plantar periosteum. Distal upward pressure should easily close the osteotomy. Palpation across the plantar aspect of the forefoot should reveal no further prominence of the affected metatarsal head.

The wound is closed in layers and a soft-tissue compressive dressing is used. Patients are allowed to walk in a postoperative bunion shoe as soon as weightbearing is tolerated. Average healing confirmed radiographically has been reported to occur at 4–7 weeks. L.S. Barouk, P. Ripstein and E. Troullec [personal communication 2001] perform a proximal oblique osteotomy which is indicated when only a small amount of dorsal elevation of the metatarsal head is desired. A longitudinal webspace incision exposes the base of the metatarsal. The osteotomy is performed in the proximal metaphysis using an oscillating saw with a very thin blade. The osteotomy starts dorsal–distal and passes as obliquely as possible, proximal and plantar. A proximal–plantar hinge is preserved, owing to the plantar curve of the proximal part of the metatarsal. This preserves the metatarsal length and its stability. The osteotomy is closed by manual elevation. Fixation is with a single 2.7-mm cannulated screw and is very stable (Figure 2d–e). Hansen prefers a dorsal closing wedge osteotomy performed in the proximal metaphysis, 1.0 cm distal to the tarsometatarsal joint. The wedge can be between 2 and 4 mm wide, and is made with a pointed rongeur. The plantar cortical bone is perforated with a 1.5-mm drill and dorsal pressure under the metatarsal head allows closure of the dorsal wedge. The amount of metatarsal head elevation is judged clinically by palpation of the metatarsal heads along the plantar side of the forefoot. The osteotomy is fixed with a 2- or 3-hole quarter-tubular tension plate. Local bone graft is applied to the osteotomy site.

Diaphyseal osteotomy

Hansen believes that the most common cause of increased weightbearing, usually of the second metatarsal, is a functionally short and hypermobile first metatarsal. Although he describes fusion of the first tarsometatarsal joint, or lengthening of the metatarsal at this joint, at times it is necessary to shorten the second metatarsal. The second metatarsal should be of equal length or shorter than the first and 1–2 mm longer than the third metatarsal. If one desires only to shorten the metatarsal, the diaphysis is approached through a dorsal longitudinal incision (Figure 3). The amount of diaphysis resected is determined using the preoperative A-P weightbearing radiograph. The periostium is elevated from that portion which will be excised. The distal cut is made first, followed by the proximal cut. The osteotomy is fixed using a four-hole quarter-tubular plate and 2.7-mm screws. The first hole is drilled 3–4 mm proximal to the osteotomy and tapped, and the plate is loosely fixed with a 2.7-mm screw. The second proximal screw is placed, the osteotomy reduced and the distal holes are drilled through the distal screw holes, which allow compression of the osteotomy site. Local bone graft is applied to the osteotomy. Postoperatively proximal and diaphyseal metatarsal osteotomies are usually immobilized in a short leg cast for about 6 weeks. However, if the osteotomy is performed only to elevate the metatarsal head, a postoperative boot may suffice. Crutches or a walker are also necessary.

Osteotomy at the neck of the metatarsal

During the past 25 years, several osteotomies of the metatarsal neck have been described. Helal [1975] performed a sliding oblique osteotomy at the neck of the metatarsal (Figure 4a). The osteotomy is made from proximal to dorsal obliquely, across the metatarsal neck distally, exiting the plantar cortex just behind the plantar condyle. An osteotome is passed through the osteotomy site to free the plantar soft tissues, allowing the head to displace dorsally and proximally. He did not use any internal fixation, preferring to allow weightbearing to determine the final position of the head. Published articles have described favorable and unfavorable results using this technique, and the osteotomy is no longer commonly used.

The dorsal closing wedge metatarsal neck osteotomy [Wolf 1973, Leventen and Pearson 1990] is performed under ankle block anesthesia with an

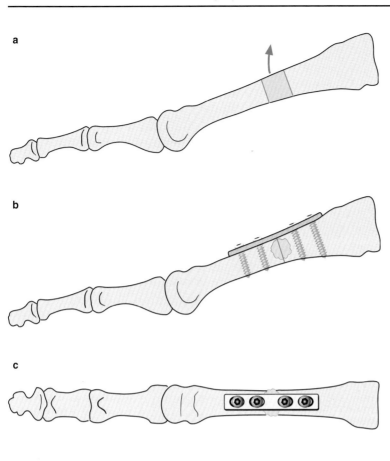

Figure 3

a. A premeasured section of diaphysis is resected; b. fixation with a 4-hole quarter tubular plate and local bone graft lateral view; c. dorsal view of fixation

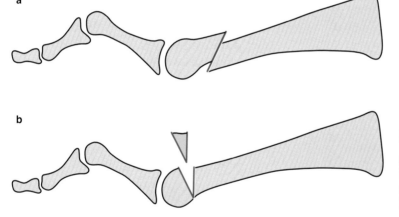

Figure 4

a. Sliding osteotomy at the neck of the metatarsal [Helal 1975]; b. dorsal closing wedge osteotomy at the neck of the metatarsal [Wolf 1973; Leventen and Pearson 1990]

Esmarch bandage around the ankle as a tourniquet. A dorsal longitudinal incision about 3 cm in length is made in the web space between the metatarsals chosen for the osteotomy (see Figure 1). The extensor tendons are retracted and the metatarsal neck is exposed sub-periosteally using small Hohmann retractors.

A V-shaped trough is cut through the dorsum of the neck transverse with the shaft and as close to the metatarsal head as possible (Figure 4b). This is done with a narrow, curved rongeur and removes about 5 mm of the dorsal cortex. The osteotomy extends through about 80% of the thickness of the neck.

The plantar cortex remains intact and is then fractured by placing upward pressure on the metatarsal head. This usually closes the dorsal wedge and elevates and redirects the metatarsal head. In this manner the osteotomy appears to be relatively stable and internal fixation is not used.

The wound is closed and a postoperative bulky dressing is applied. The patient is encouraged to walk as soon as possible in a postoperative wooden-soled shoe. This early weightbearing maintains the desired dorsal correction of the metatarsal.

Currently the most popular metatarsal osteotomy, the Weil osteotomy, will be described in detail.

Surgical management of metatarsalgia

Weil lesser metatarsal osteotomies

Metatarsalgias are a clinical expression of excessive weightbearing pressure over the lateral metatarsals. This can occur either from a more plantar position of one or more metatarsals with respect to the others (static metatarsalgia) or, more often, owing to excessive length of one or more lateral metatarsals with respect to the first metatarsal or to an adjacent metatarsal (metatarsalgia of propulsion). These appear most often in the course of the evolution of hallux valgus, which produces a syndrome of insufficiency of the first ray. Here, we exclude the metatarsalgia associated with pes cavus that requires different surgical therapies.

The clinical expression could be a syndrome of overload of the second ray with localized metatarsalgia over the head of the second metatarsal. Its evolution could pass via an acute form with effusion in the metatarsophalangeal joint of the second toe, or pass directly to a chronic form with callosity on the plantar aspect of the head of the second metatarsal associated, most often, with a clawing of the second toe. It eventually leads to articular instability and then a dislocation of the metatarsophalangeal joint of the second ray. If left untreated at this stage, a similar pattern develops over the third ray: metatarsalgia, instability, and then dislocation.

The other clinical expression is median metatarsalgia (over the median three metatarsals) which involves a round forefoot. It is characterized by a median plantar callosity associated with a clawing of the second, third and fourth toes.

Finally, metatarsalgia can appear in an isolated form, without hallux valgus, and these forms are most often associated with a short first metatarsal.

The aim of surgery is to reduce the weightbearing pressure over the overloaded metatarsal(s) but without creating a transferred metatarsalgia. Treatment will depend, above all, on the clinical symptomatology, but can be modified according to the anatomic form of the forefoot.

Anatomic forms of the forefoot

The ideal anatomic conformation of the curve of the metatarsals (Maestro's curve) is (according to a personal study of the French group 'Pied Innovation', corresponding to a study by Tanaka et al. [1995]) where one draws a line perpendicular to the second metatarsal and, taking this as a reference, the relative metatarsal lengths, in millimeters, should be:

M1	M2	M3	M4	M5
>3	0	<3	<6	<12

This represents a geometric progression of the power 2 for the lateral metatarsals (Figure 5). On the other hand, the perpendicular to the second metatarsal passing through the center of the lateral sesamoid also passes through the center of the head of the fourth metatarsal. These architectural elements constitute an ideal, but not absolute, reference for surgical correction.

The re-harmonization of the relative lengths of the metatarsals has been rendered possible by a cervicocephalic osteotomy of shortening of the lateral metatarsals described by L.S. Weil [Barouk 1994]. It is most often associated with treatment of the cause of the metatarsalgia: hallux valgus with metatarsus varus correction by a scarf osteotomy of the first metatarsal. Weil's osteotomies of the lateral metatarsals play an integral role in the comprehension and global treatment of static disorders of the forefoot.

Surgical technique for Weil's osteotomy of the lateral metatarsals

The recoil osteotomy

Principles

This is a transverse cervicocephalic osteotomy performed over the distal part of the lateral metatarsals. It allows a recoil of the metatarsal heads with conservation of their vascularity. It is situated in cancellous bone, which ensures rapid consolidation. It allows re-establishment of harmonious weightbearing over the metatarsals and a relaxation of periarticular tissues.

Approach

The approach is via a dorsal longitudinal incision over an intermetatarsal space. For multiple osteotomies, which are the most common, two incisions are necessary over the second and fourth intermetatarsal spaces, which allows an approach to two metatarsals through each skin incision (Figure 6).

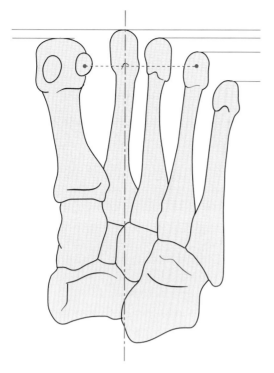

Figure 5

The ideal anatomic conformation of the curve of the metatarsals (Maestro's curve)

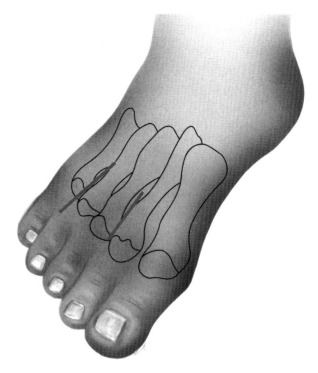

Figure 6

Two dorsal incisions to expose the distal metatarsals

Meanwhile, if for the correction of an associated hallux valgus an incision is made over the dorsum of the first intermetatarsal space for a lateral release of the first metatarsophalangeal joint, the dorsal incisions will be over the first and third spaces, completed by a lateral incision if an osteotomy of the fifth metatarsal is necessary.

Approach to the joint

Access to the joint is obtained through an incision between the two extensor tendons (longus and brevis). The incision should be proximal and end at the base of the proximal phalanx. A Hohmann retractor is placed on either side of the neck of the metatarsal and the toe is held in flexion. This maneuver is usually enough to allow exposure of the metatarsal head, but sometimes the dorsal synovial fold needs to be incised horizontally with a knife. The lateral ligaments are incised only if necessary for exposure of the metatarsal head. When multiple osteotomies are required, all the metatarsal heads are exposed before the bony sections are begun. In order to expose the distal part of the metatarsal better, a Hohmann-type retractor (Figure 7) or a hinge-type forceps is applied. This helps to protect the extensor tendons and to retract the adjacent metatarsals.

The osteotomy

This is performed with an oscillating saw using a blade of suitable size (6–10 mm in width and 3 cm in length). The beginning of the osteotomy cut is over the cartilage of the metatarsal head, 1 mm from its dorsal margin (Figure 7). This cut is as horizontal as possible, parallel to the plantar aspect of the foot. The natural tendency is to perform an osteotomy that is too vertical in the second and third metatarsals and one that is too horizontal in the fourth and fifth metatarsals. The osteotomy should measure around 2.5 cm, with a view to obtaining satisfactory contact between the two bony ends. Once the osteotomy is completed, it almost automatically produces a recoil of the head of the metatarsal.

How not to lose the head

In order to retain contact between the distal head fragment and the diaphysis proximally, it is necessary to hold the toe in flexion. In a large number of cases this is sufficient to ensure stability and allow fixation.

If the osteotomy is found to be too short, or the head fragment appears mobile, various solutions are possible:

*   The head could be held with a Chaput forceps and applied against the metatarsal shaft fragment.

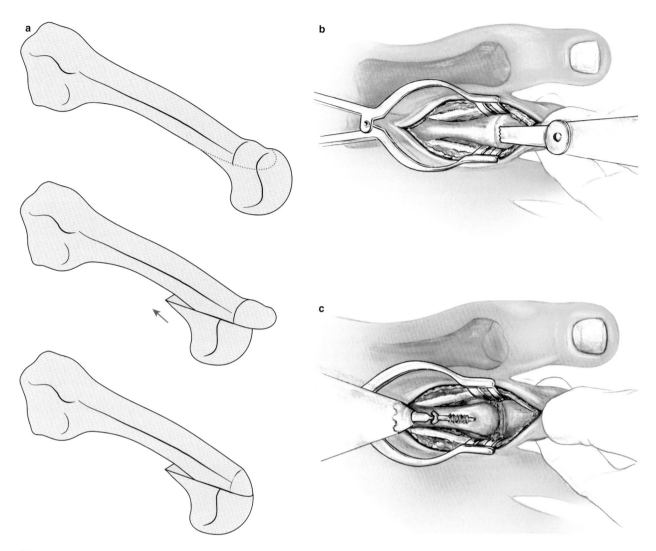

Figure 7

a. The osteotomy; b. and c. fixation with 'twist-off' screws. If twist-off screws are not used, the osteotomy can be held with a short, smooth K-wire 1.1 or 1.6 mm in diameter. A 2.0-mm cancellous screw can then be placed and the K-wire removed. This also gives excellent fixation [Davies and Saxby 1999]

This maneuver is necessary when one has to combine a recoil of the head with a lateral translation.

- The metatarsal could be held in position with a Verbuge bone-holding clamp and the toe held in flexion, allowing compression.

Extent of recoil

This is determined preoperatively from the radiographs of the forefoot in weightbearing, but in fact the amount of automatic recoil is often the best form of balance. Once the osteotomy is completed, the head automatically recoils to an extent sufficient to allow relaxation of the joint. After recoil, the position of the head must be exposed with the toe in extension, and then the toe is held in flexion, thus assuring compression between the two fragments.

Fixation

This is done with 'twist-off screws', their usual length being 14 mm for the second ray, 13 mm for the third and fourth rays and 11–12 mm for the fifth ray. For smaller feet, the dimensions are 14 mm for the second ray, 13 mm for the third, 12 mm for the fourth and 11 mm for the fifth. If contact between the two bony ends is not perfect, compression is usually produced during placement of the screw before it breaks. In case of a persistent gap after breakage the screw should be tightened further with a screwdriver.

The operation ends with resection of the visor of the helmet, i.e. the dorsal overhang of the proximal end of the metatarsal. The wound is closed in two layers, subcutaneous and skin, maintaining the toe in flexion.

*Balancing of the amount of recoil
between the different metatarsals*

When multiple osteotomies are performed, as is
most often the case, the positions of the heads of
the metatarsals can be regulated on the basis of different parameters: the preoperative calculation, the
relative lengths of the toes, and direct visualization
of the metatarsal heads.

Preoperative calculation

This gives a relative indication of the amounts of
recoil that one can carry out, this being modified as
a function of the amount of spontaneous recoil
obtained after osteotomy of the most deformed ray
(usually the second).

- The relative lengths of the toes. Once the
  osteotomy is completed, the toe should be held
  in the neutral position and its length compared
  with that of the adjacent toes. This gives a good
  indication of harmonious recoil.
- Direct visualization of the metatarsal heads. This
  is the final clinical parameter, but errors can
  occur if only this method of control is practiced.

Practical advice

Placement of Hohmann retractors is a fundamental
element in exposure of the joint. These must be
placed after a longitudinal incision is made between
the extensor longus and extensor brevis tendons.
During the osteotomy, the retractors impede the
progress of the oscillating saw at the end of the section. At that time, the retractors must be removed
and replaced by a self-retaining retractor.

In the presence of pes cavus, the tendency is to
perform an excessively vertical osteotomy, whereas
in cases of flat feet one tends to perform an excessively long osteotomy. In addition, one must take
care to avoid making an excessively long osteotomy
in the lateral metatarsals.

*Specific case: Weil' osteotomy for a
dislocation of the metatarsophalangeal joint*

In the presence of an irreducible dislocation of the
toe, after an incision between the two extensors, a
staggered section of the extensor longus and of
the extensor brevis tendons must be performed
(Figure 8): section of the extensor longus at the level
of the base of the proximal phalanx and that of the
extensor brevis at 2 cm behind the section of the
extensor longus tendon. The two extensor tendons

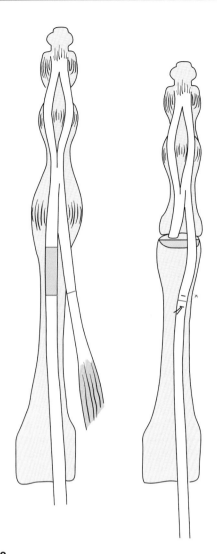

Figure 8

Weil's osteotomy for a dislocation of the metatarsophalangeal joint: tendon procedures

are retracted laterally and the articular release
effected. The latter should be done without application of force: division of the dorsal capsule with
a knife, and of the lateral capsuloligamentous
structures with a knife followed by fine scissors.
Arthrolysis is facilitated by traction along the axis of
the toe. The dislocation is progressively reduced and
the toe is held in flexion in order to expose the
metatarsal head. All brusque maneuvers are avoided
in order to prevent damage to the articular cartilage.

It is most often necessary to perform a lengthening of the extensor tendon: the proximal cut
end of the extensor longus tendon is sutured to the
distal cut end of the extensor brevis tendon, thus
producing lengthening.

Translation osteotomy

The approach to the metatarsal and the osteotomy
are identical, but the displacement of the head of

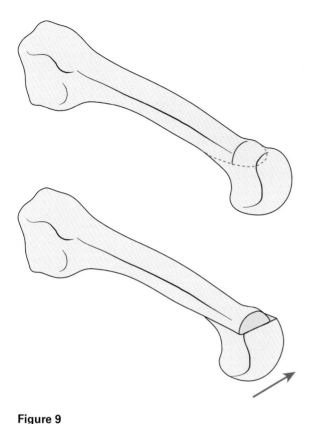

Figure 9

Translation osteotomy

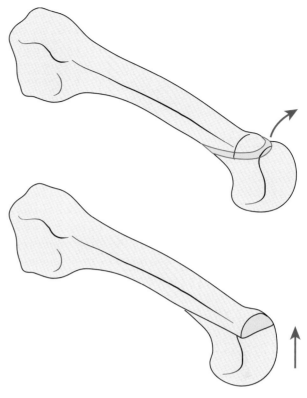

Figure 10

Elevation osteotomy. A shortening of more than 3 mm also produces a plantar depression of the metatarsal head [Trnka et al. 2001]. Therefore, in these patients a wafer of bone should be excised to prevent the plantar displacement

the metatarsal is different: it is displaced laterally or medially, most often with slight recoil (Figure 9). One must pay attention to this recoil, which can sometimes exceed expectations.

Elevation osteotomy

The difference is at the level of the osteotomy (Figure 10): either one makes two parallel cuts, removing a fine section of bone 1–2 mm wide, or one resects a wedge with its base anteriorly, with preservation of a posterior hinge that prevents an undesirable recoil.

Postoperative management

The postoperative course is very important for the quality of result, depending largely on the mobility of the lateral metatarsophalageal joints. The postoperative dressing holds the lesser toes in flexion. Passive mobilization of the metatarsophalageal joints must be started the day after surgery. The patient himself manipulates the toes in plantarflexion and dorsiflexion. During the first few days, the mobilization is limited by the dressing. The patient is allowed to stand upright the day after surgery with a walking plaster boot that is retained for 3 weeks. On

the 15th postoperative day, the dressing is discarded and re-education for the toes by the patient is increased: passive mobilization attempting to achieve maximal plantarflexion and pressing over the dorsal aspect of the proximal interphalangeal joint (and not on the end of the toe) and similar work in dorsiflexion. One must ask the patient to perform these actions in one's presence to ensure that they are performed correctly. This self-re-education should be pursued for at least 3 months.

Functional recovery

This is delayed and progressive, and can be judged only after more than a year from surgery. In patients in whom multiple osteotomies have been performed, the edema does not regress completely until 3–4 months (apart from any superimposed algodystrophy that increases the edematous period). Mobility of the metatarsophalangeal joints is acquired around the fourth month. At around 6 months, the metatarsalgias will have disappeared, the joints are supple (if everything has gone according to plan) but the active mobility of the toes is still feeble. This sensation of 'dead' toes will disappear only 1 year after surgery. The force of weightbearing on the pulps of the toes progresses over a prolonged period. Globally, these Weil's osteotomies are operations that 'age' well, the functional improvement progressing over a prolonged period of time.

Indications

The indication for a Weil osteotomy of the lateral metatarsals is, above all, clinical: the presence of mechanical pain under the head(s) of one or more metatarsals, incapacitating pain appearing while walking. An anatomic form of the forefoot not conforming to the ideal curve is not by itself an indication if there is no pain over the lateral metatarsals. The number of osteotomies to be performed is a function of the clinical picture and the anatomic conformation, the latter so as to avoid the creation of an iatrogenic pathology. Thus, several questions arise, one related to the other.

Weil's osteotomies

The number of osteotomies

This is a simple problem when one or two metatarsals are excessively long. The osteotomies are then limited to these metatarsals. At the same time, one must avoid performing an isolated osteotomy of the second ray, as the recoil, even if one wants to limit it, is always greater than what one believes it to be, and a transfer metatarsalgia over the third ray can rapidly develop.

However, most often the number of osteotomies is a function of the extent of recoil of the most affected ray and of the anatomic form of the forefoot. For metatarsalgias of mechanical origin, osteotomy of the second, third and fourth rays is the most reliable operation to avoid transfer metatarsalgias. In the presence of a dislocated metatarsophalangeal joint, the recoil often being considerable, osteotomies of the second to fifth rays may be indicated.

The amount of recoil

It can be appreciated on a preoperative anteroposterior weightbearing radiograph that the ideal result is to obtain a harmonious curve of Lelièvre with M1 = M2 > M3 > M4 > M5, with a difference in length following a geometric progression of the power 2 (curve of Maestro). This is just an estimate, as the most reliable recoil is that obtained intraoperatively by the spontaneous proximal migration of the metatarsal head after osteotomy. The amount of recoil of the adjacent metatarsals is regulated on the basis of the spontaneous recoil of the most affected ray.

Simple or thinning recoil

An osteotomy with excision of a fine section of bone is indicated essentially when one wishes to perform an isolated osteotomy of the second ray or one associated with that of the third ray. The recoil should be slightly less and the thickness of the excised section should be slightly thinner for the third rather than the second ray.

Translation

Recoil associated with translation of the metatarsal head is indicated in the presence of lateral or medial deviation of the toes: medial translation of the metatarsal head for medial deviation of the toe, and lateral translation for lateral deviation of one or more toes.

Associated procedures

At the level of the first ray

Metatarsalgias are most often associated with hallux valgus. This deformity is best corrected by a scarf osteotomy of the first metatarsal. In addition to correction of the metatarsus varus, this allows balancing of the length of the metatarsal and, eventually, lowering of the distal part.

The association of a scarf osteotomy of the first ray with a Weil's osteotomy of the lateral metatarsals raises a problem regarding the order of these procedures. One can propose a pattern: for cases with moderate hallux valgus, Weil's osteotomy followed by correction of the hallux valgus. For more severe forms of hallux valgus (hallux valgus > 40° or metatarsal I-II angle > 18°) a reliable correction of the deviation can be obtained only by a shortening scarf osteotomy. Hence, one must start with correction of the hallux valgus and regulate the recoil of the heads of the lateral metatarsals according to the recoil of the head of the first metatarsal necessary for correction of the hallux valgus.

At the level of the lesser toes

The Weil osteotomy allows spontaneous correction of supple claw deformities associated with the metatarsalgia, but sometimes a lengthening of the extensor is necessary. This is not always the case in the presence of a rigid claw, despite mobilization under anesthesia. An arthroplasty of the proximal interphalangeal joint, notably at the level of the second toe, is sometimes necessary.

On the basis of the above points, one can define a certain number of clinical patterns according to the pathology.

Depending on the pathology

Metatarsalgia of the second ray

Intermittent metatarsalgia of the second ray appearing at the end of the day or after prolonged walking is not an indication for a Weil osteotomy; the correction of the hallux valgus associated with a depressing scarf osteotomy will correct the symptoms. The indication is severe metatarsalgia that dominates the symptoms and is the main cause for consultation, the hallux valgus, even though severe, passing to a secondary position in the functional disability. Apart from an obvious disharmony of the length of the second (or second and third) ray, the indication is for an osteotomy of the second, third and fourth rays.

Instability of the second metatarsophalangeal joint

This is an elective indication for a Weil osteotomy of the three median rays associated with correction of the hallux valgus.

Dislocation of the second metatarsophalangeal joint

Here too a Weil osteotomy reliably corrects the painful anatomic problems produced by the dislocated metatarsophalangeal joint. The recoil of the head of the metatarsal required, corresponds most often to the overlap of the base of the proximal phalanx seen on the anteroposterior weight-bearing radiograph. The recoil can thus be large and necessitates and elevation osteotomy.

A rounded forefoot

Here too the indication is essentially clinical: a rounded forefoot with median plantar hyperkeratosis without pain is not an indication for metatarsal osteotomy. Only the presence of severe median plantar metatarsalgia justifies surgery on the metatarsals. The disability produced by the eventual stiffness of the metatarsophalangeal joint following surgery should be less than that caused by the metatarsalgia.

Hyperadduction of the second toe

A medial translation osteotomy of Weil of the second metatarsal, in association with medial articular release and an elongation of the extensor, allows one to obtain a reliable and durable correction of this deviation of the second toe.

Clawing of the toes

The Weil osteotomy is not the treatment for isolated clawing of the toes. As we have seen, the recoil of the metatarsal head allows correction of supple claw deformities associated with metatarsalgia without complementary surgery over the toes (this is sometimes done in the form of elongation of the extensor). The indication is metatarsalgia, and the correction of the claw is the consequence of the surgery.

Iatrogenic metatarsalgia

This could appear after surgery of the first ray, e.g. Keller's operation, producing in the long term an insufficiency of the first ray or Mayo's operation. The recoil osteotomy of the lateral metatarsals is the treatment of choice.

Metatarsalgia can also appear after inadequate surgery over the lateral ray, e.g. isolated amputation of the metatarsal head, or metatarsal osteotomies that have not restored a harmonious metatarsal curve. Here too the Weil osteotomy, aligning the metatarsal heads according to the shortest ray, would be the solution for this iatrogenic pathology.

Complications

The principal complication of the Weil osteotomy of the lateral metatarsals is stiffness of the metatarsophalangeal joints. This stiffness predominates at the level of the second ray: a slight loss of active plantarflexion of the second metatarsophalangeal joint is usual, even in the long term among the good results. There exists a compensation at the level of the proximal interphalangeal joints, causing the functional deficit to disappear. The metatarsophalangeal joint stiffness can be more severe with diminution of the plantarflexion responsible for a reduction in the contact of the pulps of the toes and a decrease in the dorsiflexion producing a painful functional disability in take-off. This complication can be avoided by strict adherence to the postoperative protocol. If stiffness appears despite this, one should not hesitate to manipulate the joints under anesthesia at around the second or third postoperative month or to perform surgical arthrolysis of the stiff joints at around 1 year.

Reflex sympathetic dystrophy is a possible complication that appears even more frequently as the osteotomies increase in number. It produces a painful edema with disability lasting several months. Paradoxically, there is practically no stiffness of the metatarsophalangeal joints in the algodystrophy that appears after Weil's osteotomies.

Results

Relief from metatarsalgia is regularly obtained (95% of cases). A transfer metatarsalgia can be superimposed in 7% of cases (personal communication by L.S. Weil, about 300 cases).

Contraindications

The presence of severe osteoporosis or of destruction of the metatarsal head constitutes a contraindication for this osteotomy.

The metatarsalgia of pes cavus is not an indication for Weil's osteotomy, nor is isolated clawing of the toes without metatarsalgia, or mild static metatarsalgia of the second ray associated with hallux valgus, as we have seen above.

Conclusion

The surgical treatment of metatarsalgia must take into account all the clinical and anatomic problems of the forefoot. It must satisfy all the criteria for orthopedic surgery: a preoperative plan for correction of the deformities, stable osteotomies fixed with strict osteosynthesis, and avoidance of iatrogenic complications that can lead to repeated, sometimes difficult, revision surgery. Anatomy must be restored and joints conserved. The shortening cervicocephalic osteotomy of the lateral metatarsals according to Weil's technique satisfies all these criteria and allows reliable treatment of metatarsalgia.

References

Barouk LS (1994) L'ostéotomie cervico-capitale de weil dans les métatarsalgies médianes. Méd Chir Pied 10: 23–33

Davies MS, Saxby TS (1999) Metatarsal neck osteotomy with rigid internal fixation for the treatment of lesser toe metatarsophalangeal joint pathology. Foot Ankle Int 20: 630–635

Dreeben SM, Noble PC, Hammerman S, et al. (1989) Metatarsal osteotomy for primary metatarsalgia: radiographic and pedobarographic study. Foot Ankle 9: 214–218

Hansen ST (2000) Functional Reconstruction of the Foot and Ankle. Philadelphia, Lippincott Williams & Wilkins, pp 397–401

Helal B (1975) Metatarsal osteotomy for metatarsalgia. J Bone Joint Surg 57B: 187–192

Helal B, Greiss M (1984) Telescoping osteotomy for pressure metatarsalgia. J Bone Joint Surg 67B: 213–217

Leventen EO, Pearson SW (1990) Distal metatarsal osteotomy for intractable plantar keratoses. Foot Ankle 10: 247–251

Mann RA (1986) Keratotic disorders of the plantar skin. In: Mann RA (ed) Surgery of the Foot. St Louis, Mosby, pp 413–466

Pedowitz WJ (1988) Distal oblique osteotomy for intractable plantar keratosis of the middle three metatarsals. Foot Ankle 9: 7–9

Sclamberg EL, Lorenz MA (1983) A dorsal wedge V osteotomy for painful plantar callosities. Foot Ankle 4: 30–32

Tanaka Y, Takakura Y, Kumai T, et al. (1995) Radiographic analysis of hallux valgus. J Bone Joint Surg 77A: 205–213

Thomas FB (1974) Levelling the tread. Elevation of the dropped metatarsal head by metatarsal osteotomy. J Bone Joint Surg 56B: 314–319

Trnka HJ, Kaider A, Kabon B, et al. (1996) Helal metatarsal osteotomy for the treatment of metatarsalgia: a critical analysis of results. Orthopaedics 19: 457–461

Trnka H-J, Nyska M, Parks BG, Myerson MS (2001) Dorsiflexion contracture after the Weil osteotomy: results of cadaver study and three-dimensional analysis. Foot Ankle Int 22: 47–50

Winson IG, Rawlinson J, Broughton NS (1988) Treatment of metatarsalgia by sliding distal metatarsal osteotomy. Foot Ankle 9: 2–6

Wolf MD (1973) Metatarsal osteotomy for the relief of painful metatarsal callosities. J Bone Joint Surg 55A: 1760–1762

Bibliography

Barouk LS (1997) New osteotomies in the forefoot and their therapeutic role. In: Valtin B (ed) Cahiers d'enseignements de la SOFCOT. Paris, Expansion Scientifique Française, Paris, pp 49–86

Leemrijse T, Valtin B, Oberlin C (1998) Vascularisation of the heads of the three central metatarsals: an anatomic study, its application and considerations with respect to horizontal osteotomies at the necks of the metatarsals. Foot Ankle Surg 4: 57–62

Valtin B (1997) Pathology of the lesser toes: a clinical study an surgical treatment. In Valtin B (ed) Cahiers d'enseignements de la SOFCOT. Paris, Expansion Scientifique Française, pp 107–119

17

The great toe sesamoids

Michael M. Stephens

Introduction

The sesamoids of the great toe, lying beneath the first metatarsal head, add height to the first metatarsal head for weightbearing and provide mechanical advantage for the lesser muscles of the hallux [Aper et al. 1994, 1996]. They are therefore essential for normal foot biomechanics. They vary in shape, size and fragmentation, i.e. they can be absent or hypoplastic, or they can be in two or more parts [Helal 1981, 1996, Wülker and Wirth 1996]. The lateral and medial sesamoids receive insertions of the lateral and medial heads respectively of the flexor hallucis brevis. They each receive a metatarsosesamoid ligament and are attached to each side of the fibrous tunnel of the flexor hallucis longus and to each other through the intersesamoid ligament. Each sesamoid has a presesamoid bursa and is attached to the base of the proximal phalanx of the hallux through the sesamophalangeal ligament. The plantar fascia inserts by separate slips into both sesamoids. The oblique head of the adductor hallucis and the deep transverse metatarsal ligament are attached to the lateral sesamoid. The abductor hallucis is attached to the medial sesamoid.

Pathology and clinical findings

In metatarsus varus and hallux valgus the metatarsal head escapes medially so that the sesamoids act only to displace laterally, with the lateral sesamoid moving to the lateral side of the metatarsal head and the medial sesamoid moving underneath the metatarsal head, eroding the intersesamoid crest of the metatarsal head. Such incongruity leads to degeneration. The sesamoids can migrate proximally if their attachment to the base of the proximal phalanx is damaged, e.g. after resection arthroplasty of the proximal phalanx of the great toe. This results in a lateral shift or transfer of pressure to the second metatarsal, due to loss of apparent height of the first ray. Transfer metatarsalgia or even stress fractures of the lesser metatarsals may follow. Elongation or rupture of the intersesamoid ligament produces sesamoid divarication, which can arise from rheumatoid arthritis or severe trauma to the first metatarsophalangeal joint [Potter et al. 1992]. Pain is commonly found under the medial or tibial sesamoid with excessive pronation and is manifested by a callosity superficial to it. The presesamoid bursa may also enlarge and give a bursitis, and is manifested by a callosity superficial to it. If the callus is point localized to this sesamoid, it is also called an intractable plantar keratosis.

Following impaction injuries the sesamoid may be crushed and fractured or the syndesmosis of partite elements damaged. As the fragments separate, that portion of the small muscles attached to the injured sesamoid becomes non-functional; for example, if the medial sesamoid is involved, the unbalanced pull of the lateral small muscles attached to the lateral sesamoid can lead to hallux valgus. Osteochondritis of the sesamoid following a crush injury has been described [Apley 1966]. A similar injury can cause chondromalacia of the articular surface, which may also arise from a tight medial portion of the plantar fascia. This initially produces a hallux rigidus, since the axis of rotation of the metatarsophalangeal joint moves plantarwards. This 'hinging' impingement produces a pit on the dorsal aspect of the metatarsal head which is seen in the early stages of hallux rigidus.

Arthropathies such as rheumatoid arthritis and gout can affect the metatarsophalangeal joint and therefore incidentally the sesamometatarsal portion of the joint. Patients with presesamoid bursitis have a doughy, tender swelling under the metatarsal head, as is commonly seen in patients with spastic diplegia, where there are excessive shear forces during the stance phase of gait and prolonged fore-foot loading due to a tight Achilles tendon.

Osteomyelitis can occur secondarily to a penetrating injury or to a neglected plantar ulcer overlying a sesamoid, particularly in diabetes mellitus patients where the pain of protection reflex is absent because of the peripheral neuropathy.

Treatment

The initial treatment of choice is conservative. In the acute injury, non-steroidal anti-inflammatory medication and avoidance of weightbearing are used first, followed by a weight-relieving insole. Physiotherapy is important for stretching the Achilles tendon and hamstrings, to reduce and shorten the time of forefoot loading, as is body weight reduction. Orthotic devices can control excessive forefoot pronation during the weightbearing cycle and therefore relieve weight on the first ray. A medial arch support with medial posting and a sesamoid cut-out will also control excessive pronation by decreasing hindfoot valgus.

A rocker sole will reduce the movement at the metatarsophalangeal joint and therefore at the sesamoid–metatarsal articulation. A metatarsal bar will shorten the weightbearing time in that area, and a metatarsal insole will decrease weightbearing on the metatarsal heads by transferring pressure to the metatarsal necks. Only when these methods of conservative treatment have failed should surgery be considered.

Surgical technique

The approaches to the sesamoids are made with particular reference to the medial digital nerve to the hallux, which lies medial to the medial sesamoid, and to the common digital nerve of the first web space and its continuation as the lateral digital nerve, which lies lateral to the lateral sesamoid. To avoid damage to these nerves it is advisable that the surgery be carried out with an ankle or thigh

tourniquet. The type of anesthesia is decided by the clinical situation, but usually general anesthesia is used.

The medial incision is the most common and safest approach to the medial sesamoid and for excision of a presesamoid bursa (Figure 1). The plantar incision is less commonly used but is the safest approach for excising the lateral sesamoid and for repairing the intersesamoid ligament (Figure 2). The medial incision (Figure 1) runs from the medial side of the distal half of the first metatarsal across the metatarsophalangeal joint and the proximal phalanx parallel to the thick plantar skin. The dorsal digital nerve will then be in the upper portion of the wound and the medial digital nerve will be in its plantar aspect. As the wound is deepened the metatarsophalangeal joint capsule is visualized, and soft-tissue dissection is then extended in this plane plantarwards. Since the capsule is attached to the medial sesamoid, continued dissection on to the plantar aspect of the medial sesamoid will expose the plantar surface of the sesamoid and the common tendon of the short flexor and abductor hallucis muscles.

The capsule blends into the proximal pole of the sesamoid and is then adherent over the plantar surface to continue distally as the medial sesamophalangeal ligament. Further soft-tissue dissection laterally will reveal the sheath in which the flexor hallucis longus tendon runs.

This incision, although on the plantar surface, heals well and is painless if there is no damage to digital nerves. The plantar incision (Figure 2) is over the same length but on the plantar surface, running in line with the flexor hallucis longus tendon, i.e. in the midportion between the medial and lateral sesamoids. In this position the medial plantar nerve to the hallux is retracted medially and the common digital nerve of the first web space is retracted laterally. This incision will expose the plantar surface of the tendons of the small muscles attached to each sesamoid proximally, their continuation as an aponeurosis adherent to the plantar surface of each sesamoid, and the medial and lateral short sesamophalangeal ligaments. Between these is the sheath of the flexor hallucis longus tendon.

The incision chosen for the surgery will dictate the positioning of the patient. With the medial approach the patient is supine with a sandbag under the contralateral buttock to rotate the leg externally. With a plantar incision the patient can be prone with the ankles in plantarflexion over a sandbag or jelly roll, or supine with the operating table in a position of maximum head-down feet-up.

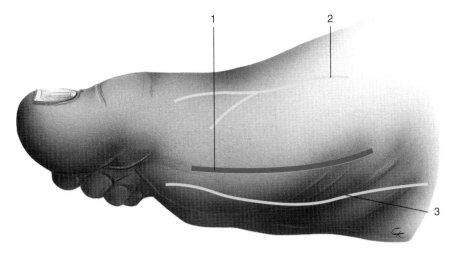

Figure 1

Medial incision for the approach to the medial sesamoid

1 Incision
2 Dorsal digital nerve
3 Medial digital nerve

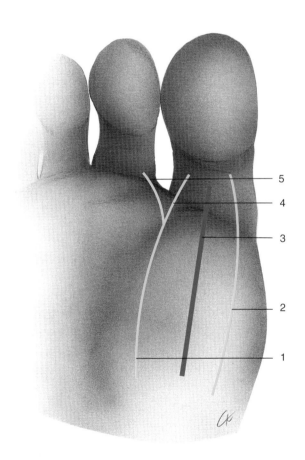

Figure 2

Plantar incision for the approach to the lateral sesamoid

1 Common digital nerve
2 Medial digital nerve to the hallux
3 Incision
4 Lateral digital nerve to the hallux
5 Median digital nerve to the second toe

In each approach the surgeon sits at the end of the table with the scrub nurse on one side and the first assistant on the other.

Partial sesamoidectomy

Partial sesamoidectomy is most commonly performed on the medial sesamoid when it becomes prominent, giving an intractable painful callus on the plantar surface. This may arise from excessive pronation, excessive plantarflexion of the first ray and clawing of the hallux. It can also occur with longstanding lateral subluxation of the sesamoids, because the medial sesamoid is no longer on the medial side of the head of the metatarsal but rather under its midportion in the area of the inter-sesamoid crest. This procedure is only a part of the management of the primary deformity. On its own it may fail, and it is often an adjunct to other weight-relieving modalities.

The procedure is performed after exposure of the medial sesamoid and its plantar surface through a medial approach, as described above. A longitudinal split is made in the plantar surface of the sesamoid through its soft-tissue envelope directly on to the sesamoid bone. Sharp dissection then separates each side as the soft tissues are elevated medially and laterally off the plantar aspect of the sesamoid. Dissection is continued until 50% of the plantar aspect of the sesamoid is exposed so that it can be resected (Figure 3) [Mann and Wapner 1992]. The value of the medial incision is that it allows the use of a fine power saw for resection, medial to lateral and parallel to the plantar weight-bearing surface (Figure 4). Once the main fragment is removed, the remainder is rounded with a burr to convert this flat surface into a surface convex proximal to distal. However, the procedure is likely to fail in the long term, unless the primary deformity, for example pronation, is not treated.

The surgical field is then lavaged with normal saline to remove bone dust and the reflected

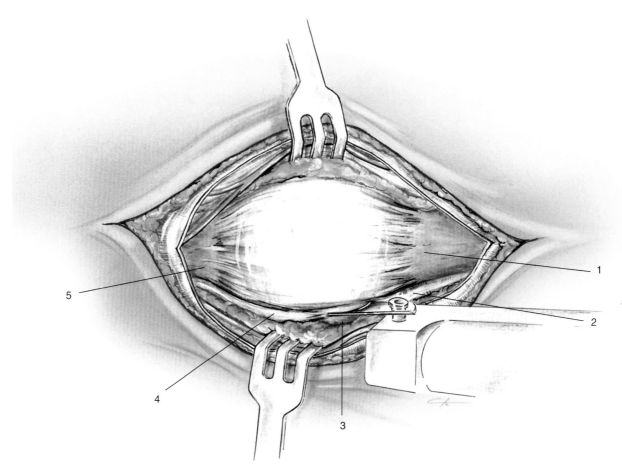

Figure 3

Partial medial sesamoidectomy, intraoperative aspect

1 First metatarsal
2 Short flexor and abductor muscle
3 Sesamoid bone
4 Sesamophalangeal ligament
5 Proximal phalanx

soft tissues are replaced over the sesamoids. Subcutaneous interrupted sutures approximate the wound edges. They must not be inserted deep, for fear of catching the cutaneous nerves. Closure is over a fine drain, or else the tourniquet is released and hemostasis obtained. The skin is closed in a routine manner and a wool and crêpe compression bandage applied. Weightbearing can commence when tolerated. High impact is discouraged for 6 weeks.

Bone grafting of sesamoid non-union

The majority of acute fractures to the sesamoids are treated conservatively and lead to union. In those patients who develop a symptomatic non-union, grafting is a successful procedure [Anderson and McBride 1997]. The approach is similar to that of partial sesamoidectomy; that is, since it commonly involves the tibial sesamoid, it is approached with a medial incision, and the plantar cortex of the sesamoid is exposed in a similar manner. In this way the non-union is identified and curetted. The defect is then packed with bone graft obtained from the medial eminence. A short leg plaster completely immobilizing the hallux is applied for 4 weeks. This is then removed and a below-knee walking cast is applied, once again immobilizing the hallux. This is removed at 8 weeks. Mobilization is then commenced with protection of the sesamoid using a weight-relieving orthotic device. Tomography then can be carried out at 10–12 weeks, which will dictate the degree of mobilization.

Excision of the presesamoid bursa

Excision is indicated for the intractable painfully enlarged bursa underneath the first metatarsal head when conservative treatment has failed. It

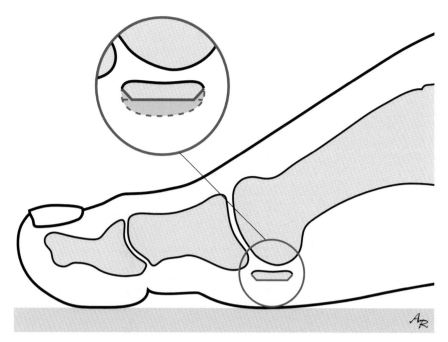

Figure 4

Bone resection in partial sesamoidectomy

may be associated with an excessively prominent medial sesamoid, and therefore bursal excision may be combined with partial sesamoidectomy. Bursitis is also found in people who have gait abnormalities, including excessive first ray pronation, excessive forefoot loading and excessive plantarflexion of the first ray associated with a clawed hallux.

Since this bursa is usually associated with the medial sesamoid, the medial incision is once again the surgical approach. However, as the bursa is often large, it may be difficult to isolate and indeed find the medial digital nerve to the hallux. In these cases extension of the wound more proximally will allow localization of this nerve proximally in normal tissues before it becomes associated with the bursa. In this way the nerve can be protected.

Once the nerve is isolated, soft-tissue dissection and separation of the bursa from surrounding tissue are obtained by blunt dissection with fine, blunt-nosed scissors. The cavity remaining is usually large and it is therefore advisable to use a drain for 12–24 h postoperatively. Closure is in the usual manner with a compression dressing. The patient must be advised prior to surgery that recurrence is not infrequent and that there is a risk of damage to the digital nerves. Once the bursa is excised, careful assessment should be made of the sesamoids because if the medial sesamoid is excessively prominent, resection of 50% of the plantar surface (partial sesamoidectomy) should be carried out.

Excision of a sesamoid

Complete excision of a sesamoid bone is now rarely indicated and should be avoided [Aper et al. 1996, Richardson 1999]. The most frequent indications are severe fragmentation, osteochondritis or chronic osteomyelitis, often associated with plantar ulceration in diabetes with peripheral neuropathy. On rare occasions excision of a sesamoid may be indicated where the primary pain source is the metatarsosesamoid joint. This is invariably associated with degeneration or with osteochondritis. Excision of either sesamoid has a high rate of iatrogenic deformity. If the medial sesamoid is excised, the hallux falls into valgus because the medial short flexor and abductor muscles become nonfunctional unless they are carefully reconstructed. If the lateral sesamoid is excised, the lateral short flexor and adductor muscles become nonfunctional and the hallux falls into varus.

The medial sesamoid is excised with ease through the medial incision and the lateral sesamoid can be excised through the plantar incision. The excision of the sesamoid should commence as for a partial sesamoidectomy, i.e. the soft tissues that cover the plantar aspect of the sesamoid are incised longitudinally and elevated off the sesamoid with sharp dissection. This is continued around the circumference of the sesamoid. It can then be enucleated. If care is taken to retain the soft tissues that cover the plantar surface of the sesamoid, they can be repaired with non-absorbable sutures to leave the short muscles in continuity with the sesamophalangeal ligaments. This means that the function of the small muscles to the great toe will remain intact.

Replacement of the sesamoid

Replacement of the sesamoids with medium-grade silicone was described by Helal [1979]. He found this useful when both sesamoids had to be removed. This technique maintains metatarsal height and prevents excessive transfer of load to the lesser metatarsals. The silicone block should be fashioned into the shape of the sesamoid, resected and carefully inserted into the defect left by its resection. To maintain its stability it is important, therefore, to repair the soft-tissue envelope over the plantar surface of the replaced sesamoids.

References

Anderson RB, McBride AM (1997) Autogenous bone grafting of hallux sesamoid nonunions. Foot Ankle Int 18: 293–296

Aper RL, Saltzman CL, Brown TD (1994) The effect of hallux sesamoid resection on the effective movement of the flexor hallucis brevis. Foot Ankle Int 15: 462–470

Aper RL, Saltzman CL, Brown TD (1996) The effect of hallux sesamoid excision on flexor hallucis longus moment arm. Clin Orthop 18: 209–217

Apley AG (1966) Open sesamoid. Proc Roy Soc Med 59: 120–121

Helal B (1979) Sesamoides du pied du sportif. In: Simon L, Claustre J, Benezis C (eds) Le Pied du Sportif. Paris, Masson p 116

Helal B (1981) The great toe sesamoid bones: the Lus or lost souls of Ushaia. Clin Orthop 157: 82–87

Helal B (1996) The accessory ossicles and sesamoids. In: Helal B, Rowley DI, Cracchiolo A, Myerson M (eds) Surgery of Disorders of the Foot and Ankle. London, Martin Dunitz, pp 357–368

Mann RA, Wapner KL (1992) Tibial sesamoid shaving for the treatment of intractable plantar keratosis. Foot Ankle 13: 196–198

Potter G, Pavlov H, Abrahams TG (1992) The hallux sesamoids revisited. Skel Radiol 21: 437–444

Richardson EG (1999) Hallucal sesamoid pain: causes and surgical treatment. J Am Acad Orthop Surg 7: 270–278

Wülker N, Wirth CJ (1996) The great toe sesamoids. Foot Ankle Surg 2: 167–174

18

Interdigital neuroma: technique of resection

Andrea Cracchiolo III

Introduction

One of the more common causes and yet one of the most overdiagnosed etiologies of forefoot pain is the condition popularly referred to as 'Morton's neuroma'. The first report on this condition is attributed to Thomas G. Morton of Philadelphia and was written in 1876 [Morton 1876]. In 1940, L.O. Betts of Adelaide described a local lesion of the digital nerve in the third web space [Betts 1940, Thomas et al. 1988]. However, the term 'neuroma' is a misnomer and the condition is often misunderstood. On microscopic examination, the swollen nerve shows atrophy of neural fibers and hypertrophy of the connective tissue elements, more consistent with an entrapment neuropathy. Most of the pathological changes are found within the bulbous portion of the nerve as it divides into its two digital branches [Lassmann 1979]. The etiology of these pathological changes is unclear but probably represents the result of anatomic factors, trauma and external pressure, as the digital nerve courses under the intermetatarsal ligament. Other names have been suggested for this condition, such as 'Morton's digital neuralgia' or 'interdigital perineural fibrosis'. However, the name 'Morton's metatarsalgia' may be most appropriate.

Diagnosis

Although there is no absolute method of making the diagnosis of an interdigital 'neuroma', several factors

can point toward this condition with certainty. First, the pain should be localized and not be a generalized metatarsalgia. It is frequently described as a burning pain or a paresthesia, and should involve either the third or the second web space [Mann and Reynolds 1983]. If it involves the first or fourth web spaces, then another diagnosis must be sought. Also, the pain should not be most severe directly under the plantar condyle of the metatarsal head, although this distinction may be difficult. The patient may give a history of pain radiating into the tibial side of the fourth toe or to the entire toe, or to the fibular side of the third toe. The condition is much more common in women. Also, the pain is usually not present at rest, but may persist following vigorous walking and running. When chronic, the pain may be more vague in location and more continuous. It may or may not be affected by wearing either athletic or fashionable shoes. Although a few patients describe a proximal radiation of the pain, radiation into the area of the ankle, the leg or more proximal is probably not related to a neuroma. The presence, or suspected diagnosis, of two neuromas in the same foot occurs rarely. Bilateral involvement occurs in about 10% of patients seen for symptoms of Morton's neuroma.

A careful physical examination of the foot with the patient seated and standing is most helpful in making the diagnosis. There may be swelling, indicated by a loss of the contour of the extensor tendon, at the dorsum of the lateral metatarsophalangeal joints. A large interdigital mass may spread the adjacent toes, usually the third and fourth. Patients with a 'neuroma' generally do not have plantar calluses. Direct palpation should first be performed on the painless areas of the forefoot. Pressure on the plantar surface directly over the common digital nerve from proximal to distal will sometimes reproduce the patient's pain when one reaches the 'neuroma' area, which is just distal to the adjacent metatarsal heads, before compressing the foot or any of the web spaces. Dorsiflexing the toe is also helpful as this makes the nerve taut. Next, each web space is compressed by squeezing dorsal and plantar, saving the third web space for last. Mediolateral compression to the forefoot is added, using the other hand. Occasionally a click [Mulder 1951] can be palpated as the mass is first forced between the metatarsal heads and then extruded. However, this sign is unreliable unless it absolutely reproduces the patient's symptoms. Each metatarsophalangeal joint is passively moved and the second, third and fourth are tested for signs of instability, to see whether the pain can be reproduced. The second and third metatarsophalangeal joints should be tested for instability. This is done by grasping the toe and attempting to sublux the base of the proximal phalanx dorsally. If this maneuver reproduces the patient's pain then the diagnosis of a 'neuroma' should be questioned. It is rare that a 'neuroma' and an unstable metatarsophalangeal joint are both symptomatic. Testing skin sensation using light touch usually gives little help in making a diagnosis.

All other tests, such as radiographs, magnetic resonance imaging (MRI) scans, ultrasonography and electrodiagnostic studies, are rarely helpful in making a diagnosis of a 'neuroma'. Any pathology that produces localized plantar forefoot pain can be confused with a 'neuroma'. Painful subluxation, usually of the second metatarsophalangeal joint, frequently gives similar symptoms to those of a 'neuroma' and is commonly undiagnosed. Other pathology, such as bursal formation in the interdigital web space, stress fractures of the metatarsal, a torn plantar plate, synovitis of a metatarsophalangeal joint, a wart, a foreign body or an early Freiberg's infraction has to be differentiated from a 'neuroma'. A diagnostic injection (Figure 1) can frequently be helpful and, if done early in the condition, may give pain relief for some time. Usually, only one web space is injected, even if two are painful. The needle is slowly directed plantarwards at the level of the adjacent metatarsal heads, and small amounts of local anesthetic solution are injected as the needle is advanced; usually about

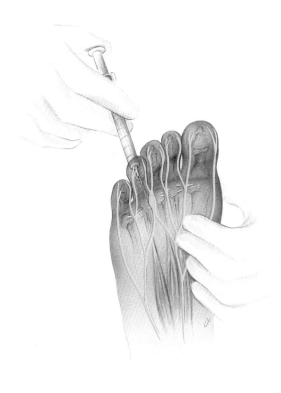

Figure 1

Injection technique for interdigital neuroma

2 ml will suffice. Frequently a resistance is felt as the needle comes against the transverse metatarsal ligament. The needle is advanced just through the ligament and another 0.5 ml is injected in this area. At this point, the patient should have experienced no significant pain, and in fact may begin to perceive some toe numbness. About 0.5 ml of a corticosteroid solution may be injected. The corticosteroid should not be injected into the fat pad and should not track back into the subcutaneous fat, as it tends to produce a small area of fat resorption. Should the injection relieve the pain completely this is evidence that something in the injected web space – whether a 'neuroma' or a bursa – is responsible for the pain. Another injection may follow about 3 weeks later. More than three injections are contraindicated as they do nothing to correct the disorder.

Treatment

Non-operative treatment

To some degree the treatment of 'neuroma' pain depends on the length of time the pain has been present and its severity. Thus pain that has been present for several weeks and is severe only occasionally may respond to non-operative care.

Non-operative treatment usually includes:

1. Modification of any standing, walking or running activity. The activity should be temporarily discontinued, altered or shortened, or the surface over which the patient may notice symptoms when running should be changed.
2. The patient's shoes should be checked for a toe box that is too narrow or too small for the forefoot.
3. A support may be placed in the shoe just proximal to the suspected area of nerve irritation, e.g. an anterior support or a metatarsal pad.
4. Analgesic or non-steroidal anti-inflammatory medication may be used. Usually drugs that do not require a physician's prescription will suffice. Stronger medications usually are not helpful and may produce only side-effects.
5. One or more web-space injections may be given.

Indications for surgery

Patients with chronic pain, especially if it is present while weightbearing and severe enough for the patient to have sought non-operative treatments which have failed, are candidates for surgery. The surgeon must clearly have evidence indicating the presence of a 'neuroma' and not operate on non-specific forefoot pain. Patients should be told that even under ideal conditions 8% of operated feet may have some residual pain, and perhaps 2% may have no relief or be worse. Patients with 'neuroma' symptoms that are localized to the second or third web space have the best results when they require surgical excision, with 80% either satisfied or satisfied with minor reservations. Patients with pain in both feet, pain in more than one web space in the same foot or pain in other than the second or third web space do not respond well to surgical excision [Friscia et al. 1991].

Surgical technique

Nerve excision

The operation to excise an interdigital neuroma is routinely done as an outpatient procedure under regional ankle block anesthesia and intravenous sedation. A tourniquet at the ankle should be used. The exposure for a primary case is most often

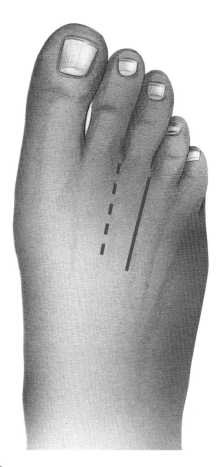

Figure 2

A dorsal longitudinal incision is made over the third web space (solid line) or over the second web space (dashed line); however, it is contraindicated to make both incisions during the same operation

through a dorsal longitudinal incision over the suspected web space, usually the third (Figure 2). The long extensor tendon is retracted laterally and does not need to be divided. However, a plantar approach has also been used (see below). Loupe magnification is helpful. Dissection is carried bluntly down to the intermetatarsal ligament (Figure 3). It is important to coagulate all potential bleeders, which are usually veins, in order not to have significant postoperative bleeding. After clearing the subcutaneous tissues, one should look for evidence of a bursa. At times a fluid-filled sac can be seen and it should be excised. Signs of previous corticosteroid injections can also be seen. It is usually easy to identify the transverse metatarsal ligament. If the interspace is not excessively narrow, a small lamina spreader can be placed between the necks of the adjacent metatarsals and this will more clearly delineate the ligament. A thickened mass surrounding the common digital nerve is seen just distal to the ligament and can be pushed into the operative field by

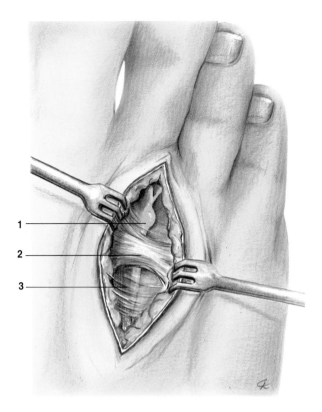

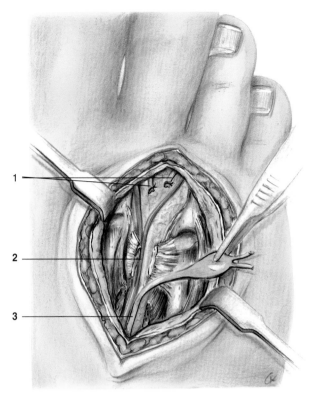

Figure 3

The transverse metatarsal ligament is easily identified. Upward pressure on the sole of the foot will usually show the 'neuroma' formation just distal to the ligament

1 Neuroma
2 Transverse metatarsal ligament
3 Common plantar digital nerve

Figure 4

Following division of the ligament, the distal digital branches of the nerve are transected. The nerve is then traced proximally and divided well within the interosseous muscle

1 Dorsal digital nerves
2 Common plantar digital artery
3 Common plantar digital nerve

pressing on the underlying plantar surface of the foot. Following epineural neurolysis, 90% of neuroma cases were found on a digital branch [Diebold et al. 1996]. This may explain why most symptoms may be present in only one toe. The transverse metatarsal ligament should be divided under direct vision and the nerve isolated. Proximal exposure is facilitated using a small right-angled retractor or clamp to pull back the dorsal interosseous muscle. Care should be taken not to confuse the lumbrical tendon or the common digital artery with the nerve. The nerve should be freed distal to the enlargement, identifying the two distal branches. These two distal branches are transected well beyond the 'neuroma' (Figure 4). It is essential to obtain wide visualization to avoid inadvertently resecting a lumbrical tendon or one of the vessels. The nerve is then traced proximally several centimeters into the non-weightbearing area of the midfoot in the area of the intrinsic muscles. Distal traction facilitates this proximal dissection. The nerve is then sharply divided proximally,

well within the interosseous muscle (Figure 4). The tourniquet is released and the wound is compressed for several minutes, then inspected for any significant bleeding vessels, which are coagulated. The skin is sutured and a compression dressing is applied.

Ligament release and epineural neurolysis

This procedure is performed under the assumption that Morton's disease is a nerve entrapment syndrome [Gauthier 1979, Diebold et al. 1996] and that decompression, as in other peripheral nerve entrapments, is sufficient to relieve symptoms. Through a dorsal longitudinal incision over the involved web space, the intermetatarsal ligament is transected. Using magnification, an epineural neurolysis is performed, without transecting the nerve. 'Good' and 'excellent' results in 83–90% of patients were reported with this technique [Gauthier 1979, Diebold et al. 1996]. Avoiding

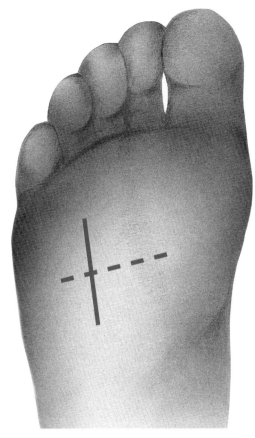

Figure 5

A suspected neuroma can also be approached through a longitudinal plantar incision (solid line) or through a transverse plantar incision (dashed line), especially in cases of revision neuroma surgery

resection of the nerve prevents loss of sensation, loss of sweat production and the development of a proximal stump neuroma.

Revision operations for Morton's metatarsalgia

Some patients with a failed primary surgical excision of an interdigital nerve present with symptoms of metatarsalgia. These patients must be fully re-evaluated to determine the true cause of their pain. One of the most frequently overlooked conditions that is confused with a neuroma is a synovitis of the metatarsophalangeal joint or an instability of the joint. However, some patients develop a painful stump neuroma (which is a true neuroma formed after the common digital nerve is resected). These patients may have had some relief – even complete

relief – of their neuroma after the primary operation, only to have localized web-space pain develop several months later. If indeed the nerve has been sectioned at a prior operation, a re-exploration should be considered. This operation should be planned as a more major foot operation. Epidural, spinal or general anesthesia and a thigh-high tourniquet are preferable. The latter will not constrict any of the structures about the foot and ankle, which aids in the exposure. Although the previous dorsal incision can still be used, the scar tissue from the previous operation may make exposure of the proximal nerve stump difficult. Therefore, a plantar incision is usually preferable [Johnson et al. 1988] and, although not essential, placing the patient in the prone position is most helpful. A plantar approach is also used by some as the preferred incision for primary operations. A longitudinal incision is made over the plantar side of the symptomatic web space (Figure 5). The incision should be carried more proximal than distal to avoid unnecessary scarring of the plantar fat pad. Most stump neuromas usually occur in the area of the metatarsal heads or the metatarsal neck areas and can be clearly found with an incision that does not traverse the weightbearing areas of the forefoot. It is best to look for the intact digital nerve proximally and trace it distally to the neuroma stump or, in the case of a primary neuroma, to the mass surrounding the nerve (Figure 6). Usually the nerve has not been transected far enough behind the weightbearing area of the forefoot. Occasionally, one may find an intact nerve, which indicates that the nerve was not resected during the first operation. The nerve should be traced far enough proximally so that it can be resected in a non-weightbearing area of the foot, whether it be a revision or a primary operation. The subcutaneous tissues and the skin are closed with interrupted sutures. The results of surgery for recurrent interdigital neuroma are far poorer than for a primary neuroma [Beskin and Baxter 1988].

Postoperative care

Following primary operations using a dorsal incision, patients are told to stay at home for a few days using a wooden-soled postoperative shoe and crutches. The compression dressing is removed after the second or third day and the incision covered with an adhesive dressing. Activities are restricted until the skin wound has healed. Generally, walking activities

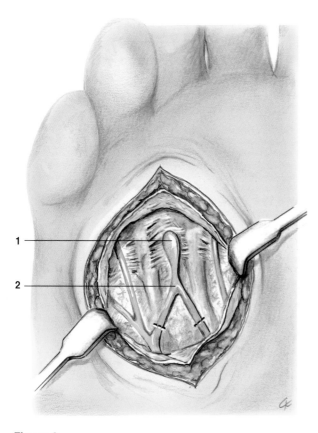

Figure 6

The intact nerve is explored proximally and then traced distally to the neuroma stump. The proximal branches of the digital nerve are excised and the remaining portion of the nerve is removed

1 Neuroma
2 Common plantar digital nerve

are restricted for about 2 weeks and running or jogging for about 4–6 weeks.

Patients having a revision operation through a plantar incision may be placed in a short leg cast which is split in the recovery room. The patient uses crutches and is partial weightbearing for 10–14 days, whereupon they return for suture removal. Patients can weightbear on the healed incision. However, if the patient is complaining of pain, a short leg walking cast is used for about another week; if the patient is relatively asymptomatic, a postoperative wooden-soled shoe or an inexpensive stiff athletic shoe can be used. Should the plantar approach be used for a primary neuroma, a compression dressing can be applied for the first week. When it appears that the incision is healing uneventfully, the patient can progress to the usual postoperative shoe.

Complications

Any possible complication associated with a soft-tissue operation on the foot can occur from this procedure. Therefore, one must discuss with the patient such potential complications as delayed wound healing, infection, hematoma formation, neurovascular damage and deep venous thrombosis as a result of using a tourniquet, complications due to the anesthesia and systemic complications of any type which may or may not be related to the operation. The most dreaded complication is the failure of the operation, with the patient having continued pain or recurrence of the original pain.

References

Beskin JL, Baxter DE (1988) Recurrent pain following interdigital neurectomy – a plantar approach. Foot Ankle 9: 34–39

Betts LO (1940) Morton's metatarsalgia, neuritis of fourth digital nerve. Med J Aust 1: 514–515

Diebold PF, Daum B, Dang-Vu V, Litchinko M (1996) True epineural neurolysis in Morton's neuroma: a 5-year follow-up. Orthopedics 19: 397–400

Friscia DA, Strom DE, Parr JW et al. (1991) Surgical treatment for primary interdigital neuroma. Orthopedics 14: 669–672

Gauthier G (1979) Thomas Morton's disease: a nerve entrapment syndrome. Clin Orthop 142: 90–92

Johnson JE, Johnson KA, Unni KK (1988) Persistent pain after excision of an interdigital neuroma – results of reoperation. J Bone Joint Surg 70A: 651–657

Lassmann G (1979) Morton's toe: clinical, light and electron microscopic investigations in 133 cases. Clin Orthop 142: 73–84

Mann RA, Reynolds JD (1983) Interdigital neuroma: a critical clinical analysis. Foot Ankle 3: 238–243

Morton TG (1876) A peculiar and painful affection of the fourth metatarsophalangeal articulation. Am J Med Sci 71: 37–45 (reprinted in Clin Orthop 142: 4–9, 1979)

Mulder JD (1951) The causative mechanism in Morton's metatarsalgia. J Bone Joint Surg 33B: 94–95

Thomas N, Nissen KI, Helal B (1988) Disorders of the lesser rays. In: Helal B, Wilson D (eds). The Foot. Edinburgh, Churchill Livingstone, pp 484–510

19

Toenail abnormalities and infections

Wendy Benton-Weil
Lowell Scott Weil Sr

Introduction

Toenail abnormalities and infections are among the most disabling disorders of the foot. The normal nail consists of the nail plate, the nail bed, the nail matrix and supporting soft-tissue structures (Figure 1). The matrix is a specialized region that synthesizes nail plate substance. It extends proximally about 5 mm underneath the proximal nail fold. Toenails grow at a rate of less than 0.1 mm a day. Growth can be influenced by circulatory disturbances, infection, nutritional abnormalities, trauma, internal and external factors, and by poor techniques of nail cutting.

The most common abnormalities of the toenails are paronychia, chronic incurvated toenails, hypertrophied toenails, onychomycosis, painful nails associated with cartilage or bony abnormalities, and subungual hematoma. Less common, but often misdiagnosed, is subungual melanoma.

Paronychia

Paronychia or infected ingrown toenail is among the most common conditions seen in a foot and ankle practice. The condition is more prevalent in young people, but may be present in all ages. The toenail of the hallux is most commonly affected, but lesser digits may be involved as well.

Often, the history relates to improper cutting of the nail – tearing the toenail instead of using sharp clippers, thereby leaving a jagged edge to penetrate the nail groove. Hereditary tendencies toward incurvated nails and shoes with tight toe-boxes are also commonly seen. If the infection becomes chronic and fails to heal, squamous cell carcinoma should be ruled out.

Individuals often present with a draining, inflamed nail lip with a deeply imbedded nail plate. The use of systemic antibiotics in such conditions is unnecessary except in the medically compromised patient. Treatment consists of removing the part of the nail plate that pierces the nail groove, which is the nidus of the infection (Figure 2). Conservative measures such as soaking for half-hour sessions with magnesium sulfate (Epsom salts) and gently pulling back on the nail lip may show some success, allowing the nail plate eventually to proceed distally. This method of treatment, however, should not be used for more than a few days. If the paronychia persists, partial nail avulsion should be undertaken.

Technique for drainage of paronychia

Following digital blockade at the base of the toe, a nail splitter is used to remove approximately 5 mm of nail plate from the offending portion (Figure 2). The nail is split from the distal portion in a proximal direction and the procedure is often completed with a small Beaver blade (no. 61 or 64). A small, straight mosquito hemostat is then used to grasp the cut portion of the nail, gripping the nail firmly at the nail root and proximal portion. This portion of nail may then be 'rolled out', removing the entire offending segment. It is not usually necessary to cut or cauterize any of the 'proud flesh' or remove any

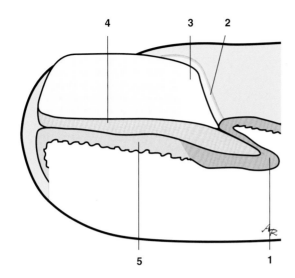

Figure 1

Anatomy of the nail

1 Nail matrix
2 Eponychium
3 Lunula
4 Nail plate
5 Nail bed

of the soft tissue following this procedure, as this just causes more bleeding and postoperative discomfort. The peripheral swelling adjacent to the infected nail will quickly reduce once the offending portion has been removed. In cases where both margins of the nail are infected, the procedure is performed on both the medial and the lateral sides. When the entire eponychium is involved (i.e. onychia), it is best to avulse the entire toenail. Following its removal, the area is packed with an antibiotic ointment and, in severe cases, a 0.5-cm gauze drain. Most patients do not require a drain and a simple sterile gauze dressing is all that is needed.

Postoperatively, patients are requested to soak the toe through the bandage for 30 min twice on the evening of the procedure and once on the following morning. By midday, they may remove the bandage and soak the toe on one more occasion. Topical use of alcohol, antibiotic ointment and good hygiene are all that is necessary thereafter. In normal, healthy patients, systemic antibiotics do not need to be prescribed following this procedure.

Chronic incurvated nails

Incision and drainage as described above are always performed first, allowing the patient a chance that the nail will grow properly and the ingrown nail will

not recur. In some cases, however, in spite of a patient's judicious efforts to cut the nail properly, chronic incurvated and painful nails can occur. The exact etiology is unknown, although tight shoes, stockings and impingement in and around the nail certainly have a great influence on the chronicity of an incurvated nail.

Although external factors have a great influence, genetic incurvated nails have been observed in many families. Onychomycosis may also cause a thickening of the nail, with resulting increased pressure in the nail grooves. Physical examination often reveals a thickened and convoluted appearance of the nail plate. The general circulatory status should always be assessed prior to any invasive procedure of the toenails. Appropriate foot care and palliative reduction of the offending portion of nail may be performed at regular intervals. A partial avulsion of the distal one-third of the nail is effective in reducing symptoms for up to 8 weeks. As the nail grows forward, however, symptoms often recur. When patients render a history of multiple infections and previous treatments, then partial surgical ablation of the nail is appropriate.

Phenol ablation for the chronically incurvated toenail

Although operative techniques for ingrown nails have been in use since the 1920s, the application of 89% phenol (carbolic acid) has now become a popular method of eradicating an ingrown toenail [Nyman 1956]. Under digital blockade, a tourniquet is placed around the base of the toe. It is essential to have a bloodless field so as not to dilute the 89% solution of phenol. Approximately 5 mm is removed from the edge of the nail toward the central portion, using a nail splitter and a small Beaver blade. Special attention is paid to avoiding injury to the eponychium. The severed portion of the nail plate is then carefully freed from the underlying nail bed and nail root, and gently lifted from the toe using a twisting method with a straight hemostat. In cases of a thickened incurvated nail, the nail root is then abraded with a small curette to remove any keratotic or fungal particles. A dry cotton swab is then used to clean and thoroughly dry the nail groove. Small swabs of cotton are dipped into the phenol and then inserted into the nail groove and rolled into the nail matrix area (Figure 3). The swab is held in place for approximately 30 s, then a second cotton swab is placed into the groove in a similar fashion. Two 30-s maneuvers are usually

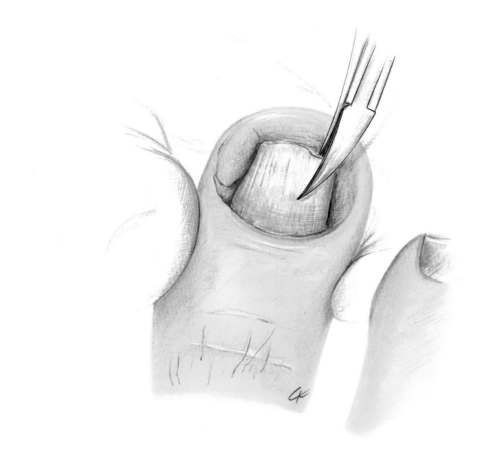

Figure 2

Paronychia with a draining, inflamed nail lip is drained, removing approximately 5 mm of nail plate from the offending portion

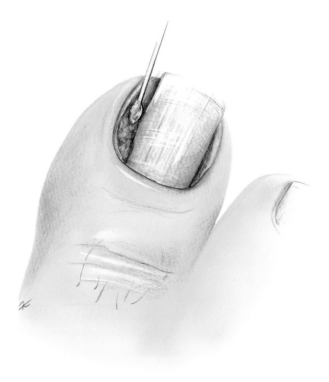

Figure 3

Chronic incurvated nails are treated by phenol ablation. An 89% solution of phenol is applied with a cotton swab following removal of approximately 5 mm of nail edge

sufficient to sterilize the nail matrix. Following phenol application, some practitioners prefer to use alcohol to rinse the nail groove. The use of a dry cotton swab and antibiotic cream packing within the nail groove may be preferable. The tourniquet is then removed and the toe wrapped in a thick gauze bandage.

The bandage is left in place until the following morning, when the patient is asked to remove the bandage and bathe the toe. Bathing is carried on twice daily and the patient is instructed to scrub the affected area vigorously, thereby providing mechanical debridement of the nail groove. Continuous use of the antibiotic cream twice daily, covered with a bandage, is all that is necessary for postoperative care. A hydrocortisone 1% cream can also be used to reduce inflammation. Postoperative oral antibiotics are not needed in the healthy patient and typically healing occurs within 14–21 days. During that time, serous drainage may back up within the nail groove, causing inflammation of the eponychium. If this occurs, the patient is instructed to clean out the nail groove vigorously and wear a loose-fitting shoe for a few days. Using the phenol method of matricectomy, success rates of over 90% can be expected with very few complications.

A small percentage of patients are sensitive to phenol, and reactions can occur. Most often these are caused by the attempt of the patient to wear a tighter shoe, thereby closing the nail grooves and not allowing for adequate drainage. This can quickly be remedied by a loose-fitting shoe and soaking three times daily.

The advantage of the phenol procedure is that no incision or suturing is needed. The patient is allowed to bathe the toe on the following day. Other incisional procedures for ablation of chronically incurvated toenails may result in an infection rate approaching 20% with significant postoperative pain, compared with the phenol procedure. Occasionally, a small barb or spicule of nail may regrow in the previously sterilized nail groove. When this occurs, it can often be removed without anesthesia and one or two drops of phenol placed into the cavity. Less commonly performed matricectomies include the use of sodium hydroxide or CO_2 laser in lieu of the phenol and alcohol.

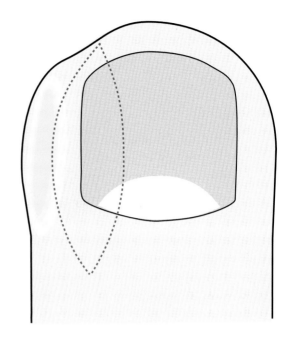

Figure 4

Incisions for Winograd procedure

Winograd procedure for hypertrophied nail lip and incurvated nail

Occasionally, along with a history of chronic incurvated nails, a patient will develop a significantly hypertrophied nail lip. If this nail lip is also painful or contributing to the pathology, a Winograd procedure may be considered.

An incision is made 5 mm into the nail plate and extended approximately 1 cm proximal to the eponychium (Figure 4). A second semi-elliptical incision is made in the hypertrophied nail fold. The incisions are carried down to the level of bone, excising the nail plate, nail matrix and hypertrophied nail lip. The nail matrix is then rasped to prevent recurrent regrowth of the nail plate. The operative site may either be sutured with simple sutures or be Steri-stripped to approximate the nail lip to the nail margin.

Hypertrophied nails

Hypertrophied nails, also known as onychauxis and onychogryphosis, often appear worse than they feel. These conditions can be caused by trauma. Dropping a heavy object on the nail may result in loss of the entire toenail, and the succeeding nail regrows much thicker. Some patients with onychogryphosis have nails 1 cm thick, which are painful when attempting to squeeze into a normal

shoe. For the most part these conditions are shoe related, in that a higher toe box will afford more comfort, and reduction of the thickness of the toenail often reduces symptoms. Palliative care consists of using a burr on a small rotary hobby drill. The nail is then ground and thinned, allowing for more comfort in footwear. Patients can use a fine wood file bought at a hardware store to reduce the thickness of their toenails. This has proved to be very successful and alleviates their symptoms at little cost. The mere presence of a hypertrophied nail should not be construed as something pathological that must be treated by avulsion or ablation. Total nail ablation is not usually recommended. Palliative treatment is preferred unless the patient absolutely insists on removing the nail. Only in patients having constant and chronic infections should nail ablation be carried out. This is done by removing the entire nail and cauterizing the nail bed and nail matrix with 89% phenol. Three to four months are required before the nail bed is completely healed. Cosmetically, the result is remarkably good. The postoperative course is similar to that for partial nail ablation. In cases of previous failures of nail ablation or surgical revisions of a badly scarred nail groove, a terminal Syme's amputation is successful in alleviating the symptoms at the cost of a disfigured and shortened toe. Surgical excision of the nail bed and matrix has been virtually abandoned.

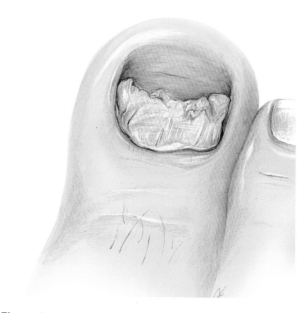

Figure 5

Onychomycosis of the hallux

Onychomycosis

Onychomycosis can be most disturbing to patients (Figure 5). Although fungal nails can be worrisome and offensive to the beholder, they truly are rarely a problem from a medical standpoint. The fungus penetrates the hyponychium and results in thickening, discoloration, onycholysis, dystrophy and/or subungual debris of the nail. Dermatophytes cause over 90% of fungal nails, the most common of which is *Trichophyton rubrum*. Superficially white nails are usually caused by *Trichophyton mentagrophtyes*. *Candida albicans*, other yeasts, and non-dermatophyte molds cause the other 10% of onychomycoses. If there is pitting involvement of the nails, psoriasis should also be considered. On some occasions the chronicity of a fungal nail condition can cause local manifestations of tinea pedis to endure; however, for the most part fungal nails are a harmless condition best treated by benign neglect rather than aggressive intervention. Many articles have been written in magazines and newspapers describing new fungal nail cures using oral medication. However, the cost is prohibitive for most people, the cure rate is less than 70% and the recurrence rate is greater than 30% following completion of a course of oral medication. Reports on the use of laser penetration of the nails followed by local medications have not been confirmed by controlled studies, and certainly avulsion of all of the toenails is a radical procedure. For those insisting on treating these conditions, the use of one of the

antifungal antibiotics for 90 days may be appropriate. Itraconazole and terbinafine appear to work best on the dermatophytes, whereas itraconazole, ketoconazole and fluconazole are most effective in *Candida* infection. Finally, in cases of pityrosporum infection the azoles are most effective. Side-effects such as liver dysfunction and drug sensitivity, as well as cost, should be considered for all.

Painful nails associated with cartilage and bony abnormalities

Conditions such as osteoma or osteochondroma often present with an unusual picture of a painful nail (see Chapter 45). This condition is often misdiagnosed as a subungual wart or periungual fibroma. Any discoloration, lump or bump, or enlargement beneath the toenail warrants two radiographic views. This is especially true in the second decade of life, when osteochondroma appears to be most prevalent. An osteochondroma and a subungual exostosis can appear similar on radiographs. Subungual exostoses usually affect adult women with a painful incurvated nail, whereas an osteochondroma usually affects males in the second and third decades. A definitive diagnosis can only be made histologically. The exostosis will have trabeculation with a fibrocartilaginous distal portion. Osteochondromas have a hyaline cartilaginous cap. Osteochondromas have a 10% malignant transformation rate. When a cartilaginous or bony lesion is discovered, aggressive removal of the bony prominence is necessary to avoid recurrence.

Technique for subungual exostosis or osteochondroma

The following approach gives a much better cosmetic result than more traditional and radical approaches. A 'fish-mouth' incision is made at the distal portion of the toe and sharp dissection is carried to the bony prominence, which is carefully dissected free from the overlying nail bed. The bony or cartilaginous prominence often penetrates through the nail bed directly into the nail plate. If this is the case, the nail plate is usually left intact to protect the bed during postoperative healing. Once the prominence is completely isolated, a large resection is undertaken, removing approximately 3–4 mm of the normal underlying bone adjacent to the lesion. This additional removal or 'saucering' of the bone will lessen the chances of recurrence. In cases of

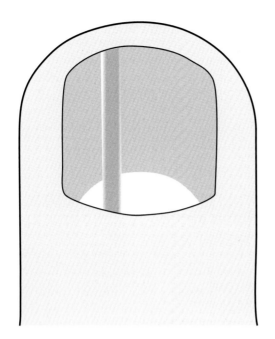

Figure 6

Pigmented band, which may be a melanoma

revision of these lesions, it is sometimes necessary to remove the entire tuft of the distal phalanx to avoid recurrence.

Subungual hematoma, black toenails and melanoma

The growing interest in physical activity and fitness has resulted in an increased incidence of black toenails and subungual hematomas. Although subungual hematoma often results directly from a traumatic episode such as a heavy object dropping on the toenail, repetitive microtrauma can also cause this condition. In traumatic cases, 25% may involve underlying distal phalanx fractures. Immediate drilling of the nail with a fine drill to release the subungual bleeding should be performed. Most often it is not necessary to anesthetize the toe, as the drilling of this area is relatively painless. Protective eyewear should be used, as often a geyser of blood comes spewing out as soon as the nail plate has been penetrated. A simpler alternative to the fine drill is using a flamed 18-gauge needle to penetrate

the nail plate. A small gauze dressing is then placed on the nail to absorb any further hematoma. The patient is allowed to bathe the following day. The nail is usually lost within 1–2 months, but a new nail grows in and pain relief is immediate. Black toenails caused by jogging, rock climbing or similar sports are a common disorder. Although often attributed to tight shoes, this condition can occur in patients with adequately sized shoes. The etiology involves a separation of the nail bed from the nail plate. A simple method of treatment uses a petroleum jelly lubricant placed directly on the toenails, covered with an athletic sock, and then a second layer of lubricant is applied on top of the sock over the toenails as well. This double layer of petroleum jelly both under and on top of the sock provides enough lubrication to avoid a black toenail.

A differential diagnosis of black toenails should include bleeding from a subungual verruca and, more importantly, malignant melanoma. A melanoma may also appear as a pigmented band (Figure 6). In Blacks and Asians pigmented bands are common and increase with age, but in Caucasians the bands should be considered pathological. Early diagnosis and biopsy are imperative.

Bibliography

Costello P (1960) Diseases of the Nails, 3rd edn. Springfield, Thomas

Daly JM, Berlin R, Urmacher C (1987) Subungual melanoma: a 25-year review of cases. J Surg Oncol 35: 107

Farrington GH (1964) Subungual hematoma: an evaluation of treatment. Br Med J 21: 742–744

Nuzuzi S, Positano R, DeLauro T (1989) Nail Disorders. Clinics in Podiatric Medicine and Surgery. Philadelphia, Saunders

Nyman SP (1956) The phenol-alcohol technique for toenail excision. J NJ Chirop 50: 5–14

Scher R, Daniel C (1990) Nails: Therapy, Diagnosis, and Treatments. Philadelphia, Saunders

Winograd AM (1929) A modification in technique of operation for ingrown toenail. J Am Med Assoc 91: 229–230

Zalas N (1980) The Nail. Jamaica, NY, Spectrum

20

Midfoot fractures and dislocations

Rudolf Reschauer
Wolf Fröhlich

Midfoot fractures

Injuries to the midfoot are rare and often neglected. These lesions represent 1% of all fractures and 2–5% of all fractures of the ankle and foot. Inadequate treatment of these injuries, which are often combined with severe soft-tissue trauma, often results in painful foot deformity and severe disturbance of gait [Rockwood and Green 1975, Chapman 1978, Goldman 1989, Klenerman 1991, Zwipp et al. 1991, DeLee 1992].

The midfoot is defined as the anatomical area between Chopart's joint and the tarsometatarsal joints, i.e. the Lisfranc joint line. It consists of the tarsal navicular, the cuboid and the three cuneiform bones. This central segment of the foot is secured by strong plantar ligaments which largely prevent motion. Biomechanically, a medial and a lateral column can be differentiated. The medial column consists of the talus, the navicular, the three cuneiforms and the medial three metatarsals. The lateral column consists of the calcaneus, the cuboid and the lateral two metatarsals. Traumatic shortening of the lateral column, e.g. in comminution of the cuboid, results in relative lengthening of the medial column. This leads to a loss of ligament function and to disturbance of foot alignment.

Midfoot fractures are generally produced by a fall from a height, the trapping of a foot between the pedals in a road traffic accident, or direct impact caused by deformation of the passenger cabin. Axial compression during deceleration or a direct force may impact the calcaneus, cuboid, navicular or the talar head.

Clinical signs and symptoms consist of pain, swelling and point tenderness at the dorsal aspect of the foot. Three standard radiographs must be obtained: a dorsoplantar radiograph tilted 20° posteriorly, a straight lateral projection of the foot, and a 45° lateral to medial oblique view of the foot.

Midfoot fractures may be divided into five groups, according to the type and the direction of the injury force [Main and Jowett 1975]: medially directed, laterally directed, longitudinal, plantarward crushing, and crush injury. Alternatively, six types may be differentiated according to the direction of the dislocating force and to the effect on bones and on ligaments [Zwipp 1994]: transligamentous, transnavicular, transcalcaneal, transtalar, transcuboidal and transnaviculocuboidal.

Treatment

All closed ligamentous injuries with subluxation or dislocation without bone involvement may be treated conservatively, if they can be reduced and are stable after reduction. Reduction is performed under spinal anesthesia using Chinese finger traps for longitudinal traction. Dislocated joints are reduced with manual pressure. In a stable injury a split below-knee cast is applied, followed

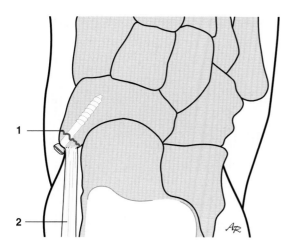

Figure 1

Tuberosity fractures of the navicular are stabilized with a small-fragment cancellous screw if displacement exceeds 3 mm

1 Fracture
2 Posterior tibial tendon

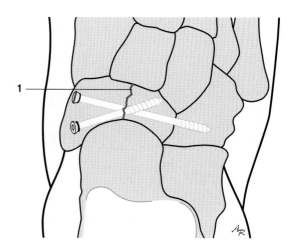

Figure 2

Displaced fractures of the navicular body are stabilized with two cancellous screws. Fixation into the cuboid is sometimes necessary

1 Fracture

by a walking cast for 6–8 weeks. All stable and undisplaced fractures are also treated conservatively. Dislocations that are unstable after reduction are stabilized with three to five percutaneous Kirschner wires, 1.4–1.8 mm in diameter, followed by cast immobilization for 6 weeks. The Kirschner wires are removed after 6 weeks. Dislocations that cannot be reduced by closed methods require open reduction. Standard incisions are longitudinal, midline, dorsal or dorsolateral.

Fracture of the navicular tuberosity

Fractures of the navicular tuberosity (Figure 1) are avulsion fractures that result from acute eversion of the foot, leading to sudden tension on the posterior tibial tendon. This fracture is usually not displaced, owing to the strong ligaments in this region. It is important to distinguish tuberosity fractures from an os tibiale externum. Displaced fractures are rare. They are found mainly in combination with compression injuries of the lateral column.

Once swelling has decreased, a short leg walking cast is applied for 6 weeks. If displacement of more than 3 mm is present, operative treatment should be considered. This is performed through a slightly curved incision placed medially over the tuberosity of the navicular. Following reduction, the fragment is stabilized with a small-fragment cancellous screw (Figure 1).

In case of a painful non-union, excision of the bony fragment is performed using the same

approach. The navicular surface is roughened and the tendon is sutured to the periosteum in the area, followed by immobilization of the foot in a below-knee cast for 4 weeks.

Dorsal chip fracture of the navicular

A dorsal chip fracture is usually produced by acute plantarflexion and inversion of the foot, resulting in a dorsal avulsion fracture of the navicular by the talonavicular ligament. This injury is often associated with a lateral ankle sprain or with fractures of the cuboid and of the anterior process of the calcaneus.

If there is no additional ligamentous instability or fracture, these injuries can be treated with a short leg walking cast for 4 weeks. As a complication, a dorsal osteophyte may develop at the navicular, and this may become symptomatic when the patient is wearing shoes. In this case, operative excision of the osteophyte is indicated.

Fracture of the navicular body

Isolated body fractures of the navicular without dislocation are rare. Displaced and comminuted fractures of the navicular body regularly occur in transtalar fracture dislocations of Chopart's joint. The degree of comminution and displacement depends on the direction and the magnitude of the resulting axial compression force. The talonavicular joint, which is the central pivot of all motions at the subtalar joint, is always involved.

Undisplaced fractures of the navicular body are treated conservatively by immobilization for 6 weeks in a below-knee walking cast. Displaced fractures require open reduction through a dorso-medial longitudinal approach over the navicular. The fracture is stabilized with two cancellous screws inserted from the medial aspect (Figure 2). Comminuted fractures are often found in transnavicular fracture dislocations. They require careful anatomic reconstruction of the medial column and of the surface of the talonavicular joint.

An 8–10-cm longitudinal incision across the talonavicular joint is used. This gives good exposure and minimizes soft tissue damage. Following exposure of the joint and of the comminuted area, the fracture must be disimpacted and the length of the medial column restored, using careful direct manipulation and valgus stress. A mini-distractor can be used to facilitate exposure of the fracture and restoration of length. The pins of the distractor are anchored in the talus and in the first metatarsal. Large dislocated fragments are reduced and temporarily stabilized with small wires. Smaller impacted fragments are pushed into the surrounding bone for reduction. In bone defects a cancellous or corticocancellous bone graft may have to be used to increase stability and to expedite union. Final fixation is achieved with Kirschner wires or with small-fragment screws. They may have to be anchored in the bones adjacent to the navicular, e.g. in the cuboid in case of a small lateral fracture fragment. A below-knee walking cast is used for 6 weeks postoperatively. Kirschner wires are removed after 6 weeks, followed by rehabilitation exercises. Full weightbearing with an arch support is achieved after 12 weeks.

Cuneiform fractures

Fractures of the cuneiform bones are rare. Displacement is unusual. The injury is usually produced by direct trauma. Pain and swelling in the area of the injury are the main symptoms.

In non-displaced fractures a short leg walking cast is used for 6 weeks, followed by a longitudinal arch support. In displaced fractures, which may be combined with tarsometatarsal dislocations, a dorsomedial approach is used for reduction, as described later.

Fractures and dislocations of the cuboid and the lateral column

Isolated fractures of the cuboid are produced by a direct force on to the lateral column. Shortening of the lateral column and ligamentous instability only rarely follow this injury. After the swelling has decreased a short leg walking cast is applied for 6 weeks.

Fractures of the cuboid with dislocation of the calcaneocuboid joint are caused by axial compression and simultaneous forefoot abduction. This mechanism results in ligamentous injury and avulsion fracture at the talonavicular joint and simultaneously compresses the cuboid between the base of the fifth metatarsal and the anterior process of the calcaneus. This injury is also referred to as a 'nutcracker' fracture [Koch and Rahimi 1991]. Surgery is usually indicated to correct shortening of the lateral column.

The incision is placed longitudinally over the calcaneocuboid joint. Injury to the sural nerve must be avoided during subcutaneous dissection. Adduction of the forefoot with a distractor, which is anchored in the fifth metatarsal and in the calcaneus, provides exposure of the joint, of the cuboid and of the anterior process of the calcaneus. The impacted fragments of the cuboidal joint surface must be elevated and disimpacted. The joint surface of the calcaneus is used as a template to reconstruct the cuboidal joint surface. Bone defects must be filled with cancellous or corticocancellous bone graft, the latter providing better stability. Large fragments are fixed with small-fragment screws which are directed parallel to the calcaneocuboidal joint surface. Alternatively, a small lateral buttress plate can be used for stabilization (Figure 3).

Postoperative immobilization in a below-knee walking cast is required for 6–8 weeks. After removal of the Kirschner wires, full weightbearing is allowed after 12 weeks, using a longitudinal arch support.

Tarsometatarsal (Lisfranc) fracture–dislocation

The tarsometatarsal joint consists of the three cuneiforms, the cuboid and the five metatarsal bones. The three medial metatarsals articulate with the three cuneiforms individually. The fourth and fifth metatarsals articulate with the cuboid. The second metatarsal is the center of the Lisfranc joint, because it reaches further proximally and is anchored between the first and third cuneiforms. No dislocation of the metatarsals can occur without involvement of the articulation between the second metatarsal and the second cuneiform.

Additional stability is provided by ligamentous structures. The bases of the second, third, fourth and

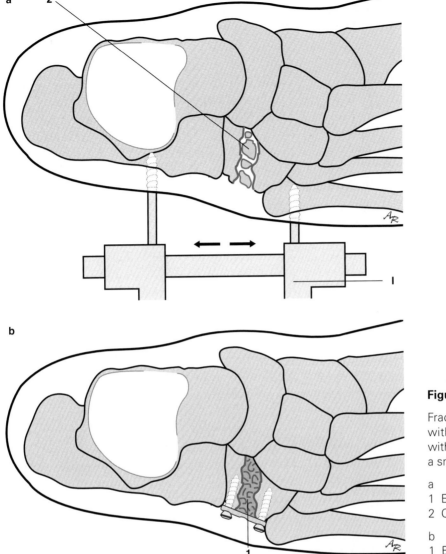

Figure 3

Fracture of the cuboid. a. reduction with an external fixator; b. fixation with corticocancellous bone graft and a small lateral buttress plate

a
1 External fixator
2 Cuboid fracture

b
1 Bone graft

fifth metatarsals are linked by transverse ligaments at the dorsal and the plantar aspect of the joint. The plantar ligaments are much stronger than the dorsal ligaments. There is no ligament between the bases of the first and second metatarsals. The four lesser metatarsals are attached to the first cuneiform by an oblique plantar and dorsal ligament, which is referred to as Lisfranc's ligament. A sudden abduction force may lead to a rupture or bony avulsion of the ligament, or to a fracture at the base of the second metatarsal, which permits lateral dislocation of the foot to occur. The first metatarsal is anchored to the first cuneiform by ligaments in an axial orientation. The insertions of the tibialis anterior, tibialis posterior and peroneus longus tendons provide additional stability. The plantar fascia, the short plantar flexor muscles and the strong plantar tarso-metatarsal ligaments prevent plantar dislocation of the tarsometatarsal joint. The dorsal ligaments of the foot are more vulnerable to injury; dorsal and lateral dislocations are therefore more common.

The branch of the dorsalis pedis artery to the plantar arterial arch is located in the first web space and is at risk in tarsometatarsal dislocations.

Etiology and pathogenesis

Tarsometatarsal injuries result from a combination of forces with rotation around the long axis of the foot. These injuries may occur with or without fracture, depending on the rotational forces that are simultaneously present.

Most tarsometatarsal dislocations are produced by indirect forces, resulting in dorsal dislocation and medial or lateral displacement of the metatarsals. A direct force, such as a weight dropped on to the foot, results in plantar dislocation of the metatarsals. Additional medial or lateral displacement may occur, depending on the direction of the injury force. Extensive soft-tissue damage and multiple associated fractures may be present.

Lateral dislocation of the forefoot can be produced by pronation of the hindfoot with a fixed forefoot [Jeffreys 1963]. Supination of the hindfoot with a fixed forefoot may result in medial dislocation of the first metatarsocuneiform joint. Complete dislocation of the forefoot may follow fractures of the second metatarsal.

Violent abduction or plantarflexion of the forefoot may also produce tarsometatarsal dislocation [Wiley 1971]. The abduction force is centered on the fixed base of the second metatarsal, leading to a fracture of the second metatarsal, followed by dislocation of the remaining metatarsals. Significant lateral displacement of the metatarsals may result in a crush fracture of the cuboid bone. Dorsal dislocation may follow axial compression of the plantarflexed foot, such as during a fall or a road traffic accident.

Pronation may initially produce isolated medial dislocation of the first metatarsal, followed by dorsolateral dislocation of the lateral four metatarsals [Wilson 1972]. This is referred to as a divergent dislocation. Supination may initially produce dorsolateral dislocation of up to four of the lateral metatarsal bones, followed by dorsolateral dislocation of all five metatarsals.

Clinical and radiographic features

Obvious deformity is usually present. This consists of forefoot equinus, forefoot abduction and prominence of the medial aspect of the midfoot. Plantar dislocation results in clawing of the toes with impaired active extension, due to relative shortening of the flexors. Gross swelling of the foot may occur within a few hours following the injury. Shortening and displacement of the forefoot may be less obvious once swelling has developed. Marked joint line tenderness and pain on passive motion are present. The dorsalis pedis pulse is often hardly palpable, and this requires Doppler examination to rule out a vascular lesion. Neurological deficits may develop, owing to swelling and compartment syndrome.

Anteroposterior, lateral and 30° oblique radiographs are taken. In normal anatomy, the interspaces between the first and fourth metatarsals are continuous with the respective intertarsal spaces at the cuneiforms and the cuboid. This relationship is disturbed in tarsometatarsal dislocations.

Classification

The following injuries can be differentiated [Hardcastle et al. 1982]:

- Type A is incongruity of the entire tarsometatarsal joint. Displacement is in one plane, which may be sagittal, coronal or combined.
- Type B is partial incongruity of the tarsometatarsal joint. Displacement is also in one plane, which may be sagittal, coronal or combined. Partial medial dislocation affects the first metatarsal either alone or in combination with the second, third or fourth metatarsals. Partial lateral dislocation affects one or more of the lateral four metatarsals.
- Type C is divergent incongruity, which may be partial or complete. On the anteroposterior radiograph the first metatarsal is displaced medially and any combination of the lateral four metatarsals is displaced laterally. Sagittal displacement also occurs in conjunction with displacement in the frontal plane.

Treatment

Restoration of a painless and stable plantigrade foot is the goal in the treatment of tarsometatarsal fracture–dislocations. Anatomic reduction is a prerequisite for normal foot function. Closed reduction must be attempted as soon as possible after the injury. Reduction will be easier the sooner it is carried out. However, an avulsed bone fragment or a trapped tendon may impede closed reduction.

Closed reduction using a wedge

The patient is placed in the supine position with the foot reaching beyond the end of the operating table. The knee is flexed 90°. The foot is placed on a wedge so that the dislocation is distal to the tip of the wedge. The tibia is stabilized manually and traction is applied to the forefoot and the toes to restore length. When the metatarsals are out to length, they are manipulated into their anatomic position by plantar pressure.

Closed reduction using the edge of the table

The patient is placed in the supine position with the knee extended. The Achilles tendon is placed over the protected edge of the table. The tibia is stabilized against the surface of the table and longitudinal traction is applied by pulling on the metatarsals

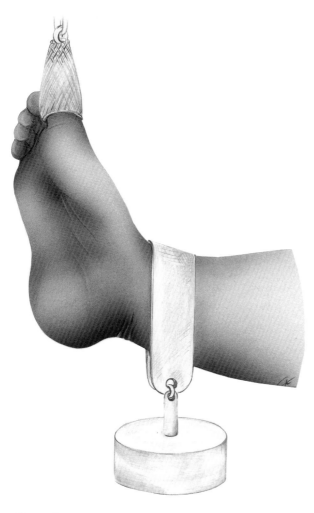

Figure 4

Reduction of tarsometatarsal dislocation with longitudinal traction

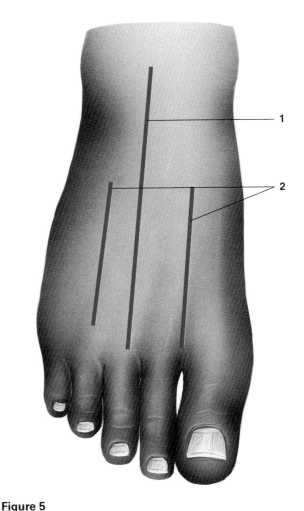

Figure 5

Skin incisions for open reduction and internal fixation of tarsometatarsal dislocations and fractures. 1. single incision; 2. double incision

distally, followed by forceful plantarflexion to achieve reduction.

Closed reduction with a traction device

The patient is positioned supine with the knee flexed. Chinese finger traps are applied to the toes (Figure 4). A counterweight of approximately 5 kg is placed around the ankle. Once the tarsometatarsal length is restored, manipulation in the dorsoplantar direction is performed.

Radiographs are obtained to document the reduction. Reduction of each of the metatarsals to their respective cuneiform or to the cuboid must be obtained.

Fixation

Once closed reduction is obtained, percutaneous Kirschner wires are required for stabilization.

Protrusion of the wires through the skin should be avoided to prevent secondary infection. In type A injuries with total incongruity one Kirschner wire is placed from the first metatarsal to the first cuneiform bone, and a second wire from the fifth metatarsal laterally to the cuboid. In type B injuries with partial displacement a single Kirschner wire is needed in displacement of the lateral segment. If the first metatarsal is displaced, the injury is grossly unstable and two wires are required. In type C injuries with divergent displacement, one or two Kirschner wires are used to stabilize the first metatarsal, with another single wire for the lateral metatarsals.

Following reduction and stabilization the foot is placed in a split short leg cast for 1 week. After 1 week a short leg cast with a well-moulded arch is applied and weightbearing is allowed. The cast and the pins are removed after 6–8 weeks. The foot is placed in a shoe with a longitudinal arch support for an additional 12 months.

Open reduction and internal fixation

Open reduction and internal fixation are indicated if anatomic reduction cannot be obtained by closed means. Under spinal anesthesia and with the patient in the supine position, the foot is placed beyond the end of the operating table. A tourniquet is applied but not inflated.

One or two longitudinal incisions are made to provide adequate exposure and to prevent skin necrosis (Figure 5). In the single incision technique a dorsal midline incision is used from the ankle joint to the distal end of the second intermetatarsal space. The subcutaneous tissues are divided with care to protect the cutaneous branches of the superficial peroneal nerve. In the double incision technique the first incision starts between the first and second metatarsals and ends proximal to the first tarsometatarsal joint. This incision provides good exposure of the first and second tarsometatarsal joints. For exposure of the remaining tarsometatarsal joints, a parallel longitudinal incision is made between the third and fourth metatarsals with a length of approximately 8 cm in a proximal direction. The interval between the two incisions must be at least 4.5 cm wide to avoid skin necrosis. When dividing the subcutaneous tissues the cutaneous branches of the superficial peroneus nerve must not be injured.

Reduction begins at the second metatarsal, which is situated between the first and third cuneiforms and provides a landmark for the adjacent metatarsals (Figure 6). The first metatarsal is reduced after the second. The extensor hallucis brevis muscle, the extensor hallucis longus and anterior tibial tendons, and the neurovascular bundle with the dorsalis pedis artery and the deep peroneal nerve are retracted medially. The extensor digitorum longus and extensor digitorum brevis tendons are retracted laterally.

If fractured, the base of the second metatarsal must be anatomically reconstructed with small Kirschner wires before it is reduced to the second cuneiform. In this case, the Kirschner wire used for stabilization of the joint is introduced longitudinally into the shaft of the second metatarsal in a distal direction to exit through the skin, and then advanced proximally into the second cuneiform. If 3.5-mm cortical screws are used for fixation of the tarsometatarsal joint, a small groove on the dorsum of the second metatarsal is made 1.5 cm distal to the joint, to avoid prominence of the screw head.

The 2.5-mm drill must be directed strictly tangential to the metatarsal into the cuneiform.

At the first metatarsal, the extensor hallucis longus tendon is retracted medially. Following anatomic reduction a Kirschner wire may be used for fixation, as mentioned above. If a cortical screw is used, temporary fixation with Kirschner wires is advised.

Following fixation of the first and second metatarsals, the third ray is exposed and stabilized in the same manner. At the fourth and fifth tarsometatarsal joints the screws must cross the cuboidometatarsal joint in a perpendicular orientation. For insertion of a screw into the fifth metatarsal an additional small stab incision is generally needed.

The skin is closed only if this is possible without undue tension. In case of marked swelling the skin is left open and the wound is temporarily covered with a skin substitute. After 4–6 days stepwise delayed closure is usually possible and a skin graft is only rarely needed.

Postoperative care

If Kirschner wires are used for fixation, a split short leg cast is applied for 10 days. At that time the skin sutures are removed and a short leg weightbearing cast is applied until 6 weeks postoperatively. The Kirschner wires are then removed and physiotherapy is begun. A support is used for the longitudinal and transverse arches of the foot until a year after the injury.

Following stable fixation with 3.5-mm cortical screws, 10–15-kg weightbearing of the foot with an arch support is allowed. In this case cast immobilization is not needed. The screws are removed after 2 months. Full weightbearing is allowed after 3 months, using an arch support.

Complications

Marked swelling with blisters on the dorsum of the foot may impede clinical diagnosis and treatment. Compartment syndrome (i.e. diminished perfusion of muscles in the tight fascial compartments) may develop, with subsequent muscle contracture and foot deformity (see Chapter 44). An immobile foot may follow unrecognized compartment syndrome.

The intertarsal and tarsometatarsal ligaments, the tibialis anterior and peroneus longus tendons and bone fragments may prevent reduction.

Insufficient cancellous bone graft, unstable fixation or early weightbearing may lead to secondary dislocation and to post-traumatic arthrosis. Primary open reduction through a midline dorsal incision provides adequate exposure for anatomical reduction.

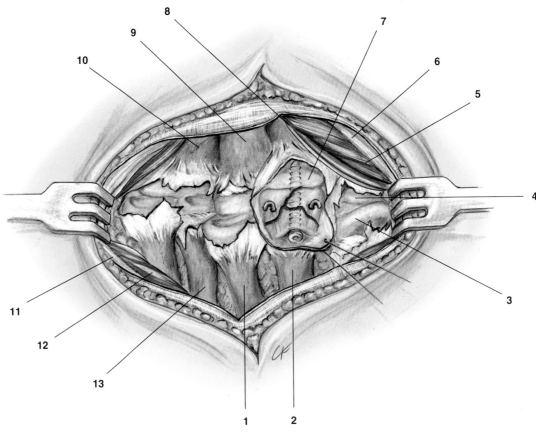

Figure 6

Open reduction of a tarsometatarsal fracture–dislocation. A fracture at the base of the second metatarsal has been stabilized with Kirschner wires. Following reduction of the second metatarsocuneiform joint, a cortical screw is inserted for fixation

1 Third metatarsal
2 Second metatarsal
3 First metatarsal
4 First cuneiform
5 Extensor hallucis brevis muscle
6 Extensor hallucis longus tendon
7 Second cuneiform
8 Neurovascular bundle
9 Third cuneiform
10 Cuboid
11 Extensor digitorum longus tendon
12 Extensor digitorum brevis muscle
13 Fourth metatarsal

Stable fixation after anatomical reduction and adequate management of the soft tissue helps to avoid complications.

Skin necrosis and hematoma may develop post-operatively. Iatrogenic injury to the dorsalis pedis artery and the final branches of the deep peroneal nerve may occur with the medial incision. Lesion of the sural nerve may occur in the lateral incision for exposure of the calcaneocuboidal joint.

Sympathetic reflex dystrophy may develop if postoperative physiotherapy is inadequate.

References

Chapman MW (1978) Fractures and fracture dislocations of the ankle and foot. In: DuVries HL, Hardcastle PH, Reschauer R, Kutscha-Lissberg E, Schoffmann W (eds) Surgery of the Foot, 4th edn. St Louis, Mosby, pp 177–183

DeLee JC (1992) Fractures and dislocations of the foot. In: Mann RA, Coughlin MJ (eds) Surgery of the Foot and Ankle. St Louis, Mosby, pp 1465–1703

Goldman F (1989) Midfoot fractures. In: Scurran BL (ed) Foot and Ankle Trauma. New York, Churchill Livingstone, pp 377–403

Hardcastle PH, Reschauer R, Kutscha-Lissberg E et al. (1982) Injuries to the tarsometatarsal joint. J Bone Joint Surg 64B: 349–356

Jeffreys TE (1963) Lisfranc's fracture–dislocation: a clinical experimental study of tarso-metatarsal dislocation and fracture–dislocation. J Bone Joint Surg 45B: 546–551

Klenerman L (1991) The Foot and Its Disorders, 3rd edn. Oxford, Blackwell, pp 220–229

Koch J, Rahimi F (1991) Nutcracker fractures of the cuboid. J Foot Surg 30: 336–339

Main BJ, Jowett RL (1975) Injuries of the midtarsal joint. J Bone Joint Surg 57B: 89–97

Rockwood CA, Green DP (1975) Fractures. Philadelphia, Lippincott, pp 1465–1473

Wiley JJ (1971) The mechanism of tarso-metatarsal joint injuries. J Bone Joint Surg 53B: 474–482

Wilson DW (1972) Injuries of the tarso-metatarsal joints. J Bone Joint Surg 54B: 677–686

Zwipp H (1994) Chirurgie des Fußes. Vienna, Springer-Verlag, pp 130–161

Zwipp H, Scola E, Schlen U, Riechers D (1991) Verrenkungen der Sprunggelenke und Fußwurzel. Hefte Unfallheilkd 220: 81–82

21 Midfoot arthrodesis

Sigvard T. Hansen Jr

Introduction

Fusion of the tarsometatarsal joints, especially at the cuneiform–metatarsal level, is a standard procedure for orthopedic surgeons with active practices in foot reconstruction.

The presence of hypermobility in the first tarsometatarsal joint and, occasionally, in the first and second intercuneiform joints is commonly associated with excessive pronation and a varus deformity in the first metatarsal and the eventual development of a hallux valgus deformity (see Chapter 5). Morton described the consequences of hypermobility in the first metatarsal segment [Morton 1935]. He believed that hypermobility is an atavistic trait and that it is the most common cause of problems in the human forefoot. In an independent paper published a year earlier, Lapidus used the same premise to propose fusion of the first cuneiform and the base of the first and second metatarsals for correction of metatarsus varus and hallux valgus deformities [Lapidus 1934].

An anatomic predisposition to hypermobility in the first metatarsal segment is not the only indication for tarsometatarsal joint fusion. The tarsometatarsal level is the most common site of neuropathic fracture–dislocation in individuals with diabetes. Even though the incidence of neuropathic foot deformity, or Charcot's foot, is less than 1%, with over 14 million diabetic patients in the USA alone, the number of individuals with dislocations is very large.

Traumatic tarsometatarsal joint dislocations (see Chapter 20) can be caused by sporting activities and motor vehicle accidents. American football is a classic mechanism of this injury and traumatic dislocations are also common in windsurfing, where the participant is required to strap the forefoot to a board. Widespread use of front-seat belts and airbags in automobiles protects the upper body during collision but leaves the feet vulnerable to a variety of injuries, including tarsometatarsal and intertarsal joint fractures and dislocations. Finally, tarsometatarsal injuries can result from industrial accidents as a consequence of falls, rollover injuries and heavy objects dropped on the foot.

Initial treatment of traumatic injuries calls for open reduction and internal fixation of the fracture or dislocation (see Chapter 20) but does not require fusion. However, a non-anatomic or unstable reduction, especially one that results from a purely ligamentous injury, is prone to the development of late arthrosis and changes in the weight-bearing axis, as described by Morton, and may require more precise reduction and fusion. Occasionally degenerative arthrosis and angulation or subluxation of the tarsometatarsal joints seem to develop for no apparent reason. Each year the author sees from one to three patients who sustained tarsometatarsal dislocations without having experienced a notable traumatic event or neuropathy. On closer examination, a tight gastrocnemius muscle, ligamentous laxity or both are frequently identified in these patients.

Arthrodesis of any of the three medial tarsometatarsal joints does not affect function because the tarsometatarsal joints are normally very stable flat joints. Other immobile joints in the foot include the intercuneiform and naviculocuneiform joints. All the bones in the midfoot, including the tarsal navicular, the three cuneiforms and the cuboid, function together as a unit controlled by the powerful posterior tibial muscle. This muscle attaches to all five bones in the midfoot as well as to the second, third and, occasionally, the fourth metatarsal bases. Thus, the first three metatarsals function as an anterior extension of the midfoot block.

The position in which the tarsometatarsal joints are fused is all-important because this determines the anatomical axis of the foot in the transverse plane and the weightbearing distribution under the metatarsal heads in the sagittal plane.

Malalignment or sagging of the naviculocuneiform joint in the absence of posterior tibial insufficiency or rupture is common with flat-foot deformities and in feet with excessive pronation. Patients with these deformities invariably have a tight heel cord or, more accurately, a tight gastrocnemius muscle. This is important to remember because heel cord or gastrocnemius lengthening is indicated in conjunction with naviculocuneiform or Lisfranc's fusions in all except post-traumatic cases.

Surgical procedures

The surgical procedures for midfoot fusions follow similar guidelines: cartilage is removed from the joints, the joints are repositioned anatomically and two screws are inserted across each joint to provide compression and rotatory control. The bone along the fusion line is opened at one or two sites with a burr and the resulting gap is filled with a shear strain-relieved cancellous bone graft.

Various combinations of midfoot arthrodesis have been used. The Miller procedure is one of the standard treatments for symptomatic flat-foot and first-degree pronation. It includes naviculocuneiform fusion and frequently fusion of the cuneiform and the first metatarsal with distal advancement of the tibialis anterior tendon [Fraser et al. 1995]. Virtually every report of the Miller operation recommends heel cord lengthening 'as needed', and it is found to be necessary in over 90% of cases. Lapidus [1934] recommended fusion of the first cuneiform and the bases of the first and second metatarsals to correct metatarsus varus and hallux valgus, combined with capsulorrhaphy of the first metatarsophalangeal joint and re-alignment of the sesamoid complex.

Arthrodesis for Lisfranc's joint dislocation

Correction of a typical chronic Lisfranc's joint dislocation (see Chapter 20) requires completely accurate anatomic re-alignment, which is greatly facilitated by meticulous preparation [Arntz et al.

1988]. The joint is exposed and debrided through two surgical approaches, the capsules are opened, and cartilage is removed prior to reduction (Figure 1). The base of the second metatarsal is reduced into the notch between the first and second cuneiforms with the help of a lateral distractor applied from the heel to the base of the fifth metatarsal, or with pointed reduction forceps (Figure 2). After the joint has been reduced, but before the first screw is inserted, the surgeon should palpate the metatarsal heads very carefully to determine whether they are all positioned at approximately the same level.

Ideally, two screws are crossed in each joint (Figure 3). They are placed so that they undermine the flap between the two dorsal incisions as little as possible. The first screw is placed from the medial side of the first cuneiform and angled at approximately 45° into the corner of the second metatarsal base. It may cross the second metatarsal and penetrate the third metatarsal for full reduction and compression of this part of the foot. After this screw has been inserted, the second screw may be placed through a trough made on the dorsal aspect of the first metatarsal. This screw runs parallel with the sole of the foot and penetrates the lower half of the first cuneiform, compressing and stabilizing the base of the first metatarsal against the first cuneiform.

The third screw is then placed through a lateral incision that is started at the lateral base of the third metatarsal. It is angled proximally and medially and enters the second cuneiform. Placement of the screw from this side allows direct observation of the third metatarsal through the incision made over the fourth metatarsal, obviating the need to lift the soft-tissue flap that covers the second metatarsal. The screws aimed into the second and third cuneiforms are inserted from the lateral side of the metatarsal shaft instead of the dorsal side to prevent the screw from sliding under the cuneiforms. Screw fixation is rarely used in the fourth and fifth tarsometatarsal joints. A screw is placed from the fourth metatarsal into the third cuneiform only when the fourth metatarsal base is unstable. When the fourth metatarsal is stable, a Kirschner wire may be used to provide adequate fixation or, if the metatarsal has not lost position, fixation may be omitted.

The surgeon must constantly monitor the level of the metatarsal heads as the screws are inserted and tightened to ensure that they stay level. The metatarsal heads may impinge on each other if one metatarsal is drawn too close against the adjacent bone.

Correction of neuropathic dislocations in patients with diabetes mellitus always requires screw fixation

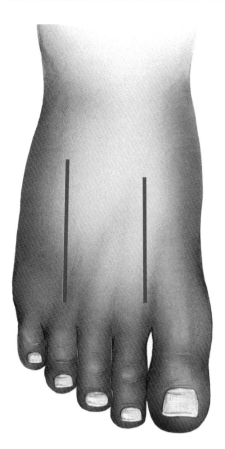

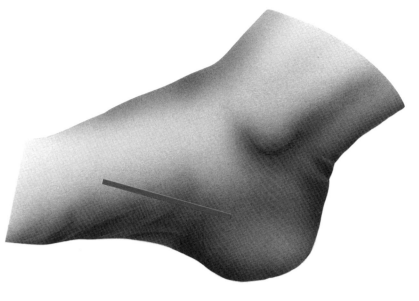

Figure 1

Incisions for midfoot arthrodesis procedures. a. one or two incisions are made on the dorsal aspect of the foot to provide access for fusion of the tarsometatarsal joints. The incisions may be extended proximally for exposure of the intertarsal joints; b. medial utility incision for arthrodesis of the naviculocuneiform joints

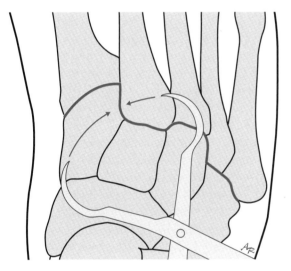

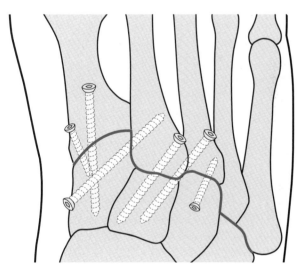

Figure 2

Arthrodesis for Lisfranc's joint dislocation. After cartilage and debris are removed from the joint, a pointed reduction forceps is inserted to reduce the base of the second metatarsal anatomically into the notch against the lateral wall of the first cuneiform

Figure 3

Screw fixation for Lisfranc's joint arthrodesis consists of 3.5- or 4-mm cortical self-tapping screws (synthes USA) that are lagged through gliding holes in the near fragment to compress the fixation

of the fourth and, occasionally, the fifth metatarsals. After one screw has been placed across each joint, the second screw is inserted to control rotation and provide more stable fixation. The second screw is

started in the cuneiform and aimed in a distal and inferior direction, toward the base of the metatarsal. A 2.7-mm screw is added on the dorsal side of the large initial screw which was placed from the first metatarsal into the cuneiform. Bone graft supplementation is always required. Divots of bone are removed or spherical holes are drilled in the joints with a burr and cancellous bone chips are packed into the gaps. Because there is minimal shear strain in the opened area, this bone graft serves the same purpose as an onlay bone graft, without producing a lump on the foot that makes shoe-fitting difficult.

First–second cuneiform arthrodesis

Fusion of the first and second cuneiforms is indicated when hypermobility is limited to these bones. This procedure is performed most commonly as part of the Lapidus procedure to treat hypermobility in the first metatarsal segment and the first tarsometatarsal joint. The joint is scraped with a curette. An arthrodesis of the first and second intercuneiform joint is fixed with two screws, one 3.5-mm and one 2.7-mm (Figure 4) placed perpendicular to one another. A shear strain-relieved bone graft is added to facilitate healing. A spherical hole approximately 7–10 mm in diameter is drilled in the central part of the joint with a burr and filled with small cancellous bone chips.

Naviculocuneiform arthrodesis

Naviculocuneiform arthrodesis is a common midfoot procedure. Miller [1927] included this arthrodesis in his treatment for flat-foot, where the tarsometatarsal joint was fused by denuding the joint and advancing the plantar capsule. Excellent results have been reported with this technique, but it is of interest to note that authors invariably recommend heel cord lengthening, which is indicated in at least 90% of cases and may account for success in treatment of the flat-foot deformity as well as of the fusion itself. Patients who have sustained severe collapse of the medial column due to rupture of the posterior tibial tendon or flat-foot due to a tight heel cord often require a naviculocuneiform arthrodesis to correct significant sagging or hypermobility in this joint. The procedure is carried out through a medial incision (see Figure 1) in the midline of the base of the metatarsal, extending towards a point about 1 cm distal to the tip of the medial malleolus. The incision is carried down just dorsal to the posterior tibial tendon. Care is taken not to transect the anterior tibial tendon coming across the first cuneiform. This tendon is carefully lifted forward and distally from the face of the

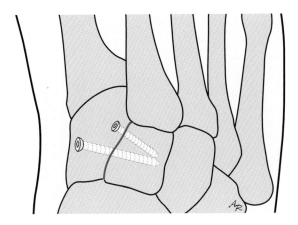

Figure 4

An arthrodesis of the first–second intercuneiform joint is fixed with two screws

first cuneiform. The dorsal and distal side of the transverse retinaculum is lifted to expose the naviculocuneiform joint and the medial proximal surface of the first cuneiform. The cartilage between the distal navicular and the proximal first and second cuneiforms is completely removed with a curved osteotome and the joint is scraped with a curette before it is drilled superficially with a 2.0 drill bit. The joint is reduced, generally by flexing the first cuneiform on to the navicular, and a pointed reduction forceps is applied across the joint. The proximal end of the forceps grasps the inferior side of the navicular tubercle and the distal end grasps the distal and superior side of the cuneiform. This maneuver flexes the cuneiform on to the front of the navicular and approximates it firmly into anatomic position.

A 3.5-mm gliding hole is drilled into the lower half of the navicular and continued into the cuneiform with a 2.5-mm drill bit. The tarsometatarsal level must not be drilled if these joints are not to be fused. The first screw (3.5 mm wide and 40 mm long) is inserted from the inferior tubercle of the navicular almost parallel to the medial border of the foot and to the dorsum of the foot (Figure 5a,b). It is aimed toward the lower half of the first cuneiform. Using the same technique, the second screw is inserted more laterally from the upper half of the navicular tubercle and aimed more laterally to enter the second cuneiform, which is more shallow and higher in the midfoot than the first. The second screw is also a 3.5-mm cortical screw that is 45 ± 5 mm long and placed with lagging, i.e. placed through a 3.5-mm gliding hole in the near bone and with a 2.5-mm tap hole in the distal bone. Placement of the fixation hardware should avoid penetration of the

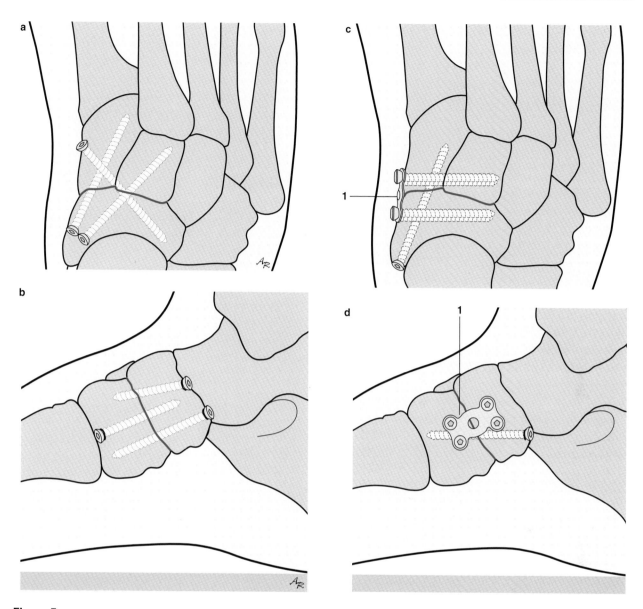

Figure 5

Arthrodesis of the navicular and the first and second cuneiforms. a. fixation with three screws, dorsal aspect; b. medial aspect; c, d. fixation with an H-plate using a supplementary position screw crossing the naviculocuneiform joint to preclude shear strain. This is similar to the most medial proximal to distal screw in a and b; c. dorsal aspect; d. medial aspect

1 H-plate

screws into the second tarsometatarsal and the talonavicular joints.

Placement of the third screw is more complex. With the foot held in dorsiflexion, the anterior tibial tendon is lifted forward and the screw is angled proximally and laterally from the middle of the first cuneiform and driven obliquely through to the lateral side of the navicular, parallel to the dorsum of the foot. This screw is 40–45 mm long, like the other two, and it is drilled in the same manner. This technique provides good compression and fixation and, when a shear strain-relieved bone graft is

added to the dorsal and inferior sides, the fusion rate is satisfactory.

Fixation with a small H-plate is an alternative technique (Figure 5c,d), which also requires technical expertise. Curettage and reduction of the two bones is carried out in the same manner as in the previous example, but fixation with an H-plate requires a wider exposure through the soft tissue.

Grafting sites for a shear strain-relieved bone graft are prepared dorsal and plantar to the joint in each case. Cancellous bone may be obtained from the calcaneus, the medial malleolus or, ideally, from the lateral proximal tibial plateau under Gerdy's tubercle.

Postoperative care

The recuperative period for all tarsometatarsal fusions ranges from 8 to 10 weeks. The foot is immobilized in a cast and weightbearing is limited to a minimal amount that provides balance during ambulation on crutches for the first 2½ weeks. After the original cast and sutures have been removed, the foot may be immobilized in a cast that allows partial weightbearing only at the heel, or – if no significant tendon balancing procedures have been done – in a cast boot. Longer cast immobilization is unnecessary when the heel cord is lengthened exclusively by the gastrocnemius slide procedure, but a cast boot should be used during the day and removed for bathing and sleeping. Ambulation is limited to protected weightbearing until radiographs taken at 8 postoperative weeks or later demonstrate early union at the fusion site. Gradual rehabilitation begins with walking and progresses to range-of-motion exercises to strengthen the ankle and stabilize the foot musculature. Walking in a swimming pool is excellent early therapy.

The screws are removed at 10–12 weeks if they are used only to stabilize a reduced joint. If screws are used for fixation of a midfoot arthrodesis, they are removed only if they cause symptoms and not before 6 months postoperatively.

Bibliography

Arntz CT, Veith RG, Hansen ST (1988) Fractures and fracture–dislocations of the tarsometatarsal joint. J Bone Joint Surg 70A: 173–181

Fraser RK, Menelaus MB, Williams PF et al. (1995) The Miller procedure for mobile flat feet. J Bone Joint Surg 77B: 396–399

Lapidus PW (1934) Operative correction of the metatarsus varus primus in hallux valgus. Surg Gynecol Obstet 58: 183–191

Miller OL (1927) A plastic flat foot operation. J Bone Joint Surg 9: 84–91

Morton DJ (1935) The Human Foot: Its Evolution, Physiology and Functional Disorders. Morningside Heights, Columbia University Press

22

The treatment of flat foot in children

Antonio Viladot Voegeli

Introduction

Flat feet are is one of the commonest reasons for consultation in pediatric orthopedic practice, and the commonest deformity in children's feet. Of these, 99% are flexible flat feet, which will only exceptionally cause problems.

In adulthood be remembered that the plantar arch is a three-dimensional structure whose shape varies according to how it is loaded. The foot of a person supine does not have the same shape as that of a person walking, running or jumping. The stability of the plantar arch is achieved by correct interaction between the bones, ligaments and musculotendinous units. Alteration or imbalance of any of these can result in a flat foot. Therefore, flat feet can be due to bony anomalies (e.g. the congenital vertical talus, tarsal coalition), a ligamentous abnormality (e.g. Ehlers–Danlos disease, Down's syndrome) or neuromuscular disease (e.g. poliomyelitis, spina bifida and cerebral palsy). Regardless of etiology, flat feet present a uniform pathological anatomy, with the primary pathology in the hindfoot and secondary changes in the forefoot.

Pathological anatomy of the hindfoot

Although a flat foot is commonly understood as loss of height of the medial longitudinal arch, what really characterizes the deformity is valgus of the heel. This results from a series of movements/displacements that take place within the tarsus (Figure 1): pronation of the talus and the calcaneus, adduction of the talus in relation to the calcaneus, which rotates externally, and plantarflexion of the talus and calcaneus, more accentuated in the latter, which moves into an equinus position.

In children this is often due to the laxity of the interosseous ligament of the subtalar joint, the spring ligament and the plantar fascia. Other contributors to the deformity are insufficiency of the tibialis posterior tendon and short/tight Achilles and peroneal tendons.

The tibialis posterior tendon, at heel rise, is responsible for bringing the hindfoot into varus, which locks the midtarsal joint, and the foot becomes a rigid structure for propulsion of the body. It is assisted by the metatarsophalangeal break and the windlass effect of the plantar fascia. Retraction of both the Achilles and the peroneal tendons contributes to the deformity, as the heel is fixed in valgus. As a result of the movements described, the talus plantarflexes and internally rotates in relation to the calcaneus, breaking the medial column of the foot by stretching the spring/calcaneonavicular ligament and the talocalcaneal navicular joint capsule.

Pathological anatomy of the forefoot

Owing to the thrust received from the head of the talus, the medial column of the foot functionally increases its length in relation to the lateral, causing

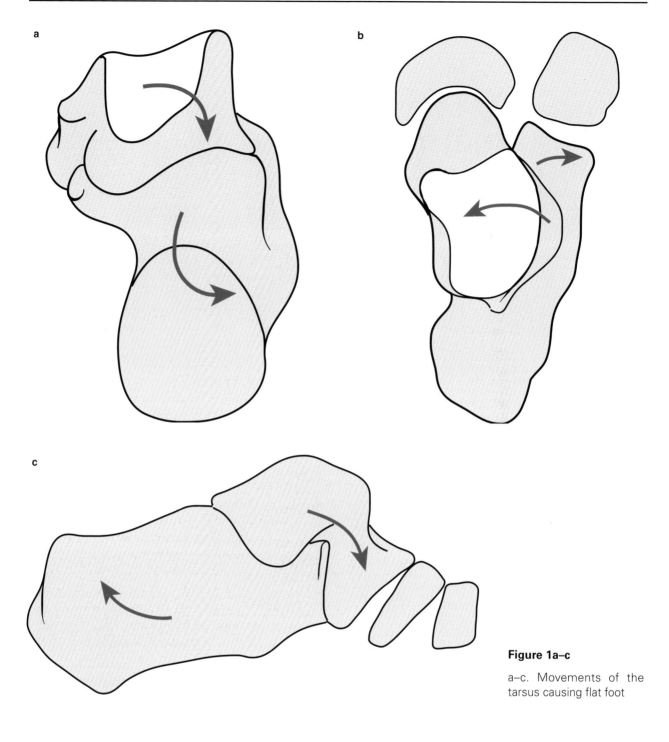

Figure 1a–c

a–c. Movements of the tarsus causing flat foot

forefoot abduction. Moreover, when the head of the first metatarsal is loaded increasingly by ground reaction since it is unstable, it allows the forefoot to supinate. Therefore, in a flat foot there are two rotating movements in opposing directions (Figure 2): hindfoot pronation and forefoot supination. Tarsal subluxations develop which are located in the talonaviculocuneiform, talonavicular and navicular–cuneiform joints. For example, in congenital vertical talus it is the talonavicular joint, and in

paralytic feet it is the navicular–cuneiform joint. In the flexible flat foot both joints are affected.

Treatment

The treatment of flat foot in children depends on both the etiology and the severity of the deformity. Most authors agree that rigid flat foot secondary to a bony abnormality should be treated surgically.

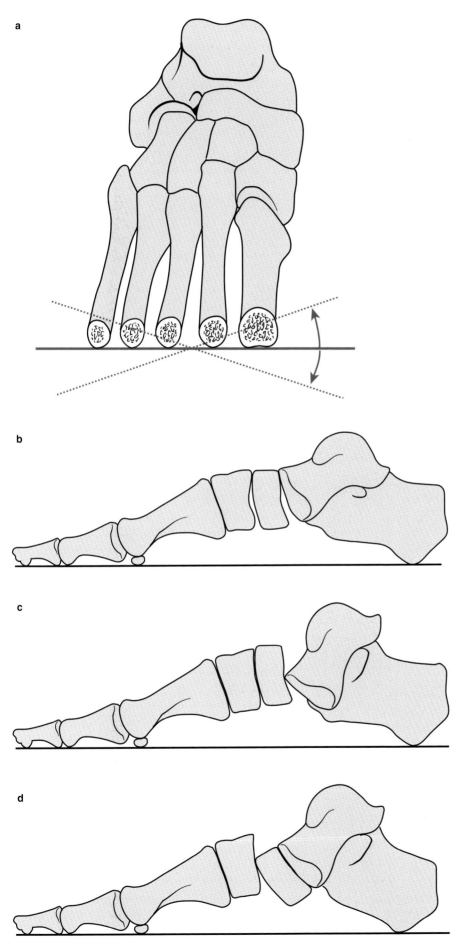

Figure 2

a–d. Double helicoid movement in flat foot. Different subluxations or dislocations. See text

The controversy arises when dealing with a flexible flat foot. (For tarsal coalition, see Chapter 27).

Treatment of the flexible flat foot

The majority of normal children below 3–4 years of age have flat feet, because the plantar arch is absent in utero and develops with growth. Its development is influenced by various factors, including the reduction of the laxity of the ligaments, and the increase of muscular strength with age. For this reason, we believe that conservative treatment, which generally gives good results, should start from the age of 5–6. When our department studied 4800 patients with flexible flat foot, only 2% had surgical treatment because the rest improved with conservative treatment.

We believe that surgical treatment for these patients is indicated in two situations: severe deformities that do not respond to conservative treatment over a minimum period of 3 years; and symptomatic flat feet with pain in the medial or lateral side of the foot, the latter due to impingement of the peroneal tendons between the lateral malleolus and the calcaneus.

For surgical correction of this type of foot, different techniques have been described: osteotomies, arthrodesis, tendon transfer, arthroereisis and/or combined techniques.

Osteotomies

Calcaneal osteotomy with medial translation of the calcaneus   Since the most characteristic deformity is a valgus heel, Koutsogiannis [1971] proposes this osteotomy to correct it. The procedure has the drawback that it is often insufficient to correct all the deformities contributing to flattening of the medial arch.

Osteotomy with lengthening of the calcaneus   As has been mentioned in relation to the pathological anatomy in this type of flat foot, we find a lengthening of the medial column and a shortening of the lateral column useful. Evans [1975] proposed his osteotomy for lengthening the calcaneus, whereby he managed to balance the two columns of the foot, restoring the plantar arch.

Osteotomy with shortening of the talus   Based on the same principles as the above, Regnauld [1986] proposed osteotomy with shortening of the neck of the talus. This is not popular, owing to concern for the vascular supply to the talus.

Arthrodesis

Miller [1927] proposed his surgical technique for correcting flexible flat foot in children based on an arthrodesis of the navicular–cuneiform and metatarsal–cuneiform joints associated with plication of the tibialis posterior tendon, but arthrodesis in the skeletally immature foot should probably be condemned, except in very severe deformity or failed reconstructive surgery.

Tendon transfer

If the heel does not go into varus on double heel rise (standing on tiptoe), if the subtalar and midfoot have a full range of movement, i.e. the tibialis posterior cannot achieve heel inversion, it is advisable to plicate/shorten the tibialis posterior tendon associated with plication of the spring ligament and the talonavicular capsule. These procedures, however, are usually combined with flexed digitorum longus transfer and a calcaneal osteotomy, as described in Chapter 23.

Arthroereisis

As indicated above, in flat foot in children there is *excess mobility* in the subtalar joint, enabling the talus to plantarflex and internally rotate in relation to the calcaneus. The aim of the technique consists of restricting this excess mobility, to prevent the medial arch from collapsing, yet conserving the *physiological mobility* of the hindfoot. An arthroereisis acts as a block to excessive valgus/external calcaneal rotation, achieved either by inserting a bone block or an implant in the sinus tarsi or using the 'calcaneus stop' technique described by Alvárez [1995]. He approached the subtalar joint laterally at the sinus tarsi and supinated the hindfoot, thereby internally rotating the calcaneus at the posterior facet. In this position, a screw was inserted vertically into the calcaneus which, as the heel attempted to move into excessive valgus, abutted against the neck of the talus, restricting excessive valgus of the hindfoot (Figure 3).

Combined techniques

Based on the studies of Grice [1952] and Miller [1927], Viladot [1965] described a technique whereby, via a double approach (medial and lateral), the talus is mobilized by positioning it in its physiological position on the calcaneus, correcting the hindfoot deformity. The correction was maintained

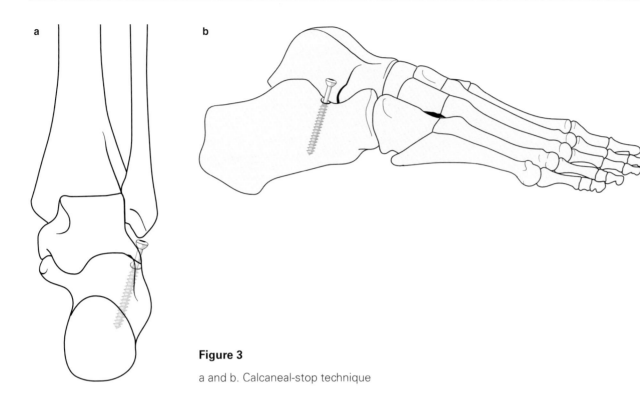

Figure 3

a and b. Calcaneal-stop technique

passively by a sinus tarsi implant. A plication of the tibialis posterior tendon gives dynamic stability. This is especially important in feet where an accessory or prominent navicular bone is the cause of an insufficiency of the tibialis posterior tendon. In most cases a lengthening of the Achilles tendon is required, which facilitates correction and prevents recurrence.

The surgical technique is performed as follows. An incision is made in the medial aspect of the foot, between dorsal skin and plantar skin, extending from the medial malleolus to the metatarsal–cuneiform joint (Figure 4a). The tibialis anterior tendon is retracted dorsally. A tendoperiosteal flap of the tibialis posterior tendon is divided, including the periosteum of the navicular (Figure 4b). An incision in the external aspect of the foot, 1 cm below and anterior to the tip of the lateral malleolus, is made and the sinus tarsi is approached by removing its soft tissues, fundamentally the retinacula and the cervical ligament (Figure 4c). The deformity is then ready for correction. A blunt instrument is inserted through the lateral incision of the sinus tarsi which passes in front of the interosseous ligament and emerges through the medial incision, just below the head of the talus (Figure 4d). A combined maneuver of supination of the hindfoot and pronation of the forefoot, repositioning the talus above the calcaneus, establishes the normal arch. If the correction is not possible the Achilles tendon

and the peroneal tendons, or a coalition, must be addressed. It is our experience that lengthening of the Achilles tendon is required in most cases.

The sinus tarsi and its canal is a cylindrical or truncated cone-shaped space between talus and calcaneus which, in the flat foot, disappears when the talus plantarflexes. Once the foot has been corrected by the above maneuver, this space is apparent and can accept an implant for an arthroereisis (Figure 5).

In the initial technique described by Viladot (Figure 4e), the arthroereisis was performed according to the ideas of Grice, with a cylinder of fibula taken from the same leg, the diameter of which was seen to match the sinus tarsi. Over time, it was noted that the fibula graft would be re-absorbed, whilst the foot would retain its correction indefinitely. The bone graft was then replaced by a cylinder of Silastic, and later by a self-stabilizing cup-shaped Silastic implant. With this technique, satisfactory results have been published for both the short and the long term [Viladot 1992, Viladot et al. 1993]. Following the same ideas, Giannini and Girolami [1985] proposed their own implant.

The author has now replaced the Silastic cup with the new Kalix® design (Nudeal, France) from Viladot et al. [2001], which is basically a metal cone that is inserted inside a trunk of polyethylene. Tightening the metal cone expands the polyethylene; this is the main benefit of this new biocompatible implant.

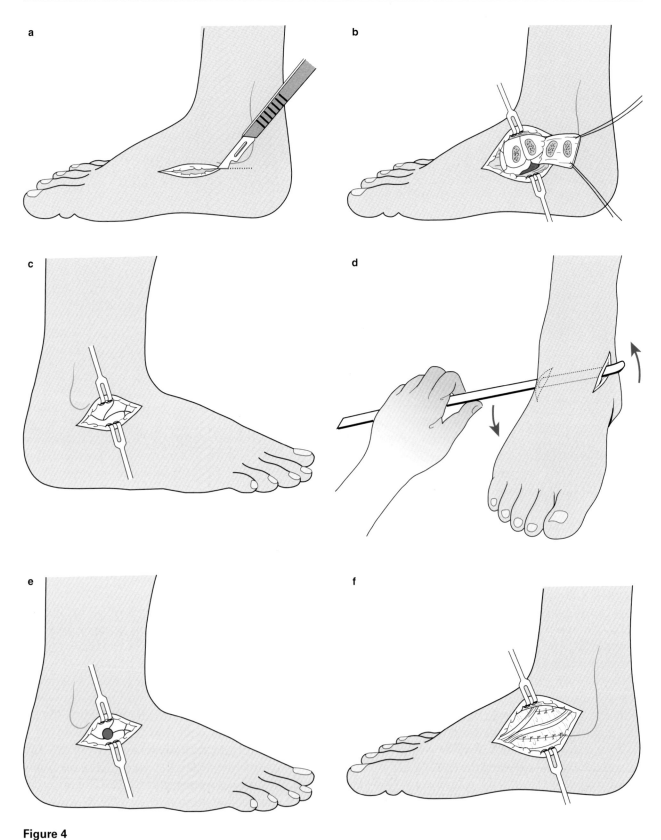

Figure 4

a–f. Double approach technique in flexible flat foot. See text

Active stabilization is considered necessary, particularly in cases where there is an accessory navicular bone causing insufficiency of the tibialis posterior tendon. This consists of advancement of the tendoperiosteal flap (Figure 4b) in a more distal position (Figure 4f) as described by Albanesse [1965], so that the tibialis posterior tendon is plicated, as is the spring ligament. We strengthen the

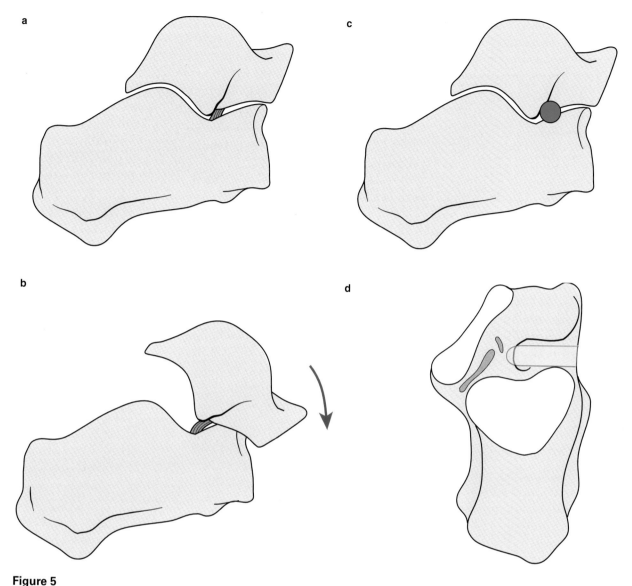

Figure 5

a. Normal talocalcaneal relation; b. relation between talus and calcaneus in flat foot. The sinus tarsi disappears; c. situation of the implant or bone graft in the sinus tarsi. Effect of arthroereisis; d. top view of the calcaneus and situation of the implant in the sinus tarsi

flap with the tibialis anterior tendon, retaining its distal insertion so as not to alter its proprioceptivity.

After skin closure, a plaster cast is applied. The sutures are removed after 10 days, and a weightbearing plaster cast is applied for 1 month. After cast removal, a medial arch support is recommended for 1 year.

Treatment of rigid flat foot

These are clearly pathological flat feet which have to be treated surgically in most cases. The majority are caused by a congenital vertical talus or tarsal coalition that develops as a painful spastic flat foot.

The former presents at birth and the latter after the age of 8 years.

Congenital vertical talus can be an isolated congenital abnormality or associated with other deformities, e.g. arthrogryposis, spina bifida, cerebral palsy or Marfan's syndrome. The diagnosis is made at birth, by the characteristic appearance of the foot: the sole is convex with a rocker-bottom appearance and the head of the talus is prominent in the sole of the foot medially.

Anatomically and pathologically, this type of foot presents as a specific deformity that requires surgical treatment. The talus has a short neck. The navicular bone is dislocated dorsally on the neck of the talus – the classic deformity. The calcaneus is in equinus and valgus. The subtalar joint is pronated and the sustentaculum tali is deformed. The Achilles, tibialis anterior, extensor hallucis longus, extensor digitorum longus and peroneal tendons are contracted and shortened. The dorsolateral ligaments are also contracted, which makes the deformity rigid. The spring ligament is lengthened and thinner, owing to the pressure from the plantarflexed head of the talus.

Surgical treatment for this type of foot is performed early, because the deformity becomes more rigid and structural with time. Surgery is influenced by the following factors. Tight muscles and tendons make the deformity rigid (Achilles, peroneal, extensor digitorum longus and extensor hallucis tendons). The talocalcaneal subluxation/dislocation can be corrected with soft tissue procedures including extensive capsulotomies if it is approached early. Later lengthening of the talus and the hypertrophy of its head make the medial column of the foot longer, so when soft-tissue correction is attempted, skeletal structures prevent correction. To achieve correction at this stage, a partial resection of the head of the talus or excision of the navicular bone is required.

Stabilization in the corrected position at surgery is essential. A Kirschner wire is used and we suture the tibialis anterior tendon to the neck of the talus, retaining its distal insertion but giving dynamic dorsiflexion to the talus. Some authors [Tachdjian 1985] propose a Grice arthrodesis to keep the talus in position, but this can result in stiffness in a child's foot.

The surgical technique is through a double approach and is performed as follows (Figure 6). We commence the procedure as for the flexible flat foot, i.e. when the tendoperiosteal flap is lifted, the talonavicular dislocation is easily visualized (Figure 6a) and extensive capsulotomies are performed with a view to later plication of the spring ligament. A lateral incision is made beneath the lateral malleolus, ascending to the lateral aspect of the ankle. Through it the Achilles and peroneal tendons are lengthened, and the common extensor to the toes and the abundant fibrous bands of the dorsum of the foot are sectioned, including the tendon of peroneus tertius.

After soft-tissue release of the calcaneal cuboid and posterior facet joint, the calcaneus is internally rotated on the talus. If the correction is not possible, owing to the relatively long medial column, the head of the talus or navicular remnant is partially resected and remodeled. Some navicular bone can be decancellated and compressed (Figure 6b). Once correction is obtained it is secured with Kirschner wires, one of which crosses the talus, navicular and cuneiform joints, another crosses the calcaneocuboid and the other the talocalcaneal joint. With this, correction is maintained of the talocalcaneal sagittal and horizontal angle (Figure 6c, d). The tibialis anterior tendon is plicated to the neck of the talus through a suture that crosses the talar neck (Figure 6c). After routine closure a plaster cast is applied for 10 days. After 10 days, the sutures are removed and a new plaster cast is applied. The Kirschner wires are removed at 6 weeks postoperatively and the foot is then casted for a further 6 weeks, to allow stabilization of the soft tissues.

Complications

The most frequent complications in children's flat foot surgery using the 'double approach' technique are:

1. Undercorrection
2. Overcorrection
3. Contracted flat foot
4. Avascular necrosis of the talus.

We saw cases of undercorrection when a silicone implant was used for the arthroereisis. In our opinion, the cause was that this material was not strong enough to resist the weight of a 12–13-year-old boy. This complication has not appeared with the implant we are using now, which is more rigid. However, we have seen a case of overcorrection. We consider that surgeons must not be too ambitious with the correction during surgery, and the size of the implant should be carefully selected.

It is our opinion that peroneal contracture is related to an insufficient removal of the soft tissues in the sinus tarsi. The retinacula and the cervical ligament are innervated structures and, if they are not completely removed, the implant may irritate them, leading to a reflex peroneal contacture.

We have had one case of talar necrosis after endoprothesis implantation. We suspect that it was caused by vascular injury during the surgical procedure. Congenital vertical talus is a very severe deformity and its principal complication is its tendency to recur. In these cases arthrodesis is the best solution.

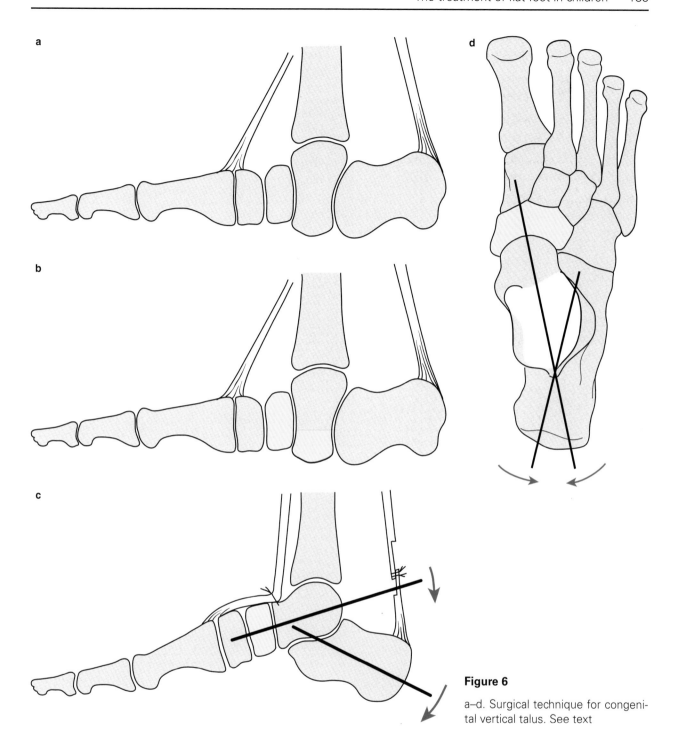

Figure 6

a–d. Surgical technique for congenital vertical talus. See text

References

Albanesse P (1965) Cited by Calgagni V

Alvárez R (1995) Calcaneo-Stop. In: Epeldegui T (ed) Flat Foot and Forefoot Deformities. Madrid, A. Madrid Vicente Ediciones

Calgagni V (1965) La solidarisation des tendons jambiers dans le traitemen du pied plat valgus. Podologie 4: 203–205

Evans D (1975) Calcaneo–valgus deformity. J Bone Joint Surg 57B: 270–277

Giannini S, Girolami M y Ceccarrellig (1985) The surgical treatment of infantile flat foot. A new expanding endo-orthotic implant. Ital J Orthop Traumatol 11: 315–322

Grice DS (1952) An extraarticular arthrodesis of the subtalar joint for correction of paralytic flat feet in children. J Bone Joint Surg 34A: 927–932

Koutsogiannis E (1971) Treatment of mobile flat foot by displacement osteotomy of the calcaneus. J Bone Joint Surg 53B: 96–100

Miller OL (1927) A plastic flat foot operation. J Bone Joint Surg 9: 84–91

Regnauld B (1986) Adult pes planovalgus. In: Regnauld B (ed) The Foot. Berlin, Springer, pp 206–208

Tachdjian M (1985) The Child's Foot. Philadelphia, WB Saunders

Viladot A (1965) Nouvelle technique chirurgique de traitement du pied plat valgus. Podologie 4: 207–208

Viladot A (1992) Surgical treatment of the child's flat-foot. Clin Orthop 283: 34–38

Viladot Voegeli A, López I, Angulo T, Crespo F y Viladot R (1993) A long term follow-up after Setrite implant for flat foot. In: Benamou PH, Montagne J (eds) Médecine et chirurgie du pied. Paris, Masson, pp 118–123

Viladot R, Viladot Voegeli A, Alvarez F (2001) Pie plano laxo infantil. In: Herrera Rodríguez A (ed) Actualizaciones en Cirugía Ortopédica y Traumatología. Barcelona, Masson

23

Flat foot in adults John Corrigan

Introduction

The adult flat foot encompasses the recently symptomatic or adult-acquired flat foot and represents failure or impending mechanical failure of the structural architecture of the foot. The asymptomatic flat foot represents a variation of normality but may predispose that foot to pathological changes, as there is greater reliance on dynamic than on static structures [Dyal et al. 1997].

The stability of the medial arch of the foot is maintained by static and dynamic structures. Colinear alignment in the sagittal plane of the bony elements of the medial arch gives skeletal stability; deviation from this alignment requires recruitment of dynamic elements to maintain structure for the foot to function to accommodate its position on uneven ground and for propulsion. The foot must fluctuate between a flexible and a rigid state. In the first half of stance from heel strike to foot flat, the hindfoot/transverse tarsal complex is unlocked and the foot is in a low energy state; it is flexible and can accommodate to the walking surface to prepare it for transition to a higher energy state at heel raise. More work is required of dynamic structures during a transition from one state to another than is required to hold a position of either of these states, because as muscles actively shorten they use approximately six times more energy than those resisting elongation. The locked position of the transverse tarsal joints occurs in the same position in all feet, but the starting position and resting position varies, depending on whether the foot is high arched, normal or flat. Because the energy differential between resting and locked is greater if the foot is flatter, there is more reliance on dynamic structures for body support and for a longer portion of stance, so more energy is required. Consequently the dynamic

elements are more vulnerable and become the initiators of failure. Since the architecture is dependent on static and dynamic factors, once failure occurs it will ultimately involve all the structural elements.

Since the skeletal structure of the foot is inherently unstable and its integrity reliant on energy input, once failure starts it will be progressive. There are many causes of acquired flat feet. The pattern of failure depends on the pathological condition as well as the premorbid foot shape. Two other factors need to be considered. Body weight determines the energy required to maintain the integrity of foot architecture, and tightness of the gastrocnemius soleus complex increases forefoot loading earlier in stance. The effects of body weight are self-evident and are commonly associated with a failure of the dynamic (posterior tibial tendon) and the static structures (plantar fascia). Maximum ankle dorsiflexion of 10° is required at the start of heel rise when the knee is in near full extension. It is at this point that gastrocnemius tightness comes into play [Aronow 2000]. However, controversy exists as to whether gastrocnemius/Achilles tendon tightness is secondary to the flat foot deformity or a primary causative factor.

Thus, failure of the medial arch arises from different foot pathology and different sites of failure produce different patterns of failure. The Lisfranc joint complex is associated with sagittal plane failure. The triad of degeneration at the second and third tarsometatarsal joints with gapping of the first tarsometatarsal joint associated with plantar fasciitis and tightness of the gastrocnemius is not an uncommon presentation. Hallux valgus with a hypermobile first ray may protect against this form of failure, as the forefoot tends to pronate. Sagittal plane failure represents failure of static structures, and treatment is directed towards these combined with release of tightness of the gastrocnemius soleus complex, i.e. corrective arthrodesis (see Chapter 8). Failure at the level of the talonavicular joint is usually secondary to posterior tibial tendon insufficiency, i.e. dynamic failure, but has been associated with spring ligament degeneration. Typically, individuals with posterior tendon insufficiency not due to systematic arthritides are overweight, have pre-existing flat feet and a tight gastrocnemius soleus complex. The direction of failure tends to be more horizontal than sagittal, owing to the lack of dynamic support from the posterior tibial tendon. Typically the first symptom is pain inferior to the medial malleolus associated with heel raise, i.e. the time of maximal energy transfer as the foot moves from its resting position to a higher energy state (stage 1 of posterior tibial tendon insufficiency [Funk et al. 1986]). Once it fails to produce the transition to the higher energy state of locking of the transverse tarsal joint, failure of static structures (spring ligament complex) occurs, giving forefoot abduction and collapse of the medial arch at the level of the talonavicular joint (stage 2). With further progression greater heel valgus is found as the calcaneus glides posteriorly, closing the sinus tarsi with impingement of the lateral talar process against the angle of Gissane. At this point, a new level of static stability is achieved, associated with lateral foot pain and calcaneofibular impingement. The foot in time becomes fixed in this position (stage 3 disease). Further progression involves the ankle with valgus tilting of the talus in the mortise and secondary degeneration (stage 4).

Treatment of gactrocnemius/ soleus contracture

Assessment and treatment of contracture of the gastrocnemius/soleus complex is an integral part of the management of flatfoot deformity and is dependent on the Silverskiold test, with dorsiflexion being measured with the knee in extension and the hindfoot neutral (valgus corrected), followed by ankle dorsiflexion and repeated with the knee in 30° of flexion. Increased dorsiflexion when the knee is flexed suggests an isolated gastrocnemius contracture. If, however, dorsiflexion of the ankle fails to achieve 5° of dorsiflexion in either knee position, it suggests contracture of the soleus component or posterior ankle structure. For the latter, Aronow [2000] recommends Achilles tendon lengthening. This is performed percutaneously using the Hoke triple-cut technique (Figure 1). For the former, a

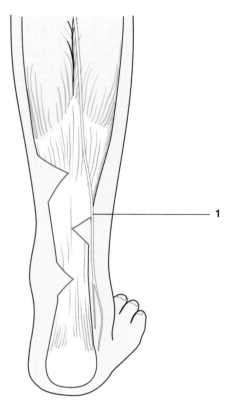

Figure 1

Triple cut Achilles tendon lengthening

1 Sural nerve

gastrocnemius recession is performed prone as an isolated procedure, but becomes more difficult when performed supine, as is necessary when combined with surgery such as posterior tibial tendon reconstruction. Placing the leg in the 'figure 4 position' aids exposure. The incision is longitudinal midline, at the level of the musculotendinous junction, protecting the short saphenous vein and sural nerve, where the interval between the soleus and gastrocnemius can be identified medially, and developed by blunt dissection. In the Vulpius technique, the aponeurosis is divided and allowed to retract proximally. The retracted aponeurosis can be sutured to the underlying soleus with two non-absorbable sutures as in the Strayer technique (Figure 2). The plantaris tendon is cut if tight. A further modification approximately 5 cm more proximal and medial to the belly of the medial head of the gastrocnemius allows the interval between the gastrocnemius and soleus to be found, where the aponeurosis is on the deep surface of the muscle and is divided transversally with a knife while leaving the overlying muscle intact (Figure 3). This has the advantage of not requiring suturing and protects the sural nerve from injury, but the saphenous nerve is at risk.

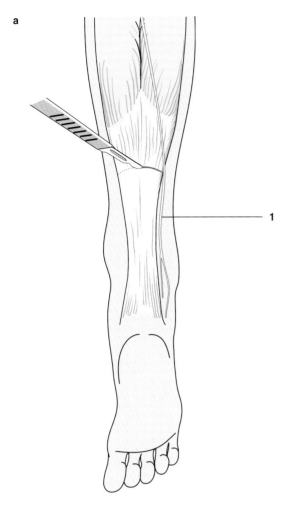

a

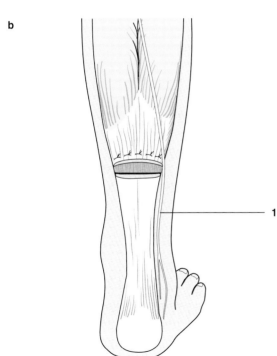

b

Figure 2

a.–b. Gastrocnemius recession (Strayer)

1   Sural nerve

Treatment of posterior tibial tendon insufficiency

Treatment depends on the stage of the pathological process and the etiology, e.g. systemic inflammatory disease process. A trial of conservative treatment such as shoe modification or an ankle–foot orthosis provides some symptomatic relief. However, posterior tibial tendon insufficiency represents a failure of an energy-based system and progression is likely. Treatments aim to maintain mobility on the hindfoot while maintaining a dynamic component to structural support; triple arthrodesis is the gold standard for fixed deformity (stage 4).

Stage 1

Stage 1 represents a failing posterior tibial tendon. Surgical treatment is designed to arrest progression and aims to remove aggravating factors, repair damage and augment the integrity of the posterior tibial tendon. Weight reduction, Achilles tendon lengthening or gastrocnemius recession and decompression of the diseased tendon with tenosynovectomy and debridement achieves this. This is followed by augmentation of its power by side-to-side anastomosis with the flexor digitorum longus (FDL) tendon.

Surgical technique

With the patient supine, a tourniquet is applied under appropriate anesthesia. Initial assessment of the gastrocnemius soleus complex is assessed by the Silverskiold test and a percutaneous Achilles tendon lengthening or gastrocnemius recession is performed as appropriate. An incision is made along the line of the posterior tibial tendon from the tuberosity of the navicular to a point inferior to the medial malleolus. The tendon sheath of the posterior tibial tendon is identified and opened in the line of the skin incision; free fluid may be found. The tendon is inspected for nodularity and intrasubstance degeneration, which is excised, and the tendon is repaired with a non-absorbable suture. A side-to-side anastomis is performed with the FDL tendon, which has been exposed through the posterior aspect of the posterior tibial tendon sheath. Toes are held in hyperextension before suturing to prevent late clawing of the lesser toes (Figure 4) [Shereff 1997]. The tendon sheath is left open and subcutaneous tissues and skin are closed. The foot is immobilized in a below-knee cast in slight inversion for 4 weeks. If there was more extensive disease requiring excision

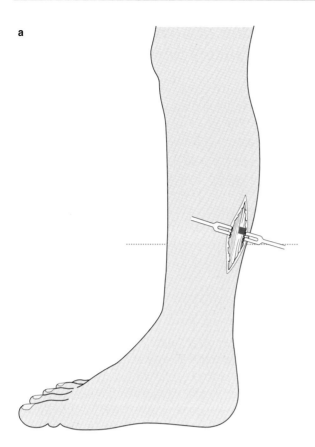

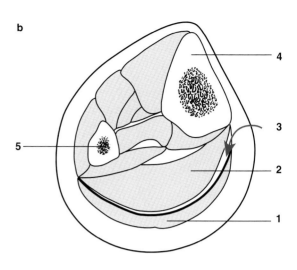

Figure 3

Gastrocnemius recession (proximal)

a. Side view with retractors opening the skin. The dotted line represents the level of the cross-section in b.

1 Gastrocnemius muscle
2 Soleus muscle
3 Exposure of space between gastrocnemius and soleus
4 Tibia
5 Fibula

of a segment of the tendon, and if direct tendon anastomosis cannot be performed without tension, a proximal lengthening of the posterior tibial tendon can be performed. With such extensive tendon involvement, and if there was a pre-existing idiopathic flat foot, then consideration should be given to treating this as stage 2, to unload the tendon.

Stage 2

In stage 2 disease by definition the posterior tibial tendon is non-functional and dynamic support has been lost; the secondary static components of the arch have started to fail. Non-operative treatment can be considered in the elderly patient with low functional demands. In the obese patient where weight control is unlikely or in the rheumatoid patient with articular involvement a triple arthrodesis, rather than reconstruction, must be considered. A prerequisite for reconstruction in stage 2 disease is full flexibility. Any fixed deformity implies that this is stage 3 disease. The aim of treatment in stage 2 disease is to restore dynamic control to the medial aspect of the foot and to overcorrect the failed static components, to create an arch that is more reliant on static components than dynamic. This reduces the work required of the dynamic reconstruction, which uses the flexor digitorum longus or

flexor hallucis longus. An alternative reconstruction uses the tibialis anterior tendon [Helal 1991]. These tendon substitutions aim to restore some medial support, but they are insufficient in themselves, as they have less strength than the intact tibialis posterior.

Abduction of the talonavicular joint and sagging of the naviculocuneiform articulation must be addressed. With the former there is shortening of the lateral column and posterior gliding of the calcaneus underneath the talus as the heel rotates into valgus. This narrows the sinus tarsi, which eventually causes impingement of the lateral process of the talus against the calcaneus at the angle of Gissane. Bony alignment must be normalized to reduce the dynamic substitution work. Reconstruction needs to be tailored to the degree of preoperative deformity. Different procedures have been described and all have merits. The medial translational calcaneal osteotomy combined with a flexor digitorum longus transfer and spring ligament plication provides a more stable structure and medializes the pull of the Achilles tendon; it produces some lengthening of the lateral column and elevation in height. In the more severe deformities it is probably insufficient, and residual sagging at the talonavicular joint persists. Lateral column lengthening as described by Evans [1975] provides more structural support by pushing the

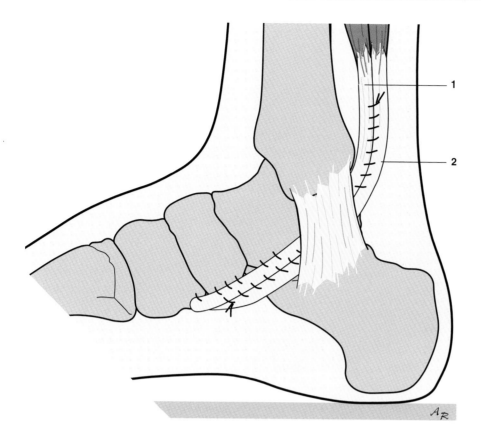

Figure 4

Flexor digitorum longus augmentation to tibialis posterior tendon

1 Tibialis posterior tendon
2 Flexor digitorum longus

navicular medially to buttress the medial arch. The posterior facet of the calcaneus, which has been displaced posteriorly by deformity, remains in this position and limits subtalar/transverse tarsal motion. Lengthening of the lateral column, when performed on adults, has been associated with degeneration of the calcaneocuboid joint. Therefore, in adults it may be preferable that lateral column lengthening be performed by distraction arthrodesis of the calcaneocuboid joint. Medial displacement osteotomy and calcaneal lengthening have been advocated by Pomeroy and Manoli [1997], who consider that the osteotomy protects the calcaneocuboid joint.

The morbidity and recovery time is dependent on consolidation of bony rather than soft tissues. Arthroereisis with insertion of a subtalar block or spacer may restore lateral column length without the prolonged recovery time associated with bony consolidation of osteotomies, but the incidence of sinus tarsi pain is a concern. It is, however, a viable option in the elderly.

Surgical technique

The detailed surgical description is confined to medial displacement osteotomies [Koutsogiannis 1971] and calcaneal lengthening [Evans 1975].

Arthroereisis and the soft-tissue procedures are carried out under general or regional anesthesia with tourniquet. The patient is supine and a roll is placed under the ipsilateral buttock. The gastrocnemius soleus tightness is assessed using the Silverskoild test and a percutaneous Achilles tendon lengthening or a gastrocnemius slide as previously described can be carried out. Attention is then directed to the lateral side of the foot (Figure 5).

Medial displacement calcaneal osteotomy

The incision line is drawn on the lateral heel. This lies posterior to the peroneal tendons, extending from the superior calcaneus deep to the Achilles tendon, ending approximately 2 cm distal to the tip of the fibula. The incision is deepened through subcutaneous tissue, care being taken to avoid the branches of the sural nerve. Dissection is carried down to the periosteum and the periosteum is split in the line of the skin incision, which is raised and dorsalaterally and inferiorly so that two small Hohmann retractors can be inserted to protect the Achilles tendon superiorly and plantar fascia inferiorly. The osteotomy is performed with an oscillating saw in line with the skin incision at an angle of 45°

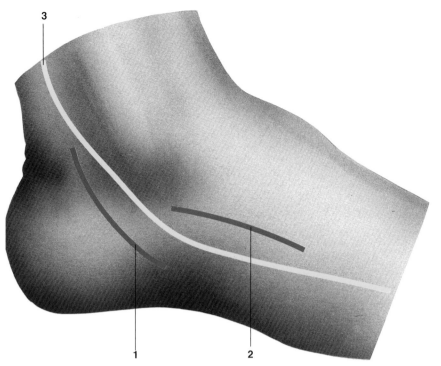

Figure 5

Lateral aspect of the foot: skin incisions

1 Incision for calcaneal osteotomy
2 Incision for calcaneal elongation osteotomy
3 Sural nerve

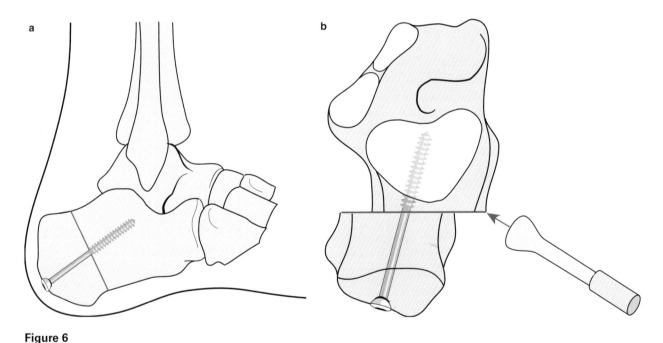

Figure 6

a.–b. Crush plasty after internal fixation of a medial displacement calcaneal osteotomy

to the plantar surface. Once the osteotomy is complete, a smooth lamina spreader is inserted into the osteotomy site so that the tips of the spreader extend to the medial side of the osteotomy. The spreader is then opened to allow soft-tissue mobilization medially. This facilitates the osteotomy to be displaced medially 0.5–1.5 cm. Care should be

taken to prevent superior migration of the posterior fragment. It is stabilized with a 7-mm cannulated screw under image intensification (Figure 6). A 'crush plasty' of the calcaneus can be performed [Schon and Bell 1996]. Closure is over a drain performed using an absorbable material and 4.0 vertical sutures to the skin.

a

b

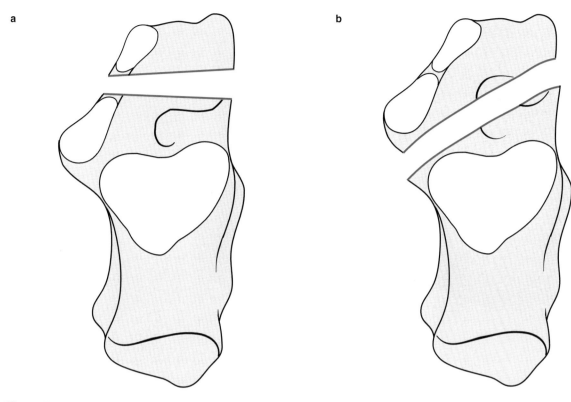

Figure 7

a. Distal calcaneal lengthening; b. proximal calcaneal lengthening

Calcaneal osteotomy with lateral column lengthening

If lateral column lengthening is planned, provision needs to be made for harvesting of a tricortical graft or using an allograft. The skin incision for the calcaneal osteotomy is extended to the base of the fourth metatarsal. The extensor digitorum brevis is elevated from the anterior calcaneus to expose the capsule of the calcaneocuboid joint. The peroneal tendons and sural nerve are elevated and the calcaneus is exposed. Hohmann retractors can be inserted superiorly and inferiorly to protect the peroneal tendon, sural nerve and plantar fascia. The calcaneocuboid joint is not opened but its position is located with a needle. The site of the osteotomy is 1.0–1.5 cm posteriorly and parallel to the calcaneocuboid joint (Figure 7). The osteotomy is directed towards the medial aspect of the foot. In certain individuals the anterior middle facets can coalesce to a single articulation, so an osteotomy anterior to the middle facet may violate it. Kundert et al. [2000] suggested directing the osteotomy posteriorly to the sustentaculum in the line of the tarsal canal. After performing the osteotomy it is distracted with a smooth spreader. If the bone is soft or tending to crush, two osteotomes can be passed side by side into the osteotomy site and the spreader placed between them. The peroneus brevis or lateral plantar fascia can be lengthened at this stage if tight. Distraction with the spreader is performed until the medial arch of the foot is formed. The size of the gap is measured. An appropriate bone block in a trapeziodal shape with the cortical bone lateral is harvested. Insertion of the bone block is facilitated by further distraction through K-wires anterior and posterior to the osteotomy site. Oversizing the graft by 1 or 2 mm on the lateral side allows for any settling and is stabilized by a 2-mm wire through the anterior process, bone block and posterior calcaneus. Closure is as for calcaneal osteotomy.

Arthroereisis

Arthroereisis is performed through a 2–3-cm incision over the sinus tarsi which is deepened to expose the extensor digitorum brevis, which is elevated. The interosseous ligament is identified and sectioned, and the sinus tarsi is cleared. A manipulating rod is then inserted into the sinus tarsi from lateral to medial to enlarge the sinus tarsi and tarsal canal. The rod allows further manipulation to rotate

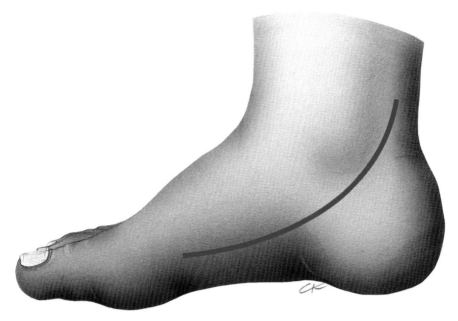

Figure 8

Medial skin incision for correction of flat-foot deformity

the calcaneus internally under the talus. Appropriate trials are inserted, to determine the size most appropriate to achieve the desired correction of the medial arch and to block heel valgus. Once the appropriate sizer has been chosen, the implant is inserted and secured, according to the individual design and methods of fixation. Subcutaneous closure is performed using a non-absorbable material and 4.0 nylon for skin. A drain is not usually required.

Soft-tissue procedures

After the lateral bony procedures are completed the roll is removed from under the ipsilateral buttock. The medial incision is marked in the line of the posterior tibial tendon (Figure 8) from the first metatarsal cuneiform joint to posterior to the medial malleolus. After incision numerous venules are encountered, especially in the distal half of the incision. The posterior tibial tendon sheath is opened and inspected for swelling, intrafascicular degeneration, scarring adhesions or complete rupture. Debridement and excision of diseased portions of the tendon are performed. The proximal tendon is tested for free excursion. If present, a primary repair may be possible with or without 'Z' lengthening. After repair, the side-to-side tenodesis of the flexor digitorum longus is performed (described earlier). If there is no excursion of the posterior tibial tendon, then the tendon is sectioned posterior to the medial malleolus. Reconstruction by tendon transfer is then indicated; this can be achieved with a flexor digitorum longus transfer or a modified Cobb procedure.

Flexor digitorum longus transfer

The tendon of the flexor digitorum longus lies posterolateral to the posterior tibial tendon. The sheath is opened and traced to the knot of Henry; here there is a plexus of veins, and bleeding following division is often difficult to control. Here both flexor digitorum and flexor hallucis longus tendons must be visualized to protect the medial plantar nerve on the plantar side. The flexor digitorum and flexor hallucis longus tendons usually have connecting fibers, so distal tenodesis is not routinely performed. The capsule of the talonavicular joint and the spring ligament need to be plicated, and this is performed using an elliptical incision to excise the lax central portion (Figure 9). The dorsal aspect of the navicular is exposed and a 4.5-mm drill hole is made dorsal to plantar approximately 1 cm lateral to its medial border. The flexor digitorum longus tendon is passed from plantar to dorsal, facilitated by placing a Chinese trap tie over the end of the tendon stump or using a Krachow-type stitch. If a 3-mm suction tube is passed through the drill hole, the suture end can be sucked into the suction tip and pulled through, followed by the tendon. The tension on the tendon transfer is such as to hold the position between rest and maximum excursion with the foot held in maximum inversion and slight plantarflexion. The tendon is sutured to the periosteum of the navicular and itself with 2.0 non-absorbable sutures (Figure 10). The strength of the reconstruction is tested by taking the foot through a full range of dorsiflexion and plantarflexion. The wound is closed in a routine manner over a drain.

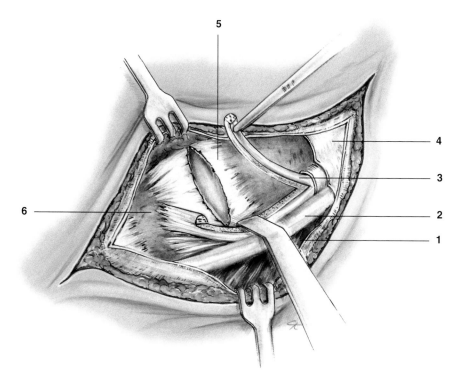

Figure 9

Following dissection of the dorsal half of the posterior tibial tendon, an incision is made in the talo-navicular joint capsule and this is plicated

1 Abductor hallucis brevis muscle
2 Flexor digitorum longus tendon sheath
3 Posterior tibial tendon (divided)
4 Flexor retinaculum
5 Talonavicular joint capsule (ellipse excised)
6 Navicular

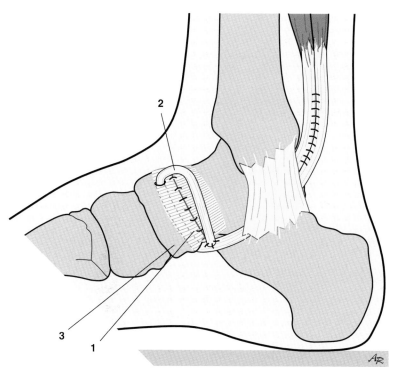

Figure 10

Flexor digitorum longus transfer. Following plication of the navicular joint capsule, the flexor digitorum longus is passed through a drill hole in the navicular. Side-to-side tenodesis is performed between the posterior tibial tendon and the flexor digitorum longus tendon

1 Talonavicular joint capsule (plicated)
2 Flexor digitorum longus transfer
3 Navicular

Modified Cobb procedure

An alternative to flexor digitorum longus transfer is to use the tibialis anterior tendon [Helal 1991]. An incision is made 10 cm proximal to the ankle joint in the line of the tibialis anterior tendon, which is exposed, and its medial half is immobilized using a tendon stripper to its insertion into the medial cuneiform. If difficulty is encountered at the level of the extensor retinaculum a separate incision is performed at this level. The separated tendon is divided and tunneled subcutaneously to the plantar aspect of the foot or passed through a drill hole in the medial cuneiform from dorsal to plantar. This gives the advantage of providing plantar support for a sagging at the naviculocuneiform joint. The tendon is then routed through the bed of the posterior tibial tendon to its proximal divided end, where an

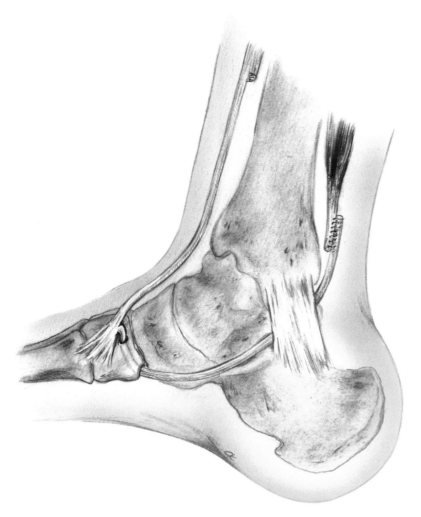

Figure 11

Modified Cobb procedure: an anastomosis is performed using a Pulvertaft weave

anastomosis is performed using a Pulvertaft weave (Figure 11) with the tension set so that the musculo-tendinous unit is taut, with the foot being held in maximum inversion and slight plantarflexion. This will allow for stretching of the fibers of the posterior tibial muscle, which have previously shortened. The talonavicular capsule and spring ligament should also be plicated. Closure is over a drain in a routine manner.

Postoperatively the dressing consists of a well-padded plaster cast with the foot in inversion and slight plantarflexion. Drains are removed after 24h. The cast is changed at 4 weeks and the foot brought into a more plantigrade position. At 6 weeks the cast is removed and a stirrup splint ankle orthosis is used for a further 6 weeks. Ten weeks after surgery the patient is commenced on inversion strengthening exercises with graduated resisted exercises and assisted heel raises using both feet with a counter or bar support, performing three sets of ten repetitions and progressing to single limb heel raises. Progress is determined by consolidation of the osteotomy. Full recovery can vary from 6 to 9 months.

Treatment of stage 3 disease

By definition stage 3 disease represents a fixed hindfoot deformity that it is not fully correctable. The fixed deformity may be confined to a single joint while the other joints remain reducible; in such cases a limited fusion may be feasible [Kelly and Easley 2001]. Any fusion must fully correct all fixed deformities determined preoperatively on clinical examination. Correction of contracture of the gastrocnemius soleus complex must be addressed at the time of surgery. Triple arthrodesis still remains the gold standard (the technique is described in Chapter 31). Pre-radiographic grade 4 disease may be found in this group, and the symptoms of ankle arthrosis may be exacerbated after a successful triple arthrodesis. A medial translational calcaneal osteotomy may be sufficient to unload the lateral ankle joint. Single and double arthrodeses can be used as an alternative, but double arthrodesis in association with posterior tibial tendon insufficiency is more prone to non-union [Mann and Beaman 1999]. For this reason supplementary

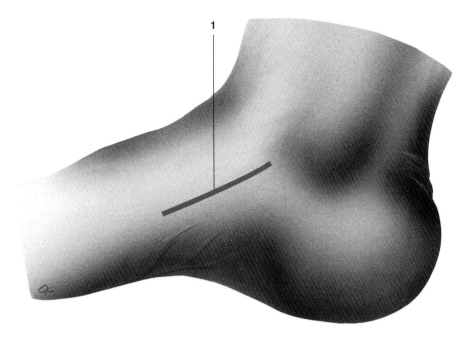

Figure 12

Medial aspect of the foot skin

1   Incision for the talonavicular arthrodesis

corticocancellous graft placed into a trough talonavicular and calcaneocuboid joints is advised when limited fusions are performed (Figure 12).

Treatment of stage 4 disease

Talar tilt of more then 2° on valgus stress radiology of the ankle joint indicates stage 4 disease. Conservative management of stage 4 disease is indicated where surgery is prohibited, or functional demands are low. Treatment of stage 4 disease is dependent on whether ankle arthrosis is symptomatic. Where the ankle arthrosis is asymptomatic then, in conjunction with triple arthrodesis, a deltoid ligament plication and medial calcaneal translational osteotomy are indicated. Where the ankle arthrosis is symptomatic then a tibiotalocalcaneal arthrodesis or a pantalar fusion are indicated. Both of these procedures are technically demanding and have the potential for complications such as skin breakdown, deep infection and malunion. Malunion is not well tolerated and deformity must be corrected as part of the procedure.

References

Aronow MS (2000) Triceps surae contractures associated with posterior tibial tendon dysfunction. Tech Orthop 15: 164–173

Dyal CM, Feder J, Deland T, Thompson FM (1997) Pes planus with posterior tibial tendon insufficiency: asymptomatic versus symptomatic foot. Foot Ankle Int 18: 85–88

Evans D (1975) Calcaneo-valgus deformity. J Bone Joint Surg 57B: 270–278

Funk DA, Cass JR, Johnson KA (1986) Acquired adult flat foot secondary to posterior tibial-tendon pathology. J Bone Joint Surg 68A: 95–102

Helal B (1990) Cobb repair for tibialis posterior tendon rupture. J Foot Surg 29: 349–352

Kelly IP, Easley ME (2001) Treatment of stage 3 adult acquired flatfoot. Foot Ankle Clin 6: 153–166

Koutsogiannis E (1971) Treatment of mobile flatfoot by displacement osteotomy of the calcaneus. J Bone Joint Surg 53B: 96–100

Kundert HP, Hintermann B, Calderrabano V (2000) Lengthening of the lateral column and reconstruction of the medial soft tissue for treatment of acquired flatfoot deformity associated with dysfunction of the posterior tibial tendon. Presented at the Calcaneal Osteotomies AFCP 2nd International Spring Meeting, Bordeaux

Mann RA, Beaman DN (1999) Double arthrodesis in the adult. Clin Orthop 365: 74–80

Pomeroy GC, Manoli A (1997) A new operative approach for flatfoot secondary to posterior tibial tendon insufficiency: a preliminary report. Foot Ankle Int 18: 206–211

Schon LC, Bell W (1996) Tips and pearls: crush-plasty of the calcaneus. Tech Orthop 11: 222–223

Shereff MJ (1997) Treatment of ruptured posterior tibial tendon with direct repair and F.D.L. tenodesis. Foot Ankle Clin 2: 281–296

24

Cavus foot deformity

Nikolaus Wülker

Introduction

Cavus foot deformity is an abnormally increased height of the longitudinal arch of the foot. This is mostly an idiopathic disorder, but undetected or obvious neurological disease may induce cavus foot deformity or contribute to it [Japas 1968, Ghanem et al. 1996]. Symptoms from idiopathic cavus foot deformity often appear during midlife and are usually related to increased focal pressures underneath the foot, most commonly at the metatarsal heads [Imhäuser 1969, Jahss 1980]. Static pain due to the abnormal foot architecture may also be present. Concomitant toe deformity often aggravates symptoms. If an underlying neurological disease is present, patients usually present during childhood or adolescence.

Diagnosis

On clinical examination, the height of the longitudinal arch of the foot is abnormally increased on the medial side. In an adult, this height is usually not higher than 3 cm. The lateral midfoot, which normally rests firmly on the ground, may also be elevated in severe cavus deformity. Hindfoot and midfoot alignment in the axial plane is usually normal, i.e. hindfoot eversion or inversion are not present and there is no more than a slight amount of forefoot adduction. Plantar callosities are common and appear particularly at the metatarsal heads – rarely under the heel. At the forefoot, the first and fifth metatarsal heads are most commonly affected, but the distribution is variable. Callosities are often extremely tender, preventing weightbearing, and

impending or complete ulceration may be present. Palpation usually reveals increased tension of the long and short extensor tendons of all toes. If advanced, this results in claw deformity of the toes, with hyperextension of the metatarsophalangeal joints and hyperflexion of the interphalangeal joints. Toe contractures develop with time, and sores from pressure against the shoe appear at the dorsum of the affected toes. Ankle dorsiflexion is often somewhat decreased, owing to tightness of the Achilles tendon, in particular if an underlying neurological disease is present. Subtalar motion is usually normal. Rearfoot and tarsometatarsal joint mobility may be normal, but is usually somewhat diminished.

Weightbearing radiographs in two planes are necessary for radiological assessment (Figure 1). On the lateral view, the axes of the talus and of the first metatarsal bone are normally parallel. In cavus foot deformity, these axes form an angle with a superior apex, and the angle between the two lines increases with the severity of the deformity. Malalignment may affect mainly the first metatarsal, or all metatarsals may be oriented plantarwards. The angle between the axes of the calcaneus and the first metatarsal bone is approximately 130° in a normal foot and is decreased in cavus foot deformity. The calcaneal pitch, i.e. the angle between the axis of the calcaneus and the ground, is physiologically between 20 and 30°. Additional deformity, in particular at the ankle and hindfoot joints, is assessed on the radiographs. Toe deformity is also often apparent on the lateral view. The dorsoplantar radiograph is used to exclude malalignment of the foot in the axial plane and bone deformity, which may be related to the etiology of cavus foot.

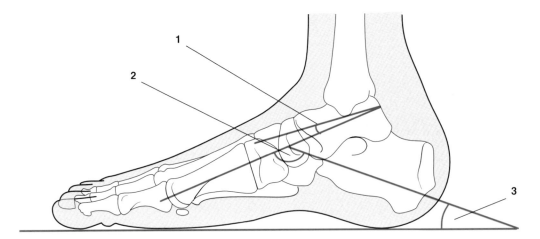

Figure 1

Measurements of cavus foot deformity on a lateral weightbearing radiograph

1   Talometatarsal angle (normal 0°);
2   Calcaneometatarsal angle (normal 130°);
3   Calcaneal pitch (normal 20–30°)

Decision making

The indication for surgery depends on the severity of symptoms. Some patients with an advanced deformity have only mild symptoms and can be treated with an orthopedic shoe with a well-moulded foot bed. Others with less advanced deformities have severe pain, usually due to metatarsalgia, and require surgical correction of their cavus deformity [Hibbs 1919, D'Souza 1997]. Surgical procedures designed for the treatment of metatarsalgia, such as distal metatarsal osteotomies, are contraindicated because they do not correct the elevation of the longitudinal arch. Corrective bone procedures should be performed after the completion of growth, unless severe deformity due to neurological disease is present. Release of the plantar fascia alone [Sammarco and Taylor 2001] is not advised and may be successful only in flexible and mild deformities, in particular in children and adolescents. Plantar fascia release in this setting may be combined with tendon transfer [Steindler 1917], e.g. of the long extensor tendons to the midfoot.

Most commonly, the apex of the cavus deformity is located between the Chopart joint and the tarsometatarsal joints, as evident on the weightbearing lateral radiograph. This is corrected with a dorsal tarsal wedge resection osteotomy [Imhäuser 1972] or its variants [Cole 1940, Coleman and Chestnut 1977, Jahss 1983]. The Chopart joint and the tarsometatarsal joints should be left intact, but the joints in between can usually not be preserved. A minor degree of forefoot supination or pronation can be corrected by rotating the osteotomy. The

plantar fascia is not routinely transected and may be helpful for tension band stabilization of the osteotomy. However, if the osteotomy cannot be closed because of increased tension of the plantar fascia, a plantar release is performed through an additional medial approach at the heel. Achilles tendon tightness must to be corrected simultaneously, if present. Additional toe deformities are corrected according to their severity.

If metatarsal malalignment affects only the first metatarsal, i.e. if the axes of the talus and of the remaining metatarsals are parallel, the deformity is corrected with a dorsal closing wedge first metatarsal osteotomy [Siffert et al. 1966, Swanson et al. 1966]. A claw deformity of the great toe often has to be corrected simultaneously.

Less frequently, hindfoot malalignment is responsible for cavus deformity. In these patients, the talometatarsal angle is normal but the calcaneometatarsal angle is increased, i.e. an increased pitch of the calcaneus causes the deformity. This requires a calcaneal osteotomy with superior displacement of the posterior tuberosity fragment [Jones 1927, Dwyer 1975]. Additional procedures at the toes, plantar fascia or Achilles tendon are not usually required in this setting.

If significant heel varus is present, the deformity is more a club foot than a cavus foot. In adults, this usually requires a triple arthrodesis [Samilson 1976] or rarely a corrective calcaneal osteotomy.

General contraindications, such as peripheral vascular disease or severe neurological disability, must be observed.

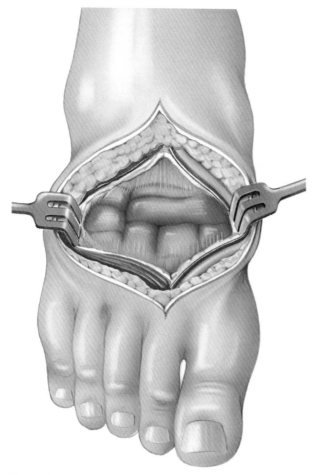

Figure 2

Surgical exposure for dorsal tarsal wedge resection osteotomy

Operative technique

The patient is placed on the operating table in the supine position with an adequate wedge support under the ipsilateral pelvis. General or spinal anesthesia is preferable; an ankle block alone is usually not adequate. The leg is exsanguinated and a thigh tourniquet is applied. A prophylactic single-dose antibiotic may be given.

Dorsal tarsal wedge resection osteotomy

This is the most commonly used bone procedure to correct cavus foot deformity. A 6–8-cm longitudinal incision extends from the anterior aspect of the ankle joint distally between the second and third rays to mid-metatarsal level. The subcutaneus tissues are divided with care to protect the cutaneous branches of the superficial peroneal nerve. A plane

is identified between the long extensor tendons to the second and third toes. The extensor digitorum brevis muscle is identified, elevated subperiosteally and retracted with the tendon of the peroneus brevis laterally. The tendons of the extensor hallucis longus, the tibialis anterior and the dorsalis pedis artery are retracted medially (Figure 2).

Hohmann retractors are placed around the tarsal bones and the anatomy is securely identified. In particular the level of the Chopart joint and of the tarsometatarsal joints must be seen. The first osteotomy is performed just distal to the Chopart joint and parallel to the joint surface, i.e. perpendicular to the bottom of the foot (Figure 3). An oscillating saw may be used initially, but the osteotomy should carefully be completed with an osteotome in order to avoid injury to the plantar structures. The distal part of the foot is slightly plantarflexed in order to ensure that the osteotomy through the navicular and through the cuboid is complete. However, the periosteum on the plantar aspect of the osteotomy should remain intact, to enhance stability once the osteotomy is closed.

The second osteotomy is made further distally, but preferably proximal to the tarsometatarsal joints. The location of the second osteotomy depends on the degree of the deformity, because the size of the wedge to be removed is proportionate to the amount of forefoot equinus that is to be corrected. The angle between the two osteotomies corresponds to the talometatarsal angle on the preoperative weightbearing radiograph. The second osteotomy must be aimed so that it exits at the plantar margin of the first osteotomy.

The wedge is closed by dorsiflexion of the forefoot. If this is not possible without undue force, the soft tissues at the plantar aspect of the osteotomy should be carefully mobilized. This usually allows closure of the wedge. If excessive tension is still present, the plantar fascia is released through a separate medial incision at the heel (see below). Additional bone resection is not advised as this will shorten the foot. If a rotational supination or pronation deformity is present between the forefoot and the heel, this is simultaneously corrected by adding the appropriate corrective rotation at the osteotomy site.

Fixation of the closed wedge osteotomy is best achieved with large bone staples inserted through the dorsum of the foot (Figure 4). The staples may sometimes have to reach proximally across the Chopart joint or distally across the tarsometatarsal joints. This is acceptable as long as they are removed once the osteotomy has healed.

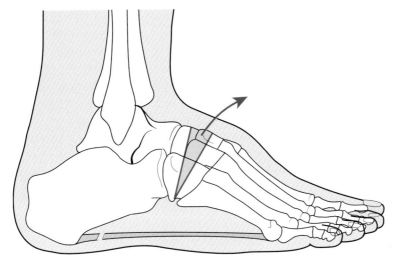

Figure 3

Dorsal tarsal wedge resection osteotomy. A bone wedge with a dorsal base is resected between the Chopart joint and the tarso-metatarsal joints. The size of the wedge corresponds to the degree of cavus deformity on preoperative weightbearing radiographs

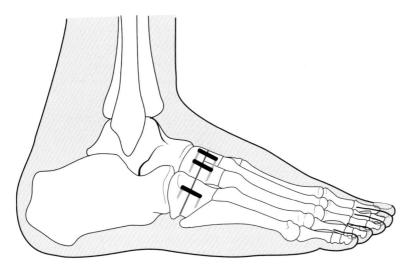

Figure 4

The dorsal tarsal wedge resection osteotomy is best stabilized with large bone staples on the dorsal side

Alternatively, compression screws across the osteotomy may be used, but they also generally cross the adjacent joints and should be removed following consolidation of the osteotomy. Fixation with wires is generally less stable. An intraoperative radiograph or fluoroscopy are recommended to secure complete correction of the deformity.

The extensor tendon sheaths and retinaculum are closed with interrupted absorbable sutures. Skin closure is routine. A split below-knee cast is applied under anesthesia.

Additional toe correction or Achilles tendon lengthening may have to be performed as needed (see below).

Basal first metatarsal osteotomy

The approach is through a dorsomedial incision centered over the base of the first metatarsal bone.

Round retractors are inserted around the bone. The first tarsometatarsal joint is identified in order to avoid injury to its articular surfaces. The osteotomy is carried out preferably with a power saw. A proximal cut is made parallel to the tarsometatarsal joint through two-thirds to three-quarters of the metatarsal base (Figure 5). The distal cut is made obliquely to meet the plantar end of the first osteotomy. The distance between the osteotomies depends on the severity of the deformity and on the size of the foot. It is usually around 4 mm. The wedge is closed by dorsiflexing the forefoot and cracking the plantar cortex of the metatarsal. Stable internal fixation is advised and this is best achieved with dorsal bone staples or with a tension band wire loop. Only the skin is closed with interrupted sutures.

Additional correction at the great toe may have to be performed as needed (see below).

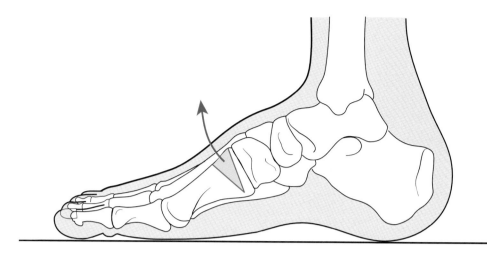

Figure 5

Basal first metatarsal osteotomy

Calcaneal osteotomy

An oblique incision is made laterally over the body of the calcaneus behind the peroneal tendons. The peroneal tendon sheath should not be opened. The subcutaneous tissues are divided and the periosteum is removed from the lateral calcaneal surface with a periosteal elevator. The origin of the plantar fascia and of the short flexor muscles at the tuber of the calcaneus are exposed. An extensive plantar release is usually necessary to allow sufficient displacement of the calcaneus. Round retractors are inserted superiorly and inferiorly around the calcaneus. The calcaneofibular ligament is sectioned and the peroneal tendons are retracted anteriorly.

The osteotomy may be initiated with an oscillating saw but must cautiously be completed with an osteotome, in order to avoid injury to the neurovascular structures medial to the calcaneus. The location of the osteotomy is midway between the posterior margin of the subtalar joint and the posterior border of the calcaneus (Figure 6). The orientation of the osteotomy is midway between the longitudinal axis of the calcaneus and the vertical axis of the foot. Once the surrounding periosteum has been sufficiently released, superior displacement of the posterior calcaneal fragment should be possible, usually 1–2 cm, depending on preoperative measurements, to restore a normal calcaneometatarsal angle. A thick threaded pin may have to be inserted into the posterior fragment to facilitate manipulation.

Once adequate correction is obtained, the pin is advanced into the body of the calcaneus for temporary fixation. One or two large cancellous screws are used for permanent stabilization. They are oriented perpendicular to the osteotomy. Care must be taken to avoid penetration of the screws into the subtalar

joint, and intraoperative radiography is advised. Washers may have to be used in soft bone, but excessive protrusion of the screw heads must be avoided. The calcaneofibular ligament and the peroneal tendon sheath are sutured with absorbable thread and the skin is closed. A split below-knee cast is applied under anesthesia.

Additional procedures at the toes or at the Achilles tendon are not usually necessary.

Plantar release

This procedure is rarely carried out alone and is usually used in conjunction with bone procedures, if required. The incision begins medially at the posterior calcaneal tuberosity and extends halfway along the inferior aspect of the calcaneus. The subcutaneous tissues are divided in line with the skin incision. The superficial and deep surfaces of the plantar fascia are separated from the fat and muscles. The abductor hallucis muscle is released from its origin at the calcaneus. A generous portion of the plantar fascia is excised throughout its breadth. The short flexor and plantar muscles are divided extraperiosteally from their origin at the calcaneus and stripped distally. The short plantar, long plantar and calcaneonavicular ligaments are sectioned if further correction is required. A wound drain may have to be inserted. The wound is usually closed in one layer. A split below-knee cast is applied under anesthesia.

Correction of toe deformity

Toe malalignment in cavus foot deformity is particularly common at the great toe and is due to excessive tension of the long extensor tendon. Treatment is by

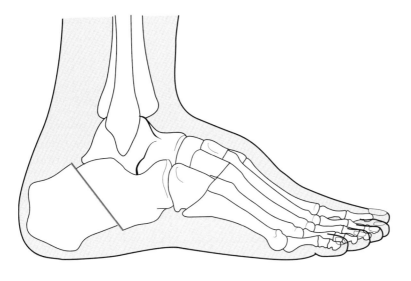

Figure 6

Calcaneal osteotomy

transfer of this tendon to the metatarsal head. This is performed through a longitudinal dorsal incision. At the great toe, the extensor tendon is guided through a horizontal drill hole at the first metatarsal head, from lateral to medial. The tendon must be under moderate tension in the neutral foot position. At the lesser toes, fixation of the tendon to the soft tissues at the dorsum of the metatarsal head is usually adequate. Additional capsular release at the metatarsophalangeal joint, with transection of the short extensor tendon if necessary, and condylectomy of the proximal phalanx or arthrodesis of the (proximal) interphalangeal joint may be necessary, if contractures are present.

Postoperative treatment

Postoperatively, the foot is elevated in a below-knee splint. After a few days, ambulation without weightbearing is allowed as swelling of the foot permits. Sutures are removed after 2 weeks and a non-weightbearing below-knee plaster cast is used for 6 weeks. The cast must be well moulded, with the foot in the corrected position. A lateral radiograph in the cast must be obtained. Six weeks postoperatively, the cast is removed and radiographs in two planes are taken to assess the position and the consolidation of the osteotomy. Subsequently, a weightbearing cast is applied until 12 weeks postoperatively. Following cast removal, intensive physiotherapy is initiated to restore ankle and hindfoot joint motion and a normal gait pattern. Regular shoes can be used and insoles or plantar pads are prescribed only if plantar pressure symptoms persist in the corrected position of the foot. The metal

implants are not removed in older patients, if they do not cross the Chopart and tarsometatarsal joints. Otherwise, hardware removal is after approximately 1 year.

Results and complications

The goal of cavus foot correction is to restore a normal longitudinal arch and a pain-free, physiological plantar pressure pattern. The former is generally achieved if adequate operative technique is used, but a number of patients will have slight residual symptoms even several years after the procedure [Wülker and Hurschler 2002]. Some pain on weightbearing often persists, even if it is generally clearly improved compared to preoperatively. This is mostly diffuse discomfort at the mid- or hindfoot, or residual plantar pressure pain.

Complications include delayed wound healing and deep infection, which are no more common than with other hindfoot procedures. Neurovascular injury may occur but is usually limited to sensory disturbance at the dorsum of the foot and at the toes. Non-union of the osteotomy is most common with the dorsal tarsal wedge resection osteotomy, but does not always cause symptoms and rarely requires revision. Implants should be removed to avoid breakage.

Overcorrection, and in particular undercorrection, may occur and should be avoided by meticulous measurements on preoperative radiographs and intraoperatively. The risk of deep vein thrombosis and pulmonary embolism is increased during postoperative cast immobilization, and prophylactic anticoagulants should be administered.

References

Cole WH (1940) Treatment of claw foot. J Bone Joint Surg 22: 895–908

Coleman SS, Chestnut WJ (1977) A simple test for hindfoot flexibility in the cavovarus foot. Clin Orthop 60: 123

D'Souza LG (1997) Cavus foot deformity. In: Wülker N, Stephens M, Cracchiolo A (eds) An Atlas of Foot and Ankle Surgery. London, Martin Dunitz, pp 181–190

Dwyer FC (1975) The present status of problem of pes cavus. Clin Orthop 106: 254

Ghanem I, Zeller R, Seringe R (1996) The foot in hereditary motor and sensory neuropathies in children. Rev Chir Orthop Rep Appar Mot 82: 152–160

Hibbs RA (1919) An operation for claw foot. J Am Med Assoc 73: 1583–1585

Imhäuser G (1969) Die operative Behandlung des stakren Hohlfußes und des Ballenhohlfußes. Z Orthop 106: 488–494

Imhäuser G (1972) Podiumsgespräch Arbeitskreis 'Hohlfuß'. Z Orthop 110: 833–838

Jahss MH (1980) Tarsometatarsal truncated wedge arthrodesis for pes cavus and equinovarus deformity of the fore part of the foot. J Bone Joint Surg 62A: 713

Jahss MH (1983) Evaluation of the cavus foot for orthopaedic treatment. Clin Orthop 181: 52–63

Japas LM (1968) Surgical treatment of pes cavus by tarsal V osteotomy. J Bone Joint Surg 50A: 927

Jones AR (1927) Discussion on treatment of pes cavus. Proc Roy Soc Med 20: 1117–1132

Samilson RL (1976) Crescentric osteotomy of os calcis for calcaneo cavus feet. In: Bateman JE (ed) Foot Science. Philadelphia, WB Saunders, pp 18–25

Sammarco GJ, Taylor R (2001) Cavovarus foot treated with combined calcaneus and metatarsal osteotomies. Foot Ankle Int 22: 19–30

Siffert RS, Forster RI, Nachamie B (1966) Beak triple arthrodesis for correction of severe cavus deformity. Clin Orthop 45: 103

Steindler A (1917) Stripping of os calcis. Surg Gynecol Obstet 24: 617

Swanson AB, Browne HS, Coleman JD (1966) The cavus foot: concepts of production and treatment by metatarsal osteotomy. J Bone Joint Surg 48A: 1019

Wülker N, Hurschler C (2002) Cavus foot correction in adults by dorsal closing wedge osteotomy. Foot Ankle Int 23: 344–347

25

Chronic heel pain: surgical management

William C. McGarvey

Introduction

Inferior heel pain may be the most common problem seen by orthopedic surgeons specializing in the foot and ankle. A host of etiologies have been suggested, including metabolic, systemic, traumatic, or even neoplastic disorders (Table 1). However, inferior heel pain is most often attributed to degeneration at the insertion of the plantar fascia on the calcaneus, entrapment of the first branch of the lateral plantar nerve or the concomitant existence of both. Factors previously thought to be contributory to painful heel syndrome, such as obesity, gender, lifestyle, or the presence and size of the heel spur, are not predictive. In a non-athletic population, inferior heel pain has been attributed to the initiation of an exercise program, periods of unusual or excessive activity or idiopathic spontaneous occurrences. More athletic individuals are affected by errors in training, or unsuitable footwear or training surfaces. A thorough history and physical examination are the most important diagnostic tools. The patients usually report pain in the plantar medial heel, worse with the first few steps in the morning or upon rising after prolonged sitting. Pain frequently diminishes after activity has begun but may not completely resolve. Some will have worsening pain aggravated by prolonged walking or standing on hard surfaces. Physical findings include tenderness at the calcaneal insertion of the plantar fascia on the medial tubercle. Additionally, many patients will have tenderness along the course of the first branch of the lateral plantar nerve and have a

Table 1   Sources of heel pain

1. *Heel pain syndrome*
   Plantar fasciitis
   First branch of lateral plantar nerve entrapment
   Inflammation of short flexor origin
   Inferior calcaneal bursitis
   Plantar heel spur

2. *Fat pad atrophy*

3. *Arthritides*
   Rheumatoid arthritis
   Reiter's syndrome
   Ankylosing spondylitis
   Psoriatic arthritis

4. *Trauma*
   Soft-tissue contusion, repetitive trauma
   Stress fracture
   Acute fracture
   Puncture wound
   Plantar fascia rupture

5. *Miscellaneous*
   Benign tumors
   Malignant tumors (primary and metastatic)
   Infection
   Metabolic (diabetes, crystalline arthropathies, Paget's disease)

6. *Vascular*
   Peripheral vascular disease

7. *Secondary*
   Extremity injuries leading to abnormal gait, compensatory stresses
   Radiculopathy

positive Tinel's sign in this area. Provocative measures such as pronation and abduction of the foot or simultaneous dorsiflexion of the toes and ankle are occasionally helpful. Radiographs will *sometimes* show a plantar spur but this is not considered an etiological factor. In confusing cases, adjunctive testing with either electrodiagnostic studies or bone scans is helpful. Usually these are more useful in eliminating other sources of pathology, e.g. lumbar radiculopathy or calcaneal stress fracture.

Once diagnosed, painful heel syndrome is most often treated successfully by non-operative means. In fact, 90% of patients will respond to conservative measures at an average of 11 months from the onset of this pain. Non-operative treatment includes stretching of the heel cord and of the plantar foot structures for 10-s intervals 8–10 times a day. Also helpful are viscoelastic heel cushions or other orthotic modifications, such as heel wedges or arch supports, and night splinting. Medical treatments such as short courses of anti-inflammatory drugs or cortisone injections are sometimes useful. In recalcitrant cases, immobilization using various taping or strapping techniques or even casting has been helpful.

Even after exhaustive non-surgical treatment, 10% of patients will still complain of heel pain. After all other causes of heel pain have been ruled out, surgical management via partial plantar fasciotomy with nerve release may be indicated. Contraindications include other sources of heel pain, such as metabolic or systemic disease, lumbar radicular pain, peripheral neuropathy, tarsal tunnel syndrome and various rheumatological disorders.

Anatomy

It is important for the surgeon to be familiar with the pertinent anatomy and potential variations, in particular with the nerves that supply the heel (Figure 1).

The medial calcaneal branches usually arise proximally from the tibial nerve, are frequently multiple, and travel posterior to the area of the planned incision.

The first branch of the lateral plantar nerve in most cases originates just distal to the line connecting the medial malleolus with the calcaneal tuberosity. It dives deep to the abductor hallucis muscle and travels plantarwards between the taut deep fascia of the abductor hallucis and the medial caudal margin of the quadratus plantae muscle, where it is thought to become entrapped. It then proceeds in a

horizontal path laterally toward the abductor digiti quinti between the quadratus plantae above and the flexor digitorum brevis below. Most anatomy texts describe the nerve traversing at the level of the midfoot; however, more recent anatomic studies have revealed that it travels much more proximally, at the region just anterior and superior to the origin of the flexor digitorum brevis, i.e. on top of the heel spur, if one is present. Studies have also revealed that this nerve is probably mixed, containing sensory fibers for the calcaneal periosteum and plantar fascia as well as motor fibers to the quadratus plantae, flexor digitorum brevis and abductor digiti quinti.

Treatment

Surgical technique

The patient is placed in the supine position on the operating table. A contralateral hip roll along with slight flexion of the hip and knee will facilitate external rotation and improve access to the desired area of the foot. The procedure is performed most frequently under regional anesthesia. A tourniquet may be used but is not mandatory.

A 3–4-cm oblique incision is made on the medial heel over the proximal portion of the abductor hallucis muscle (Figure 2). The incision should traverse a vertical line extending down just posterior to the medial malleolus and parallel the course of the first branch of the lateral plantar nerve. The incision is situated anterior to the sensory branches of the medial calcaneal nerve, but aberrant nerves, if encountered, should be preserved.

Sharp dissection proceeds until the superficial abductor fascia is encountered, at which point a self-retaining retractor is inserted. The interval between this fascial covering and the medial border of the plantar fascia is then identified. If necessary, a small portion of plantar fascia may be excised for better delineation of the plane between it and the deep abductor fascia. However, in most cases the plantar fascia is identified by sliding a freer along its medial border to encounter its plantar surface.

Once oriented, the surgeon divides the superficial fascia of the abductor hallucis muscle with a no. 15 blade and retracts the muscle belly superiorly, exposing the deep fascial layer (Figure 3). The deep fascia is divided sharply to the extent that the muscle is retracted. This will function to decompress the area in which the nerve is compressed between the taut fascia of the abductor hallucis and the medial border

a

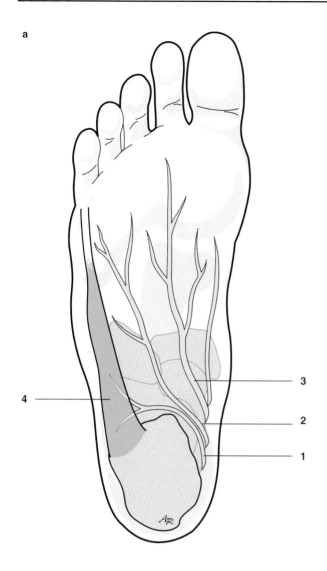

b

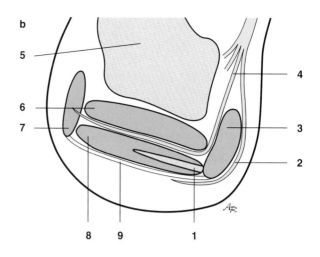

Figure 1

Normal heel anatomy. a. plantar aspect, b. cross-section

a
1 First branch of lateral plantar nerve
2 Lateral plantar nerve
3 Medial plantar nerve
4 Abductor digiti quinti muscle

b
1 Heel spur (if present)
2 Medial calcaneal nerve
3 Abductor hallucis muscle
4 First branch of lateral plantar nerve
5 Calcaneus
6 Quadratus plantae muscle
7 Abductor digiti quinti muscle
8 Flexor digitorum brevis muscle
9 Plantar fascia

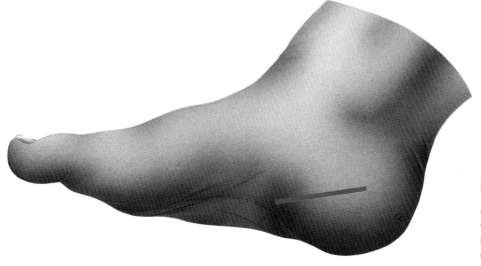

Figure 2

An oblique incision is used over the medial heel at the proximal portion of the abductor hallucis muscle

of the quadratus plantae muscle as the nerve changes its course from vertical to horizontal on its way to the abductor digiti quinti muscle. The deep fascia of the abductor hallucis muscle is thick and usually of two layers, being directly over the neurovascular bundle.

The surgeon should visualize the perineural fat before proceeding. It is not necessary to dissect out the nerve as this only increases the risk of bleeding and thrombosis of the vessels, along with perineural scarring and devascularization. The abductor hallucis

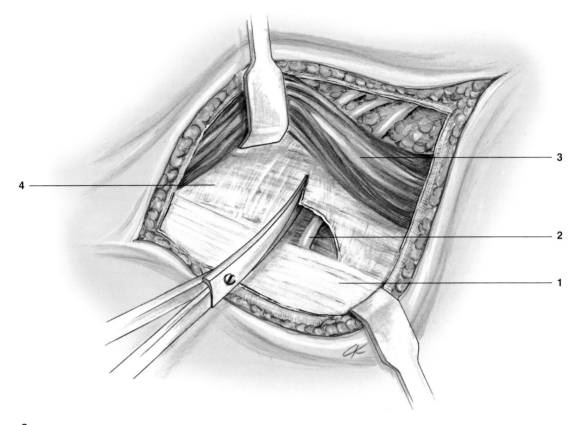

Figure 3

Part of the plantar fascia is resected, as necessary, and the nerve is released

1 Plantar fascia
2 First branch of lateral plantar nerve
3 Abductor hallucis muscle
4 Abductor hallucis deep fascia

is now retracted inferiorly, and again the thick deep fascia is incised to complete its division. The course of the nerve can now be checked by inserting a freer or small hemostat behind the abductor hallucis to palpate any remaining tight bands.

Attention is then directed to the plantar fascia to inspect for chronic inflammatory changes and thickening. If these findings are present, a partial plantar fasciectomy may be performed. It is helpful at this point to reposition the self-retaining retractor more inferiorly to maximize visualization into the wound. The no. 15 blade is used to excise a rectangular portion of full-thickness plantar fascia measuring 4–5 mm longitudinally and approximately one-third to one-half the width of the entire plantar fascia (Figure 4).

Should the patient have symptoms along the entire plantar fascia, as determined preoperatively, it may be beneficial to perform a complete fasciotomy after gaining good visualization of the entire width of the plantar fascia.

Routine excision of the plantar heel spur is not performed for several reasons. First, there is no direct evidence that implicates the spur as a reproducible source of heel pain. Second, resection of the exostosis requires a generous dissection of muscle and fascia which, in turn, increases the postoperative pain and prolongs the recuperative period. Last, an overaggressive resection of bone may lead to a calcaneal stress reaction or frank fracture, leading to further debilitation of the patient. If, however, a heel spur is present and is felt to be involved in compressing the nerve, it may be removed. This can be done by carefully separating the fibers of the flexor digitorum brevis with the freer and retracting both above and below the bony exostosis. It should be remembered that the first branch of the lateral plantar nerve lies directly superior to the bony shelf along the muscle, and is at risk. A rongeur is usually sufficient to grasp most of the spur and remove it until the inferior calcaneus is smooth.

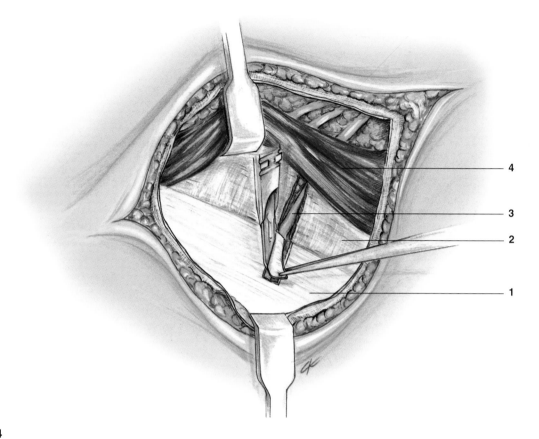

Figure 4

A rectangular portion of full-thickness plantar fascia is excised if chronic inflammatory changes and thickening are present

1   Plantar fascia
2   Abductor hallucis deep fascia
3   First branch of lateral plantar nerve
4   Abductor hallucis muscle

Prior to closure the course of the nerve is checked once again to affirm a free course into the plantar side of the foot. The wound is irrigated and single-layer superficial closure is performed with 3–0 nylon interrupted horizontal mattress sutures. A bulky compressive dressing is then applied to the heel and ankle.

Postoperative care

The postoperative dressing is maintained for 3 days and then changed by the patient to a lighter wrap. The patient should elevate the foot for the majority of the first 48 h postoperatively, getting up only when absolutely necessary. Crutches are generally used for 4–5 days and weightbearing can commence on the third day with the support of a postoperative shoe.

Compression and a light covering are continued along with the postoperative shoe for 2 weeks, after which time the sutures are removed. Patients may then begin gradually to discontinue the bandage and progress to wearing a jogging or other type of shoe with a soft heel pad. By 3 weeks most patients are able to tolerate stationary bicycling, and are walking or even running 1 month from their procedure. The average length of time to full recovery is 3 months, with a range of 1 month to 6 months or beyond in rare cases.

Complications

Complications of the surgical treatment of heel pain include bleeding, infection and wound healing problems. In the specific procedure described above, inadvertent transection of the medial calcaneal nerve branch can leave an area of numbness along the medial plantar heel. This can be avoided by placing the incision properly and taking care to dissect gently at the superior wound margin. Excessive bleeding may lead to hematoma formation and perineural scarring. Careful gentle dissection along with meticulous hemostasis will reduce the incidence of this complication, as will the addition of a compressive postoperative dressing and limited weightbearing in the immediate postoperative period.

Resecting too much plantar fascia can lead to stress transfer to the lateral foot. Good visualization is important to resect the desired width of fascia and avoid this problem. Should stress transfer occur, strapping, taping or even cast immobilization will be of benefit to hold the foot in the proper position until a stabilizing scar forms. Removal of the heel spur also carries inherent risks. Although it is a rare problem, surgeons must be aware that a stress riser may be created by overexuberant removal of bone at the inferior calcaneus, leading to a fracture. Treatment involves limitation of activities and at times avoidance of weightbearing.

Reflex sympathetic dystrophy, now known as complex regional pain syndrome, is an unfortunate, frequently unpredictable and unpreventable result of any surgery, but is a particular concern in operations involving nerve decompressions. Fortunately it occurs only rarely. Therefore, careful surgical technique and a limited dissection must be employed along with a thorough awareness of the anatomy of this area. Should the surgeon suspect the development of reflex sympathetic dystrophy, an early aggressive approach with a variety of treatment modalities is the best management plan.

Alternative methods in the treatment of heel pain

Not all clinicians believe that heel pain originates in the plantar foot. Some are of the opinion that the main culprit in the creation of the painful heel is a tight Achilles tendon. Although this has not been proved, there is good evidence that an overtaut Achilles tendon can, at the very least, contribute to the origination and continuance of plantar heel pain. Many successful conservative modalities are directed, at least in part, to gradual stretching of the Achilles tendon. It is with little surprise, therefore, that recent focus has been directed at surgical lengthening of the Achilles tendon in the treatment of plantar fasciitis.

Most surgeons who are performing these procedures prefer a gastrocsolius recession in the method described by Strayer or a similar technique. In this way, the muscular attachment of the heel cord is undamaged and the strength preserved while allowing greater length and flexibility. Step-cut recessions, like that described by Hoke, have been suggested to weaken the integrity of the tendon and are purported to provide the patient with more weakness.

Recently, non-invasive treatment of plantar fasciitis has been proposed with the concept of 'orthotripsy'. Extracorporeal shock wave therapy has gained wide acceptance as a reasonable step in the presurgical approach and conservative management of heel pain originating purely from chronic, recalcitrant plantar fasciitis. With short treatment times and mild post-procedure discomfort, success rates reported at an average of 65–70% for first treatment and a negligible complication rate, shock wave therapy carries great expectation and promise for the future treatment of this sometimes difficult treatment entity. Further clinical trials and longer-term follow-up are necessary to gain a better understanding of the ultimate usefulness of this management tool.

Endoscopic plantar fascia release

Endoscopic plantar fascia release (EPFR) has gained increasing popularity. Its reported advantages are a smaller incision and quicker recovery time. Preliminary reports, mostly in the podiatric literature but also by some orthopedists, suggests that the method is just as efficacious as an open procedure. However, the blind insertion of the trocar still causes problems. Neurovascular structures – particularly those that deviate somewhat from standard anatomy – are at great risk. Unfortunately, numerous patients are now seen who suffer from neuritic complications of this procedure.

Additionally, owing to the limited visibility through the endoscope, there is the propensity to cut too little or too much of the plantar fascia. If too little is released, the patient will at least have recurrent symptoms. Inadvertent release of too much plantar fascia can lead to load transfer to the outside of the foot, resulting in lateral foot pain secondary to stress overload and possibly even midfoot collapse, a potentially devastating sequela. These problems are not easily treated and frequently do not respond well to conservative orthotic management.

Also, if the patient manifests inferior heel pain syndrome, an endoscopic release addresses only a portion of the problem. Nerve decompression is not possible through this technique and therefore limitations exist with regard to its ability to relieve this condition. It is the author's belief that endoscopic plantar fascia release may have a role in the treatment of some forms of plantar fasciitis, but the surgeon must have experience as well as a good functional awareness of the pertinent anatomy. In addition, the surgeon must be aware of the limitations of this procedure and particularly its potential hazards.

Since the publication of the last edition of this text, the safety and efficacy of EPFR have improved dramatically. This is now a commonly performed procedure, but still carries a rather steep learning curve. The procedure should be reserved for those individuals with isolated plantar fasciitis and no concomitant pathology. Surgeons opting for this method of treatment should be well acquainted with the patient's diagnosis as well as the technique.

Further reading

Baxter DE (1994) Release of the nerve to the abductor digiti quinti. In: Johnson KA (ed) Master Techniques in Orthopaedic Surgery. New York, Raven Press, pp 333–340

Baxter DE, Pfeffer GB (1992) Treatment of chronic heel pain by surgical release of the first branch of the lateral plantar nerve. Clin Orthop 279: 229–236

Baxter DE, Pfeffer GB, Thigpen M (1989) Chronic heel pain treatment rationale. Orthop Clin North Am 20: 563–568

Davis PF, Severud E, Baxter DE (1994) Painful heel syndrome: results of non-operative treatment. Foot Ankle 15: 531–535

Davis TJ, Schon LC (1995) Branches of the tibial nerve: anatomic variations. Foot Ankle 16: 21–29

Lutter LD (1986) Surgical decisions in athletes' subcalcaneal pain. Am J Sports Med 14: 481

Rondhuis M, Hudson A (1986) The first branch of the lateral plantar nerve and heel pain. Acta Morphol Neurol Scand 24: 269–280

Schon LC (1993) Plantar fascia and Baxter's nerve release. In: Myerson MS (ed) Current Therapy in Foot and Ankle Surgery. St Louis, Mosby, pp 177–182

26

Tendon transfers

Kaj Klaue
Jean Pfändler
Mathias Speck
Martin Beck

Definitions

The following conventions are used in this chapter [Sarrafian 1993]:

- **extension:** movement of any joint within a plantigrade foot which results in lifting the distal bone of the joint
- **flexion:** movement of any joint within a plantigrade foot which results in lowering the distal bone of the joint
- **eversion:** static axial deviation of the foot towards the lateral (internal rotation of the foot about its long axis)
- **inversion:** static axial deviation of the foot towards the medial (external rotation of the foot about its long axis)
- **pronation:** active action on to the foot rotating it towards the medial (internal rotation of the foot about its long axis)
- **supination:** active action on to the foot rotating it towards the lateral (external rotation of the foot about its long axis)

TS   triceps surae (Achilles tendon)
TA   tibialis anterior
TP   tibialis posterior
FDL   flexor digitorum longus
EDL   extensor digitorum longus
FHL   flexor hallucis longus
EHL   extensor hallucis longus
PB   peroneus brevis
PL   peroneus longus
PT   peroneus tertius

Introduction

The hindfoot and midfoot areas contain a multidirectional joint complex, its movement controlled mainly by ten extrinsic muscle tendons (Figure 1). For phylogenetic reasons, motor units for flexion are partly associated with those for supination, and extensors are often associated with pronators. This is due to the fact that during evolution the foot underwent a 90° eversion from its prehensile to a weightbearing function [Hinrichsen et al. 1994]. In comparison with the hand, which is phylogenetically older than the human foot, the range of mobility of joints within the foot is generally smaller, resulting in a smaller amplitude of excursion of the extrinsic tendons. In consequence the transmission of force by the extrinsic tendons has much greater significance.

Because of the multiarticular anatomy of the hindfoot and midfoot, some bones have no muscular attachment and are thus bypassed by one or more extrinsic tendons. The most important among these is the talus. More than 70% of the surface of the talus is covered with articular cartilage.

From a functional standpoint, the extrinsic tendons may be divided into flexors and extensors, mainly in relation to the ankle joint (Figure 2). Their moments of rotation in relation to the ankle joint are shown in Table 1 [Sarrafian 1993]. There appears to be a functional imbalance between flexors and extensors, with flexors having more total power than extensors. Extrinsic tendons may also be divided into supinators and pronators, mainly in relation to the talocalcaneonavicular joint (Figure 3). Their

a

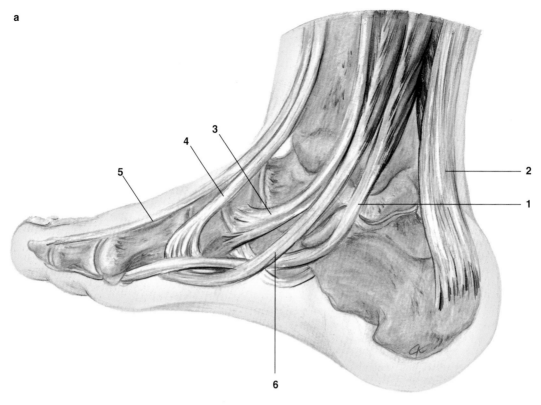

b

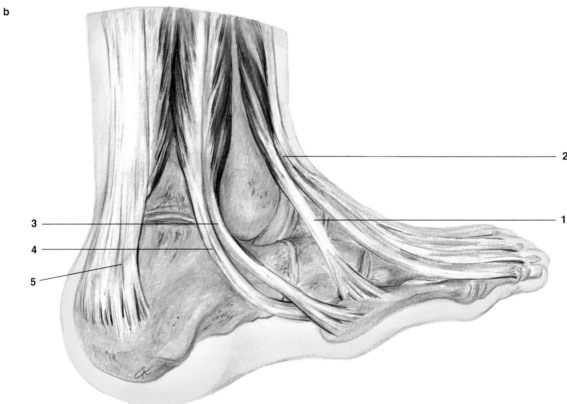

Figure 1

Extrinsic tendons at the foot and ankle. a. posteromedial
aspect; b. posterolateral aspect

a
1 FHL
2 TS (Achilles tendon)
3 TP
4 TA

5 EHL
6 FDL

b
1 PT
2 EDL
3 PB
4 PL
5 TS (Achilles tendon)

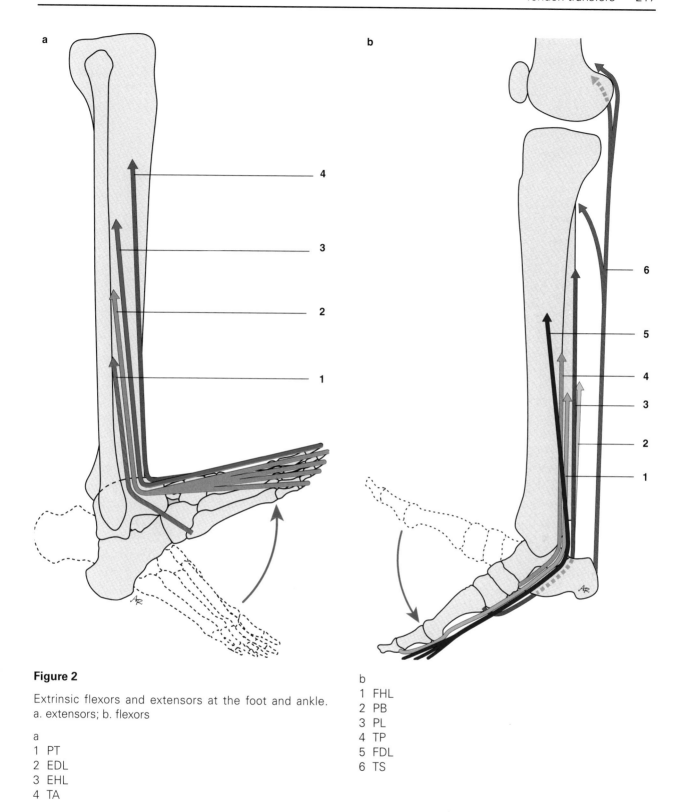

Figure 2

Extrinsic flexors and extensors at the foot and ankle.
a. extensors; b. flexors

a
1 PT
2 EDL
3 EHL
4 TA

b
1 FHL
2 PB
3 PL
4 TP
5 FDL
6 TS

moments of rotation are shown in Table 2. The tibialis anterior is quoted as both pronator and supinator. This muscle is active in two directions because of the proximity of its bony insertion to the axis of rotation. There appears to be a functional imbalance between supinators and pronators, with supinators having more total power than pronators

[Sarrafian 1993]. This muscular imbalance corrects the static imbalance created by eccentric loading of the foot by the center of gravity of the body during weightbearing. The effects of physiological muscular imbalance become apparent in patients with prolonged bed rest and without other foot pathology, if no prophylactic physiotherapy is

Table 1   Moments of rotation of the extrinsic tendons in relation to the ankle joint [Sarrafian 1993]

Tendon	Moment of rotation (N m)
Flexor tendons	
Achilles tendon	164
Flexor digitorum longus	3.9
Tibialis posterior	3.9
Peroneus longus	3.9
Peroneus brevis	2.9
Flexor hallucis longus	8.8
Extensor tendons	
Tibialis anterior	25
Extensor hallucis longus	3.9
Extensor digitorum longus	7.8
Peroneus tertius	4.9

performed: contractures will fix the foot in flexion (pes equinus) and inversion (pes supinatus).

Functional muscular imbalance may occur secondary to malformation, e.g. in neurological disorders, and following trauma. Interestingly, secondary malalignment, such as in the hindfoot, may recur despite operative correction with an arthrodesis [Wetmore and Drennan 1989].

Muscle tendon transfers aim at rebalancing the lost equilibrium in functioning joints or after joint fusion. In this chapter, various indications are described in relation to the available tendon transfers. These indications are based on the personal experience of the senior author. A combination of transfers is performed in approximately 35% of cases. The prerequisite for adequate treatment is a thorough clinical assessment of all individual extrinsic muscles. In some instances electroneurographic studies may be required. Thorough planning must be performed preoperatively, taking into account that any muscle tendon transfer causes the muscle to lose about 10–30% of its power. Therefore, alternative transfers may have to be considered, as there is more than one theoretical rebalancing plan for every condition.

After partial amputation of the foot the stabilizing function of the extrinsic musculature is markedly disturbed. Significant changes in levers behind and in front of the ankle joint increase the natural imbalance and are likely to cause post-traumatic equinus and varus deformity of the stump. Early rerouting of the tendons is advocated to avoid such a course. In the tarsometatarsal amputation, transfer of both the peroneus tendons to the lateral and dorsal aspect of the foot, together with the extensor digitorum longus (EDL) and the extensor hallucis longus (EHL), may

prevent the deformity. In addition, lengthening of the Achilles tendon should be performed.

The basic principles of tendon transfers were described in the 1920s [Lange 1928].

Restoring extension

Indications for these procedures include post-traumatic drop foot, pes equinus and cerebral palsy.

Ankle joint

Tibialis posterior tendon transfer to first or second cuneiform

The most popular and efficient technique to recover active extension of the ankle joint is the tibialis posterior (TP) tendon transfer to the dorsum of the foot (Figure 4). Harvesting this tendon may cause significant static instability at the midfoot. Therefore, the transferred TP tendon must simultaneously be replaced with a flexor digitorum longus (FDL) transfer. This is performed through the same surgical approach.

Through a longitudinal incision of about 8 cm, centered on the navicular tubercle, the entire insertion of the TP tendon is dissected and harvested, reaching as far distally as the fibers go along the bone. Below and parallel to this tendon runs the FDL, which is harvested at the tendon chiasma with the flexor hallucis longus (FHL), after section of the 'master's knot' of Henry. The distal segment of the FDL tendon can be left free, owing to its physiological cross-links with the stronger FHL, which takes over toe flexion.

Through a second incision about 15 cm proximal to the tip of the medial malleolus, the TP muscle and tendon are identified behind the FDL, which is more superficial at this level. If no adhesions from previous surgery are present, the tendon can be pulled out without difficulty.

The posterior surface of the interosseous membrane is palpated through the same medial incision and without detaching the periosteum. The membrane is perforated with a curved clamp in a distal direction. The canal thus created measures about 8 cm in length and is centered approximately 5 cm distal to the level of mobilization of the muscle.

A third incision is made at the front of the lower leg, over the lateral border of the tibialis anterior (TA) tendon. Behind its tendon sheath, staying on the tibial side and on top of the periosteum, the perforation of the interosseous membrane is completed obliquely in a proximal direction. The tendon is

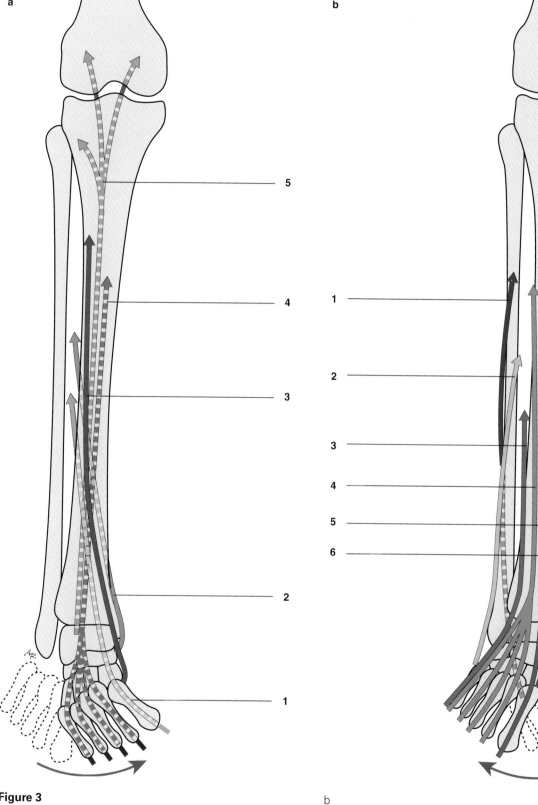

Figure 3

Extrinsic supinators and pronators at the foot and ankle. a. supinators; b. pronators

a
1 FHL
2 TP
3 TA
4 FDL
5 TS

b
1 PL
2 PB
3 PT
4 EDL
5 EHL
6 TA

Table 2 Moments of rotation of the extrinsic tendons in relation to the foot plate and the subtalar joint axis [Sarrafian 1993]

Tendon	Moment of rotation (N m)
Supinator tendons	
Achilles tendon	48
Flexor digitorum longus	7.8
Tibialis anterior	9.8
Tibialis posterior	18
Flexor hallucis longus	7.8
Pronator tendons	
Peroneus longus	17
Peroneus brevis	13
Extensor digitorum longus	7.8
Peroneus tertius	4.9
Extensor hallucis longus	1
Tibialis anterior	2.9

passed through this oblique path to the subcutaneous layer. Staying subcutaneously, the TP tendon is then pulled to the desired midfoot area at the cuneiforms, depending on the inversion–eversion stability of the foot. In order to conserve all available subtalar and talocalcaneonavicular mobility, the tendon should not be split to be anchored at two insertions.

Anchorage is performed within a bone tunnel at the superior portion of one of the cuneiform bones. The passing suture is pulled through the bottom of the cuneiform. The bone tunnel accommodates the TP tendon coming from the dorsum of the foot and the FDL coming from the medial side. The two tendons are secured with transosseous sutures at both ends of the tunnel. At the end of the procedure, the foot should spontaneously come to lie in the neutral position, in both sagittal and frontal planes.

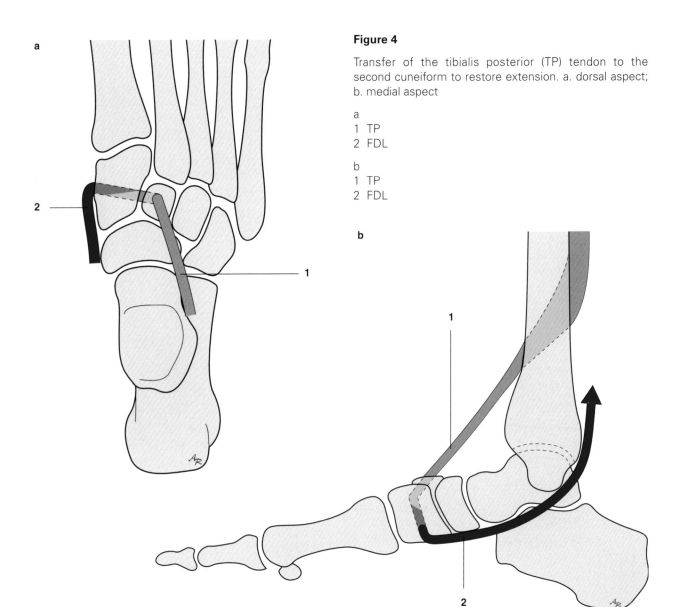

Figure 4

Transfer of the tibialis posterior (TP) tendon to the second cuneiform to restore extension. a. dorsal aspect; b. medial aspect

a
1 TP
2 FDL

b
1 TP
2 FDL

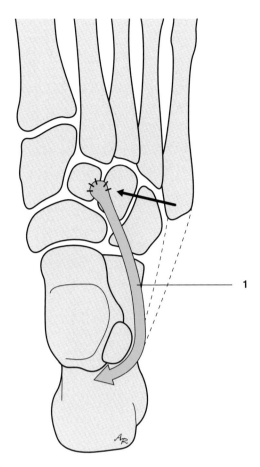

Figure 5

Transfer of the peroneus brevis (PB) tendon to the second cuneiform to restore extension

1 PB

Peroneus brevis tendon transfer to the second cuneiform

If both the peroneus brevis (PB) and peroneus longus (PL) muscles are functional and if sufficiency of the TP tendon transfer alone is questionable, the PB can be tenotomized at its insertion at the fifth metatarsal and transferred subcutaneously around the lateral aspect of the fibula on to the cuneiforms (Figure 5).

Extensor digitorum longus/hallucis longus to the midfoot

If the drop foot is accompanied by hyperextension and dorsal subluxation of the metatarsophalangeal joints, this may be due to increased tension of the long extensors of the toes (recruitment principle of the extensors). This often results in hammer or claw toe deformity, because the long extensors and flexors act in synergy, shortening the toes like an accordion.

This condition can be addressed with tenotomies of the EHL, the EDL or both, which are transferred

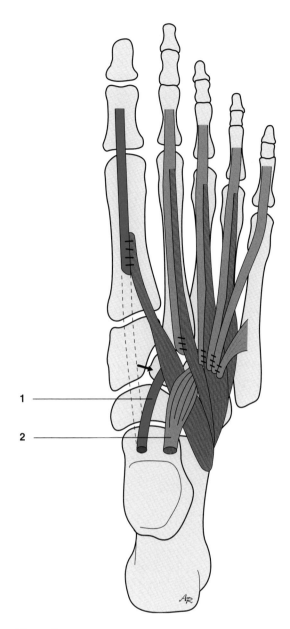

Figure 6

Transfer of the extensor digitorum longus (EDL)/hallucis longus (EHL) to the midfoot to restore extension

1 EHL
2 EDL

on to the cuneiforms (Figure 6). This technique is similar to the TP transfer. Split tendon transfers significantly limit subtalar mobility and are not recommended. Additional imbalance of pronation or supination can be corrected by choosing the appropriate insertion site of the transfer.

First tarsometatarsal joint

Pes cavus of the anterior type may be associated with hyperflexion of the first tarsometatarsal joint.

This deformity can be passively corrected by PL tenotomy and transfer to the lateral side of the foot (see below: restoring pronation).

In neurological disorders, simultaneous lengthening of the Achilles tendon should be considered.

Restoring pronation

Indications for procedures to restore pronation include Charcot–Marie–Tooth disease, congenital clubfoot and post-traumatic pes supinatus.

Talocalcaneonavicular joint

Imbalance is due to dysfunction of the PB and the PL or to more subtle imbalance between the PL and the PB. Insufficient extensors, in particular the EDL and peroneus tertius (PT), may also contribute to this condition. Correction by tendon transfer will provide either additional extension or additional flexion at the ankle joint.

Tibialis anterior tendon transfer to the third cuneiform

Tibialis anterior (TA) tendon transfer to the third cuneiform (Figure 7) is very effective in congenital clubfoot where the TA tendon must be lengthened. Three approaches are required.

1. Through a medial incision at the first tarsometatarsal joint, the entire tendon is harvested and mobilized.
2. A second incision above the ankle joint is made to pull the tendon out of its sheath. No kinking or soft tissue impingement may occur at this location. The tendon is pulled straight to the desired insertion, e.g. to the third cuneiform.
3. A third incision on the dorsum of the foot is used to pull the tendon through the subcutaneous tissue and through the tunnel which is drilled from the third to the first cuneiform, where the first incision is located. The tendon is secured with transosseous sutures at the two openings of the tunnel.

In a modified technique, which may be used in severe inversion deformity, the TA tendon is transferred on to the peroneus tertius (PT) tendon. This technique is recommended if the PT tendon has adequate strength compared to the TA tendon.

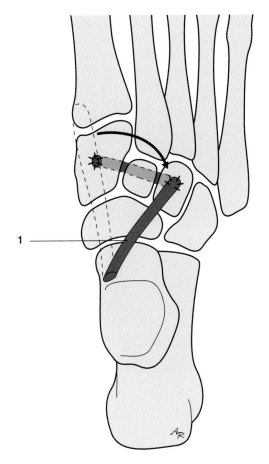

Figure 7

Transfer of the tibialis anterior (TA) tendon to the third cuneiform to restore pronation

1 TA

Flexor hallucis longus transfer to the peroneus brevis tendon

Flexor hallucis longus transfer to the PB tendon (Figure 8) has been applied in Charcot–Marie–Tooth disease and in clubfoot in which the adduction component at the calcaneocuboidal joint was a significant part of the deformity. Three surgical approaches are needed in this technique [ST Hansen, 1990, personal communication].

1. The FHL is harvested following incision of the 'master's knot' on the medial plantar aspect of the foot. This allows re-attachment of the distal leg of the tendon on to the FDL to minimize loss of flexion power of the great toe.
2. A posterolateral vertical incision, as in the posterolateral approach to the ankle, is used to identify the musculotendinous junction of the FHL and to pull out its tendon. At the level of the posterolateral corner of the subtalar joint, the PB tendon sheath is widely opened at

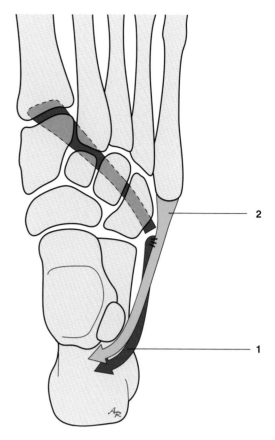

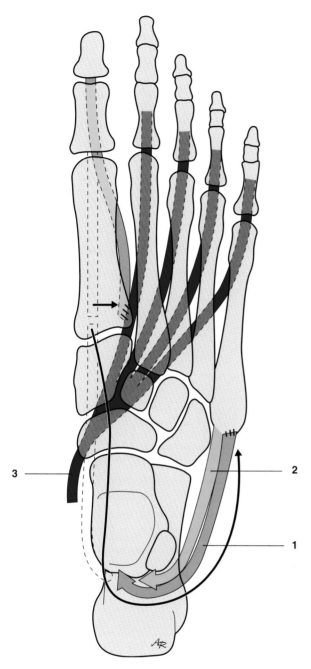

Figure 8

Transfer of the flexor hallucis longus (FHL) to the peroneus brevis (PB) tendon to restore pronation

1 FHL
2 PB
3 FDL

its posterior inferior aspect. Lateral opening should be avoided, owing to the risk of tendon dislocation.

3. At the insertion of the PB, the tendon sheath is opened and the FHL tendon is passed side-to-side with the PB. The length of the FHL tendon is just sufficient to buttonhole it through the PB tendon.

Figure 9

Transfer of the peroneus longus (PL) to the peroneus brevis (PB) tendon to restore pronation

1 PL
2 PB

Peroneus longus transfer to the peroneus brevis tendon

Transfer of the peroneus longus to the PB (Figure 9) is one of several techniques of transfer between these two tendons. Tenotomy of the PL reduces the medial arch of the foot through flexion release at the base of the first metatarsal. Augmentation of the PB with the PL enhances active pronation of the midfoot.

The approach is by an incision 5 cm long and proximal to the base of the fifth metatarsal. The PB tendon is mobilized plantarwards in order to visualize the PL, which reflects medially beneath the cuboid. Tenotomy is performed at this location and the proximal leg of the PL is sutured through a buttonhole within the PB.

Restoring flexion

Conditions requiring the restoration of flexion include poliomyelitis, pes talus, cerebral palsy and hammer toes.

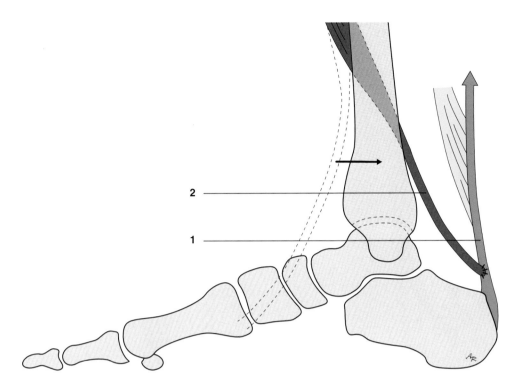

Figure 10

Transfer of the tibialis anterior (TA) tendon to the Achillies tendon (TS) to restore flexion

1 TS
2 TA

Ankle joint

Tibialis anterior tendon transfer to the Achilles tendon

In cerebral palsy, weakness of the quadriceps is often accompanied by weakness of the calf muscles, which results in a typical gait with flexed knees and extended ankles. In poliomyelitis, weak calf musculature may cause secondary deformities of bones, e.g. vertical calcaneus, and of joints, e.g. at the posterior subtalar joint. Tenotomy of the TA relieves one of the deforming forces, which causes extension of the tarsometatarsal joint. In addition, transfer of the TA tendon to the Achilles tendon and/or to the calcaneus redirects muscle power to foot flexion and to push-off (Figure 10).

Three surgical approaches are necessary: one at the insertion of the TA for harvesting of the tendon, a second approach above the ankle joint to prepare the interosseous passage, and a third posterolateral approach to advance the tendon on the lateral aspect of the FHL muscle to the tuber of the calcaneus. Anchorage of the TA is either to the Achilles tendon or through the calcaneus.

Flexor hallucis longus transfer to the Achilles tendon

The very effective transfer of the flexor hallucis longus to the Achilles tendon (Figure 11) represents not only a mechanical improvement during push-off, but also a biological plastic procedure. The FHL has a

moment of approximately 10 N m and thus is one of the most powerful ankle joint flexors. It is also in optimum mechanical alignment with the Achilles tendon. In addition, a significant width and volume of the muscle belly regularly reaches the posterior aspect of the subtalar joint. This helps to diminish chronic tendinitis of the Achilles tendon, chronic infection after surgery or compromised vascular supply at this particular location [Klaue et al. 1991].

Peroneus brevis/longus transfer to the Achilles tendon

Mechanical power at push-off can be added by transfer of one peroneus tendon to the Achilles tendon. If the PB is chosen for this transfer, the distal PB stump must be fixed to the medial reflection of the PL near the cuboid (Figure 12). If the PL is chosen for the transfer (Figure 13), attention must be given to the stability of the medial column. Generally, the distal stump of the PL should be transferred to the insertion of the PB.

A significant pronation or supination effect may result, depending on the insertion site at the calcaneus.

First tarsometatarsal joint

Flexor hallucis longus transfer to the base of the first metatarsal

Hyperextension of the first tarsometatarsal joint may be a striking deformity in cerebral palsy with

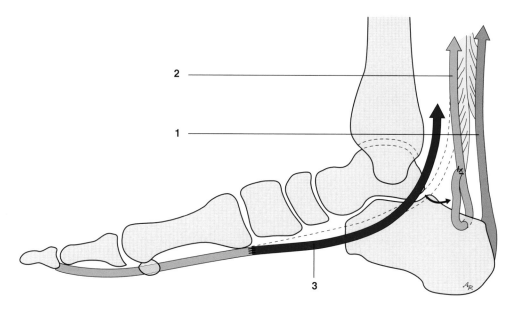

Figure 11

Transfer of the flexor hallucis longus (FHL) to the Achilles tendon (TS) to restore flexion

1 TS
2 FHL
3 FDL

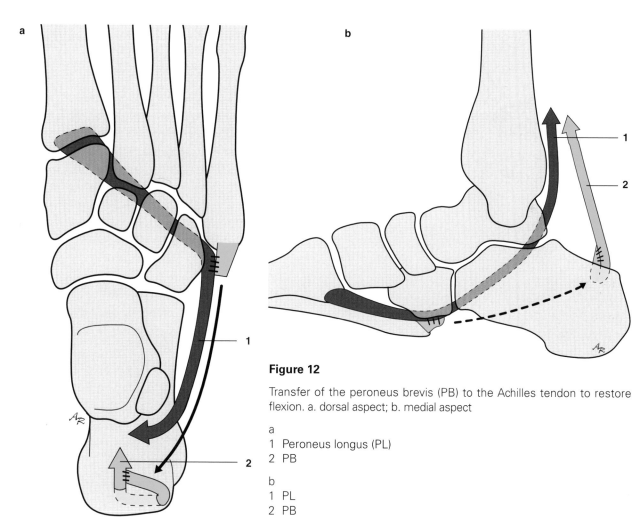

Figure 12

Transfer of the peroneus brevis (PB) to the Achilles tendon to restore flexion. a. dorsal aspect; b. medial aspect

a
1 Peroneus longus (PL)
2 PB

b
1 PL
2 PB

overuse of the TA. In minor deformity with a deficient anteromedial buttress and without hypermobility of the first ray, transfer of the FHL (Figure 14) will actively restore the forefoot weightbearing pattern. The FHL tendon is transferred to the base of the first metatarsal rather than more distally, for two reasons. First, the tendon is more effective with a small lever arm at the tarsometatarsal joint, which has a more or less plane surface. Second, the main blood supply to the distal part of the first metatarsal enters the bone at

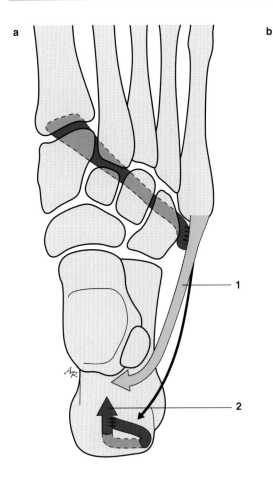

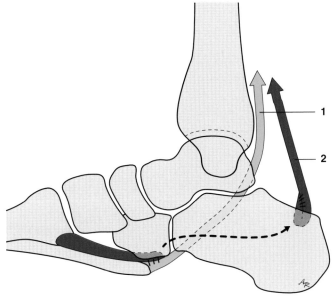

Figure 13

Transfer of the peroneus longus (PL) to the Achilles tendon to restore flexion. a. dorsal aspect; b. medial aspect

a
1 Peroneus brevis (PB)
2 PL

b
1 PB
2 PL

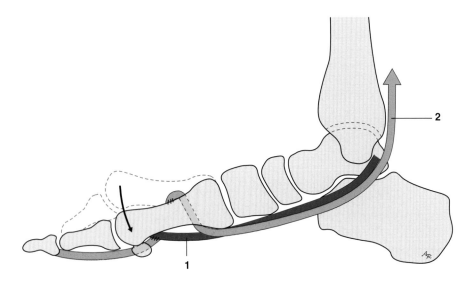

Figure 14

Transfer of the flexor hallucis longus (FHL) to the base of the first metatarsal to restore flexion at the first tarsometatarsal joint

1 Flexor digitorum longus (FDL)
2 FHL

the plantar aspect of the subcapital region; this would be unnecessarily compromised by surgical dissection.

Metatarsophalangeal joints

Flexor digitorum longus and brevis transfer to the dorsal aspect of the proximal phalanx

Hyperextended metatarsophalangeal joints are often part of the hammer toe deformity. This deformity

may be due to plantar plate destruction at the metatarsophalangeal joints and to dysfunction of the intrinsic musculature of the foot, followed by extrinsic imbalance. Failure to flex the proximal phalanx leads to hyperflexion of the middle and distal phalanges, due to the tension of the FDL. Furthermore, the EDL tendon expands to the lateral aspect of the metatarsophalangeal joints. Therefore, there is no strong counterforce to extension of the proximal phalanx.

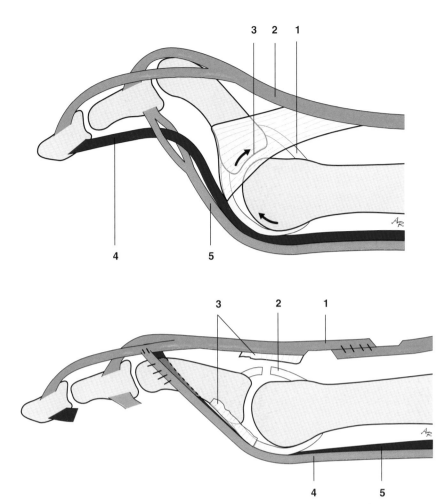

Figure 15

Transfer of the flexor digitorum longus (FDL) and brevis (FDB) to the dorsal aspect of the proximal phalanx to restore flexion at the metatarsophalangeal (MTP) joint. a. preoperatively; b. postoperatively

a
1 MTP joint capsule
2 Extensor digitorum longus (EDL)
3 EDL extension to the MTP joint capsule
4 FDL
5 FDB

b
1 EDL
2 MTP joint capsule
3 EDL extension to the MTP joint capsule
4 FDB
5 FDL

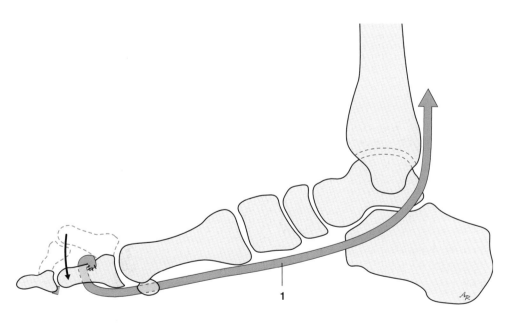

Figure 16

Transfer of the flexor hallucis longus (FHL) tendon to the proximal phalanx to restore flexion of the great toe

1 FHL

Correction by tendon transfer (Figure 15) aims at rebalancing the flexion/extension mechanism, bearing in mind that weightbearing is more important than mobility. The FDL and the FDB are harvested either through a longitudinal dorsal approach with tenotomy of the EDL, or through a lateral approach.

Pulled back to the level of the proximal phalanx, the tendon may be brought to the dorsum of the proximal phalanx either on one side alone, or split in two legs along both sides of the bone. Complete manual reduction of the metatarsophalangeal joint is a prerequisite for this transfer. This often requires

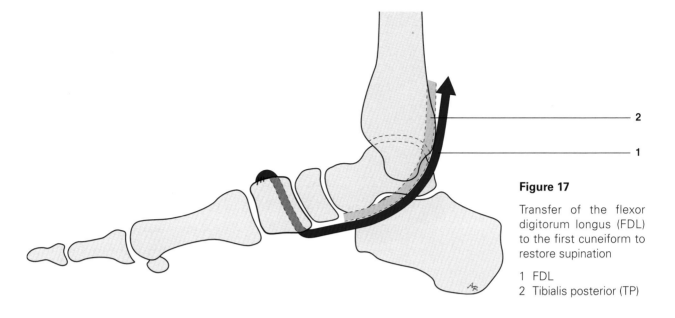

Figure 17

Transfer of the flexor digitorum longus (FDL) to the first cuneiform to restore supination

1 FDL
2 Tibialis posterior (TP)

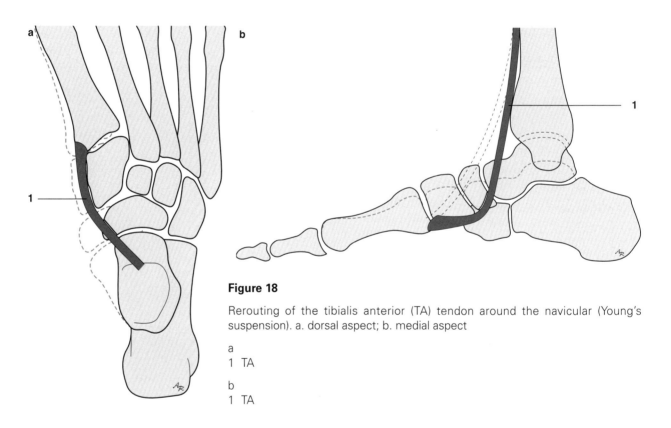

Figure 18

Rerouting of the tibialis anterior (TA) tendon around the navicular (Young's suspension). a. dorsal aspect; b. medial aspect

a
1 TA

b
1 TA

extensive debridement, especially of the medial and lateral expansions of the EDL on to the proximal phalanx.

Flexor hallucis longus tendon transfer on to the proximal phalanx

Flexor hallucis longus tendon transfer to the proximal phalanx (Figure 16) corresponds to the above-mentioned transfer in the lesser toes. Hammer toe deformity of the great toe is often associated with a neurological problem. At the great toe, the bones are large enough to accommodate the tendon within a drill hole through the diaphysis of the proximal phalanx.

Restoring supination

Indications for procedures to restore supination include congenital pes planus valgus and chronic rupture of the TP tendon.

Restoring active supination, i.e. inversion by muscle power, with tendon transfers alone does not generally suffice to re-establish physiological static conditions of the foot and ankle. Bone procedures, such as osteotomies and arthrodeses, are usually necessary to restore normal foot morphology. Tendon transfers may also add flexion or extension power.

Talocalcaneonavicular joint

Flexor digitorum longus transfer to the first cuneiform

Tibialis posterior tendon insufficiency occurs either congenitally or following chronic rupture due to degeneration or inflammation. Optimum active correction is achieved using the FDL, which is located close to the TP from the lower leg to the midfoot (Figure 17). Harvesting the FDL does not jeopardize toe flexion, owing to the anatomical anastomosis between the FHL and the FDL in the midfoot area, which is able to substitute the FDL force.

Rerouting of the tibialis anterior tendon around the navicular (Young's suspension)

Young's suspension (Figure 18) has been popular for the correction of hypermobile flat-foot in children. The indication must be considered carefully: the break of the sagittal talometatarsal axis must be distal to the navicular.

Peroneus brevis tendon transfer to the peroneus longus

Transfers between the two peroneus tendons have been discussed above. The PB transfer to the PL helps to stabilize the medial arch of the foot in hypermobile flat feet. In neurological conditions, it may be combined with a FHL transfer to the base of the first metatarsal. The transfer thus reinforces foot flexion. If the foot is hypermobile at the midfoot region and has no tendency to varus deformity of the hindfoot, hypermobility may be stabilized by simple tenodesis of the PL and the PB at the insertion site of the PB, without tenotomy.

References

Hinrichsen KV, Jacob HJ, Jacob M et al. (1994) Principles of ontogenesis of leg and foot in man. Anat Anz 176: 121–130

Klaue K, Masquelet AC, Jakob RP (1991) Soft tissue and tendon injury in the foot. Curr Opin Orthop 2: 519–528

Lange F (1928) Die Fussdeformitäten. In: Lehrbuch der Orthopädie, 3rd edn. Jena, Fischer

Sarrafian SK (1993) Anatomy of the Foot and Ankle, 2nd edn. Philadelphia, JB Lippincott

Wetmore RS, Drennan JC (1989) Long-term results of triple arthrodesis in Charcot–Marie–Tooth disease. J Bone Joint Surg 71A: 417–422

27

Resection of tarsal coalitions

Greta Dereymaeker

Introduction

Tarsal coalition is a fibrous, cartilaginous or osseous fusion of two or more tarsal bones. Calcaneonavicular and talocalcaneal coalitions are the most common types. Talonavicular coalitions are third in frequency of occurrence. Other coalitions, less frequent and of less clinical importance, have been reported: calcaneocuboid, cubonavicular and naviculocuneiform. More recently, even more distal coalitions have been reported [Tanaka et al. 2000] as case reports. Tarsal coalitions were found in remains of ancient people and were first described more than 200 years ago. An association of spastic and rigid flat foot with calcaneonavicular coalition and with medial talocalcaneal coalition was first described at the beginning of the 20th century.

In the vast majority of cases tarsal coalition represents a congenital anomaly, as a consequence of autosomal dominant inheritance [Bohne 2001], but it can also be acquired. Older theories proposed incorporation of accessory intertarsal ossicles as a cause of tarsal coalition. This hypothesis does not explain the presence of the anomaly before birth, which has been demonstrated. It is now believed that the coalition is a result of failed differentiation and segmentation of primitive mesenchyme. This gene can be of variable penetrance, resulting in subclinical cases of tarsal coalition.

If the tarsal coalition is acquired, it is usually secondary to trauma. Other possible causes are degenerative joint disease, rheumatoid arthritis and infection.

The talus normally articulates with the calcaneus at three distinct joint surfaces: the posterior, the middle and the anterior facets. The middle and anterior facets may be partially or completely united. Talocalcaneal coalition occurs mainly at the medial side. The coalition is most frequently situated at the level of the middle facet just in front of the sinus tarsi, i.e. at the posterior aspect of the sustentaculum tali. It is less frequent at the level of the posterior facet. The anterior talocalcaneal facet is rarely involved.

There is no true articulation between the calcaneus and the navicular bone. Calcaneonavicular coalition is usually a union of the anterior facet of the calcaneus with the navicular and can be up to 1 cm wide. These coalitions may occur bilaterally. Talonavicular, calcaneocuboid and cubonavicular coalitions occur only sporadically and are often bilateral.

Several classification systems have been proposed. Classification is best based on the anatomic description of the coalition [Tachdjian 1985]. Coalition may occur as an isolated anomaly or as part of a more complex deformity. Coalitions may also be classified according to the type of connective tissue uniting the involved tarsal bones. The term 'syndesmosis' is applied when two bones are united by fibrous tissue. If cartilaginous tissue is present, the coalition is termed a 'synchondrosis' and an osseous coalition is a 'synostosis'. Combinations of tissue types may be seen, especially in talocalcaneal coalitions. More attention is paid now to 'complete' or 'partial or incomplete' coalitions as this influences the clinical symptoms and final outcome of treatment. This differentiation is made by computed tomography (CT) scan or magnetic resonance imaging (MRI).

It is difficult to know the exact incidence in the general population because many asymptomatic tarsal coalitions exist. The overall incidence is probably about 1%. Calcaneonavicular and talocalcaneal coalition represent 90% of all coalitions. Since the introduction of CT scanning, talocalcaneal coalition appears to be diagnosed more frequently than calcaneonavicular coalition. Talonavicular coalitions are the third most common type.

Tarsal coalition is more frequently seen in the presence of a flat-foot deformity than in any other type of postural hindfoot pathology. Tarsal coalition has therefore been considered to be a cause of peroneal spastic flat foot. Recent studies, however, have demonstrated that many patients with tarsal coalition do not have peroneal spasm or flat feet [Stormont and Peterson 1983, DeVriese et al. 1994]. There are many causes of peroneal spastic flat foot other than tarsal coalition [Outland and Murphy 1960, Cowell 1972, Jayakumar and Cowell 1977, Harper 1981].

If a rigid flat foot is present in talocalcaneal and calcaneonavicular coalitions, this is due to loss of normal subtalar joint rotation. With motion between the talus and the calcaneus reduced to zero, the midtarsal joint loses its gliding capacity and assumes a more hinge-like movement. This motion accounts for the navicular overriding the talus, elevating the dorsal capsule and periosteum [Mosier and Asher 1984]. The ensuing reparative process may cause beaking of the talus, which may be observed on radiographs.

In talocalcaneal coalition, a cavovalgus foot deformity may also be present. This is due to pronation–abduction in the talonavicular and calcaneocuboid joints, to compensate for hindfoot valgus. Restriction of subtalar motion may be compensated for by increased laxity of the ankle ligaments, leading to recurrent ankle sprains [Harris 1955].

If massive or combined tarsal coalitions are present in early childhood, a ball and socket ankle joint may develop, owing to lack of screw movement in the hindfoot.

Clinical and radiographic findings

Patients with tarsal coalition present at age 8–18 years. The age at presentation appears to be approximately 3–4 years after ossification of the tarsal coalition. However, some patients may report that minor symptoms had existed for several years. Calcaneonavicular coalition ossifies between 8 years and 12 years of age, and symptoms usually appear at age 13–14 years [DeVriese et al. 1994]. Talocalcaneal coalition ossifies at 12–16 years of age and the average age at presentation of symptoms is 18 years. Talonavicular coalition ossifies at 3–5 years of age and patients usually present at 8 years [Cowell and Elener 1983].

The onset is usually insidious, sometimes precipitated by minor trauma such as an ankle sprain or a fall. Other precipitating factors may be an increase in body weight or physical activity and accelerated growth of the foot.

Tarsal coalitions may be totally asymptomatic and be an accidental radiographic finding [Outland and Leonard 1974; Murphy 1960]. In symptomatic cases, pain is localized in the hindfoot and midfoot and aggravated by walking over uneven terrain, prolonged standing, jumping or participating in athletics. Rest relieves the pain. In talonavicular coalition, pain is mainly localized at the anterolateral aspect of the foot, directly over the coalition. In talocalcaneal coalition the pain is situated more deeply, at the medial aspect of the subtalar joint. Histopathological study of non-osseous tarsal coalition revealed that the pain in tarsal coalition is not mediated by nerve elements at the coalition itself, but is caused by a mechanical abnormality that results especially from incomplete coalition [Kumai et al. 1998].

Decreased range of motion of the affected joint on examination often suggests a tarsal coalition. In calcaneonavicular coalition, motion of the subtalar joint may be diminished, but is usually not completely obliterated. Inversion and especially eversion of the midtarsal joint is usually limited. In talocalcaneal coalition, subtalar motion is markedly reduced. Increased tibiotalar motion due to ankle joint instability must not be mistaken for subtalar motion.

Static foot deformities are common in tarsal coalitions. The foot may be in a rigid valgus position. Medial talocalcaneal coalition may cause a cavovalgus abduction deformity. Calcaneonavicular coalition mainly leads to a planovalgus deformity. When children present with a planus or a planovalgus foot, which is painful or has a restricted range of motion, tarsal coalition should always be considered.

Spasm of the peroneal musculature may be present, but this neither confirms nor excludes the diagnosis of tarsal coalition. Spasticity is generally tonic, as opposed to the chronic spasm in neuromuscular disease. Occasionally, the anterior and posterior tibial muscles are in spasm and may cause varus deformity of the foot [Stuecker and Bennett 1993].

Radiographic evaluation is always needed to confirm the diagnosis. Routine anteroposterior, lateral and oblique radiographs will reveal coalitions between the talus and the navicular and between the calcaneus and the cuboid. Later weightbearing radiographs demonstrate typical signs of tarsal coalition: talonavicular beaking [Conway and Cowell 1969] may be present in talonavicular and in talocalcaneal coalitions. In the latter, the 'C' sign represents increased trabeculation under the sustentaculum tali [Lateur et al. 1994]. In calcaneonavicular coalition the 'anteater's nose sign' represents a tubular elongation of the anterior process of the calcaneus [Oestreich et al. 1987].

Several special radiographic views were recommended in the past. However, these views are technically difficult and coalitions may easily be missed if the projection is not entirely correct. Consensus now exists that a CT scan with coronal [Hochman and Reed 2000] and axial (approximately 45° to the horizontal plane) views is the 'gold standard' in diagnosing a tarsal coalition and remains the more cost-effective diagnosing modality, superior to MRI [Emmery et al. 1998]. The sections should not be thicker than 2 mm, in order not to miss the coalition. CT accurately delineates the coalition and allows measurement of the size of the bridge, which is of importance for preoperative planning. Flattening of the lateral talar process, loss of the subtalar joint space and secondary degenerative changes may be present. Degenerative arthritis of adjacent joints can also be found. If other causes for ankle pain are also entertained, MRI can be performed and provide nearly equivalent accuracy for detecting tarsal coalition.

Treatment

Treatment of tarsal coalition is necessary only when it is or becomes symptomatic. The great majority of cases of talocalcaneal and calcaneonavicular coalition can be treated conservatively. A painful hindfoot without a severe static deformity can be treated with an insole and physiotherapy. If irreversible muscle spasms cause a static deformity, immobilization in a corrective cast, applied under anesthesia, for 4 or 5 weeks may give sufficient pain relief. This can be followed by treatment with an insole to keep the foot in the correct position. Surgical resection of the tarsal coalition is recommended in young individuals with persistent symptomatic feet and limited hindfoot motion, as long as there are no signs of osteoarthritis. However, more recently, Cohen et al. [1996] reported succesful resection of calcaneonavicular coalition in an adult population.

Surgical technique

Calcaneonavicular coalition

Calcaneonavicular resection is performed through an oblique incision over the anterior part of the sinus tarsi (Figure 1a). The inferior portion of the extensor retinaculum is split in the direction of its fibers, and the muscle belly of the extensor digitorum brevis is stripped from its proximal origin distally, following the anterior part of the calcaneum medially. This exposes the upper part of the calcaneus and the plantar side of the navicular with the calcaneonavicular coalition. Resection of the bar is begun at the calcaneal side, in the notch between the talar head, the cuboid and the navicular (Figures 2, 3 and 4). An osteotome with a width of approximally 1 cm is used, and this is directed plantarwards.

A second osteotome is placed parallel to the first at the plantar side of the navicular bone. This osteotome is advanced approximately 1 cm into the bone, then directed to converge with the calcaneal osteotome. Once the plantar border of the calcaneonavicular is divided, the coalition will become loose. The osteotomes are removed and the coalition is mobilized and removed with a periosteal elevator or a rongeur. Motion of the subtalar joint and of the midtarsal joints is assessed, especially pronation and supination. More bone may have to be resected so there is no impingement between the calcaneus, navicular, talus, cuboid and the medial intermediate cuneiform. An oblique radiograph is taken intraoperatively to ensure that enough bone has been removed. The resected area may be marked with a metal wire prior to taking the radiograph. As a general rule, enough bone is resected to visualize 1 mm of adjacent articular surfaces.

If the extensor brevis muscle is sufficiently large, it can be interposed into the resection and fixed with sutures, which are tied over a button at the plantar side of the foot. The postoperative treatment consists of a cast, with avoidance of weightbearing for 2 weeks, and with weightbearing for another 2–3 weeks. The suture button is removed at 5 weeks postoperatively.

If the extensor digitorum brevis muscle is too small for interpositioning, it is attached in its anatomic origin and the gap is filled with a free fat graft from the buttock. The skin is closed and a posterior splint is applied for 2 weeks. Exercises are performed out of the cast twice a day or on a continuous passive motion machine, starting the first

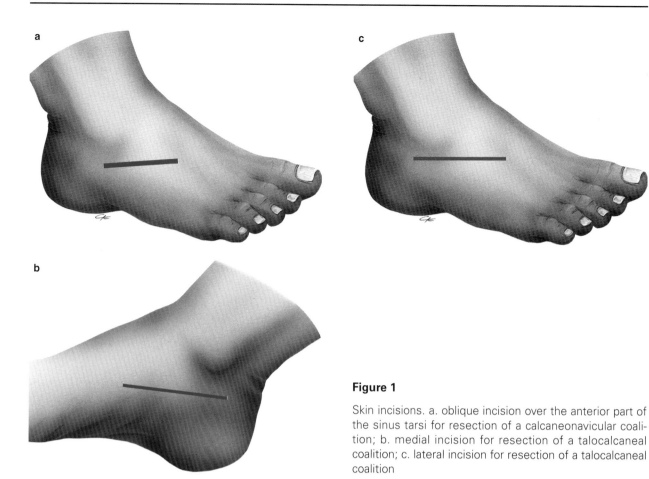

Figure 1

Skin incisions. a. oblique incision over the anterior part of the sinus tarsi for resection of a calcaneonavicular coalition; b. medial incision for resection of a talocalcaneal coalition; c. lateral incision for resection of a talocalcaneal coalition

postoperative day. Walking on crutches with plantar contact for 4–5 weeks is recommended.

Talocalcaneal coalition

Talocalcaneal coalitions can be resected through either a medial or a lateral approach. If the coalition is situated at the posterior facet only a medial approach can be used.

Medial approach   A transverse incision is made at the level of the subtalar joint, about 1.5 cm posterior and 1 cm inferior to the tip of the medial malleolus, continuing anteriorly over about 5 cm (Figure 1b). The subcutaneous tissue is divided in the same direction. The tibialis posterior tendon is retracted dorsally and the flexor hallucis and neurovascular bundle plantarwards (Figure 3). The tarsal coalition is located with a needle under fluoroscopic control. This is not always easy, especially when a severe fixed valgus deformity of the talocalcaneal complex is present. In these cases one will first localize the anterior point of the posterior facet and the posterior point of the head of the talus and then follow the lower margin of the neck of the talus posteriorwards to the medial facet. When the coalition is

encountered it is resected with an osteotome, care being taken not to damage the articular joint surfaces. A 6–7-mm wide segment of the coalition is resected so that the base of the coalition is countersunk below the level of the existing bone surface. Subsequently, motion of the subtalar and midtarsal joints is assessed. When the tarsal coalition is situated at the level of the sustentaculum, care must be taken not to remove too much bone. In the case of a severe valgus deformity of the hindfoot, it is helpful, after having made the first cut, to open the talocalcaneal joint by inserting a medium lamina spreader from the lateral side (see lateral approach) in the sinus tarsi and correct the subtalar valgus deformity before resecting bone block of the coalition. For containment of the valgus correction, inserting a sinus tarsi spacer is recommended [DeVriese et al. 1994]. This can give some discomfort in the first 2 postoperative months, but better remoulding in the long term. For correction of the abduction of the midtarsal joints, reefing of the distal portion of the spring ligament is usually added by the author. The spacer is removed after about 18 months. Early motion on a continuous passive motion machine and mobilization on crutches for 4–6 weeks are advised postoperatively.

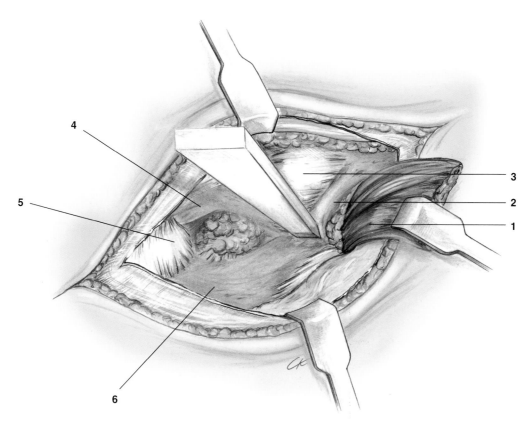

Figure 2

Resection of a calcaneonavicular coalition through a lateral approach. An osteotome is inserted into the calcaneal side of the coalition

1 Extensor digitorum brevis muscle
2 Calcaneonavicular coalition
3 Talonavicular joint capsule
4 Talus
5 Subtalar joint capsule
6 Calcaneus

Lateral approach   The lateral approach is recommended if there is a large coalition involving the complete medial facet of the subtalar joint. The skin incision is centered over the sinus tarsi (see Figure 1c). The superficial tissues are divided in line with the skin incision. After the contents of the sinus tarsi have been removed, the medial facet of the subtalar joint can be visualized. Usually the coalition is localized at the anterior medial border of the sinus tarsi. Opening the posterior subtalar joint should be avoided, if possible. A medium-sized lamina spreader is inserted and gently retracted. This will provide a good view of the coalition. The coalition is divided horizontally with an osteotome at the lower (calcaneal) border (Figure 4). After this maneuver, the lamina spreader can be opened further. The coalition can then be completely removed at the talar side. To reduce the valgus of the hindfoot, a sinus tarsi spacer can be introduced.

This keeps the hindfoot reduced and prevents recurrence of the bar. The spacer is best removed after 18 months. After closure of the skin, a well-moulded below-knee cast is applied. Two weeks postoperatively the sutures are removed and a below-knee walking boot is applied for a period of 3–4 weeks. Rehabilitation of normal gait may take 6–9 months.

Subtalar/triple arthrodesis

When signs of degenerative arthritis are present, resection of the tarsal coalition can no longer be performed. In these cases a triple arthrodesis with correction of the static foot deformity is performed (see Chapter 31).

Fibrous talocalcaneal coalition in adults without degenerative arthritis of the adjacent joints can be treated by subtalar arthrodesis alone.

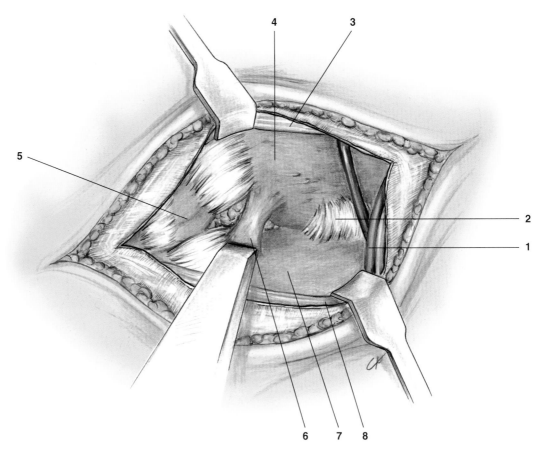

Figure 3

Medial approach for resection of a talocalcaneal coalition

1 Neurovascular bundle
2 Subtalar joint capsule
3 Tibialis posterior tendon

4 Talus
5 Navicular
6 Talocalcaneal coalition
7 Calcaneus
8 Flexor hallucis longus tendon

A corticocancellous bone graft should be interposed to keep the midtarsal joints in the normal position. Calcaneonavicular and bony talocalcaneal coalitions with signs of degeneration at the adjacent joints should always be treated with a triple arthrodesis.

Complications

When performing the lateral approach, there is always a chance of damaging a branch of the superficial peroneal nerve, which lies just underneath the skin. The nerve needs to be gently retracted anteriorly.

Care must be taken not to enter adjacent facets with the osteotome when the coalition is resected. This can cause serious damage to the articular cartilage. The coalition itself has to be removed completely to prevent its recurrence. This is probably the most frequent complication and is usually due to insufficient removal of bone.

A good correction of the static deformity is another important factor and must be checked after resection of the coalition. If the correction is poor it may be necessary to resect more bone, especially in calcaneonavicular coalition, to obtain unrestricted motion at Chopart's joint. More attention has to be paid to the necessary supplementary soft-tissue or bony procedures, as simple resection of the coalition is not always a guarantee of static deformity correction. In particular, the severe planovalgus biomechanics of the foot need to be well understood before these surgical procedures are started.

More recently, as more tarsal coalitions have been diagnosed, the author has seen too agressive resections in order to gain enough motion. This can lead to even greater biomechanical problems for the adolescent than the previous exsisting tarsal coalition. Only arthrodesis can salvage these iatrogenic problems. Triple or subtalar arthrodesis may be used as salvage procedures.

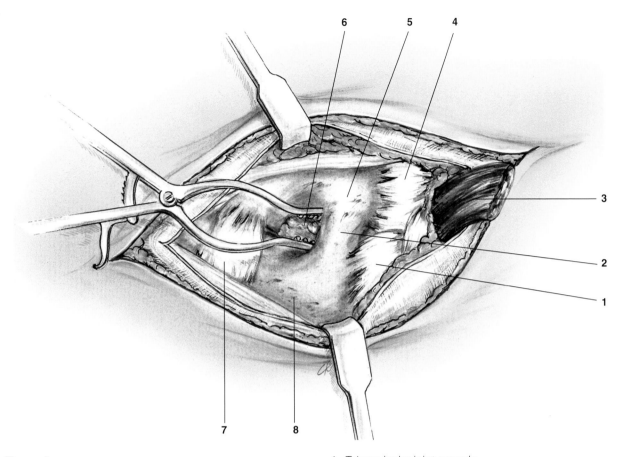

Figure 4

Lateral approach for resection of a talocalcaneal coalition

1 Calcaneocuboid joint capsule
2 Talocalcaneal coalition
3 Extensor digitorum brevis muscle

4 Talonavicular joint capsule
5 Talar neck
6 Sinus tarsi
7 Subtalar joint capsule
8 Calcaneus

References

Bohne WH (2001) Tarsal coalition. Curr Opion Pediatr 13: 29–35

Cohen BE, Davis WH, Anderson RB (1996) Success of calcaneonavicular coalition resection in the adult population. Foot Ankle 17: 569–572

Conway JJ, Cowell HR (1969) Tarsal coalition: clinical significance and roentgenographic demonstration. Radiology 92: 799–811

Cowell HR (1972) Talocalcaneal coalition and new causes of peroneal spastic flatfoot. Clin Orthop 85: 16

Cowell HR, Elener V (1983) Rigid painful flatfoot secondary to tarsal coalition. Clin Orthop 177: 54–60

DeVriese L, Dereymaeker G, Molenaers G, Fabry G (1994) Surgical treatment of tarsal coalitions. J Pediatr Orthop Part B 3: 96–101

Ehrlich MG, Elmer EB (1991) Tarsal coalition. In: Jahss M (ed) Disorders of the Foot and Ankle, 2nd edn. Philadelphia, Saunders, pp 921–938

Emmery KH, Bisset GS 3rd, Johnson ND, Nunan PJ (1998) Tarsal coalition: a blinded comparison of MRI and CT. Pediatr Radiol 28: 612–616

Harper MC (1981) Traumatic peroneal spastic flatfoot. Orthopaedics 5: 466

Harris RI (1955) Rigid valgus foot due to talocalcaneal bridge. J Bone Joint Surg 37A: 169

Harris RI, Beath T (1948) Etiology of peroneal spastic flat foot. J Bone Joint Surg 30B: 624

Hochman M, Reed MH (2000) Features of calcaneonavicular coalition on coronal computed tomography. Skeletal Radiol 29: 409–412

Jayakumar S, Cowell HR (1977) Rigid flatfoot. Clin Orthop 122: 77

Kulik SA Jr, Clanton TO (1996) Tarsal coalition. Foot Ankle 17: 286–296

Kumai T, Takakura Y, Akyiama K, et al. (1998) Histopathological study of nonosseous tarsal coalition. Foot Ankle 19: 525–531

Lateur LM, Van Hoe LR, Van Ghillewe KV, et al. (1994) Subtalar coalition: diagnosis with the C-sign on lateral radiographs of the ankle. Radiology 193: 847–851

Leonard MA (1974) The inheritance of tarsal coalition and its relationship to spastic flat foot. J Bone Joint Surg 56B: 520

Lusby HLJ (1959) Naviculo-cuneiform synostosis. J Bone Joint Surg 41B: 150

Mosier KM, Asher M (1984) Tarsal coalitions and peroneal spastic flatfoot. J Bone Joint Surg 66A: 976–983

Oestreich AE, Mize WA, Crawford AH, Morgan RC (1987) The 'anteater nose', a direct sign of calcaneonavicular coalition on the lateral radiograph. J Paediatr Orthop 7: 709–711

Outland T, Murphy ID (1960) The pathomechanics of peroneal spastic flat foot. Clin Orthop 16: 64

Stormont DM, Peterson NA (1983) The relative incidence of tarsal coalition. Clin Orthop 181: 26–36

Stuecker RD, Bennett JT (1993) Tarsal coalition presenting as a pes cavo-varus deformity: report of three cases and review of the literature. Foot Ankle 14: 540–544

Tachdjian ML (1985) The Child's Foot. Philadelphia, Saunders

Tanaka Y, Takakura Y, Sugimoto K, Kumai T (2000) Non-osseous coalition of the medial cuneiform–first *metatarsal* joint: case report. Foot Ankle 21: 1043–1046

Wechsler RJ, Schweitzer ME, Deely DM, et al. (1994) Tarsal coalition: depiction and characterization with CT and MR imaging. Radiology 193: 447–452

28

Osteochondritis of the foot: surgical treatment

David Grace

Introduction

The term 'osteochondritis' has historically been applied to a variety of different pathological conditions that can afflict the growing or mature skeleton. In children and adolescents, the foot is especially prone to these conditions. The continued use of the term is unfortunate, however, as it is too imprecise to describe accurately the underlying pathological process. Osteochondritis implies inflammation of bone and its adjacent articular or ossifying cartilage. Although some degree of inflammatory response may be present in these conditions, it only appears secondary to the primary cause. The primary cause is usually avascular necrosis, trauma or overuse, either alone or in combination. To confuse matters further, eponymous titles exist for many of these conditions [Köhler 1908, 1923, Sever 1912, Freiberg 1914].

Osteochondritis has been described in about 50 different locations in the body [Siffert 1981]. Osteochondritis of the navicular is usually referred to as Köhler's disease; it is similar to Perthes' disease of the hip. Calcaneal apophysitis or Sever's disease of the heel is similar to Osgood–Schlatter disease of the knee. Osteochondritis dissecans, which is seen most commonly in the knee, may also affect the talar dome (see Chapter 35) and the metatarsal heads. Osteochondritis of the metatarsal heads, most commonly at the second ray, is referred to as Freiberg's disease or Köhler II disease.

Osteochondritis of the metatarsal heads

Freiberg [1914] described six patients in whom the second metatarsal head appeared to be crushed. The etiology of this condition is still in debate. It is generally felt that ischemic necrosis of the metatarsal head is the most likely cause. However, it is not clear whether this is a consequence of arterial insufficiency or of trauma [Smillie 1957], or if both of these factors need to be present to initiate the condition. Whatever the cause, the metatarsal head becomes softened and this starts dorsally in the subchondral bone. Bony collapse follows.

Freiberg described the process as an 'infraction', a term that does not adequately describe the condition of the metatarsal head when it is seen at surgery. This term may also be confused with 'infarction', which suggests that the process is unequivocally avascular necrosis. Therefore, the use of the term 'infraction' should be abandoned.

Five stages in the evolution of the condition have been described:

1. Fissure fracture
2. Bone absorption
3. Further absorption with sinking of the central portion
4. Loose body separation
5. Flattening, deformity and arthrosis of the metatarsophalangeal joint.

Chondrolysis and dorsal cratering with expansion and flattening of the metatarsal head and secondary degenerative changes may occur rapidly. The patient is almost invariably an adolescent. The condition is commonest between the ages of 15 years and 18 years. In 68% it affects the second metatarsal head, in 27% the third and in 5% the fourth or fifth metatarsal heads. It is sometimes bilateral. It occurs rarely in adjacent metatarsals [Norton and Eyres 1998] and may occur sequentially [Brown et al. 1996]. The pain often begins insidiously, so that when the patient presents for treatment the condition is often quite advanced radiographically. The pain is felt in the region of the affected metatarsal head, and clinical examination shows tenderness and swelling of the metatarsophalangeal joint. Movements of the toe, particularly forced dorsiflexion, also cause pain in the joint.

The diagnosis is readily apparent on the plain radiographs, but in early cases, isotope bone scanning or magnetic resonance imaging (MRI) may be necessary. If the condition is left untreated, its natural history may be progression to osteoarthritis of the joint. However, many cases recover symptomatically. Expansion and flattening of a metatarsal head on radiographs during adult life are commonly an incidental finding.

The treatment of the condition depends on the severity of the symptoms, on the age of the patient and on the stage of the disease. In early cases, where symptoms are minimal and radiographic changes are minor, simple immobilization is the treatment of choice [Smillie 1957]. A below-knee cast can be worn for several weeks. However, the majority of patients have bony collapse of the metatarsal head at the time of initial presentation, and therefore some sort of operative intervention is usually necessary.

Surgical technique

The following procedures may be used in the treatment of Freiberg's disease, depending upon the stage of the disease:

- Debridement and synovectomy
- Bone grafting
- Shortening osteotomy at the metatarsal shaft
- Dorsal closing wedge osteotomy at the metatarsal neck or head
- Removal of the metatarsal head
- Removal of the base of the proximal phalanx
- Implant arthroplasty.

Debridement, synovectomy and cheilectomy

Debridement and synovectomy [Smillie 1957] are accomplished through a short, dorsal, longitudinal incision centered directly over the affected metatarsophalangeal joint (Figure 1). The extensor tendons are retracted towards the lateral side of the foot and the dorsal capsule is incised transversely. A synovectomy is performed and loose chondral or bony fragments and any other debris are removed (Figure 2). The dorsal crater is curetted, and sometimes its base is drilled to allow some regeneration by fibrocartilage. Bone spurs are removed from the dorsal, medial and lateral aspects of the joint using small rongeurs. This is similar to a cheilectomy undertaken for degenerative changes in the first metatarsophalangeal joint. The subcutaneous fat is closed with two or three absorbable sutures, and the skin is closed over a suction drain to avoid hematoma formation.

Bone grafting

Bone grafting was originally advocated only for the treatment of early disease before there was too much deformity of the metatarsal head. The surgical approach is the same as that described above. A cortical window is made in the dorsal aspect of the metatarsal neck. Bone graft, which can be harvested from just above the medial malleolus, is impacted into the dorsal aspect of the metatarsal head to elevate the subchondral bone and restore a more normal, rounded contour to this part of the head. It is also intended to stimulate osteoneogenesis by creeping substitution, thus restoring vascularity to the bone as well as preventing collapse.

This operation is not widely used, as it is technically difficult and may damage the already compromised metatarsal head. Furthermore, there is the potential for donor site morbidity.

Osteochondritis of the metatarsal heads

Osteotomies

Osteotomy is the treatment of choice in the typical symptomatic adolescent case. Two types of osteotomy have been described: first, a dorsal closing wedge osteotomy through the neck [Kanse and Chen 1989, Kinnard and Lirette 1989, Chao et al. 1999] or head [Gauthier and Elbaz 1979] of the metatarsal; and second, a shortening osteotomy of the distal shaft. A dorsal closing wedge osteotomy of the metatarsal neck leaves the dorsal crater

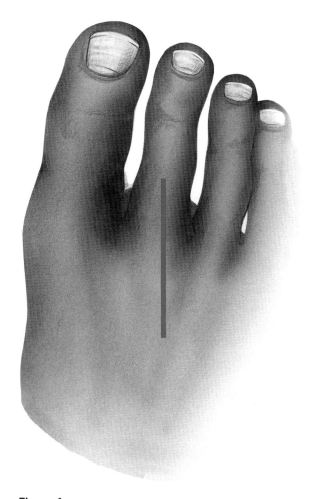

Figure 1

Skin incision for arthrotomy of the second metatarsophalangeal joint. Some surgeons prefer a curved or zig-zag incision to avoid any possible tethering or contracture

undisturbed and is technically simple (Figure 3). A dorsal longitudinal incision is made over the head and neck of the metatarsal and the joint is approached as described previously. A debridement can be carried out at the same time. To fashion the osteotomy, two small bone levers are placed subperiosteally on either side of the narrowest part of the metatarsal neck. A dorsal wedge of bone of approximately 40° is removed using a micro-oscillating saw. An attempt is made to keep the plantar cortex intact in order to hinge the osteotomy for additional stability. This hinge should be at the level of the narrowest part of the metatarsal neck and should not extend too far distally, otherwise it will encroach upon the plantar condyles. With the osteotomy fully closed, two crossed Kirschner wires are inserted dorsal–distally to plantar–proximally. They are bent over and left below the skin. Alternatively, a figure-of-eight wire may be used. It will be immediately apparent that the joint space is

widened because of the shortening that has occurred. This reduces the pressure within the joint, and also displaces the eroded cartilage from contact with the base of the proximal phalanx. The osteotomy also partially defunctions the whole ray. The wound is closed around a suction drain and the patient is allowed to heel-walk the following day. Most patients are fully weightbearing within 2 weeks. The osteotomy readily unites within 4–6 weeks and the Kirschner wires can then be removed. The author has used this procedure in over 20 cases with gratifying results.

Dorsal closing wedge osteotomy within the metatarsal head itself (Figure 4) is technically more difficult and less commonly used. The dorsal crater is excised and the osteotomy fixed with a figure-of-eight wire.

For the shortening osteotomy, a dorsal longitudinal approach is made over the distal shaft of the metatarsal, and a section of bone approximately 4 mm in length is removed. The bone ends are apposed and a small fragment plate and screws are applied (Figure 5). The plate is removed after a minimum of 12 months. Although normal movement is usually not restored at the metatarsophalangeal joint, this procedure was reported to result in an apparent remodeling of the normal shape of the metatarsal head with improved congruity between it and the proximal phalanx [Smith et al. 1991].

Removal of the metatarsal head

Resection of the metatarsal head was suggested for advanced cases of Freiberg's disease [Giannestras 1973]. However, most foot surgeons agree that this should be avoided, because it simply transfers excessive loads to the adjacent metatarsals. This leads to the formation of intractable plantar keratosis, which can be very painful for the patient and is difficult to treat. For this reason, removal of the metatarsal head is not recommended.

Removal of the base of the proximal phalanx

Partial resection of the proximal phalanx has been used to treat osteochondritis of the metatarsal head [Trott 1982]. This would seem to be a better option for the treatment of advanced cases of Freiberg's disease with degenerative changes, since it preserves the metatarsal head while removing the source of pain. However, loss of the concavity at the proximal phalanx usually results in postoperative toe deformity with dorsiflexion and shortening. This can be offset by surgical syndactyly to the adjacent

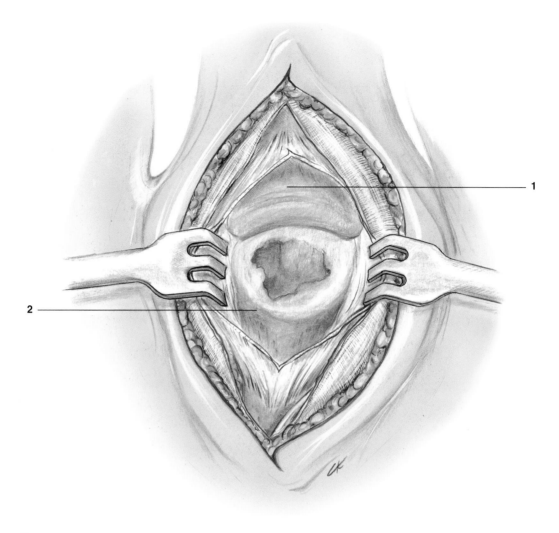

Figure 2

Typical intraoperative appearance with chondrolysis and dorsal cratering as well as expansion and flattening of the metatarsal head

1 Proximal phalanx
2 Metatarsal head

toe, which is a more extensive procedure and has the disadvantage of potentially defunctioning the toe.

Implant arthroplasty

Implant arthroplasty should be confined to elderly patients with advanced joint destruction because of uncertainty over the long-term results of silicone implants and the possibility of developing silicone synovitis. Replacement is either a single- or a double-stem design, the latter being generally more successful. The double-stemmed designs are either ball-shaped or cylindrical spacers, or alternatively possess a hinge.

Perioperative antibiotic cover is required because of the small risk of infection. The joint is exposed through a short, dorsal, longitudinal incision and approximately two-thirds of the metatarsal head is resected, with trimming of the plantar condyles. A thin shaving is also taken off the base of the proximal phalanx. The intramedullary canals are entered using a small bone awl, and are enlarged using power burrs until the holes are of sufficient size and shape to admit the rectangular stems. The implant is then inserted with the flexural concavity on the dorsal aspect of the joint. Titanium grommets are now recommended to protect the shoulder section of the implant in an attempt to reduce synovitis [Swanson et al. 1991].

Several authors [Cracchiolo 1996, Tillmann 1996] have discontinued the use of implant arthroplasty since they have found no advantages compared with resection arthroplasty in this situation.

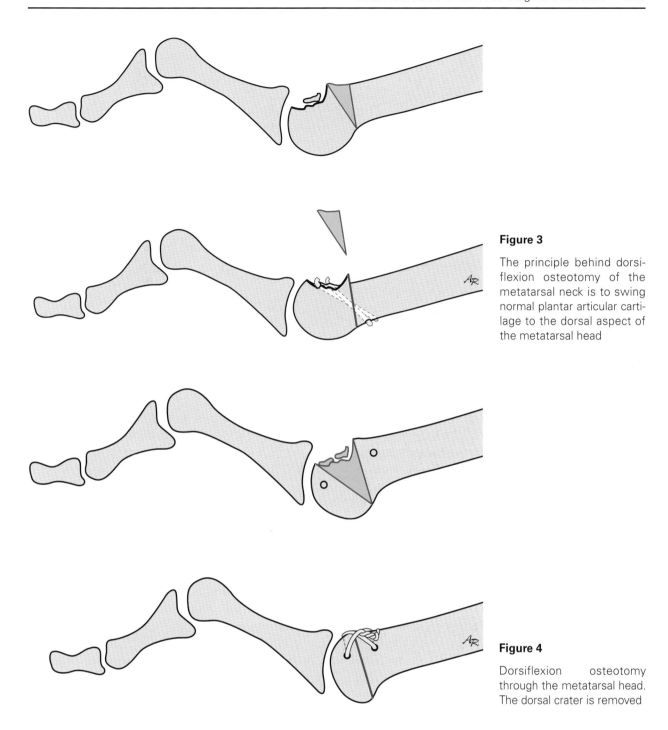

Figure 3

The principle behind dorsiflexion osteotomy of the metatarsal neck is to swing normal plantar articular cartilage to the dorsal aspect of the metatarsal head

Figure 4

Dorsiflexion osteotomy through the metatarsal head. The dorsal crater is removed

Osteochondritis of the tarsal navicular

In 1908, Köhler described an osteochondritis of the tarsal navicular bone. It was originally thought to be caused by tuberculosis or some other unknown inflammatory disease. It is now apparent that it is due to avascular necrosis. Fragmentation and collapse of the bone are visible radiographically, although many of these abnormal radiographic appearances have been shown to be due to normal variance [Waugh 1958]. This is because the navicular sometimes ossifies from multiple ossification centers, giving the bone a somewhat irregular outline on radiographs. It is speculated that the condition starts as a combination of mechanical and vascular vulnerability. The navicular is the last bone of the foot to ossify and may therefore be more susceptible than the others to the effects of weightbearing. The condition affects mainly boys, with a male to female ratio of 6.5 to 1 [Karp 1937]. It occurs at a slightly later age in boys and this supports the theory of mechanical compression of the bone. It is possible that the arterial supply is thus cut off from a large single ossific nucleus, leading to the changes described.

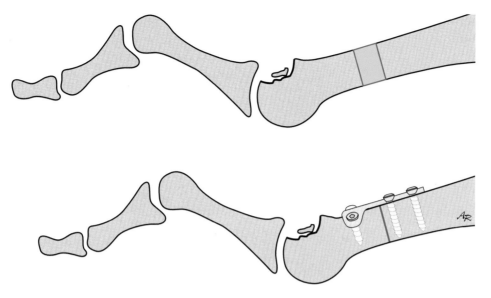

Figure 5

Shortening the metatarsal shaft in the treatment of osteochondritis of the metatarsal head, followed by mini-plate fixation

In a typical case, a child aged 3–6 years presents with pain in the foot and limping. There may be tenderness and slight swelling overlying the bone. As stated earlier, the radiographs should not be considered abnormal if there appears to be more than one ossific center. The hallmark of diagnosis is an obvious radiological abnormality in association with symptoms. In extreme cases the navicular appears flattened, with fragmentation and sclerosis. The differential diagnosis includes a painful accessory navicular, although it is very uncommon for this condition to present at such an early age, as it is usually seen in adolescents. Similarly, stress fractures of the navicular usually occur at a later age. Osteoid osteoma and juvenile rheumatoid arthritis must not be overlooked.

If untreated, the natural history of the condition is for fairly rapid revascularization, with a subsequent return to normal bone texture. This occurs much more readily in the navicular than in the femoral head following Perthes' disease, since there is no epiphyseal plate in the navicular to act as a barrier to the ingress of new blood vessels. The initial treatment therefore simply requires restriction of physical activities with immobilization of the foot in a plaster cast. This is necessary not only to relieve pain, but also to reduce the effects of impact on the navicular, which sits like a nut in a nutcracker with the forces of ground reaction. Hence, the shape of the bone is preserved. The cast should be well moulded around the arch and is worn for 6–8 weeks. A walking cast is just as effective as avoiding weightbearing. Surgical treatment is never indicated in children.

There is some controversy concerning possible long-term sequelae following the condition in childhood. Some authors have been unable to

demonstrate any adverse long-term effects of the disorder [Williams and Cowell 1981]. However, adult patients with flattened, irregular navicular bones could easily represent cases of previous avascular necrosis. Adult cases with fragmentation of the navicular due to previous avascular necrosis and unilateral talonavicular sag with early degenerative arthritis have been described [Scranton and Rowley 1996]. Patients such as these have usually received conservative treatment over a number of years with arch supports and anti-inflammatory medications.

Other adults may present acutely or subacutely with pain due to a sagittal stress fracture through the thinned sclerotic central portion of the navicular. The shape of the bone in these cases can be highly abnormal, having the radiograph and MRI scan appearance of central narrowing and peripheral extrusion, as if it has been squashed.

At this late stage, even without a fracture, degenerative changes are usually advanced, indicating a pan-navicular arthrodesis. It should be remembered that this involves fusing six joints: talonavicular, naviculo-medial, middle, lateral and two cuneocuneiform.

Osteochondrosis of the first metatarsal head

Uncommonly, adolescents and young adults may damage the articular surface of the first metatarsal head, usually while engaged in sports. If this injury occurs, the articular cartilage may separate from the underlying subchondral bone. This may produce only minimal symptoms and probably heals without the patient ever having sought medical attention. In some, however, the cartilage may separate, producing a flap of loose articular cartilage which causes pain and synovitis, and may be a precursor of hallux rigidus later on. In other patients, the initial lesion may be an osteochondral fragment similar to osteochondritis dissecans in the knee or ankle. Again, some of these may heal themselves, but in others, early degenerative changes can sometimes appear quite rapidly. These changes may go on to produce flattening of the first metatarsal head and osteophytes in early adult life.

Diagnosis is difficult in the early stages of this condition. The patient, typically a soccer player, will complain of pain on kicking a ball, or inability to last to the end of a match. There may be some tenderness and slight swelling over the first metatarsophalangeal joint. Plain radiographs occasionally show a lucent subchondral defect at the apex of the metatarsal head. If radiographs are normal, investigations may include MRI, isotope bone scanning, computed tomography and rarely arthrography. If the diagnosis is still uncertain, the joint may require surgical exploration or arthroscopy. Excision of chondral flaps or osteochondral fragments, combined with drilling holes in the base or burring the bone down to healthy subchondral bone may promote healing, as it does in other joints such as the knee or ankle.

Miscellaneous osteochondritides in the foot

Osteochondrosis may affect the sesamoid bones (see Chapter 17). Rarely, the epiphysis at the base of the proximal phalanx of the hallux is bifid, or may show irregular ossification. Osteochondritis has also been described at the base of the fifth metatarsal and is thought to represent a traction apophysitis due to tension created by the pull of the peroneus brevis. Finally, involvement of isolated tarsal bones such as the medial and intermediate cuneiforms has been described.

References

Brown JN, Haq A, Smith TWD (1996) Sequential unilateral Freiberg's disease. Foot 6: 86–87

Chao KH, Lee CH, Lin LC (1999) Surgery for symptomatic Freiberg's disease: dorsal closing wedge osteotomy in 13 patients followed for 2–4 years. Acta Orthop Scand 70: 483–486

Cracchiolo A III (1996) The rheumatoid foot and ankle. In: Helal B, Rowley DI, Cracchiolo A, Myerson MS (eds) Surgery of Disorders of the Foot and Ankle. London, Martin Dunitz, pp 443–451

Freiberg AH (1914) Infraction of the second metatarsal bone. A typical injury. Surg Gynecol Obstet 49: 191–193

Gauthier G, Elbaz R (1979) Freiberg's infraction. A subchondral bone fatigue fracture: a new surgical treatment. Clin Orthop Rel Res 142: 93–95

Giannestras NJ (1973) Foot Disorders: Medical and Surgical Management, 2nd edn. Philadelphia, Lea & Febiger, pp 421–423

Kanse P, Chen SC (1989) Dorsal closing wedge osteotomy for Freiberg's disease. J Bone Joint Surg 71B: 889

Karp MG (1937) Köhler's disease of the tarsal scaphoid. J Bone Joint Surg 19: 84–96

Kinnard P, Lirette R (1989) Dorsiflexion osteotomy in Freiberg's disease. Foot Ankle 9: 226–231

Köhler A (1908) Über eine häufige bisher anscheinend unbekannte Erkrankung einzelner kindlicher Knochen. Münchner Med Wochenschr 55: 1923

Köhler A (1923) Typical disease of the second metatarsophalangeal joint. Am J Roentgenol 10: 705–710

Norton MR, Eyres KS (1998) Acute Freiberg's disease in adjacent metatarsals. Foot 8: 230–232

Scranton PE, Rowley DI (1996) Osteochondritides. In: Helal B, Rowley DI, Cracchiolo A, Myerson MS (eds) Surgery of Disorders of the Foot and Ankle. London, Martin Dunitz, pp 785–792

Sever JW (1912) Apophysitis of the os calcis. NY Med J 95: 1025

Siffert RS (1981) Editorial comment: the osteochondroses. Clin Orthop 158: 2–3

Smillie IS (1957) Freiberg's infraction. J Bone Joint Surg 39B: 580

Smith TW, Stanley D, Rowley DI (1991) Treatment of Freiberg's disease. A new operative technique. J Bone Joint Surg 73B: 129–130

Swanson AB, de Groot Swanson G, Maupin BK et al. (1991) The use of a grommet bone liner for flexible hinge implant arthroplasty of the great toe. Foot Ankle 12: 149–155

Tillmann K (1996) Rheumatoid forefoot surgery. In: Helal B, Rowley DI, Cracchiolo A, Myerson MS (eds) Surgery of Disorders of the Foot and Ankle. London, Martin Dunitz, pp 457–466

Trott AW (1982) Developmental disorders. In: Jahss MH (ed) Disorders of the Foot, vol. 1. Philadelphia, WB Saunders, pp 200–211

Waugh W (1958) The ossification and vascularisation of the tarsal navicular and their relation to Köhler's disease. J Bone Joint Surg 40B: 765–777

Williams G, Cowell H (1981) Köhler's disease of the tarsal navicular. Clin Orthop 158: 53–58

29

Calcaneus fractures: open reduction and internal fixation

Hans Zwipp
Stefan Rammelt
Johann Marian Gavlik

Introduction

Few injuries have seen such dramatic changes in treatment as calcaneus fractures. In a remarkable review, Goff [1938] described no fewer than 41 different operative treatment methods for calcaneus fractures. High infection rates and inadequate fixation devices have led to a decline in calcaneus surgery in the mid-20th century, many surgeons advocating primary or secondary subtalar arthrodesis instead. The unsatisfying functional results after conservative treatment of intra-articular calcaneus fractures [James and Hunter 1983] and the routine availability of computed tomography (CT) scanning for diagnosis have resulted in a re-appraisal of the surgical approach [Sanders 1992, Benirschke and Sangeorzan 1993, Zwipp et al. 1993]. Today open reduction and internal fixation is favored by most surgeons, although the strategy is still a matter of debate [Rammelt and Zwipp 2004]. However, there are no uniform criteria for fracture classification and outcome assessment, which hampers comparison between different studies and makes general conclusions on the topic difficult.

Because of the vulnerable and highly specialized soft-tissue cover of the calcaneus, the soft-tissue conditions are highly predictive in fracture outcome. Calcaneus fractures are regularly associated with considerable soft-tissue damage. Therefore, timing of surgery and careful treatment of associated soft-tissue injuries is as important as proper fracture

reduction. The use of local and free microsurgical soft-tissue coverage has greatly contributed to the treatment of higher-degree open fractures of the calcaneus, which still have a guarded prognosis with a high incidence of deep infections and even amputation of the foot [Brenner et al. 2001]. Since most calcaneal fractures occur in male industrial workers, the sequelae of these injuries have a considerable socioeconomic impact [Sanders 2000].

Anatomy and biomechanics

The calcaneus (os calcis) is the largest bone of the foot. It makes up the whole posterior part of the longitudinal foot arch and the lateral foot column. Moreover, it acts as a strong lever arm during walking, standing and crouching, with the largest tendon of the human body attached to it, transmitting the force of the triceps surae muscle to the foot. The external and internal bony architecture of the calcaneus is unique, with a cortical shell of varying thickness and a vaultlike trabecular pattern of the cancellous bone that reflects the axial compression forces that transmit the body weight through the calcaneus to the calcaneal tuberosity and the forefoot. This leaves a neutral triangle with sparse trabeculae that is prone to impaction of the posterior facet in calcaneus fractures. Conversely, the trabeculae are condensed beneath the posterior facet of the subtalar joint, forming the 'thalamic portion' of the calcaneus. The cortical bone is especially thin at the lateral side of the calcaneus, which leads to lateral bulging in the majority of calcaneal fractures. Along the neck of the calcaneus the cortical layer is thick, forming Gissane's crucial angle with a normal value of 120–145° in the lateral radiographic projection [Sarrafian 1993, Zwipp 1994]. Further posteriorly the cortical bone forms the tuberosity joint angle described by Böhler, which is the most frequently used measurement for the vault function of the calcaneus in the lateral view and thus the quality of restoration of the anatomical shape after calcaneal fractures. The individual values of Böhler's angle vary considerably between 25 and 40°. For that reason lateral radiographs of the contralateral (uninjured) side are recommended for exact assessment of reduction [Zwipp 1994].

Four bony processes emanate from the calcaneal body. The tuberosity is the strong posterior point of weightbearing. The Achilles tendon is attached to its dorsoproximal part, whereas the inferior part, which can be further divided into a medial and a lateral process, anchors the plantar aponeurosis, the flexor retinaculum and several intrinsic foot muscles. The sustentaculum tali has a strong cortical architecture that makes it the most stable part of the calcaneus. It is connected to the talus via strong ligamentous structures, the medial and lateral talocalcaneal ligaments. The flexor hallucis longus tendon runs beneath its inferior border and conveys a dynamic press-fit force to the sustentaculum that preserves the anatomical position in relation to the talus even if the sustentaculum is fractured. The peroneal trochlea represents the smallest bony process of the calcaneus and is located along its lateral side. The peroneal tendons are guided by the peroneal sulcus (grooves located above and below the peroneal trochlea) and the distal peroneal retinaculum. The anterior process serves as a strong buttress leading to the navicular and cuboid bones, which are attached to it via the strong bifurcate and dorsal calcaneocuboidal ligaments. At the inferior aspect of the anterior process lies the small anterior tuberosity that is separated from the calcaneocuboidal joint by the coronoid fossa.

Three of the four joint surfaces are located on the superior aspect of the calcaneus and represent facets of the subtalar joint complex that articulates with the talus. The largest of them is the convex posterior facet. The concave middle facet and the anterior facet, which is flat, are merged in about one-fifth of all cases [Zwipp 1994]. The posterior facet is separated from the smaller anterior and middle facets by a groove called the sulcus calcanei. Together with the inferior surface of the talus the calcaneus forms the canalis tarsi medially and the sinus tarsi at its widened lateral portion. Within the sinus tarsi lies the strong talocalcaneal interosseous ligament complex, which consists of five parts: the lateral and medial roots of the inferior extensor retinaculum, the oblique talocalcaneal ligament, the ligament of the tarsal canal and the external talocalcaneal 'cervical' ligament [Sarrafian 1993]. The biconcave, saddle-shaped calcaneocuboid joint surface is relatively large and important for the range of motion in the Chopart joint as well as for the static function of the lateral buttress of the foot.

The subtalar joint acts in close coupling with the ankle joint and strongly influences the performance of the more distal foot articulations. It is essentially a mitered hinge between the talus and the calcaneus, with a single axis that passes from medial to lateral at an angle of approximately 16° in the transverse plane and approximately 42° in the horizontal plane, with considerable individual variations [Mann 1999]. The subtalar joint complex allows a considerable inversion/eversion movement of the hindfoot, which is essential for shock absorption during heel strike as well as rigidity of the foot during push-off. It also allows adaptation of the foot on uneven ground at foot flat. During heel strike the calcaneus goes into rapid eversion and the longitudinal foot arch flattens. The subtalar joint converts the internal rotation of the tibia into pronation at the level of the Chopart joint, making it more flexible at that stage. This appears to be an entirely passive process that depends on the configuration of the joint facets as well as their capsular and ligamentous support [Mann 1999]. During foot flat the subtalar joint demonstrates progressive inversion, transforming the midfoot into a more rigid structure. At push-off the calcaneal inversion reaches its maximum and the whole foot is transformed into a rigid lever arm. It follows from the above that, if either subtalar joint congruity or calcaneal anatomy is destroyed in the wake of calcaneus fractures, the whole gait cycle is considerably disturbed, leading to the many observed functional impairments, especially after conservative management.

Fracture mechanism

Fractures of the calcaneus are typically produced by axial force. The vast majority result from a fall from a height or from motor vehicle accidents, i.e. heavy deceleration. Men are afflicted four to five times as often as women [Zwipp et al. 1993, Sanders 1992].

Important factors affecting fracture morphology are the amount and direction of the impacting force, the foot position during the accident, the muscular tone of the calf and plantar muscles and the mineral content of the bone [Zwipp 1994].

The vertical load axis of the leg (and the talus) lies medially to the longitudinal axis of the calcaneus. The typical primary fracture line [Essex-Lopresti 1952] beginning at the angle of Gissane is a result of the eccentrically directed vertical axial force and the diverging longitudinal axes of the talus and the calcaneus, which form an angle of about 25–30°. The impacting force of the lateral talar process exerts a wedge-like action on the calcaneus, forcing the subtalar joint into eversion. The sustentaculum tali is sheared off the body of the calcaneus. The result of this sagittal plane fracture are two main fragments: a superomedial (sustentacular) and a posterolateral (tuberosity and body) portion. The foot position at the time of impact determines the course of this primary fracture. With the hindfoot in eversion the fracture line runs laterally, creating a large superomedial fragment. With the hindfoot in inversion the fracture line lies more medially, sometimes producing isolated fractures of the sustentaculum [Zwipp 1994]. The fracture mechanism consistently results in a lateral wall blow-out ('bulging'), leading to impingement of the soft tissues around the fibular tip and the peroneal tendons.

If the energy of the impact is not completely exhausted, secondary fracture lines develop, beginning at the posterior aspect of the subtalar joint [Essex-Lopresti, 1952]. In joint depression-type fractures the secondary fracture line runs downward posterior to the impacted posterior facet, only marginally touching the tuberosity. In tongue-type fractures the secondary fracture line extends longitudinally into the tuberosity, probably owing to a strong active pull of the Achilles tendon [Zwipp 1994], resulting in a complex deformity of the hindfoot, neutralizing and sometimes even reversing the tuberosity joint angle.

The fundamental clinical observations of Essex-Lopresti [1952] were validated by experimentally created calcaneal fractures [Wülker and Zwipp 1986]. Although a great variety of joint depression and tongue-type fractures were created, the primary and secondary fracture lines and resulting main fragments are relatively constant [Zwipp 1994, Sanders 2000]. Additional fracture lines may extend anteriorly and lead to a division in the sustentacular fragment or the calcaneocuboid joint, forming anterior process and anteromedial facet fragments. CT analysis of over 200 cases consistently demonstrated

five main fragments (tuberosity, sustentaculum, posterior facet, anterior process and anteromedial facet) with a maximum of three fractured joint surfaces [Zwipp 1994].

Special fracture types are avulsions of the bifurcate ligament at the superomedial tip of the anterior process by forced inversion of the foot and fractures of the superior aspect of the tuberosity produced by a violent contraction of the gastrocnemius–soleus muscle complex, resulting in an avulsion of the Achilles tendon insertion (the so-called 'beak fractures'). Direct lateral impaction results in extra-articular fractures of the tuberosity; medial force may generate isolated fractures of the medial tubercle of the tuberosity. Isolated compression fractures of the anterior process may occur as a component of fracture–dislocations at the midtarsal (Chopart's) joint.

Diagnosis and classification

Typical features of calcaneal fractures are swelling of the hindfoot and ankle region, hematoma and pain below the malleoli. The calcaneus is tender to palpation over the heel. Further symptoms are the impossibility of weightbearing in the affected leg, reduced ability to pro- and supinate the foot, and most often bulging and valgus deformity of the hindfoot. In case of any doubt, radiographic examination has to be carried out, especially in polytraumatized patients, where these injuries are still frequently overlooked. This is particularly true for isolated sustentacular fractures. Continuous assessment of the soft-tissue status is indispensable, since blister formation may develop within a few hours and, with severe fragment pressure from the inside, skin necrosis must be avoided. These factors delay surgical repair and may provoke soft-tissue breakdown or even infection, further worsening the final outcome. Furthermore, with severe soft-tissue swelling a compartment syndrome has to be ruled out, especially the deep calcaneal compartment containing the quadratus plantae muscle and the lateral plantar nerve [Manoli and Weber 1990].

Standardized radiographs include axial and lateral views of the calcaneus supplemented by a dorsoplantar view of the foot. Anteroposterior films of the ankle joint are obtained to see the amount of fibulocalcaneal abutment and medial talar subluxation in blow-out fractures. If surgery is indicated, plain radiographs of the contralateral (unaffected) foot are useful in assessment of the normal shape of the hindfoot, since there are remarkable individual differences (especially Böhler's angle). Oblique views of the subtalar joint (Brodén series) show the extent of subtalar joint involvement. The foot is placed in neutral flexion and internal rotation of 45°, while the X-ray tube is angled at 10–40°, the former showing the posterior, the latter the anterior portion of the subtalar joint. While the information from these views can be deduced more precisely by CT scans, the technique is useful for intraoperative assessment of reduction [Sanders 1992].

If an intra-articular fracture is suspected, axial and coronal CT scans have to be carried out. These allow for a three-dimensional analysis of fracture morphology, exact involvement of the joint facets and precise therapeutic planning. Furthermore, the modern classification systems of calcaneus fractures are based partly or solely on CT scanning.

The most widely used classification is that by Sanders [1992], which is based purely on the amount of fracture lines in the coronal CT scans. Extra-articular fractures are classified as Sanders I, one fracture line as Sanders II, two fracture lines as Sanders III and three or more fracture lines as Sanders IV. Laterally situated fracture lines are encoded with the letter A, intermediate with B and medial ones with the letter C. Zwipp introduced a 12-point fracture scale that reflects the number of fragments (2–5) and involved joint surfaces (0–3) as well as the extent of soft-tissue trauma and accompanying fractures of neighboring bones (additional 4 points). This classification proved to have a predictive value of 86% in a greater patient population [Zwipp 1994].

Treatment

Indications for and timing of surgery

The authors' preference is that all intra-articular fractures with joint displacement of more than 1 mm and extra-articular fractures with a hindfoot varus of more than 5°, hindfoot valgus of more than 10° or considerable flattening, broadening or shortening of the hindfoot (more than 20%) should be treated operatively. General contraindications to surgery are generally severe neurovascular insufficiency, poorly controlled insulin-dependent diabetes mellitus, poor compliance and severe systemic disorders with a poor overall prognosis or immune deficiency. Age over 65 years represents only a relative contraindication, depending on the patient's overall condition and functional demand.

The soft-tissue conditions and associated injuries are crucial for the timing of surgery. The treatment of open fractures and closed fractures with compartment syndrome or severe incarceration of the soft tissues are emergency procedures. Open fractures are treated with initial debridement of the wound, which is typically situated medially, temporary closure with skin substitutes, minimally invasive fracture reduction and K-wire fixation supplemented by an external fixator. After 48–72 h a second look with repeated debridement is carried out and the type of soft-tissue coverage determined. A standard internal fixation is performed after soft-tissue consolidation, mostly within 10–14 days. Alternatively, in patients with good overall condition, an early internal fixation within 120 h may be supplemented by a local or free flap procedure for definite wound closure, in order to reduce infection rates and allow for early functional treatment [Brenner et al. 2001]. In polytraumatized patients with compartment syndrome of the foot, a classic dorsomedian dermatofasciotomy is carried out, releasing the skin, dorsal fascia and distal extensor retinaculum. The deep calcaneal compartment is released by a separate hindfoot incision similar to that used for a plantar fascia release [Sanders 2000]. Alternatively, a medial compartment release is performed. In polytraumatized patients this procedure is followed by a medial external transfixation; in monotraumatized patients with compartment syndrome, release of the hematomas is followed by a standard osteosynthesis.

The vast majority of calcaneus fractures are accompanied by considerable soft-tissue compromise, representing Tscherne grade II closed soft-tissue damage. Therefore, delayed osteosynthesis is preferred after the swelling has markedly decreased, usually within 10 days. However, surgery should not be delayed beyond 2 weeks after the injury, especially in cases with total hindfoot collapse, to avoid shrinking of the skin and soft-tissue contracture leading to higher complication rates [Rammelt and Zwipp 2004].

Preoperatively, the patient is restricted to bed-rest. The injured limb is elevated and ice is applied to the foot. To reduce soft-tissue swelling further, the use of non-steroidal anti-inflammatory drugs (NSAIDs) and enzymatic drugs, as well as emptying the venous plexus with venous pump training, is useful. Patients are administered low-molecular-weight heparin.

Surgical approach

Open reduction and internal fixation of intra-articular calcaneus fractures aims at restoration of the anatomical shape of the calcaneus, anatomic reconstruction

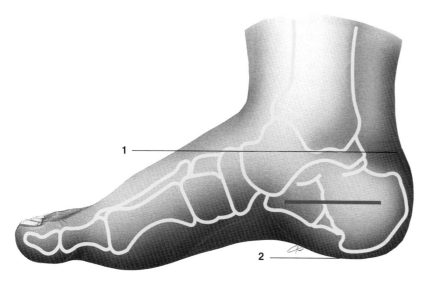

Figure 1

Medial approach to the calcaneus. The incision lies exactly halfway between the tip of the medial malleolus (1) and the medial edge of the sole (2). It is mostly done straight, but may also be performed in a lazy-S fashion

of all affected joint surfaces and stable osteosynthesis without joint transfixation to allow early active and passive movement.

For open reduction of calcaneal fractures a multitude of surgical approaches have been advocated. They include lateral, medial and combined medial–lateral approaches. The extended lateral approach today represents the standard approach for displaced intra-articular fractures of the calcaneus [Benirschke and Sangeorzan 1993, Zwipp et al. 1993, Sanders 2000]. This approach allows direct visualization and reconstruction of the destroyed lateral wall of the calcaneus, and the posterior and facet of the subtalar joint and the calcaneocuboid joint. With the medial approach [McReynolds 1982] only indirect reduction of the displaced posterior facet is possible. This is therefore mainly used in simple (two-part) extra-articular fractures with relevant varus/valgus deformity or subtalar dislocation fractures and in rare cases of medial wall blow-out [Zwipp et al. 1993]. The hazard of medial approaches lies in the possible destruction of the nearby neurovascular bundle containing the posterior tibial artery, vein and nerve. A modified medial approach ('sustentacular approach') [Zwipp 1994] is suggested for isolated sustentacular fractures or in addition to the extended lateral approach with fragmentation of the medial facet in more complex intra-articular calcaneus fractures.

Because of the critical soft-tissue conditions, minimally invasive treatment options for selected fracture patterns have gained increased attention for fluoroscopically and arthroscopically assisted procedures over recent years [Tornetta 1998, Gavlik et al. 2002]. In addition, limited approaches and percutaneous osteosynthesis are employed with critical soft-tissue conditions, in polytraumatized patients and selected younger patients with contraindications to open surgery [Zwipp et al. 1993].

Medial approach

The medial approach [McReynolds 1982] to the calcaneus allows no control over joint congruity of the posterior facet and only indirect reduction of the main fragments. The patient is placed on the operating table in a supine position. A tourniquet is placed on the thigh of the injured leg. The incision is made horizontally or as a lazy-S cut in line with the skin creases, about 8–10 cm, exactly halfway between the tip of the medial malleolus and the sole (Figure 1). The cutis, subcutis and fascia are dissected. The neurovascular bundle is carefully prepared, marked and held away with a Penrose drain (Figure 2a). The abductor hallucis longus muscle is retracted downward, whereas the flexor hallucis longus tendon is only identified and left in place. The sustentacular fragment of the calcaneus is now fully visualized with preparation down to the periosteum. A cancellous 6.5-mm Schanz screw with handle is introduced after stab incision and drilling into the tuberosity. The tuberosity fragment can now be reduced under axial pull against the sustentacular fragment and the anterior process. If correct anatomical reconstruction of the medial wall is achieved, the result is fixed temporarily with 1.6–2.0 mm K-wires. It is useful to introduce two parallel K-wires from the inferior aspect of the tuberosity fragment into the sustentacular fragment and two K-wires from the posterior aspect of the tuberosity fragment into the anterior process of the calcaneus. Temporary transfixation may exceed the joint lines, if necessary. Definite fixation is

a

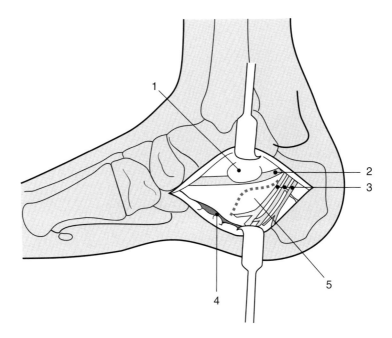

b

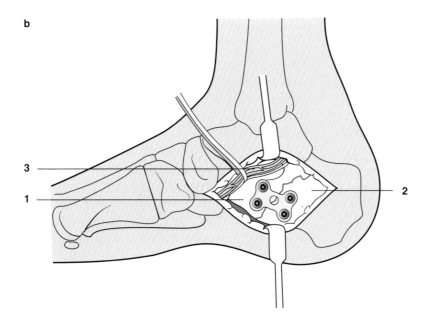

Figure 2

a. Exposure of the medial aspect of the calcaneus. The sustentaculum tali (1) is identified with the flexor hallucis longus tendon (2) running beneath within its sheath. Care has to be taken not to injure the tibialis posterior neurovascular bundle (3). The abductor hallucis brevis muscle (4) is retracted from the medial wall of the calcaneus which is covered by a fascia (5); b. after indirect reduction of the main sustentacular (1) and tuberosity fragments (2) a plate is applied to the medial wall of the calcaneus in an anti-glide fashion. The tibialis posterior neurovascular bundle (3) is held aside with a soft strap

achieved with a small anti-glide 'cervical' H-plate and four 3.5-mm cortical screws, of which one should run into the sustentacular fragment, one into the processus anterior fragment and two into the tuberosity fragment (Figure 2b). It is advisable to contour the H-plate according to the individual form of the medial wall of the calcaneus to prevent any gliding of the fragments when fastening the screws. Correct reduction and extra-articular position of the screws are controlled by intra-operative standard radiographs.

Sustentacular approach

This approach excludes the hazards of neurovascular damage compared to the McReynolds approach [Zwipp 1994]. It may be recommended in isolated sustentacular fractures as well as a supplement to the extended lateral approach in complex intra-articular fractures with fragmentation of the medial facet. The patient is placed on the operating table in a supine position. A tourniquet is placed on the thigh of the injured leg. The incision is made

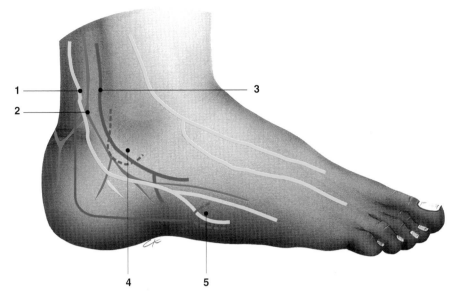

Figure 3

Extended lateral approach to the calcaneus. The incision is boomerang-shaped and respects the course of the sural nerve (1), the lesser saphenous vein (2) and the lateral calcaneal artery (3). The tip of the lateral malleolus (4) and the tuberosity of the fifth metatarsal base (5) serve as landmarks for the incision

longitudinally about 3 cm long parallel to the sole of the foot, 1–2 cm distal and anteriorly to the tip of the medial malleolus directly over the palpable sustentaculum. The nearby running tendons and the posterior tibial neurovascular bundle are only identified and left in place. The sustentaculum is identified. The medial facet is reduced to the corresponding facet of the talus and two long (about 50–60 mm) 3.5-mm compression screws are introduced into the sustentaculum tali along its axis into the main tuberosity fragment. Correct reduction and extra-articular position of the screws are controlled by intraoperative standard radiographs.

Extended lateral approach

This standard approach is most useful with displaced intra-articular calcaneus fractures that involve the posterior facet, which is fractured in 96% of cases [Benirschke and Sangeorzan 1993, Zwipp 1994] and will therefore be described in detail. Surgery is usually carried out under general anesthesia. The patient is placed on a radiolucent operating table, allowing intraoperative fluoroscopy, in a lateral decubitus position on the non-injured side; alternatively the prone position is used. A tourniquet is applied to the thigh of the injured leg, the leg is draped free and a sterile tape is applied to the toes. The tourniquet (200–300 mmHg) is used only for joint reconstruction in the absence of an additional acute compartment syndrome.

The skin incision is boomerang-shaped over the lateral aspect of the heel, running between the lateral malleolus and the posterior and inferior borders

of the heel, respectively (Figure 3). It is rounded slightly at the angulation. With respect to the blood supply to the lateral aspect of the heel via the lateral calcaneal artery [Freeman et al. 1998], the incision is placed vertically close to the Achilles tendon and horizontally where the skin lines become visible when pushing from the plantar surface [Zwipp et al. 2004]. With fragmentation of the anterior process or calcaneocuboidal joint involvement, the incision is continued towards the tip of the fifth metatarsal base (Figure 3). The subcutaneous layer is then dissected in a strict vertical fashion, beginning from the angle of the incision until the lateral wall of the calcaneus becomes visible. Care has to be taken to save the sural nerve as well as the lesser saphenous vein in the proximal incision. When extending the subcutaneous dissection distally to visualize the calcaneocuboidal joint, the peroneal tendons are identified. The tendons are mobilized within their sheath, in order to prevent postoperative adhesions, and gently held back with a blunt retractor. The tendon sheath is detached only from the peroneal tubercle.

After the incision is extended to full length, the calcaneus is prepared epiperiosteally until the subtalar joint becomes visible. The distal retinaculum of the peroneal tendons and the fibulocalcaneal ligament are detached subperiosteally. In this manner a full-thickness cutaneous flap is produced that can be held back temporarily with K-wires introduced into the lateral process of the talus and the cuboid or non-resorbable threads [Benirschke and Sangeorzan 1993] (Figure 4). The use of sharp distractors has to be avoided. All structures within the flap will return to their anatomical position at the end of surgery, when

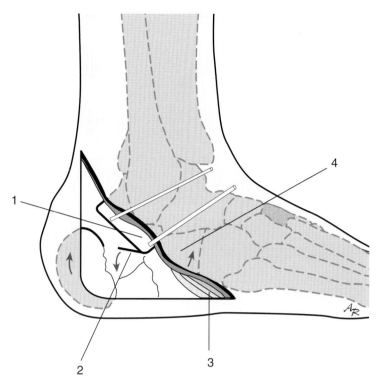

Figure 4

Exposed lateral wall of the calcaneus. K-wires are introduced into the lateral process of the talus (1) to gently hold away the full-thickness cutaneous flap. The depressed posterior facet fragment (2) is identified and shell-like lateral bulge fragments are removed temporarily. The peroneal tendons (3) are mobilized within their sheaths, if exposure of a fractured anterior process (4) becomes necessary

the flap is folded back. With careful preparation, neither circulation nor nerve supply within the flap will be disturbed by the en bloc dissection, because it preserves both the peroneal artery and the sural nerve. If the bulged fragment of the lateral wall is only loosely fixed to the central portion it is retracted inferiorly or turned around temporarily to achieve better visualization. The latter is most often necessary also for the lateral part of the depressed posterior facet (intermediate fragment) in Sanders type III fractures. The primary fracture line is identified at the angle of Gissane. For correct visualization it may be necessary to remove some fibrous tissue and the fat pad from the sinus tarsi.

When all fracture fragments are identified after copious lavage, the first and crucial step to restore the anatomical shape of the calcaneus is the mobilization of the tuberosity fragment with the Westhues maneuver (Figure 5). This maneuver also allows better visualization and easier elevation of the depressed posterior facet fragment(s). A 6.5-mm cancellous Schanz screw with handle is introduced into the tuberosity after stab incision and drilling. Under direct visualization of the subtalar joint space the handle is moved downward in order to bring the tuberosity fragment back to its correct position. At the same time, varus or valgus malalignment is corrected.

The posterior facet is now reduced in a step-wise fashion from medial to lateral (Figure 7). In cases of

deep impaction, it may be loosened and elevated with a sharp elevator. Should the medial portion of the posterior facet be tilted laterally it must be reduced congruently to the inferior joint surface of the talus first and fixed with a 2.0 K-wire introduced from plantar into the talus. In a second step the depressed lateral, and if present intermediate, portions of the posterior facet are elevated and fixed with 2.0 K-wires to the sustentaculum. If an intermediate fragment is present, the K-wires are drilled through the medial wall and pulled back from medially to the lateral edge of this fragment onto which the lateral fragment is now reduced. The K-wires are now drilled back to lateral. The K-wires are introduced 5 mm below the joint surface and are directed 10° superiorly towards the talus and 15° anteriorly towards the midfoot. The resulting articular block is then fixed to the initially mobilized tuberosity fragment (Figure 6c).

The whole posterior fragment can now be brought into alignment with the anterior process fragment to reconstruct the crucial angle (Figure 6d). To visualize the anterior process fully it is sometimes necessary to split or even to dissect the talocalcaneal interosseous ligament, especially if it retracts the processus anterior fragment, thus rendering reduction impossible [Zwipp 1994]. Additional K-wires are now introduced along the longitudinal and vertical axes of the calcaneus (Figure 6d). With extremely unstable fractures temporary fixation is extended to the talus and

a

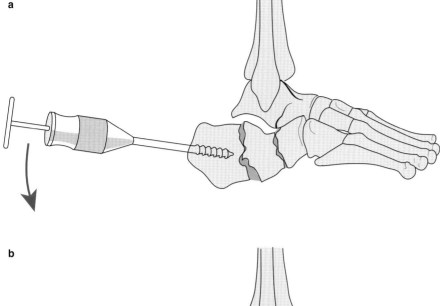

b

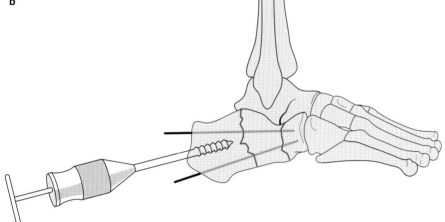

Figure 5

a, b. Reduction of the main tuberosity fragment with a Schanz screw introduced percutaneously (Westhues maneuver). The tuberosity joint (Böhler's) angle is restored and varus/valgus malalignment is corrected

cuboid. If the main fragments are large enough, it is always advisable to use two parallel K-wires in order to achieve better stabilization. Should a fifth fragment be present, the so-called anterior facet fragment, the calcaneocuboidal joint has to be reduced congruently and the fragment, is fixed with two additional K-wires. The exact restoration of the calcaneus is controlled also by an image intensifier, including oblique views into the subtalar joint space corresponding to the Brodén views. 3D fluoroscopy is most helpful for this step.

In the authors' preference, the quality of reduction of the crucial posterior joint facet is controlled by open subtalar arthroscopy after K-wire fixation to evaluate the areas inaccessible to the eye [Rammelt et al. 2002]. A small diameter arthroscope (2.3 mm/30° arthroscope) is introduced into the exposed subtalar joint 2–4 mm posterior to the angle of Gissane, or alternatively into the posterior rim of the posterior facet resembling the anterior and posterior lateral portals. The joint is irrigated manually with a blunt cannula. The introduction of the arthroscope is facilitated by applying varus stress to the heel

through the Schanz screw introduced into the calcaneal tuberosity, while care is taken not to exert too much tension with the screw handle in order not to displace the K-wires. The posterior facet is inspected for remaining incongruities or minor loose osteochondral fragments. If an intra-articular step is found, the position of the posterior facet should be corrected immediately, thus preventing painful postoperative conditions or the need for further surgery [Rammelt et al. 2002]. After joint reduction the tourniquet is opened.

In most cases the elevation of the depressed lateral portion of the posterior facet leaves a subthalamic defect zone resulting from impaction of this fragment into the neutral triangle. However, the need for defect filling, either with bone grafting from the ipsilateral iliac crest or with bone substitutes, is controversial. A comparative study did not show superior results with bone grafting than without [Longino and Buckley 2001]. While some authors deny the necessity for defect filling completely and refer to the regenerative capacities of cancellous bone [Stephenson 1987, Sanders 1992],

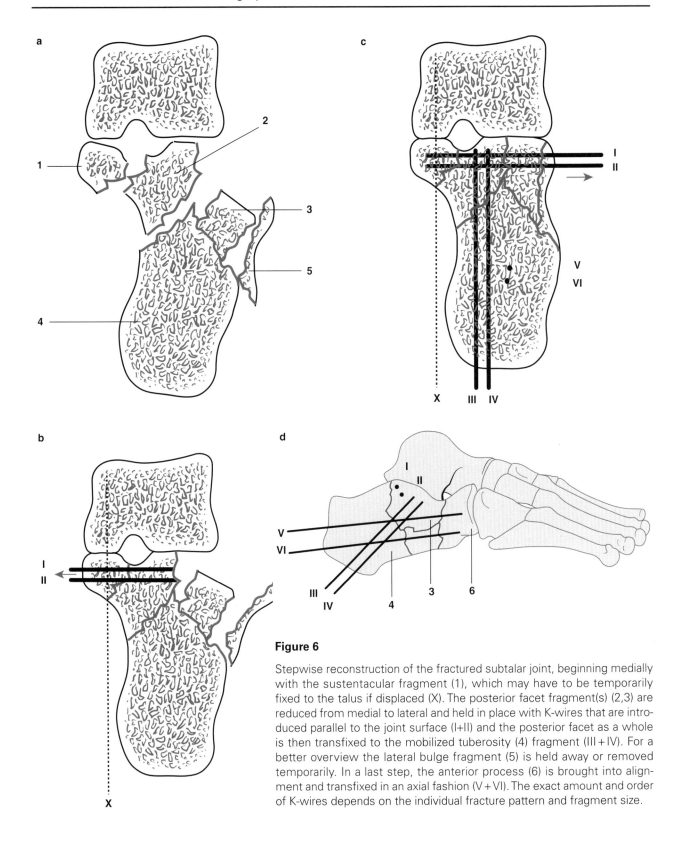

Figure 6

Stepwise reconstruction of the fractured subtalar joint, beginning medially with the sustentacular fragment (1), which may have to be temporarily fixed to the talus if displaced (X). The posterior facet fragment(s) (2,3) are reduced from medial to lateral and held in place with K-wires that are introduced parallel to the joint surface (I+II) and the posterior facet as a whole is then transfixed to the mobilized tuberosity (4) fragment (III+IV). For a better overview the lateral bulge fragment (5) is held away or removed temporarily. In a last step, the anterior process (6) is brought into alignment and transfixed in an axial fashion (V+VI). The exact amount and order of K-wires depends on the individual fracture pattern and fragment size.

others use bone grafting for greater defects (>1 cm³) in highly unstable fractures [Benirschke and Sangeorzan 1993, Zwipp et al. 1993]. The use of interlocking plates may obviate the need for bone grafting completely [Zwipp et al. 2004].

Internal fixation is completed with the use of an anatomically shaped plate affixed to the restored lateral wall of the calcaneus. The use of several plates has been advocated, such as 3.5-mm reconstruction plates, one or two (double or triple) H-shaped plates, a single Y-shaped plate, some irregularly shaped plates, and interlocking plates [Rammelt and Zwipp 2004]. In most studies a sufficient degree of stability can be achieved with the use of a single lateral plate that is contoured and affixed to the calcaneus with 3.5-mm cortical or cancellous screws (Figure 7). An anatomic stainless steel plate with interlocking screws recently introduced is used for more unstable fracture patterns [Zwipp et al. 2004]. Two of the screws should be directed into the sustentaculum tali, two or three into the tuberosity and two into the anterior process close to the calcaneocuboid joint. One or two additional screws may be placed outside the plate in order to obtain ideal positioning into the sustentaculum tali or a severely displaced anterior process, anterior facet or tongue fragment. The K-wires and Schanz screw are removed. The correct anatomical restoration, joint congruency and extra-articular position of the screws are documented by standard radiographs: a dorsoplantar view of the foot, lateral and axial views of the hindfoot, including a 20° Brodén view. After careful hemostasis the skin is closed in layers. With considerable bleeding from the cancellous bone, a collagen sponge is introduced epiperiosteally. A sterile compression dressing is applied to the foot and postoperatively a below-the-knee split plaster cast is applied to the injured leg.

Bilateral approaches

In rare cases of destruction of the medial joint facet in comminuted fractures a combined medial–lateral approach, as proposed by Stephenson [1987], seems beneficial. However, this approach is associated with an increased incidence of wound edge necrosis. An alternative is the combination of the extended lateral approach with a sustentacular approach [Zwipp 1994].

Primary subtalar arthrodesis

Some authors hold that anatomical reconstruction is not possible in highly comminuted fractures (Sanders type IV) and therefore advocate primary subtalar arthrodesis in these cases [Sanders, 1992, 2000]. This procedure must be combined with reconstruction of heel height and width in order to achieve a plantigrade foot. After reconstruction of the anatomical shape of the calcaneus and plate fixation as described above, all remaining cartilage is removed from the joint surfaces and arthrodesis is achieved with autologous bone graft and one or two 6.5–8.0-mm cancellous bone lag screws. Alternatively, secondary arthrodesis may be performed after primary standard osteosynthesis, if painful subtalar arthritis develops, since asymptomatic ankylosis may occur. Also in these cases, primary open reduction reduces soft-tissue strain and

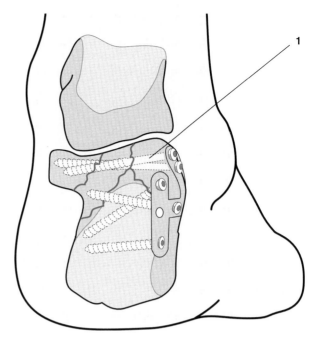

Figure 7

Internal fixation is achieved with an anatomical calcaneus plate that is attached to the restored lateral wall with six to eight cortical screws. At least two screws are introduced into the thalamic portion (1) and directed towards the sustentaculum tali. The tuberosity and processus anterior fragments are fixed with at least two screws each. The K-wires are removed gradually

alleviates the arthrodesis procedure that may be performed in situ [Zwipp 1994].

Minimally invasive percutaneous osteosynthesis

To minimize minor and major wound complications after open reduction and internal fixation, percutaneous reduction and screw osteosynthesis have gained increased attention over recent years. However, closed reduction and minimally invasive osteosynthesis carries the risk of inadequate reduction of the subtalar joint. Therefore, percutaneous osteosynthesis is most suitable for less complex fracture patterns (Sanders type II) [Tornetta 1998, Gavlik et al. 2002]. Limited approaches are also indicated with patients in a critical overall condition (such as polytraumatized patients) or with extremely damaged soft tissues, as discussed above [Zwipp 1994].

The patient is placed on a radiolucent operating table in a lateral decubitus position on the non-injured side. Reduction of the main tuberosity fragment is carried out with percutaneous leverage as in open reduction and internal fixation. The screw is placed centrally into the main portion of the fragment parallel to the upper aspect of the tuberosity and directed to the most distal aspect of the displaced posterior facet. After loosening the impacted fragments with medial/lateral stress, the handle is moved downward in order to bring the tuberosity fragment back into alignment with the main sustentacular fragment (Westhues maneuver, Figure 8a). Additional varus or valgus malalignment is reduced with lateral or medial movement of the handle, respectively (see also Figure 5). The amount of correction of the tuberosity joint angle and varus/valgus deformity is controlled fluoroscopically. In case of residual bulging of the lateral wall, manual compression is carried out bilaterally to reduce any remaining broadening of the calcaneus. If the posterior facet is displaced as a whole (two fragments, tongue-type Sanders IIC fractures), proper reduction of the calcaneal tuberosity is usually sufficient to achieve anatomical reduction. In more complex fracture patterns (three or four fragments, Sanders IIA and IIB) the separate lateral posterior facet fragment has to be manipulated percutaneously with additional Kirschner wires. In cases of impaction, the lateral posterior facet fragment is brought up to the joint level with a pestle or sharp elevator introduced percutaneously while the anterior process fragment may have to be pushed downward (Figure 8a,b). Joint congruity is controlled with high-resolution fluoroscopy – preferably 3D – and arthroscopically [Rammelt et al. 2002]. The anterolateral or posterolateral portal can be used for arthroscopically assisted joint reduction, depending on the fracture location.

In isolated calcaneus fractures screw osteosynthesis is generally preferred to K-wire transfixation, since it provides sufficient stability and allows for early mobilization. The fragments are fixed with three to six cannulated cortical screws introduced percutaneously via stab incisions (Figure 8c). One or two screws are placed into the thalamic portion, parallel to the posterior facet, towards the sustentaculum tali. The exact number and position of screws depends on the individual fracture pattern. With extension of the fracture line into the calcaneocuboid joint, the anterior process fragments are fixed under fluoroscopic control. In cases with severely compromised soft tissues or in polytraumatized patients, K-wires are used instead of screws and are supplemented by tibiometatarsal transfixation or three-point distraction (calcaneal tuberosity, talar head and navicular or medial cuneiform) with an external fixator. The same may apply for polytraumatized patients, when the duration of surgery must be kept to a minimum until definite osteosynthesis

becomes feasible. If no internal fixation is done, K-wires and external fixation devices are removed after 10–12 weeks.

Postoperative management

The goal of postoperative care is early mobilization of the patient. Physical therapy is directed towards early regaining of the full range of motion in the ankle, subtalar and Chopart joints. While the exact postoperative protocol varies from surgeon to surgeon, the following may serve as a guideline.

The injured foot is placed postoperatively in a split non-weightbearing below-the-knee plaster cast for 8–10 days. The patient is told to press the sole of the injured foot against the plaster cast about ten times an hour in order to empty the venous plexus of the foot and reduce swelling. Continuous passive motion of the ankle and subtalar joint is begun the first postoperative day. Physical therapy begins with active and passive, pain-restricted range-of-motion exercises in the ankle and subtalar joints on the second postoperative day. The desired motion is best achieved by describing a circle with the great toe. Mobilization of the foot and ankle is supplemented by isotonic and isometric exercises of the affected leg, including proprioceptive training and neuromuscular facilitation. The patient is mobilized on crutches with partial weightbearing of the injured leg on the third to fifth postoperative day.

The suture material is removed after 8–10 days and the patient mobilized in his custom shoe. Weightbearing is limited to 15–20 kg for 6 weeks (in comminuted fractures up to 12 weeks). For the whole period the patient must undergo an extensive physical therapy program including active range-of-motion exercises, manual mobilization of the hindfoot and lymphatic drainage, to obtain a good functional outcome. The patient should abstain from active sports and heavy loading of the injured foot for at least 4 months postoperatively. Special rehabilitation programs are usually not necessary. The hardware can be removed about 1 year after surgery. In case of stiffness at the subtalar joint this may be combined with subtalar arthrolysis, consisting of intra- and extra-articular debridement of the subtalar joint [Rammelt et al. 2002].

Hazards and complications

Early complications of operative treatment can be minimized by careful preparation, which includes

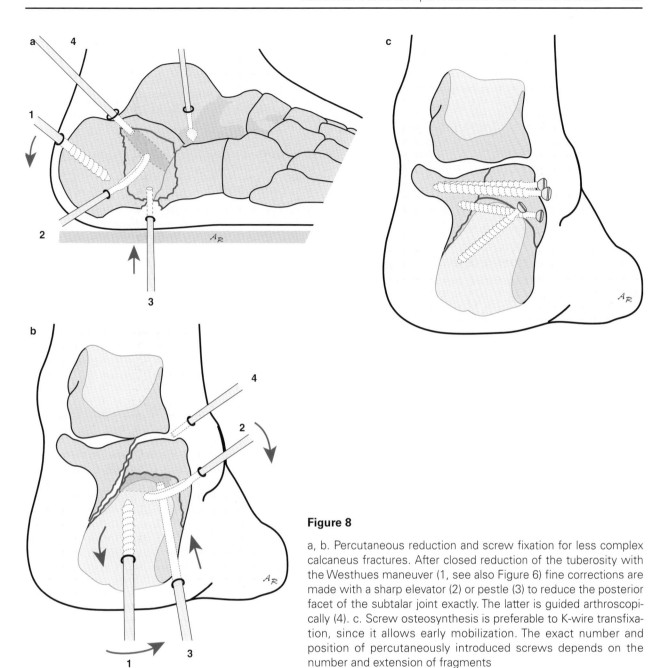

Figure 8

a, b. Percutaneous reduction and screw fixation for less complex calcaneus fractures. After closed reduction of the tuberosity with the Westhues maneuver (1, see also Figure 6) fine corrections are made with a sharp elevator (2) or pestle (3) to reduce the posterior facet of the subtalar joint exactly. The latter is guided arthroscopically (4). c. Screw osteosynthesis is preferable to K-wire transfixation, since it allows early mobilization. The exact number and position of percutaneously introduced screws depends on the number and extension of fragments

the correct approach, identification of neurovascular structures, perpendicular incision, no sharp distracters and strict atraumatic operation technique. Single-shot intravenous antibiotics should be administered in cases of open fractures and with severe closed soft-tissue damage. Injuries to the cutaneous nerves most frequently afflict the sural nerve laterally and the posterior tibial nerve medially. These lesions usually result in hypesthesia and are treated conservatively except for neuroma formation, for which excision is advised [Sanders 2000]. The most frequently observed postoperative complication is superficial wound edge necrosis, which is seen in 2–10% of cases after standard osteosynthesis via an extended lateral approach [Benirschke and

Sangeorzan 1993, Zwipp et al. 1993]. The incidence increases considerably to 27% with a bilateral approach [Stephenson 1987]. Superficial breakdown of the wound margins usually heals spontaneously with the application of dry dressings. Superficial infections are treated with local revision and immobilization. Subcutaneous hematoma is treated initially with leg elevation and ice dressings. If there is no regression, aspiration or surgical revision is indicated in about 5% to prevent infection or skin necrosis [Zwipp et al. 1993]. The application of a collagen sponge over the lateral wall of the calcaneus after internal fixation may reduce the incidence of subcutaneous hematomas, since most hemorrhage occurs from the cancellous bone.

Deep soft-tissue and bone infections occur in 1.3–7% [Benirschke and Sangeorzan 1993, Zwipp et al. 1993]. Radical surgical debridement and aggressive antimicrobial therapy is the treatment of choice; second and third looks have to be done until wound swabs are negative. If infection persists the calcaneal plate has to be removed and replaced by screw osteosynthesis. Antibiotic beads are inserted temporarily. If chronic post-traumatic osteomyelitis develops despite all these measures, subtotal or total calcanectomy is inevitable. If soft-tissue coverage cannot be achieved even after conditioning with synthetic skin substitutes or continuous suction, free flaps have to be considered in order to control infection and to avoid protracted courses [Brenner et al. 2001]. Non-union is very rare after stable internal fixation and can be treated with bone grafting and fixation using 6.5-mm cancellous screws. Overall, in greater series, good to excellent results could be achieved in more than two-thirds of cases with open reduction and internal fixation of displaced intra-articular calcaneus fractures [Sanders 1992, Benirschke and Sangeorzan 1993, Zwipp et al. 1993, 2004].

References

Benirschke SK, Sangeorzan BJ (1993) Extensive intraarticular fractures of the foot. Surgical management of calcaneal fractures. Clin Orthop 292: 128–134

Brenner P, Rammelt S, Gavlik JM, Zwipp H (2001) Early soft tissue coverage after complex foot trauma. World J Surg 25: 603–609

Essex-Lopresti P (1952) The mechanism, reduction technique, and results in fractures of the os calcis. Br J Surg 39: 395–419

Freeman B, Duff S, Allen P, et al. (1998) The extended lateral approach to the hindfoot. Anatomical basis and surgical implications. J Bone Joint Surg (Br) 80: 139–142

Gavlik JM, Rammelt S, Zwipp H (2002) Percutaneous, arthroscopically-assisted osteosynthesis of calcaneous fractures. Arch Orthrop Trauma Surg 122: 424–428

Goff CW (1938) Fresh fractures of the os calcis. Arch Surg 36: 744–765

James ET, Hunter GA (1983) The dilemma of painful old os calcis fractures. Clin Orthop 177: 112–115

Longino D, Buckley RE (2001) Bone graft in the operative treatment of displaced intraarticular calcaneal fractures: is it helpful? J Orthop Trauma 15: 280–286

Mann RA (1999) Biomechanics of the foot and ankle. In: Coughlin MJ, Mann RA (eds) Surgery of the Foot and Ankle. St Louis, Mosby, pp 1–35

Manoli A 2nd, Weber TG (1990) Fasciotomy of the foot: an anatomical study with special reference of release of the calcaneal compartment. Foot Ankle 10: 267–275

McReynolds JS (1982) Trauma to the os calcis and the heel cord. In: Jahss MH (ed) Disorders of the Foot. Philadelphia, WB Saunders, 1497

Rammelt S, Gavlik JM, Barthel S, Zwipp H (2002) The value of subtalar arthroscopy in the management of intra-articular calcaneus fractures. Foot Ankle Int 23: 906–916

Rammelt S, Zwipp H (2004) Calcaneus fractures: facts, controversies and recent developments. Injury 35: 443–461

Sanders R (1992) Intra-articular fractures of the calcaneus: present state of the art. J Orthop Trauma 6: 252–265

Sanders R (2000) Displaced intra-articular fractures of the calcaneus. J Bone Joint Surg 82A: 225–250

Sarrafian SK (1993) Anatomy of the Foot and Ankle. Philadelphia, JB Lippincott

Stephenson JR (1987) Treatment of displaced intra-articular fractures of the calcaneus using medial and lateral approaches, internal fixation, and early motion. J Bone Joint Surg 69A: 115–130

Tornetta P, 3rd (1998) The Essex-Lopresti reduction for calcaneal fractures revisited. J Orthop Trauma 12: 469–473

Wülker N, Zwipp H (1986) Fracture anatomy of the calcaneus with axial loading. Foot Ankle Surg 2: 155–162

Zwipp H, Tscherne H, Thermann H, Weber T (1993) Osteosynthesis of displaced intraarticular fractures of the calcaneus. Results in 123 cases. Clin Orthop 290: 76–86

Zwipp H (1994) Chirurgie des Fußes. Vienna, Springer Verlag

Zwipp H, Rammelt S, Barthel S (2004) Calcaneus fractures – open reduction and internal fixation (ORIF). Injury 35 (Suppl 2): 46–54

30

Talus fractures: open reduction and internal fixation

Suguru Inokuchi

Introduction

Talus fractures are not only rare but are also difficult to treat. The majority of fractures occur at the neck of the talus. Fractures of the body and of the head are less common. Because 60% of the surface of the talus is covered by articular cartilage and no tendons or muscles attach to it, there are only a few sites where feeding arteries can enter. The feeding artery along the interosseous talocalcaneal ligament is damaged in fracture–dislocations of the neck of the talus, and aseptic necrosis of the body tends to occur. If aseptic necrosis develops, the trochlear portion of the talus collapses under the weight of the body and degenerative arthrosis develops at the ankle joint and the subtalar joint, with pain and limitation of range of motion as sequelae. Since articular surface incongruity and contracture also cause degenerative arthrosis, anatomical reduction and rigid internal fixation, which allow early postoperative motion, are essential. Even though the anterior and middle subtalar joints and the posterior subtalar joint curve in opposite directions and are separated by the tarsal canal, they have a common axis of rotation, and from a functional standpoint are regarded as a single joint. Thus, although fractures of the neck of the talus pass through the talar canal and are extra-articular, they require the same anatomical reduction as intra-articular fractures.

Even though the diagnosis is usually evident on plain radiographs, computed tomography in the axial and frontal planes is often helpful for the classification of the fracture and the choice of treatment.

Classification

Fracture–dislocations of the neck of the talus are most common and have been classified according to the displacement of the fracture fragments [Hawkins 1970]. This classification is of particular value with regard to the incidence of aseptic necrosis. Type 1 injuries are non-displaced fractures of the talar neck, which may be impacted and quite stable. In type 2 injuries, the posterior subtalar joint is subluxed or dislocated. The talocalcaneal ligaments are disrupted, which impedes anatomic reduction of the fracture. In type 3 injuries, there is additional dislocation of the ankle joint. A large percentage of type 3 fractures are open injuries. In type 4 injuries, the talonavicular joint is also dislocated [Canale and Kelly 1978].

Talar body fractures are less common. They may be classified as osteochondral lesions, shear fractures of the body of the talus, posterior process fractures, lateral tubercle fractures and crush injuries of the talar body [Sneppen et al. 1977]. Fractures of the head of the talus are also uncommon. They occur as impacted compression fractures or as sagittal or oblique fractures, which usually involve the talonavicular joint.

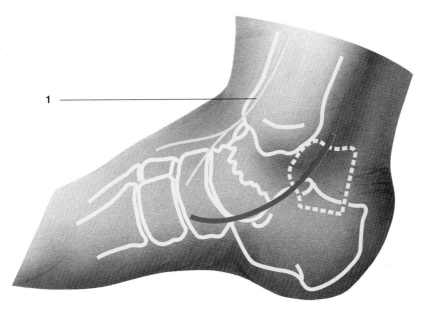

Figure 1

The skin incision reaches from the tuberosity of the navicular bone to behind the medial malleolus

1 Saphenous nerve

Treatment

Indications for surgery

Type 1 fractures of the talar neck are generally treated conservatively [Dunn et al. 1966]. Type 2 and other fracture–dislocations of the talar neck are indications for surgery [Szyszkowitz et al. 1985, DeLee 1992]. Immediate reduction may be required if there is significant displacement, compromising the surrounding soft tissues and neurovascular structures. Subtalar subluxation sometimes reduces naturally, but it may be associated with comminuted bone fragments in the talar canal and require surgery.

Osteochondral lesions of the talar body are usually re-attached by arthroscopy [Beck 1991]. The remaining talar body fractures are treated according to the same principles as talar neck fractures. Owing to the involvement of the ankle and the subtalar joint, open reduction and internal fixation should be used whenever there is any displacement of the fracture fragments. Talar head fractures should also be anatomically reduced and stabilized, if there is any significant displacement and if the talonavicular joint is involved. Alternatively, small fracture fragments may be excised.

Surgical technique

The patient is placed in the supine position and a pneumatic thigh tourniquet is applied. The hip joint is flexed and externally rotated, the knee slightly flexed, and the medial malleolus of the ankle joint is turned so that it faces up. Surgery is performed under general or spinal anesthesia.

Surgical approach

The skin is incised from the tuberosity of the navicular bone over the tip of the medial malleolus to the posterior margin of the tibia (Figure 1). If osteotomy of the medial malleolus is not necessary (see below), the skin incision is stopped at the tip of the medial malleolus. Caution is required to avoid injuring the saphenous nerve, the great saphenous vein and the tibialis posterior tendon when making the incision. If the descending branch of the greater saphenous vein impedes exposure of the subcutaneous tissue, it is ligated and sectioned.

In type 3 or 4 fracture–dislocations of the neck and fracture–dislocations of the body it may be necessary to perform an osteotomy of the medial malleolus, to ensure an adequate exposure of the surgical field. The flexor tendon retinaculum is opened and the tibialis posterior muscle is displaced, the anterior margin and the posterior margin of the base of the medial malleolus are exposed through small capsular incisions (Figure 2), and the angle between the roof of the ankle joint and the articular surface of the medial malleolus is palpated with a narrow periosteal elevator. A 3.2-mm hole is drilled in the tip of the medial malleolus parallel to its articular surface, in order to re-attach the medial malleolus after the procedure. The position of the osteotomy is marked on the surface of the medial malleolus. The osteotomy of the medial malleolus is performed with the bone saw pointing slightly distally towards the angle of the medial side of the ankle articular surface, at a right angle to the drill hole. The medial malleolus is then reflected distally with

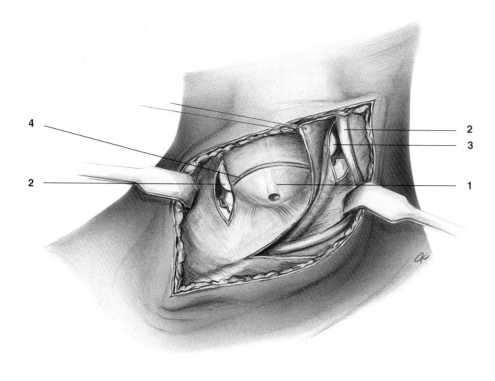

Figure 2

If an osteotomy of the medial malleolus is needed for exposure, the skin incisions are mobilized, small incisions are made in the joint capsule and the anterior and posterior margins are dissected through small incisions. A drill hole is made in the tip of the medial malleolus parallel to its articular surface. The flexor tendon retinaculum is opened, and the tibialis posterior tendon is retracted posteriorly

1 Drill hole in medial malleolus
2 Anterior and posterior margins of tibia
3 Posterior tibial tendon
4 Osteotomy

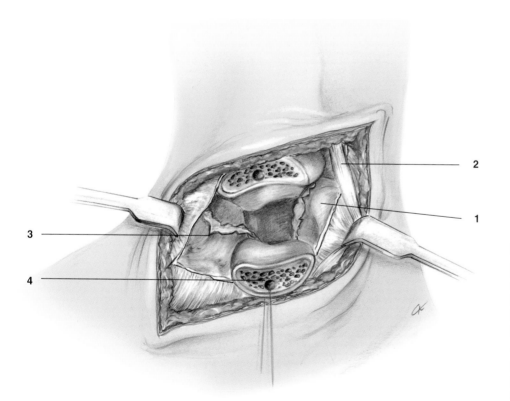

Figure 3

Following osteotomy of the medial malleolus, the talus fracture and the ankle joint space are exposed

1 Talar body fragment
2 Posterior tibial tendon
3 Talar neck fragment
4 Medial malleolus

the deltoid ligament serving as the fulcrum, and a nylon suture is passed through the bone hole as a landmark. The fracture surface in the talus, the articular surface of the tibia and of the lateral malleolus, and the posteriorly displaced body of the talus can be visualized (Figure 3).

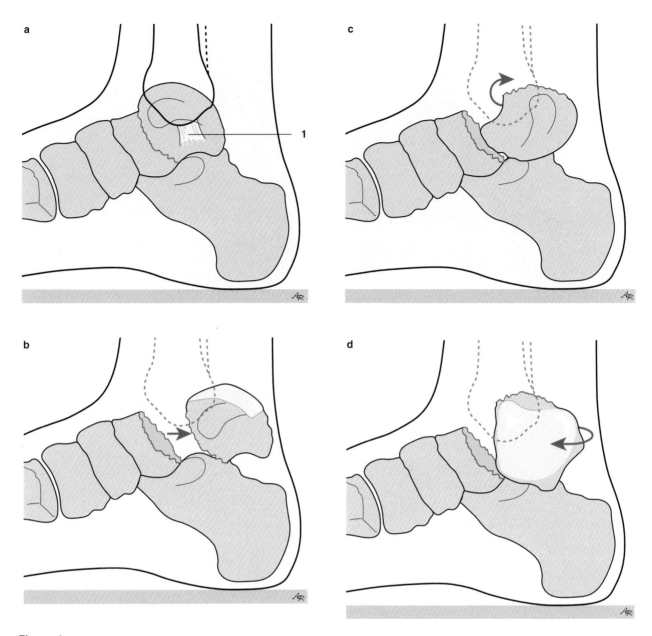

Figure 4

Dislocation of the body fragment. a. original position; b. posterior displacement; c. posterior rotation; d. external rotation. Reduction is performed in the reverse order (d to a)

1 Deltoid ligament

Reduction

With the deltoid ligament as the fulcrum, the fragment of the talar body is displaced from the ankle joint space posteriorly and rotated posteriorly and externally. The fracture surface is turned so that it faces superiorly and the trochlear surface so that it faces medially. The body fragment is often positioned posterior to the medial malleolus and superomedial to the tuberosity of the calcaneus (Figure 4).

Reduction is performed in the reverse order, by internal and anterior rotation with the deltoid

ligament as the fulcrum. The ankle is plantarflexed to relax the flexor tendons. With the trochlea facing up, the area between the Achilles tendon and the tibia is pushed in. The ankle joint is dorsiflexed while pulling the calcaneus inferiorly and pushing the fragment of the body anteriorly in the direction of the ankle joint space. If it is difficult to grasp the calcaneus during reduction, traction can be exerted on the tuber calcanei with a Kirschner wire. During this maneuver, care is taken not to injure the remaining deltoid ligament and the blood vessels feeding the body of the talus, which course along it [Pennal

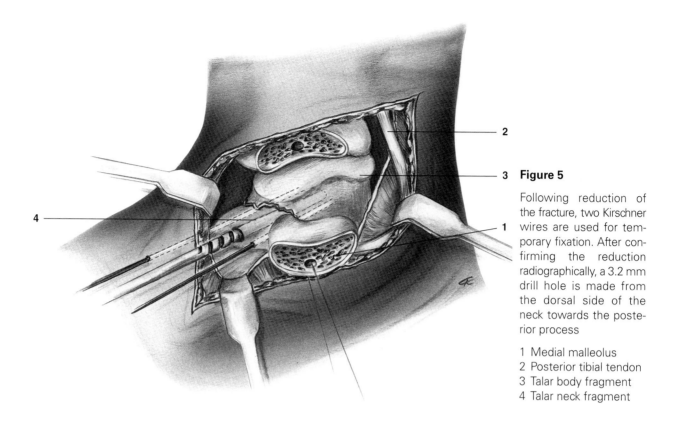

Figure 5

Following reduction of the fracture, two Kirschner wires are used for temporary fixation. After confirming the reduction radiographically, a 3.2 mm drill hole is made from the dorsal side of the neck towards the posterior process

1 Medial malleolus
2 Posterior tibial tendon
3 Talar body fragment
4 Talar neck fragment

1963]. The deltoid ligament, which is attached to the fragment of the body, must never be severed even if reduction is difficult.

This maneuver is followed by thorough examination of the fracture and irrigation, and by removal of clotted blood and small bone fragments that might impede reduction. The Achilles tendon, the tibialis posterior tendon, the flexor digitorum longus tendon and the flexor hallucis longus tendon may block the bone fragments in the body of the talus and interfere with reduction. In this case, the tibialis posterior tendon is detached from its insertion at the navicular bone with a bone fragment attached, and the other flexor tendons are sectioned in a Z-shaped fashion.

When the body of the talus has been repositioned in the ankle joint, the fracture surfaces are reduced anatomically. Because there are few anatomic landmarks to verify the reduction of neck fractures, it is easy to leave the talus in rotation deformity. However, when the fracture line passes through the anteromedial aspect of the trochlea, this serves as a good indicator for reduction. If the talus fracture is comminuted and complete reduction is uncertain, congruence can be achieved at the ankle joint and the posterior subtalar joint surfaces by pronation and supination of the subtalar joint while simultaneously pressing on the body of the talus and the calcaneus through the sole of the foot. In type 4 lesions, only the alignment of fracture surfaces can

be used as an indicator for reduction, because the head of the talus is dislocated as well.

Internal fixation

Following reduction, the fracture should be temporarily stabilized with two 1.5-mm Kirschner wires (Figure 5). One wire is inserted so that it passes from the anterior portion of the navicular bone through the talonavicular joint toward the posterior margin of the lateral malleolus. The other wire is inserted at the superomedial aspect of the talonavicular joint and directed toward a slightly more medial position in the posterior process of the talus. At times, an additional posterolateral incision must be made (Figure 6) and a Kirschner wire inserted into the talus from posterolateral to anteromedial. The ankle joint and the subtalar joint are moved passively at this point to reconfirm reduction. Once reduction appears to be adequate, this is confirmed by intraoperative radiographs in two planes. If a cannulated malleolar screw is used, radiography is performed following insertion of the guide wires. Stainless steel malleolar screws or cannulated titanium malleolar screws are used for internal fixation (Figure 7). The site of insertion in talar neck fractures is at the posterolateral border of the talonavicular joint. After perforating the insertion area with a small round chisel, a 3.2-mm drill hole is

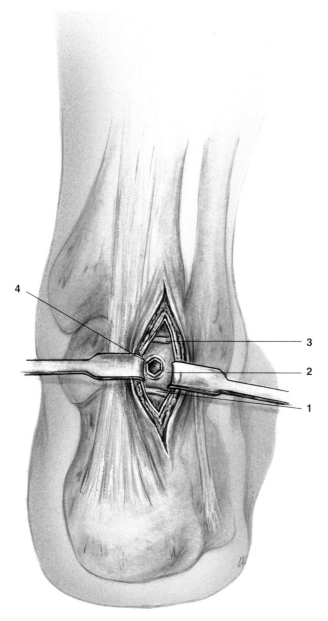

Figure 6

An additional posterolateral approach may be necessary for insertion of a screw from posterolateral to anteromedial

1 Subtalar joint
2 Talus
3 Ankle joint
4 Fixation screw

advanced toward the posterior process of the talus. The length of the drill hole is determined with a depth gauge, and compression fixation is achieved with a malleolar screw that is 5 mm shorter than the measured length. If adequate compression fixation is obtained, both Kirschner wires are removed. If the fracture surface is comminuted and compression is not optimal, a second screw is inserted

from anteromedial or from posterolateral, or the Kirschner wire inserted into the neck of the talus may be left in place to prevent rotation. In talar neck fractures, the break occurs in a perpendicular plane to the long axis of the neck of the talus. In talar body fractures the break occurs in a perpendicular plane to the long axis of the trochlea. In talar body fractures, the screw is inserted more lateral to medial, i.e. along the long axis of the trochlea, compared with screw placement in neck fractures. More rigid fixation can be achieved by making a small incision on the lateral aspect of the ankle joint anterior to the lateral malleolus and inserting another Kirschner wire or malleolar screw into the anterolateral margin of the trochlea in the direction of the posterior process. Alternatively, the posterior process of the talus can be exposed from a posterior lateral malleolar incision and a malleolar screw be inserted into the posterolateral margin of the trochlea toward the neck of the talus (see Figure 6).

Body fracture

Body fractures occur at a more posterior site than neck fractures. The anteromedial approach and osteotomy of the medial malleolus are required to reveal the fracture site and to reduce the dislocated fracture. However, it is difficult to fix the body fracture rigidly using only the screw inserted from the anteromedial aspect. The body fracture is perpendicular to the long axis of the foot, whereas the neck fracture is perpendicular to the long axis of the talus (Figure 8b). The screw inserted from the anteromedial side of the neck cannot pass the fracture plane vertically and should be inserted from the anterolateral aspect of the neck to achieve this (Figure 8).

Closure

Thorough irrigation is performed so that no bone fragments are left within the joint space. The reflected medial malleolus is returned to its anatomical position and the previously drilled hole is used to fix it with a malleolar screw (Figure 9). If sufficient pressure cannot be achieved, an additional Kirschner wire is inserted parallel to the screw, to prevent rotation. If the tibialis posterior tendon has been detached from the navicular, it is re-attached through a drill hole. If tendons were sectioned, they are repaired. After returning the flexor tendons to their anatomical position, the flexor tendon retinaculum is closed loosely.

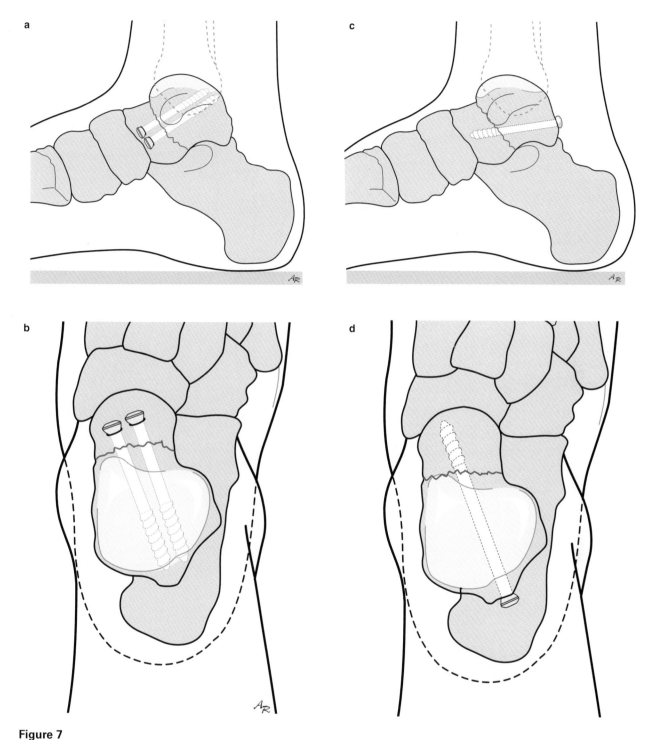

Figure 7

Compression fixation is generally achieved with cannulated titanium malleolar screws. a. screw placement from antero-medial to posterolateral, medial aspect; b. superior aspect; c. screw placement from posterolateral to anteromedial, medial aspect; d. superior aspect

The tourniquet is released. After adequate hemostasis, the subcutaneous tissue and the skin are sutured. A padded plaster splint is applied and wrapped with an elastic bandage, providing compression.

Postoperative care

If postoperative magnetic resonance imaging (MRI) is available, cannulated titanium malleolar screws alone should be used for internal fixation. An MRI

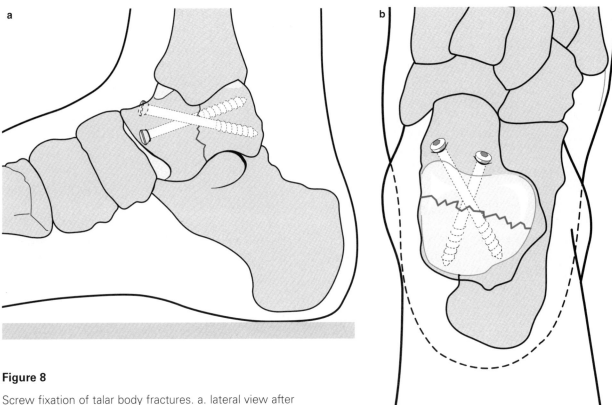

Figure 8

Screw fixation of talar body fractures. a. lateral view after
fixation; b. superior view after fixation

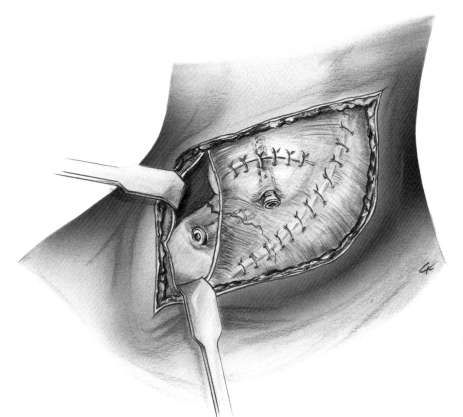

Figure 9

The medial malleolus is returned
to its anatomical position, and
stabilized with a cannulated titanium malleolar screw. The flexor
tendon sheath is closed

examination is performed in the early postoperative period, and the images are checked for low-signal areas that suggest aseptic necrosis of the talus. If none can be found, aseptic necrosis is unlikely. If a low-signal area is present, the patient is followed by both conventional radiography and MRI for early detection of aseptic necrosis.

If rigid internal fixation was achieved, active ankle joint motion is started 1 week after surgery. If fixation is inadequate, motion is started 3 weeks postoperatively. Frontal radiographs of the ankle joint are taken 3–6 weeks after surgery. The absence of subchondral bone atrophy of the trochlear articular surface of the talus in spite of subchondral bone atrophy at the distal end of the tibia suggests aseptic necrosis [Hawkins 1970]. If subchondral bone atrophy at the trochlea is present, and if bone union is confirmed on radiographs 9–12 weeks after the operation, partial weightbearing is started, and full weightbearing is permitted 3 weeks later. Active motion without weightbearing is continued during this period.

If subchondral bone atrophy has not occurred even 12 weeks postoperatively, and if sclerosis in the trochlear area of the talus is observed, a diagnosis of aseptic necrosis of the body of the talus is made. A weight-relieving appliance is prepared, and non-weightbearing motion of the ankle joint is continued while awaiting resumption of perfusion to the talus. This is confirmed by the bone atrophy shadow expanding from the attachment site of the deltoid ligament, the lateral process, the posterior tubercle or the fracture site. The strength of the body of the talus is lowest at the time when circulation resumes, and it tends to collapse. Therefore, careful monitoring is required during this period. Blood flow may resume up to 3 years after the injury.

Complications

Aseptic necrosis of the talus is the most common complication following talus fractures [Gillquist et al. 1974]. Its frequency ranges from 10% in type 1 talar neck fractures to 70% in severely displaced fractures of the neck or the body. The incidence is related to the severity of fracture displacement, to the amount of soft-tissue dissection during surgery and to the time between injury and reduction. Aseptic necrosis may result in segmental or total collapse of the talar dome, or it may revascularize over a period as long as 2–3 years. If the body of the talus collapses, it is resected and a fusion of the tibia to the distal portion of the talar neck [Blair 1943] or arthrodesis between the tibia and calcaneus is performed. Malunion may occur if inadequate reduction of the fracture is accepted. Degenerative arthrosis of the ankle joint or the subtalar joint may ensue if anatomic reduction of the joint surfaces was not achieved. Non-union is an uncommon complication, but bone healing may be delayed for 6–12 months after the injury.

References

Beck E (1991) Fractures of the talus. Orthopäde 20: 33–42

Blair HC (1943) Comminuted fractures and fracture dislocations of the body of the astralgus. Am J Surg 59: 37–43

Canale ST, Kelly FB (1978) Fractures of the neck of the talus. J Bone Joint Surg 60A: 143–156

DeLee JC (1992) Fractures and dislocations of the foot. In: Mann RA, Coughlin MJ (eds) Surgery of the Foot and Ankle. St Louis, Mosby, pp 1539–1600

Dunn AR, Jacobs B, Campbell RD (1966) Fractures of the talus. J Trauma 6: 443–468

Gillquist J, Oretorp N, Stenstrom A et al. (1974) Late results after vertical fracture of the talus. Injury 6: 173–179

Hawkins LG (1970) Fractures of the neck of the talus. J Bone Joint Surg 52A: 991–1002

Pennal GF (1963) Fractures of the talus. Clin Orthop 30: 53–63

Sneppen O, Christensen SB, Krogsoe O et al. (1977) Fracture of the body of the talus. Acta Orthop Scand 48: 317–324

Szyszkowitz R, Reschauer R, Seggl W (1985) Eighty-five talus fractures treated by ORIF with five to eight years of follow-up study of 69 patients. Clin Orthop 199: 97–107

31

Triple arthrodesis Nikolaus Wülker

Introduction

Triple arthrodesis is an arthrodesis of the subtalar joint, the talonavicular joint and the calcaneocuboid joint. This technique was commonly used in the first half of the 20th century to treat foot deformity caused by poliomyelitis. Since then, poliomyelitis has largely receded and congenital hindfoot deformity, post-traumatic conditions, degenerative and inflammatory diseases of the hindfoot joints have become the most common indications for triple arthrodesis. In addition, operative planning and technique have become more refined and only joints directly involved in the disease process are now usually fused. This has led to the common use of isolated arthrodesis of the subtalar joint and of the talonavicular joint, and less frequently of the calcaneocuboid joint. Arthrodeses of two hindfoot joints, such as the 'double arthrodesis' of the talonavicular joint and the calcaneocuboid joint, or a combined arthrodesis of the subtalar joint and the calcaneocuboid joint, are also commonly used.

The main indication for triple arthrodesis is a rigid foot deformity. In a flexible deformity, preference is generally given to soft-tissue procedures and tendon transfers (see Chapter 26). Triple arthrodesis is performed following the completion of growth of the foot and should not be used in children or adolescents.

The position and the mobility of the heel largely determine whether a triple arthrodesis must be used to treat complex foot deformity, or if individual hindfoot joints can be preserved. In congenital hindfoot deformity, e.g. following clubfoot deformity during infancy, the calcaneus is most commonly in inversion, with restricted motion of the subtalar joint. This varus malalignment of the hindfoot generally requires a triple arthrodesis. Equinus deformity of the foot with correct varus–valgus alignment of the heel and sufficient subtalar motion is usually due to plantar-flexion deformity of the calcaneus and/or cavus deformity of the midfoot, as is commonly seen in paralytic conditions and in neuromuscular disease. Plantarflexion deformity of the calcaneus can often be corrected sufficiently by lengthening the Achilles tendon and incising the capsules of the ankle and of the subtalar joint, in adults as well as in children. Cavus foot deformity generally requires a tarsometatarsal osteotomy and incision of the plantar fascia (see Chapter 24). However, triple arthrodesis is usually not necessary. Tarsometatarsal osteotomy with resection of a dorsal wedge cannot be used to correct equinus deformity of the calcaneus, as this will result in a rocker-bottom foot.

Post-traumatic hindfoot deformity, such as following calcaneus fractures, most often involves eversion and broadening of the heel and restriction of subtalar motion. This can usually be treated with an isolated subtalar arthrodesis. If the anterior process of the calcaneus is involved, additional fusion of the calcaneocuboid joint may be required. Triple fusion is rarely necessary. More complex hindfoot trauma may result in a stiff and deformed hindfoot with degenerative arthrosis of the involved joints and necessitate triple arthrodesis.

Rheumatoid arthritis, which often involves a combination of hindfoot joints, is a common indication for triple arthrodesis. The hindfoot is generally everted, but this may be due to deformity at the ankle joint rather than the subtalar joint. Owing to the progression of the disease, triple arthrodesis is often preferable to isolated fusion of individual hindfoot joints, even if the hindfoot is in normal alignment.

Triple arthrodesis is also used in older patients with symptomatic flatfoot deformity. The talus is generally in increased plantarflexion and the talar head may become prominent at the plantar–medial aspect of the foot. The calcaneus is generally everted. Degenerative arthrosis commonly develops at the hindfoot joints. Flatfoot deformity in the elderly may also be due to posterior tibial tendon insufficiency. Reconstruction of the tendon is an alternative to triple arthrodesis, but the results are less predictable.

Clinical and radiographic appearance

Comprehensive examination of the foot and ankle is necessary prior to triple arthrodesis. During gait, it must be noted whether the heel touches the ground and to what degree normal toe-off is possible. The position of the heel is examined from behind, the patient having the heel down as far as possible and standing tiptoed. Painful callosities at the sole of the foot must be noted. In residual equinovarus deformity they are particularly common at the lateral border of the foot and under the fifth metatarsal head.

Examination of joint motion and position is of particular significance at the subtalar joint. This is evaluated with the ankle in one hand of the examine, while the heel is everted and inverted with the other hand. Tightness of the Achilles tendon is assessed with forced dorsiflexion of the foot. The condition of the soft tissues may be compromised in post-traumatic deformity or following previous surgery. The presence of both pedal pulses, capillary filling and any evidence of peripheral vascular insufficiency must be noted and documented.

Plain radiographs of the entire foot and ankle in two planes are obtained. The lateral radiograph should be in maximum forced dorsiflexion of the foot, to evaluate the tightness of the Achilles tendon and the flexibility of the hindfoot deformity. An oblique view of the hindfoot, directed from dorsolateral to plantar–medial, is often helpful for better visualization of the talonavicular and the calcaneocuboid joints, which are otherwise obscured by the adjacent bones. An axial view of the heel may yield information concerning varus/valgus alignment of the calcaneus, if this cannot sufficiently be determined clinically. If further evaluation is needed, a computed tomography (CT) scan is most helpful. This should be performed in an axial and coronal plane. Other tomographic techniques, such as magnetic resonance imaging (MRI), are less helpful.

Indications for surgery

Orthotic appliances and orthopedic shoes may relieve symptoms, particularly in a mild deformity. Non-operative treatment, including anti-inflammatory medication and physiotherapy applications, should be attempted especially in older patients, and triple arthrodesis should be performed only if symptoms persist and if foot function is markedly impaired. In young patients following completion of growth, surgery may be indicated more readily, i.e. if the heel does not touch the ground when standing or walking, even when symptoms are relatively mild. Often, simultaneous Achilles tendon lengthening is indicated if there is a marked plantarflexion deformity of the calcaneus on lateral radiographs with the foot in maximum dorsiflexion.

Treatment

If marked equinus deformity of the calcaneus is present, Achilles tendon lengthening should be performed prior to triple arthrodesis. This must also include excision of the dorsal capsules of the ankle and of the subtalar joint. The foot can be used as a lever arm to bring the ankle joint forcefully into dorsiflexion.

Residual equinus deformity of the calcaneus is corrected with the triple arthrodesis by excising bone from the inferior aspect of the distal talus and/or from the superior aspect of the distal calcaneus. This approach has been widely used in the past without Achilles tendon lengthening [Lambrinudi 1927]. However, bone resection can be markedly reduced if the Achilles tendon is lengthened.

Arthrodesis of the subtalar joint is performed first. The main concern is to correct varus or valgus malalignment of the calcaneus. The former requires excision of a laterally based bone wedge; the latter often mandates insertion of an iliac crest bone graft. The alignment of the calcaneus following excision of the subtalar joint is assessed intraoperatively by palpation and by inspection. Intraoperative radiographs at this stage are not usually necessary. Internal fixation is not used until the position of all three joints has been corrected.

The calcaneocuboid joint is then resected through the same skin incision, followed by resection of the talonavicular joint through a separate dorsomedial skin incision. Bone is removed from the anterior process of the calcaneus and from the head of the talus, until optimal approximation of the bone resection surfaces on the medial and lateral side is attained.

Owing to the three-dimensional architecture of the hindfoot, bone contact at the arthrodeses may be less optimal than in isolated arthrodesis of individual hindfoot joints. Roughening of the bone resection surfaces with an osteotome or, less commonly, insertion of a bone graft can usually sufficiently improve bone contact. If at this time there is still a residual equinus deformity of the calcaneus, this should not be corrected at the talonavicular and calcaneocuboid joints, as it may result in a postoperative rocker-bottom deformity. Instead, bone should be removed distally from the undersurface of the talus and from the upper surface of the calcaneus. Alternatively, a bone graft can be used in the posterior part of the posterior facet to correct residual equinus of the calcaneus.

Stable internal fixation should be used to prevent pseudarthrosis [Wülker and Flamme 1996], even though additional postoperative immobilization in a plaster cast will be necessary in almost all cases.

Surgical technique

The patient is placed supine with the operated side elevated on a pillow, to facilitate access to the dorsolateral aspect of the foot. General anesthesia or spinal anesthesia should be used so that a bone graft can be obtained from the iliac crest on the operated side, should this become necessary. A thigh tourniquet is applied and the leg is exsanguinated. Prophylactic antibiotics are administered prior to inflation of the tourniquet. The ipsilateral iliac crest is draped free.

Achilles tendon lengthening and capsulotomy

A longitudinal 10–13-cm dorsomedial skin incision is made along the medial side of the Achilles tendon (Figure 1a). The subcutaneous tissues are divided and hemostasis is performed. The paratendineum is divided longitudinally. Following complete dissection of the tendon from its insertion to the musculotendinous junction, two blunt elevators are placed underneath the tendon and a Z-plasty is performed (Figure 1b). It is best to use a longitudinal incision in the frontal plane, exiting posteriorly at the proximal end of the Z and anteriorly at the distal end. The tendon flaps are covered with moist sponges and held away from the wound. Retractors are placed into the fatty tissue underneath the tendon. The incision is carried to the posterior aspect of the ankle joint and of the subtalar joint. Some fat may

have to be resected to obtain optimal exposure. The joint capsules are incised horizontally with a scalpel and removed with a rongeur, including the medial and lateral corners. When releasing the subtalar joint, the flexor hallucis longus tendon must be identified and protected. It is important to ascertain by digital palpation that all constricting structures have been released. One can usually feel and hear constrictures break when the foot is forcefully brought into maximum dorsiflexion. Closure of the Achilles tendon Z-plasty is not performed until after the triple arthrodesis.

Resection of the subtalar joint

A curved incision from slightly posterior and proximal to the tip of the lateral malleolus to the base of the fifth metatarsal bone is used (Figure 2a). The sural nerve passes plantarwards of the incision. The subcutaneous tissues are divided and hemostasis is performed. The peroneal tendon sheath is divided and the tendons are retracted posteriorly. The subtalar joint is opened (Figure 3) and the joint capsule and the surrounding soft tissues are removed with a rongeur, including the contents of the tarsal canal anteriorly. A 1-cm osteotome is inserted into the subtalar joint to lever open the joint surfaces. In severe joint contracture, the osteotome may have to be hammered medially several times until a significant gap between the joint surfaces can be obtained. A laminar spreader is inserted into the joint. The remaining joint cartilage and the subchondral bone are removed with an osteotome, curettes and a rongeur, so that the medial border of the joint surface becomes visible.

In significant inversion deformity of the calcaneus, bone is removed laterally from the talus and the calcaneus, until the position of the calcaneus is in approximately 7° of valgus (Figure 4). One must be sure that the calcaneus does not impinge against the tip of the lateral malleolus. In eversion deformity of the calcaneus, the joint is opened with a laminar spreader until a correct position of the calcaneus is attained. In slight eversion deformity, it may suffice to elevate the cancellous bone of the talus and of the calcaneus with an osteotome to fill the resulting gap. In more significant deformity, an iliac bone graft of corresponding size must be obtained (Figure 4). This should be a wedge-shaped tricortical graft, which is inserted with the three cortical layers oriented in a vertical direction and tapped into place. The bone graft should be obtained only after the resection of all three joints is completed and an optimum correction of foot alignment is

a

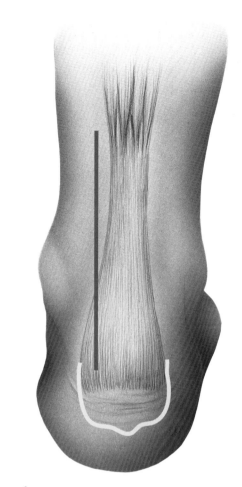

b

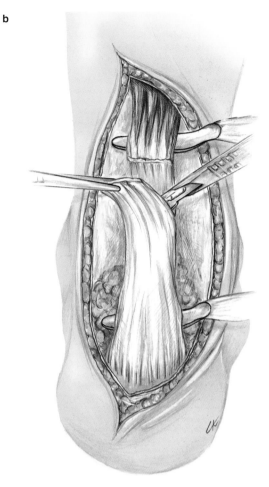

Figure 1

Achilles tendon lengthening. a. a longitudinal incision is made medial to the Achilles tendon; b. following division of the paratendineum, a Z-plasty is performed

attained. One must be sure that the skin can be closed without undue tension following the correction of heel alignment. It may be preferable to leave a valgus deformity partially uncorrected to avoid postoperative skin necrosis.

If the foot is still in significant equinus deformity following Achilles tendon lengthening and capsulotomy, bone is removed from the anterior process of the calcaneus superiorly and from the head and the neck of the talus inferiorly (Figure 5). In a very rigid deformity, complete correction of calcaneal alignment may be possible only following resection of the talonavicular and the calcaneocuboid joint.

Internal fixation at the subtalar joint is delayed until after all three joints have been prepared.

Resection of the calcaneocuboid joint

The anterior process of the calcaneus, the calcaneocuboid joint and the proximal part of the cuboid are exposed by extending the previous lateral incision. The extensor digitorum brevis muscle is dissected from the superior aspect of the calcaneus and from the joint with an elevator and retracted distally. The insertion of the peroneus brevis tendon at the fifth metatarsal base must be preserved. The joint capsule and the ligamentous structures between the cuboid and the calcaneus are incised vertically and removed with a rongeur, exposing the superior and lateral aspect of the joint. A narrow osteotome is inserted into the joint and used to spread the joint surfaces apart as far as possible. A lamina spreader is then inserted. The joint surfaces and the subchondral bone are removed, taking as little bone as possible. In complex hindfoot deformity, sufficient bone contact with the forefoot in anatomical alignment can usually be obtained only following resection of the talonavicular joint. Internal fixation is not used until all three joints have been prepared.

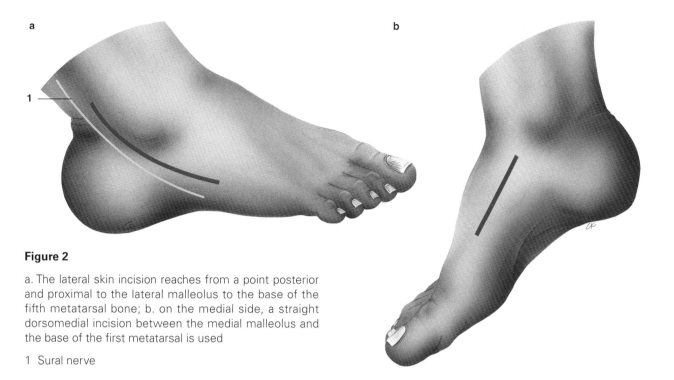

Figure 2

a. The lateral skin incision reaches from a point posterior and proximal to the lateral malleolus to the base of the fifth metatarsal bone; b. on the medial side, a straight dorsomedial incision between the medial malleolus and the base of the first metatarsal is used

1   Sural nerve

Resection of the talonavicular joint

A skin incision is made from just anterior to the medial malleolus straight to the base of the first metatarsal bone (Figure 2b). The subcutaneous tissues are divided and the dissection is carried to the talonavicular joint. The capsule is incised with a scalpel and removed with a rongeur. The joint space is opened with an osteotome until a lamina spreader can be inserted. The joint surfaces and the subchondral bone are removed with an osteotome and with a rongeur. The entire joint surface must be removed, including its lateral portion. Following adequate resection, one should be able to see the resected calcaneocuboid joint laterally.

Following resection of the talonavicular joint, an attempt is made to bring the bone surfaces of all joints into contact and to position the calcaneus in slight eversion and the forefoot in neutral. If the foot does not reach a plantigrade position, additional bone must be resected between the talus and the calcaneus. If the resection surfaces at the talonavicular and the calcaneocuboid joint cannot be sufficiently approximated, small amounts of bone are resected until sufficient contact is obtained. In a severe deformity it may be best to create one flat bone surface through the talonavicular and the calcaneocuboid joint with a long sawblade or an osteotome.

Various grafting techniques have been designed to improve bone contact at the arthrodesis site, such as grafts inlaid into the joint or slotted across the joint, and rotating dowel grafts [Cracchiolo 1988]. They are not usually employed by the author. Extra-articular arthrodesis of the subtalar joint [Grice 1952] should not be used as part of the triple arthrodesis [Ross and Lyne 1980].

Internal fixation

The subtalar joint is best stabilized with one 6.5-mm partially threaded cancellous bone screw, which is inserted from the dorsal aspect of the talar neck into the tuber of the calcaneus (Figure 6). This is generally done through the incision used for arthrodesis of the talonavicular joint. The orientation of the screw should be approximately perpendicular to the subtalar joint. A washer may have to be used in soft bone. The threads of the screw must be completely on the calcaneal side so that compression of the arthrodesis is attained.

At the calcaneocuboid joint, the arthrodesis is oriented almost perpendicular to the lateral aspect of the calcaneus and the cuboid. Therefore, screw fixation is usually not feasible and large bone staples should be used (Figure 6). There is usually enough room for two staples, one inserted from the lateral aspect and one from dorsolateral.

The talonavicular joint lends itself to stabilization with cancellous bone screws, owing to its curved configuration. In an isolated arthrodesis of the talonavicular joint, one or two 6.5-mm or 4.0-mm

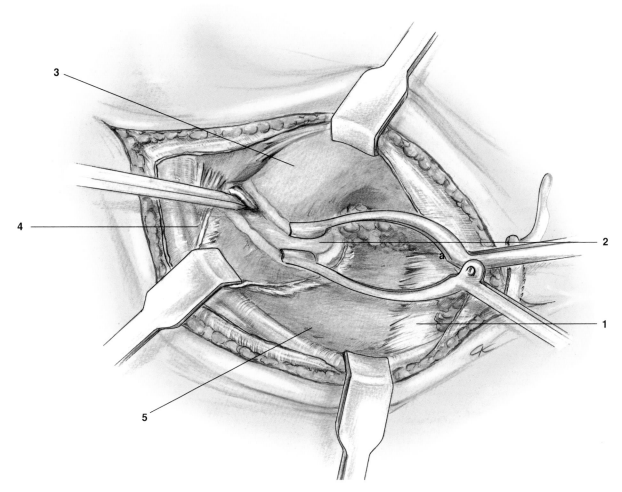

Figure 3

Following retraction of the peroneal tendons and exposure of the subtalar joint, the joint surfaces are removed with an osteotome

1 Calcaneocuboid joint capsule
2 Subtalar joint
3 Talus
4 Peroneal tendons
5 Calcaneus

partially threaded cancellous screws are inserted from dorsomedial to plantar lateral into the talar neck. In a triple arthrodesis the screws can also be advanced into the calcaneus, which may facilitate screw placement. Washers should be used in soft bone. In congenital deformity the navicular may be too small and the bone may be too soft for screw placement. Rather than placing the screws in a position where the screw heads may disturb motion at the naviculocuneiform joint, large bone staples should be used (Figure 6). Generally, their prongs are positioned parallel to the bone resection surface, and one staple is inserted from the dorsal aspect, one from the medial aspect and one from in-between.

Closure

The tourniquet is deflated and intraoperative radiographs are taken while a compression dressing is applied. Hemostasis is performed following wound irrigation. Remaining bone graft is placed around the arthrodesis sites (Figure 7), in particular in the region between the subtalar joint and the calcaneocuboid joint. If no iliac bone graft was obtained, small amounts of bone can usually be acquired by partially breaking the cortical layer anterior to the subtalar arthrodesis with an osteotome, and from the lateral aspect of the calcaneus.

Suction drains may be placed medially and laterally. On the lateral side, the peroneal tendons are repositioned behind the lateral malleolus and the retinaculum is closed. The skin is closed with interrupted sutures. In patients with preoperative valgus deformity, there may be unacceptable tension on the skin edges. This may be relieved by careful subcutaneous mobilization of the skin. However, it may be preferable to leave a valgus deformity

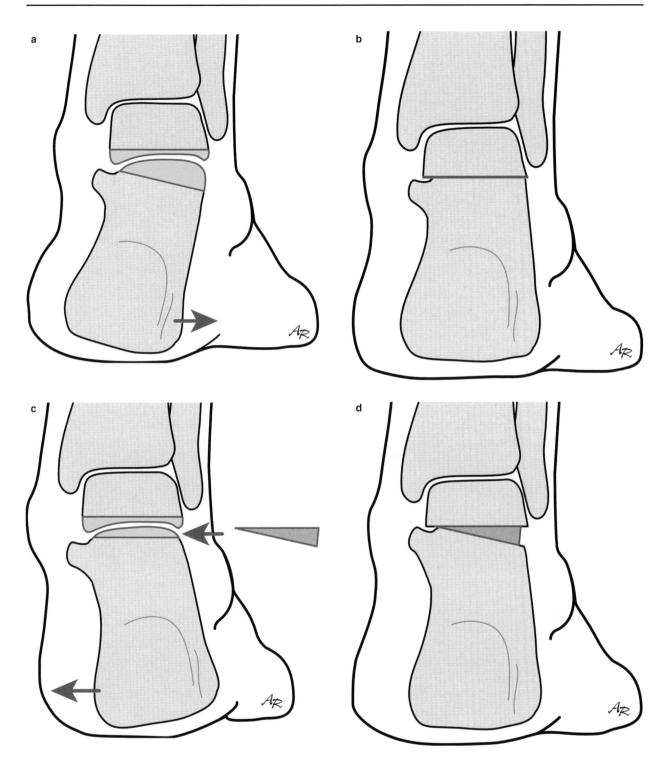

Figure 4

Correction of hindfoot deformity. a, b. inversion deformity is corrected by removal of a laterally based bone wedge from the subtalar joint; c, d. eversion deformity by insertion of an iliac crest bone graft

uncorrected and have less tension on the skin. Medially, the periosteum and the fascia are closed in one layer with interrupted sutures. The skin is also closed with interrupted sutures. A bulky soft compression dressing is applied and the lower leg is placed in a posterior plaster splint.

Postoperative treatment

Bed-rest with the operated leg elevated is usually necessary for a few days to prevent swelling. Subsequently, the patient is allowed to ambulate short distances on crutches. Once wound healing has

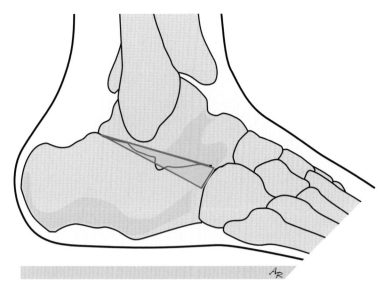

Figure 5

Equinus deformity that remains after Achilles tendon lengthening is corrected by removal of bone between the anterior portions of the talus and the calcaneus, rather than by a dorsal bone wedge resection more anteriorly, as the latter may result in a rocker-bottom foot

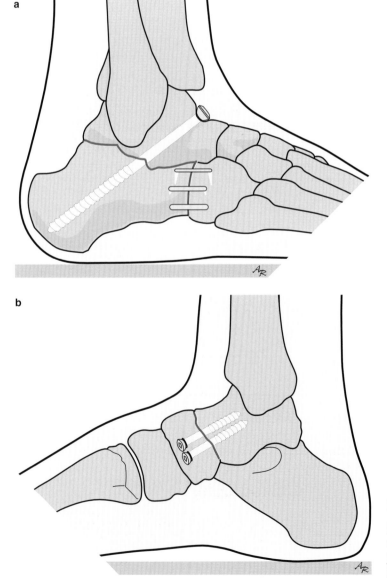

Figure 6

For fixation, a cancellous screw is used at the subtalar joint, two screws at the talonavicular joint and bone staples at the calcaneocuboid joint. a. lateral aspect; b. medial aspect

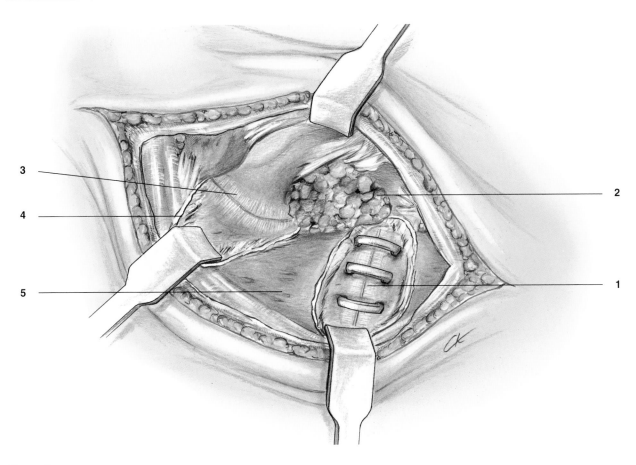

Figure 7

Bone graft is inserted between the talar neck and the anterior process of the calcaneus, and the cortical layer is broken with an osteotome to promote bone healing. Bone staples are used for fixation of the calcaneocuboid joint

1 Calcaneocuboid joint (fused)
2 Bone graft
3 Subtalar joint (fused)
4 Peroneal tendons
5 Calcaneus

occurred at approximately 2 weeks postoperatively, the sutures are removed and a lower leg non-weight-bearing plaster cast is applied. Wound healing may be delayed, particularly at the lateral wound. Six weeks postoperatively, the cast is removed and radiographs are taken. Bony union is often difficult to ascertain on radiographs at this time. If the alignment of the arthrodeses has been maintained, the foot is mobilized and the patient is returned to full weightbearing over the following 2 weeks. Orthotic appliances and orthopedic shoes are not usually necessary and should be prescribed only if normal and pain-free ambulation is not attained after 3 months.

Complications

Delayed wound healing on the lateral side is a common complication, especially if a valgus deformity of the heel was corrected. This may result in skin necrosis, followed by deep infection. Meticulous intraoperative handling of the soft tissues on the lateral side, in particular careful placement of sharp retractors, may prevent this complication. The skin must not be closed with undue tension.

Non-union is not an uncommon complication, in particular if no or insufficient internal fixation techniques are used. Screw fixation is the preferred method of stabilization. Degenerative arthritis at the ankle and at the tarsometatarsal joints occurs in a number of patients. This may be evident radiographically, but few patients have symptoms.

Bibliography

Angus PD, Cowell HR (1986) Triple arthrodeses. A critical long-term review. J Bone Joint Surg 68B: 260–265

Atar D, Grant AD, Lehman WB (1990) Triple arthrodesis. Foot Ankle 11: 45–46

Banks HH, Green WT (1958) The correction of equinus deformity in cerebral palsy. J Bone Joint Surg 40A: 1359–1379

Cracchiolo A (1988) Operative technique of the ankle and hindfoot. In: Helal B, Wilson D (eds) The Foot. Edinburgh, Churchill Livingstone, pp 1205–1244

Cracchiolo A, Pearson S, Kitaoka H, Grace D (1990) Hindfoot arthrodesis in adults utilizing a dowel graft technique. Clin Orthop 257: 193–203

Dekelver L, Fabry G, Mulier JC (1980) Triple arthrodesis and Lambrinudi arthrodesis: literature review and follow-up study. Arch Orthop Trauma Surg 96: 23–30

Evans D (1975) Calcaneo-valgus deformity. J Bone Joint Surg 57B: 270–278

Graves SC, Mann RA, Graves KO (1993) Triple arthrodeses in older adults. J Bone Joint Surg 75A: 355–362

Grice DS (1952) An extra-articular arthrodesis of the subastralgar joint for correction of paralytic flat feet in children. J Bone Joint Surg 34A: 927–940

Jahss MH (1980) Tarsometatarsal truncated-wedge arthrodesis for pes cavus and equinovarus deformity of the fore part of the foot. J Bone Joint Surg 62A: 713–722

Johnson KA (1990) Hindfoot arthrodeses. Instr Course Lect 39: 65–69

Klaue K, Hansen ST (1994) Principles of surgical reconstruction of the mid- and hindfoot. Eur J Foot Ankle Surg 1: 37–44

Lambrinudi C (1927) New operations on drop-foot. Br J Surg 15: 193–200

Mann RA (1992) Arthrodesis of the foot and ankle. In: Mann RA, Coughlin M (eds) Surgery of the Foot and Ankle. St Louis, Mosby, pp 673–713

McCluskey WP, Lovell WW, Cummings RJ (1989) The cavovarus foot deformity. Etiology and management. Clin Orthop 247: 27–37

Nieny K (1905) Zur Behandlung der Fußdeformitäten bei ausgeprägten Lähmungen. Arch Orthop Unfallchir 3: 60–64

Ross PM, Lyne ED (1980) The Grice procedure: indications and evaluation of long-term results. Clin Orthop 153: 194–200

Sammarco GJ (1988) Technique of triple arthrodesis in treatment of symptomatic pes planus. Orthopaedics 11: 1607–1610

Sangeorzan BJ, Smith D, Veith R, Hansen ST Jr (1993) Triple arthrodesis using internal fixation in treatment of adult foot disorders. Clin Orthop 294: 299–307

Scranton PE Jr (1987) Treatment of symptomatic talocalcaneal coalition. J Bone Joint Surg 69A: 533–539

Soren A, Waugh TR (1980) The historical evolution of arthrodesis of the foot. Int Orthop 4: 3–11

Tang SC, Leong JC, Hsu LC (1984) Lambrinudi triple arthrodesis for correction of severe rigid drop-foot. J Bone Joint Surg 66B: 66–70

Williams PF, Menelaus MB (1977) Triple arthrodesis by inlay grafting – a method suitable for the undeformed or valgus foot. J Bone Joint Surg 59B: 333–336

Wülker N, Flamme C (1996) Rückfußarthrodesen. Orthopäde 25: 177–186

32

Reconstruction of lateral ankle instability

Roderick Coull and Michael M. Stephens

Introduction

Injuries to the ankle's lateral ligament complex are common, particularly during sports and recreational activities. The lateral ligament complex is composed of four main ligaments: the anterior talofibular, the calcaneofibular, the posterior talofibular and the lateral talocalcaneal. The calcaneofibular ligament spans both the ankle and the subtalar joints (Figure 1). The lateral talocalcaneal ligament spans the subtalar joint, while the remainder spans the tibiotalar joint.

Approximately two-thirds of acute ankle sprains are isolated injuries to the anterior talofibular ligament [Broström 1964]. With more severe ankle inversion, the calcaneofibular ligament is also injured. The posterior talofibular ligament is an extremely strong structure and is rarely injured except in cases of complete ankle dislocation.

Chronic instability is not always the result of previous acute ankle sprains but may evolve from repetitive varus stress causing attenuation of the lateral ligaments.

Clinical and radiological assessment

Acute injuries of the lateral ligaments present with pain and difficulty on weightbearing following an injury sustained to the hindfoot while in inversion and some plantarflexion. Swelling is localized anterior and distal to the lateral malleolus. By 36–48 h after the injury there is ecchymosis on the lateral side of the ankle giving rise to a distinct line of bruising just above the junction of the lateral plantar skin.

Patients with chronic lateral ankle instability present with symptoms of recurrent sprains, of giving way, and of difficulty accommodating to uneven surfaces. Instability symptoms are particularly troublesome for athletes and dancers. Pain associated with chronic instability may be due to secondary pathology such as synovitis, impingement from anterior tibial spurs, peroneal tenosynovitis or tendon tears and osteochondral talar lesions [O'Farrell et al. 1996, DiGiovanni et al. 2000].

Clinical evaluation includes stress testing by means of the anterior drawer and talar tilt tests. The anterior drawer test is performed supine with the knee flexed. The heel is cupped with one hand and drawn forward, internally rotating the talus, while the distal tibia is stabilized with the other hand. In addition to noting increased laxity compared to the contralateral normal side, a sulcus sign or dimple may be present over the anterior talofibular ligament as the lax ligament and skin are sucked inwards by the effect of negative pressure within the ankle joint [Aradi et al. 1988]. The inversion stress test is perfomed by placing an inversion and internal rotation stress on the plantarflexed ankle and comparing it to the opposite ankle. When positive, this test may be associated with apprehension from the patient.

If there is doubt about the diagnosis clinically, stress radiographs are performed. Normal anterior

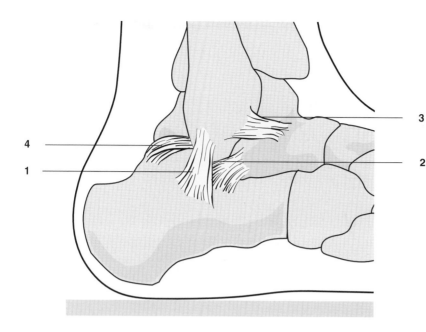

Figure 1

The lateral collateral ligaments of the ankle

1 Calcaneofibular ligament
2 Lateral talocalcaneal ligament
3 Anterior talofibular ligament
4 Posterior talofibular ligament

translation of the talus in the uninjured ankle joint averages 7 mm and normal talar tilt 5° [Karlsson et al. 1989]. A 10° difference in talar tilt compared to the normal side indicates a significant ligamentous instability. Talar tilt greater than 20° is a reliable indicator of a tear of both anterior talofibular and fibulocalcaneal components of the lateral ligament [Black 1977].

Evaluation of these patients should include consideration of additional subtalar instability. The calcaneofibular ligament is one of the main stabilizers of the subtalar joint [Pisani 1977], as is the lateral and interosseous talocalcaneal ligament, injury to which often accompanies lateral ligament injuries [Allieux 1979]. With an apparently convincing history of ankle instability associated with unconvincing clinical and radiological findings, the diagnosis of subtalar instability should be considered, particularly when proprioceptive rehabilitation has failed. Tenderness may be present in the sinus tarsi or more proximally over the posterior facet of the subtalar joint. During stress testing, if inversion of the heel is clinically excessive and disproportionate to the amount of radiological talar tilt, then there is subtalar laxity [Stephens 1994]. Opening of the lateral aspect of the subtalar joint on a Broden's view of the posterior facet during stress testing is only seen in cases of gross subtalar laxity.

Surgical reconstruction in these cases must address stabilization of the subtalar joint by reconstruction of the calcaneofibular ligament and incorporation of the extensor retinaculum, which also stabilizes the subtalar joint, into the repair [Stephens and Sammarco 1992].

Indications for operative treatment

The large majority of acute lateral ligament tears are treated non-operatively. Surgical repair should be considered only in the high-performance athlete with a grade III injury, i.e. a complete rupture of the ligament indicated by severe swelling, hematoma and tenderness with positive anterior drawer and talar tilt tests. Stress testing in the acute setting is difficult, owing to pain, and should be either delayed for 2 weeks or performed under local or general anesthesia. Alternatively, magnetic resonance imaging (MRI) has now been shown to be 90% accurate in diagnosing ruptures of the anterior talofibular and calcaneofibular ligaments [Verhaven et al. 1991].

In chronic instability, surgery is indicated when the patient has failed to stabilize the ankle sufficiently following an intensive rehabilitation program including peroneal muscle strengthening, proprioceptive training and Achilles tendon stretches.

Surgical reconstruction for acute lateral ligament tears

Acute injuries may be either midsubstance tears or bony avulsion injuries from the fibular origin or talar insertion. For the bony avulsions, osteosynthesis is dependent on the size of the bony fragment. When the avulsion fragment is too small to permit internal

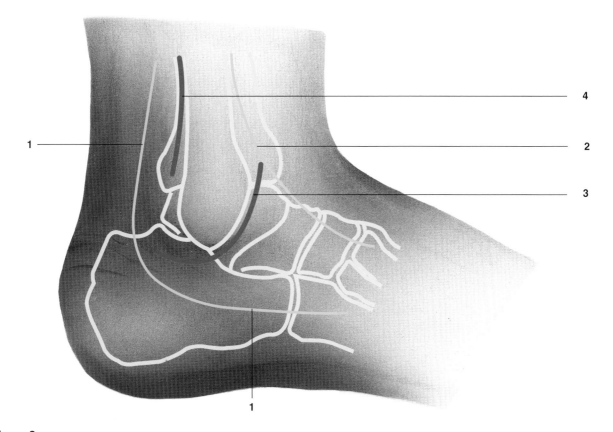

Figure 2

Incisions for acute and chronic repairs

1 Sural nerve
2 Lateral branch of superficial peroneal nerve
3 Incision for acute repair, Broström repair and distal incision for modified Chrisman–Snook repair
4 Proximal incision for modified Chrisman–Snook repair

fixation it should be excised and the ligament re-attached through drill holes or suture anchors.

The operation [Yamamoto 1998] is performed with a thigh tourniquet. A large sandbag is placed under the ipsilateral buttock to rotate the leg sufficiently internally for access to the lateral structures. Prior to incision the lateral branch of the superficial peroneal nerve is identified using the fourth toe flexion sign [Stephens and Kelly 2000]. A J-shaped incision is made around the lateral malleolus (Figure 2). During subcutaneous dissection, care is taken to avoid injuring the sural nerve posteriorly and the lateral branch of the superficial peroneal nerve anteriorly. Blunt dissection leads to the torn ankle joint capsule. Blood within the joint is evacuated. The anterior talofibular ligament, which is intracapsular, may be easily identified in a fresh injury, because the capsule itself will be torn from the distal fibula and tibia. The anterior talofibular ligament usually tears at a point near the middle or

close to the fibula. In young patients, the fibers avulse with a small bone fragment from the fibula. The joint must be inspected for intra-articular injuries, such as a talar osteochondral fracture. Loose bodies of bone or cartilage are removed. The peroneal tendon sheath is opened below the fibula, in order to retract the tendons laterally and permit viewing of the calcaneofibular ligament.

Midsubstance tears of the anterior talofibular ligament and the calcaneofibular ligament are repaired with the same technique: the ends of the torn ligaments are approximated as near as possible to their original anatomical position with interrupted 2-0 absorbable monofilament sutures [Broström 1966] (Figure 3a). At the time of suture, the ankle is placed in valgus and the foot is placed in eversion, abduction and neutral plantarflexion. If two ligaments are torn, the calcaneofibular ligament is repaired first because it is the most difficult to visualize, followed by the anterior talofibular ligament.

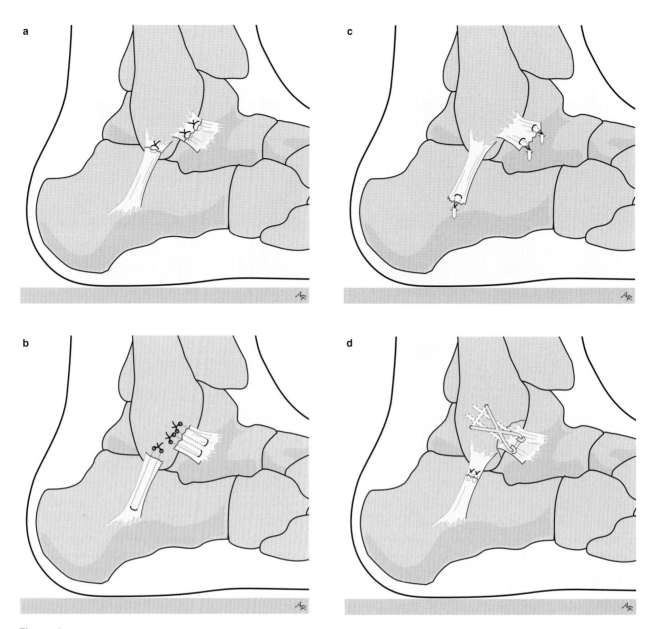

Figure 3

Repair of acute ligament tears. a. midsubstance tears are repaired anatomically; b. tears close to the fibula are tied to the periosteum through two 1.2-mm drill holes at their origin at the lateral malleolus;. c. in tears near the insertion at the talus or the calcaneus, the torn ligament is attached to its anatomic insertion site with bone anchors and sutured to the periosteum; d. avulsion fractures are reduced anatomically and fixed with tension-band wires

In tears of the anterior talofibular ligament and the calcaneofibular ligament close to the fibula, the ligaments are sutured to the periosteum of the fibula through two 1.2-mm drill holes at their point of origin at the lateral malleolus, using absorbable monofilament sutures (Figure 3b). In a tear of the anterior talofibular ligament close to the talus, the ligament is attached with bone anchors to its anatomic insertion site and sutured to the periosteum (Figure 3c), or the sutures are passed from the anatomic insertion site through two 1.2-mm drill holes to the medial side of the talus and tied over a button.

A similar technique may be used in a tear of the calcaneofibular ligament close to the calcaneus.

In avulsion fractures with a small bone fragment, the fragment is excised and the ligament is sutured to the thick periosteum around its anatomic origin, or to the tip of the fibula through drill holes, as previously described. Large bone fragments are reduced and fixed anatomically with a screw or using tension-band wiring with two 1.2-mm Kirschner wires and a 0.8-mm wire loop (Figure 3d).

The ankle joint capsule is repaired with absorbable sutures. The peroneal tendons are relocated into the tendon sheath and it is closed. The wound is closed in layers with absorbable sutures and the skin is sutured with subcuticular or interrupted nylon sutures.

Postoperatively, the patient is immobilized in a splint for 1 week. After the swelling subsides, a short leg walking cast is applied for 4 weeks, with the ankle in neutral position. After removal of the cast, patients wear an ankle brace to limit inversion. An active physiotherapy program is started, which consists of active and assisted-active plantarflexion and dorsiflexion exercises, with no inversion. Eight weeks after surgery, active inversion exercises are begun with more vigorous plantarflexion and dorsiflexion exercises of the lower leg muscles (especially the peroneals) and proprioception exercises. For athletes, muscle strengthening and proprioception exercises with a balance board are essential. The patients may return to sports 10–12 weeks after surgery.

Surgical options for reconstruction of chronic instability

Numerous reconstructive procedures have been described for the treatment of chronic lateral ankle instability. These operations fall into two categories: anatomical repairs such as the Broström, and the non-anatomical procedures usually using a peroneus brevis tenodesis, e.g. the Chrisman–Snook procedure [Snook et al. 1985].

Independent long-term reports of the Broström, Watson–Jones and Chrisman–Snook procedures are comparable, with 85–90% good and excellent results [Hamilton et al. 1993, Sugimoto et al. 1998, Sammarco and Idusuyi 1999]. However, both clinical and cadaveric studies comparing the Broström repair to the non-anatomical procedures have shown both greater stability and less restriction of ankle motion in the Broström groups [Liu and Baker 1994, Krips et al. 2000]. The long-term results of the Evans procedure have been suboptimal [Rosenbaum et al. 1997, Nimon et al. 2001].

We favor the Broström anatomical repair whenever possible, reserving the Chrisman–Snook tenodesis for revision of failed anatomical repairs and for cases when anatomical repair is not possible. Both procedures will be described. On the rare occasion of a failed Chrisman–Snook repair, the use of the lateral third of the Achilles tendon to reconstruct the lateral ligament has been described [Thornes and Stephens 1999].

The Broström repair with Gould modification

The superficial and deep anatomical structures surrounding the lateral ligament complex are illustrated (Figure 4).

The patient is placed supine with a large sandbag under the buttock to internally rotate the leg 45°. A thigh tourniquet is used. A J-shaped incision is made around the lateral malleolus (Figure 2). Care is taken to identify the lateral branch of the superficial peroneal nerve in the subcutaneous layer and the nerve is retracted medially. The superior band of the inferior extensor retinaculum is identified and mobilized distally to expose the anterior talofibular ligament. The retinaculum should not be incised, as it is used for attachment to the distal fibula as the final step of the reconstruction [Gould et al. 1980]. This is particularly important in cases of additional subtalar instability, as the retinaculum is a stabilizer of the subtalar joint.

The peroneal tendons overlie the calcaneofibular ligament. To gain adequate access to the calcaneofibular ligament, the peroneal tendon sheath is opened and the tendons are retracted inferiorly. If the superficial peroneal retinaculum is incised to aid mobilization of the tendons, this structure must be repaired to prevent peroneal tendon subluxation.

The attenuated anterior talofibular ligament is then incised in a curvilinear fashion to leave a substantial cuff of ligament attached to the lateral malleolus. This incision is continued posteriorly also incising the calcaneofibular ligament with a cuff (Figure 5). To shorten and hence tighten the lateral ligaments, multiple strong absorbable monofilament sutures are use to double-breast the ligament in 'a vest over pants' fashion. These sutures are tied while the hindfoot is held in maximum eversion, external rotation and dorsiflexion. Finally the superior border of the extensor retinaculum is sutured to the periosteum of the lateral malleolus to reinforce the repair (Figure 6). The repair is gently stressed by inverting the hindfoot to check the integrity of the reconstruction.

The skin is closed with a subcuticular suture over a superficial drain and a below-knee plaster cast applied with the hindfoot everted. The patient mobilizes partially weightbearing for 6 weeks, following which rehabilitation is commenced, concentrating on optimizing proprioception, regaining peroneal muscle strength and Achilles tendon stretches. The patient can usually return to sports training 12 weeks following surgery.

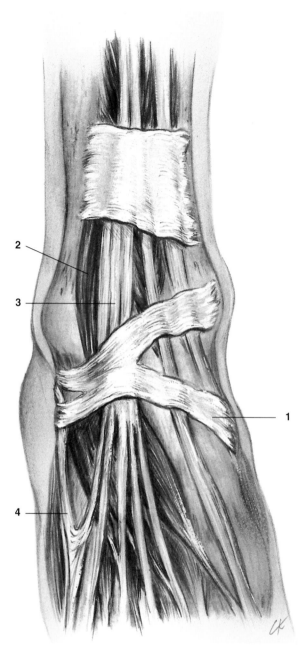

Figure 4

The superficial anatomy of the lateral aspect of the ankle

1 Extensor retinaculum
2 Peroneus tertius
3 Extensor digitorum longus
4 Peroneus brevis

The modified Chrisman–Snook repair

When the quality of the residual attenuated ligaments is too poor to support an anatomical repair, or there is a history of a previous Broström repair, we recommend a peroneus brevis tenodesis based on the Chrisman–Snook procedure [Snook et al.

1985]. Chrisman and Snook used a split peroneus brevis graft as a modification to the Elmslie procedure (in which a fascia lata graft was used) to reconstuct the anterior talofibular and calcaneofibular ligaments [Elmslie 1934]. Sammarco and DiRaimondo [1988] further modified the bony tunnels used by Chrisman and Snook by adding a third vertical tunnel in the talus in order to reconstruct the lateral talocalcaneal ligament and create a more anatomical anterior talofibular ligament and calcaneofibular ligament reconstruction. This reconstruction will be described.

Two incisions are required (Figure 2). The distal incision is a J-shaped incision distal to the lateral malleolus identical to that described for the Broström procedure. The proximal incision is required to harvest the split peroneus brevis tendon from its musculotendinous junction. A short longitudinal incision is made along the posterior border of the fibula to a point 2 cm above the lateral malleolus. The sural nerve is identified and protected. The peroneus longus, which overlies the peroneus brevis, is retracted posteriorly and the musculotendinous junction of the peroneus brevis is identified. The proximal extent of the incision is determined by the position of the musculotendinous junction. The brevis tendon is split upwards to the musculotendinous junction, where the half with the longest tendon component is divided from the muscle belly (Figure 7a), from which it is mobilized by sharp dissection. Attention is now turned to the distal incision.

Following the distal J-shaped incision (Figure 2), the lateral branch of the common peroneal and the sural nerves are identified and protected. The sural nerve can usually be found at a point 1.5 cm posteroinferiorly to the tip of the lateral malleolus. The superior peroneal retinaculum and peroneal tendon sheath are incised to expose both peroneal tendons. The peroneus longus is retracted posteroinferiorly. A tendon passer is used to retrieve the split peroneus brevis graft into the distal wound and the split is carefully propagated distally, leaving both halves of the tendon attached to the fifth metatarsal base. A suture is passed through the end of the tendon to aid its retrieval through the bony tunnels. The graft is set aside in a moist swab.

The sinus tarsi is exposed by detaching the extensor digitorum brevis proximally. The contents of the sinus tarsi are left undisturbed. The anterolateral ankle joint capsule is identified and incised to expose the anterior border of the lateral facet of the talar dome. The remnant of the insertion of the anterior talofibular ligament is identified in the axilla between

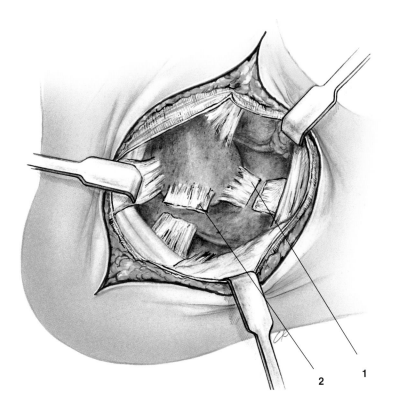

Figure 5

Anterior talofibular ligament (1) and calcaneofibular ligament (2) incised, leaving cuff of ligament attached to the fibula

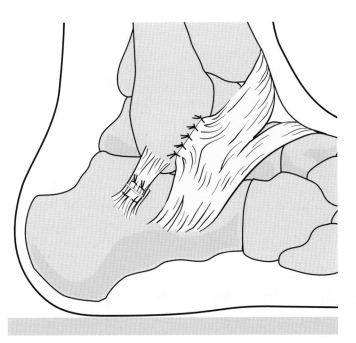

Figure 6

Repair reinforced by attaching the mobilized extensor retinaculum to the lateral malleolus

the lateral articular surface and the cartilage of the dome of the talus. From this point a 4.5-mm drill hole is made proximal to distal into the roof of the sinus tarsi. Using a tendon passer the graft is passed through this drill hole from distal to proximal.

An oblique 4.5-mm drill hole is made through the lateral malleolus from proximal–anterior to distal–posterior, connecting the origins of the anterior talofibular and calcaneofibular ligaments with a minimum bony bridge of 1 cm. The graft is then

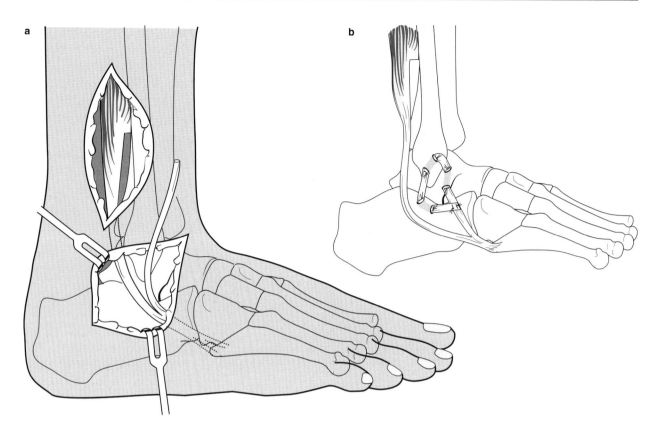

Figure 7

The modified Chrisman–Snook procedure a. graft harvesting; b. final position of tenodesis

passed through the fibula from anterior to posterior, running in the same direction as the anterior talofibular ligament. With the foot everted, externally rotated and dorsiflexed, the tendon graft is sutured to the fibular tunnels with absorbable monofilament sutures.

A third tunnel is made at the approximate insertion site of the original calcaneofibular ligament. By retracting the peroneals inferiorly and dissecting distally along the lateral wall of the calcaneum, a vertical ridge of bone can usually be located at the calcaneofibular ligament insertion. Two drill holes are made on either side of this ridge with a minimum connecting cortical bridge of 1 cm. The two drill holes are connected with curved curettes of sequentially increasing size. The free end of the graft is then returned to the fibular groove and passed deep to the peroneal tendons and passed through the calcaneal drill hole from posterior to anterior (Figure 7b). Again, sutures are placed between the graft and the adjacent soft tissues while the foot is held in the corrected position. This stage of the reconstruction duplicates the calcaneofibular ligament.

Finally, the free end of the graft is sutured back on to itself anterior to the fibular tunnel, further stabilizing the subtalar joint. We use a strong absorbable suture, e.g. #1-PDS (Polydioxanone, Johnson and Johnson Ltd.) for the tenodesis. The superficial peroneal retinaculum is repaired and the wound is closed over a suction drain.

A walking cast is applied with the foot plantgrade and in mild eversion. The patient mobilizes non-weightbearing for the first 2 weeks, followed by weightbearing as tolerated for a further 4–6 weeks. Rehabilitation is then commenced as for the Broström repair.

Complications

The commonest complications are infection, wound necrosis, nerve injury and venous thrombosis. Careful identification and protection of the sural and lateral branch of the superficial peroneal nerve are imperative. Thromboprophylaxis should be used for high-risk patients.

In the modified Chrisman–Snook procedure fracture of the roof of the bone tunnels can occur. This is avoidable by ensuring a cortical bridge of 1 cm between each end of the tunnel. Talocalcaneal ligaments within the sinus tarsi should be preserved, as they contribute to the proprioceptive function of the hindfoot.

Prolonged immobilization may contribute to the development of reflex sympathetic dystrophy, particularly in young women (see further, the findings of Coull et al. [2003]).

References

Allieux Y (1979) Contribution à l'étude biomécanique des contraintes ligamentaires au cours des entorses de la cheville. In: Simon L, Chaustre J, Benezi C (eds) Le Pied du Sportif. Paris, Masson, pp 6–10

Aradi AJ, Wong J, Walsh M (1988) The dimple sign of a ruptured lateral ligament of the ankle: brief report. J Bone Joint Surg 70B: 327–328

Black H (1977) Roentgenographic consideration of the ankle. Am J Sports Med 5: 238–242

Broström L (1964) Sprained ankles: anatomic lesions in recent sprains. Acta Chir Scand 128: 483–495

Broström L (1966) Sprained ankles: VI. Surgical treatment of chronic ligament ruptures. Acta Chir Scand 132: 551–565

Coull R, Raffiy T, James LE, Stephens MM (2003) Open treatment of anterior impingement of the ankle. J Bone Joint Surg 85B: 550–553

DiGiovanni BF, Fraga CJ, Cohen BE, Shereff MJ (2000) Associated injuries found in chronic lateral ankle instability. Foot Ankle Int 21: 809–815

Elmslie RC (1934) Recurrent subluxation of the ankle joint. Ann Surg 100: 364–367

Gould N, Seligson D, Gassman J (1980) Early and late repair of lateral ligament of the ankle. Foot Ankle 1: 84–90

Hamilton WG, Thompson FM, Snow SW (1993) The modified Broström procedure for lateral ankle instability. Foot Ankle 18: 144–150

Karlsson J, Bergsten T, Lansinger O, Peterson L (1989) Surgical treatment of chronic lateral instability of the ankle joint. Am J Sports Med 17: 268–273

Krips R, van Dijk CN, Halasi T et al. (2000) Anatomical reconstruction versus tenodesis for the treatment of chronic instability of the ankle joint. Knee Surg Sports Traumatol Arthrosc 8: 173–179

Liu SH, Baker CL (1994) Comparison of lateral ankle ligamentous reconstruction procedures. Am J Sports Med 22: 313–317

Nimon GA, Dobson PJ, Angal KR et al. (2001) A long-term review of a modified Evans procedure. J Bone Joint Surg 83B: 14–18

O'Farrell D, McCabe JP, Curtin B et al. (1996) Use of magnetic resonance imaging and scintigraphy for diagnosis of osteochondral fractures in acutely sprained unstable ankles. Foot Ankle 2: 209–214

Pisani G (1977) Il complesso legamentoso periastragalico. Chir Piede 1: 559–561

Rosenbaum D, Becker HP, Sterk J et al. (1997) Functional evaluation of the 10-year outcome after modified Evans ankle instability. Foot Ankle Int 18: 765–771

Sammarco GJ, DiRaimondo CV (1988) Surgical treatment of lateral ankle instability syndrome. Am J Sports Med 16: 501–511

Sammarco GJ, Idusuyi OB (1999) Reconstruction of the lateral ankle ligaments using a split peroneus brevis tendon graft. Foot Ankle Int 20: 97–103

Snook GA, Chrisman OD, Wilson TC (1985) Long-term results of the Chrisman–Snook operation for reconstruction of the lateral ligaments of the ankle. J Bone Joint Surg 67A: 1–7

Stephens MM (1994) Hindfoot laxity – ankle or subtalar joint or both? Foot Dis 1: 111–115

Stephens MM, Kelly PM (2000) Fourth toe flexion sign: a new clinical sign for identification of the superficial peroneal nerve. Foot Ankle Int 21: 860–863

Stephens MM, Sammarco GJ (1992) The stabilizing role of the lateral ligament complex around the ankle and subtalar joints. Foot and Ankle 13: 130–136

Sugimoto K, Takakura Y, Akiyama K et al. (1998) Long-term results of Watson–Jones tenodesis of the ankle. J Bone Joint Surg 80A: 1587–1596

Thornes BS, Stephens MM (1999) Revision lateral ankle ligament reconstruction using Achilles tendon graft: a case report. Foot Ankle 5: 267–270

Verhaven EFC, Shahabpour M, Handelberg FWJ (1991) The accuracy of three-dimensional MRI in the diagnosis of ruptures of the lateral ligaments of the ankle. Am J Sports Med 19: 583–585

Yamamoto H (1998) Repair of acute lateral ankle ligament tears. In: Wülker N, Stephens MM, Cracchiolo A III (eds) Atlas of Foot & Ankle Surgery. London, Martin Dunitz, pp 271–275

33

Tarsal tunnel release

Yoshinori Takakura

Introduction

Tarsal tunnel syndrome is an entrapment neuropathy which occurs as a result of compression of the tibial nerve in the tunnel formed by the tarsal bones and the flexor retinaculum in the posteroinferior area of the medial malleolus of the ankle joint [Keck 1962, Lam 1962]. The tibial nerve in the tarsal tunnel divides into several terminal branches (Figure 1).

The two major branches of the tibial nerve are the medial and lateral plantar nerves. The other smaller branches are the two medial calcaneal branches; the first is a sensory branch to the medial side of the heel and the second is a mixed sensorimotor nerve branch to the abductor digiti quinti muscle [Mann 1974]. The clinical features of this syndrome are characteristic pain at the medial malleolus radiating to the sole and heel, paresthesia, dysesthesia and hyperesthesia in the distribution of the terminal branches of the tibial nerve. Its incidence is low in comparison with the carpal tunnel syndrome, and few papers have been published on this subject. Axonal demyelinization due to ganglion, exostosis, direct pressure by trauma or post-traumatic bleeding, tumors and varicose veins have been mentioned as the causes of this condition. Systemic factors, such as abnormalities of the endocrine system and neurological diseases, are other possible causes. However, cases that do not present obvious abnormal findings (idiopathic) have been reported [Keck 1962, DiStefano et al. 1972]. In most patients requiring operative tarsal tunnel release, a space-occupying lesion is found [Takakura et al. 1991, Nagaoka and Satou 1999]. Ganglia developing in the tarsal tunnel are relatively common, and they may be found in patients having no obvious clinical swelling or lump. Patients with a talocalcaneal coalition have an exostosis of the talus or calcaneus which puts pressure on the nerve.

Diagnosis

Diagnosis of tarsal tunnel syndrome is based on the patient's symptoms, physical examination including Tinel's sign, the sensory disturbances and the electromyographic findings. Sensory disturbance, including hyperalgesia or hypoesthesia, usually occurs in the area of the medial plantar nerve, less commonly in the area of the medial and lateral plantar nerves, and rarely only in the lateral plantar nerve distribution or along the whole sole of the foot. When there is a mass, the contents are examined by aspiration. If it is a ganglion, the diagnosis is easily made by its clear, viscous contents. Electrodiagnostic tests typically reveal reduced sensory nerve conduction velocity, reduced amplitude and increased duration of the motor evoked potentials and distal motor latency [Edwards et al. 1969, Kaplan and Kernahan 1981]. Abnormalities have been found in 84% of patients with a clinical diagnosis of tarsal tunnel syndrome [Takakura et al. 1991]. Most patients have a decreased or even undetectable sensory conduction velocity, and this is more useful than distal motor latency.

Treatment

Indication for operative treatment

Conservative treatment is employed initially, using local steroid injections and a variety of orthoses. If the condition fails to respond to conservative

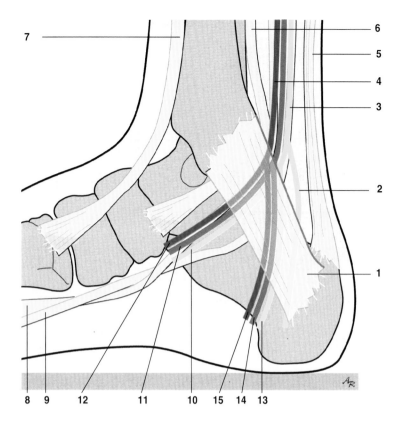

Figure 1

Anatomy of the tarsal tunnel

1 Flexor retinaculum
2 Medial calcaneal branch of tibial nerve
3 Tibial nerve
4 Posterior tibial vein
5 Achilles tendon
6 Tibialis posterior tendon
7 Tibialis anterior tendon
8 Flexor digitorum longus tendon
9 Flexor hallucis longus tendon
10 Medial plantar nerve
11 Medial plantar artery
12 Medial plantar vein
13 Lateral plantar nerve
14 Lateral plantar artery
15 Lateral plantar vein

treatment and the subjective symptoms are of sufficient magnitude, a tarsal tunnel release procedure is indicated. If there is a space-occupying lesion, it should be excised early, rather than continuing with conservative treatment.

Surgical technique

Operative tarsal tunnel release is performed with the patient in the supine position. Spinal anesthesia is preferable. A tourniquet is applied around the proximal thigh to minimize intraoperative bleeding. A curved skin incision is made from a point 5 cm proximal to the posterior aspect of the medial malleolus parallel to the posterior border of the tibia and the margin of the medial malleolus to midway between the tip of the navicular and the abductor hallucis muscle (Figure 2).

The incision is deepened through the subcutaneous tissue and fat. The proximal and distal portions of the flexor retinaculum are exposed. The tendon sheath of the tibialis posterior muscle is palpated behind the posterior margin of the tibia. The tendon sheath of the flexor digitorum longus and the bundle of the artery, vein and nerve are located behind the posterior tibial tendon. The retinaculum is carefully released along the posterior margin of the posterior tibial tendon sheath (Figure 3).

If there is a significant space-occupying lesion, e.g. a large ganglion, exostosis or neoplasm in the tunnel, the tibial nerve is often compressed between the lesion and the retinaculum. In such a patient the retinaculum should be released first at its proximal or distal portion, leaving the space-occupying lesion in place. When dissecting out this area, a curved clamp should be placed between the retinaculum and the underlying tissues to avoid accidental injury to the neurovascular bundle.

The proximal part of the tibial nerve is carefully identified by blunt dissection. It is traced distally through the tarsal tunnel where it divides into the three terminal branches. If there is a ganglion or there are osteophytes caused by a talocalcaneal coalition in the tunnel, the tendon of the tibialis posterior and flexor digitorum longus should be retracted anteriorly and the neurovascular bundle carefully retracted posteriorly. Any ganglion or bony eminence is isolated from the surrounding tissues and carefully excised. The ganglia in the tarsal tunnel generally originate from the deltoid ligament, the tendon sheaths of the flexor digitorum longus and the flexor hallucis longus, or from the talocalcaneal joint. It is necessary to ligate the stem of the ganglia at their origin because they may recur. A bony prominence should be excised until the normal cartilage layer can be recognized.

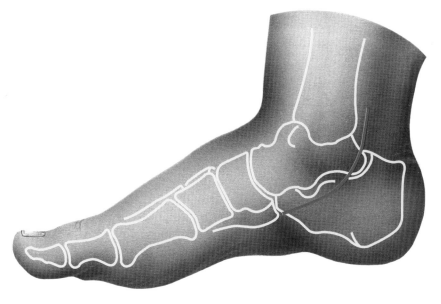

Figure 2

The curved incision is carried parallel to the posterior border of the tibia and the margin of the medial malleolus to end at the navicular

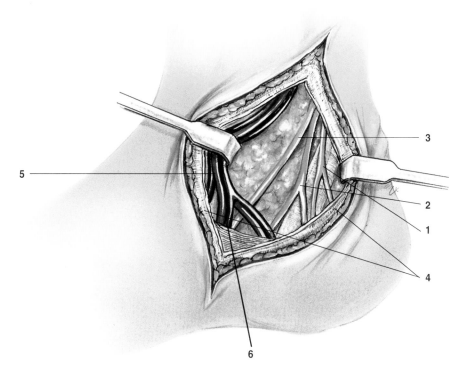

Figure 3

The flexor retinaculum is carefully released along the posterior margin of the posterior tibial tendon sheath

1 Medial calcaneal branch of tibial nerve
2 Lateral plantar nerve
3 Medial plantar nerve
4 Flexor retinaculum
5 Posterior tibial artery and vein
6 Abductor hallucis muscle

After the space-occupying lesion has been removed from the tunnel, the tibial nerve can easily be followed further distally. The medial plantar nerve is traced distally around the tendon sheath of the flexor digitorum longus and is followed beneath the abductor hallucis until it passes through a fibrous tunnel. The passage of the medial plantar nerve through its fibrous tunnel in the abductor hallucis should be observed. If the tunnel is tight, some fibrous tissue should be released. It is sometimes also necessary to identify the medial plantar nerve distally and trace it back proximally underneath the vessels that are covering it. At times, some of the veins should be ligated, if they are thought to be a factor in compression of the nerve.

The lateral plantar nerve is traced distally by blunt dissection to observe its passage behind the abductor hallucis muscle. It is often necessary to excise a portion of the dorsal half of the origin of this muscle from the calcaneus, because this forms a dense, fibrous band which may constrict the nerve. After the tibial nerve and its terminal branches are traced carefully again, the tourniquet is released.

Any bleeding must be controlled. When the tourniquet is released, the nerve is inspected for adequate capillary filling along its course. If some parts of the nerve do not reveal a good pink color, vascular constriction must be suspected. It is then necessary to explore the nerve again and release the epineurium. The retinaculum is not closed, to avoid constricting the nerve. If there is still some minor bleeding following hemostasis, the wound may be closed over a drain. The wound is then closed in layers.

Postoperative care

Postoperatively, a short leg plaster cast is used for 2 weeks to prevent bleeding and pain. Full weightbearing on the operated leg is allowed after 2 weeks. In patients with excision of osteophytes from a tarsal coalition, full weightbearing and full range-of-motion exercises are allowed after 4 weeks.

Complications

When the contents of the tumor are aspirated, the tibial nerve and its branches are sometimes injured. Therefore, repeated punctures should be avoided. A ganglion often recurs if the stem is not ligated at its origin. When a space-occupying lesion is present, such as a ganglion, a bony eminence from a talocalcaneal coalition or a neoplasm, satisfactory results with complete relief of the symptoms are usually obtained. However, if the interval

between the onset of symptoms and operative release in cases with a space-occupying lesion is more than 10 months, recovery of the nerve is poor. Therefore, patients with a definite space-occupying lesion should be operated on early. If there is no specific etiology for the tarsal tunnel syndrome, some cases obtain little or no relief of the symptoms [Pfeiffer and Cracchiolo 1994]. When no specific cause can be identified in spite of thorough examination, surgery should be delayed and conservative treatment continued.

References

DiStefano V, Sack JT, Whittaker R, Nixon JE (1972) Tarsal tunnel syndrome: review of literature and two case reports. Clin Orthop 88: 76–79

Edwards WG, Lincoln CR, Bassette FH, Goldner JL (1969) Tarsal tunnel syndrome: diagnosis and treatment. J Am Med Assoc 207: 716–720

Kaplan PR, Kernahan WT (1981) Tarsal tunnel syndrome: an electrodiagnostic and surgical correlation. J Bone Joint Surg 63A: 96–99

Keck C (1962) The tarsal tunnel syndrome. J Bone Joint Surg 44A: 180–182

Lam SJS (1962) Tarsal tunnel syndrome. Lancet 2: 1354–1355

Mann RA (1974) Tarsal tunnel syndrome. Orthop Clin North Am 5: 109–115

Nagaoka M, Satou K (1999) Tarsal tunnel syndrome caused by ganglia. J Bone Joint Surg 81B: 607–610

Pfeiffer WH, Cracchiolo A (1994) Clinical results after tarsal tunnel decompression. J Bone Joint Surg 76A: 1222–1230

Takakura Y, Kitada C, Suginoto K et al. (1991) Tarsal tunnel syndrome: causes and results of operative treatment. J Bone Joint Surg 73B: 125–128

34

Peroneal tendon dislocation Nikolaus Wülker

Introduction

Dislocation of the peroneal tendon is a rare but striking condition. Most commonly, the long peroneal tendon dislocates anteriorly and laterally on to the lateral surface of the distal fibula; less commonly, the short peroneal tendon is affected; rarely, both peroneal tendons are affected.

Peroneal tendon dislocation is caused by a sudden intrinsic or extrinsic force, or a combination of both. Dislocation has often been reported in skiers [Tourne et al. 1995]. The supposed mechanism is intrinsic dislocation by sudden activation of the peroneal muscles, e.g. during a fall. With the foot held in its position in a boot, tension on the peroneal tendons at their angulation around the distal fibula causes a force in an anterior direction. This force may be sufficient to cause dislocation, especially if the foot is held in dorsiflexion by the boot and if the restraining mechanism of the tendons is weakened by an anatomic abnormality. A similar intrinsic mechanism can occur when the mobile foot is pulled into maximum eversion by the peroneal tendons. Extrinsic dislocation may be caused by forceful passive supination of the foot, e.g. during a traffic accident, but the precise mechanism of dislocation is usually less clearly defined in these patients.

Of all peroneal tendon dislocations, 20–40% are considered idiopathic, with no history of previous trauma. The etiology may be insufficient strength of the peroneal retinaculum or an abnormally convex posterior surface of the fibula.

In an acute dislocation, the tendons usually have been relocated by the patient by active or passive movement of the foot before they are seen by a physician. Only some tenderness and swelling may be present at the posterior aspect of the distal fibula and diagnosis may be difficult. However, there is a high likelihood of recurrence, which appears not to be related to the type of treatment of the acute dislocation. Young athletic individuals appear to be more likely to have a recurrence. Usually, no repeated trauma is necessary and many patients are able spontaneously to dislocate and relocate their tendons by the time they are seen by a physician.

Subluxation, i.e. displacement of the tendon on to the posterolateral edge of the fibula but not beyond it, is a variant of dislocation. Diagnosis is more difficult, because patients often complain merely of vague pain or ankle instability without a feeling of tendon displacement. Treatment of acute and of recurrent subluxation does not differ from that of complete dislocation.

Normal and pathological anatomy

From their musculotendinous junction at the lower leg, the peroneal tendons course distally at the posterior surface of the fibula and then anteriorly to their anatomic insertions, i.e. the first and second metatarsal and medial cuneiform for the peroneus longus tendon and the base of the fifth metatarsal bone for the peroneus brevis tendon. At their angulation at the tip of the fibula, the peroneus longus tendon is situated posterior and lateral; the peroneus brevis tendon is anterior and medial.

The peroneal tendons are restrained in their positions by the peroneal tendon retinaculum, which has strong horizontal fibers from the dorsal lateral aspect of the distal fibula to the tibia. It extends 4–6 cm proximally from the tip of the fibula. Additional restraint is provided by the bony contour of the posterior fibular surface, but this is clearly less significant than the peroneal retinaculum [Orthner et al. 1989]. A groove is created by a lateral bony ridge, at the insertion area of the peroneal tendon retinaculum. The height of this ridge and hence the depth of the groove varies considerably between individuals. Anatomy studies have produced variable results [Mabit et al. 1996], but it must be assumed that a groove is present in most individuals. Absence of a sulcus may be related to the occurrence of dislocation of the peroneal tendons. Finally, the peroneal tendons are restrained by a fibrocartilaginous rim of various dimensions, which is located medial to the fibular insertion of the retinaculum at the fibula, thereby deepening the peroneal tendon groove.

In recurrent dislocation, the avulsed peroneal tendon retinaculum and periosteum have developed into a pouch, which involves more or less of the lateral surface of the distal fibula. The fibrocartilaginous rim is usually avulsed together with the retinaculum to form the inner surface of the pouch. The fibular surface within the pouch takes on a shiny appearance as evidence of repeated tendon dislocation into this area.

Splitting of the peroneal tendons or peroneal tenosynovitis are often observed. However, they rarely require treatment. Other pathologies are less common, e.g. rupture of the peroneal retinaculum, or avulsion of the retinaculum from the fibrocartilaginous rim.

Various stages of peroneal tendon dislocation can be defined on the basis of pathological findings (Figure 1). Grade 1 is stripping of the retinaculum and periosteum from the fibula and the cartilaginous rim; grade 2 is avulsion of the cartilaginous rim off the fibula, together with the retinaculum and periosteum; and grade 3 is an additional avulsion of a small bone fragment, either from the fibula together with the cartilaginous rim or from the tibia at the posterior retinacular insertion.

Indications for surgery

The acute dislocation is not an indication for surgery. Immobilization and non-weightbearing according to symptoms will result in stable tendons and a fully functional ankle in a number of patients. Surgical reconstruction is reserved for recurrent, symptomatic instability. Only elderly and less physically active patients will tolerate continuous episodes of dislocation and relocation. All others, and in particular athletic patients, should undergo surgical stabilization following their third dislocation.

Preoperatively, ankle radiographs in two planes are routinely required. In addition, computed ankle tomography or magnetic resonance imaging should be obtained to assess the posterior fibular surface and tendon pathology. Tangential retromalleolar radiographs are now less commonly used.

A number of surgical procedures have been described. The ultimate goal of surgery is the restoration of normal anatomy, with a sufficiently tight peroneal retinaculum, a fibrocartilaginous rim attached to the fibula and a peroneal groove of sufficient depth at the posterior fibular surface. The precise technique to achieve this goal can be decided only intraoperatively, once the full extent of the pathology is visualized. Non-anatomic reconstructions, which divert the tendons or adjacent ligaments from their normal positions, are not strongly recommended.

There are only few contraindications to surgery, in particular insufficient blood perfusion of the extremity, or poor skin condition.

Surgical technique

A 6–8-cm incision is made just posterior to the distal end of the fibula, angled slightly anteriorly round the tip of the fibula (Figure 2). Care is taken during subcutaneous dissection in order not to injure the sural nerve, which may be located in the area of the incision. Skin retraction must be used with caution and sharp rake retractors should not be used, to avoid postoperative wound edge necrosis. The peroneal retinaculum is exposed and separated from the subcutaneous fatty tissues with a small cotton swab. Laxity of the retinaculum is often evident when this is elevated with a forceps.

The peroneal retinaculum is divided directly at its insertion into the fibula. Reflection of the retinaculum in a posterior direction exposes the peroneal tendons. The peroneus longus, the peroneus brevis or both are pulled laterally with a blunt retractor; they are dislocated from their anatomic positions on to the lateral surface of the distal fibula. Reduction is usually easily achieved by supination of the foot.

A number of pathologies may be observed: laxity of the peroneal retinaculum is always present. Remnants of the fibrocartilaginous rim may be seen at the original position of the rim at the dorsolateral edge of the distal fibula or at the inner surface of the elevated retinaculum, giving it a similar appearance to a capsulolabral avulsion at the shoulder. However, the rim is often completely dissolved in patients with frequent recurrences. Rarely, a small bone fragment is avulsed

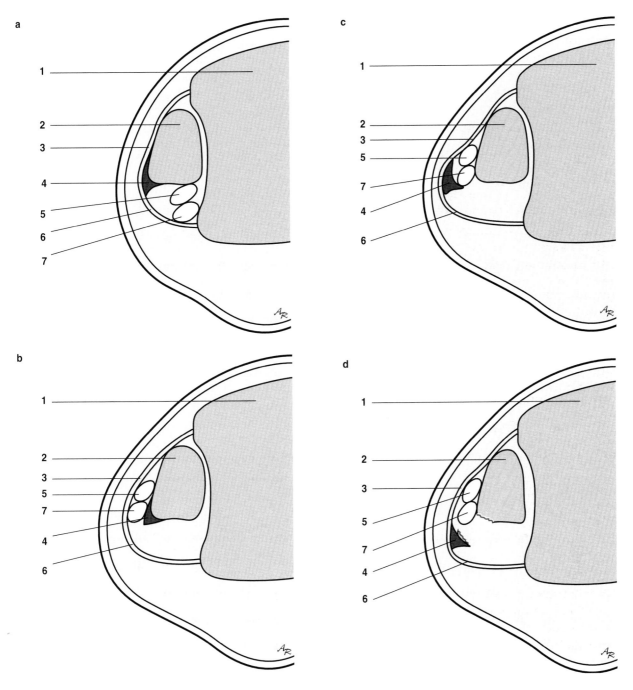

Figure 1

Stages of peroneal tendon dislocation: a. normal anatomy; b. grade 1: stripping of the retinaculum and periosteum from the fibula and the cartilaginous rim with dislocation of the tendons; c. grade 2: avulsion of the cartilaginous rim off the fibula, together with the retinaculum and periosteum; d. grade 3: avulsion of a small bone fragment

1 Tibia
2 Fibula
3 Periosteum
4 Fibrous rim
5 Peroneus longus tendon
6 Retinaculum
7 Peroneus brevis tendon

off the fibula together with the fibrocartilaginous rim. The periosteum is elevated from the lateral surface of the distal fibula, creating a dislocation pouch in continuity with the avulsed retinaculum. The

lateral aspect of the fibula takes on a shiny appearance as evidence of repeated dislocations. No bone ridge or an insufficient ridge may be seen and palpated at the posterior fibular surface, with no or

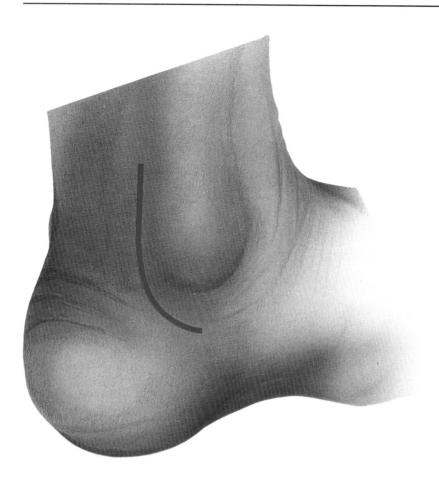

Figure 2

Skin incision for reconstructive procedures in peroneal tendon dislocation

only a shallow sulcus for the peroneal tendons. The normal, anatomic depth of the sulcus is 2–5 mm. Pathology at the tendons, such as peroneal tenosynovitis or tendon splitting, is often observed but does not seem to affect the results of treatment.

Anatomic reconstruction

Reconstruction entails reefing of the peroneal retinaculum and the creation of a peroneal groove, if this is abnormally shallow.

The peroneal retinaculum is reefed by creating a flap from the central portion of the retinaculum, with a width of approximately 2–3 cm (Figure 3). The posterior insertion of the flap remains attached to the tibia. The anterior edge is tagged with non-absorbable stay sutures at its corners. A slit of corresponding length is made in the distal fibula in a posterior to anterior direction. Preferably, an oscillating saw is used for this purpose. The entry point of the slit is just medial to the posterior fibular bone ridge. The slit must have an appropriate thickness to accommodate the flap; two immediately adjacent saw cuts may be necessary. The bone edges at the posterior opening of the slit are carefully smoothed with a rongeur. The tag sutures of the flap are led

through the slit from posterior to anterior, using a thin wire loop or other instrument. Adequate tension on the flap can then be created by pulling the sutures anteriorly. Stability of the peroneal tendons is assessed by attempting to pull them in a lateral direction with a blunt retractor. If the retinacular tissue does not have sufficient strength, reinforcement with the peroneus brevis tendon, with a strip of Achilles tendon or with the plantaris longus tendon has been used, but the author has not found this to be necessary. Once sufficient tension of the flap is attained, the tag sutures are fixed through bone at the posterior or anterior aspect of the fibula. Additional sutures may be inserted if the retinacular flap is long enough to emerge from the anterior opening of the bone slit. The remaining peroneal retinaculum superior and inferior to the flap is closed with thin, absorbable sutures, with some reefing to create an additional restraint to dislocation of the peroneal tendons. This reconstruction is sufficient for treatment of recurrent peroneal tendon dislocation if no bone deformity and an abnormally shallow or absent peroneal tendon groove is present.

If intraoperative inspection reveals a flat or convex posterior fibular surface with no bony barrier for the peroneal tendons, the technique described above is

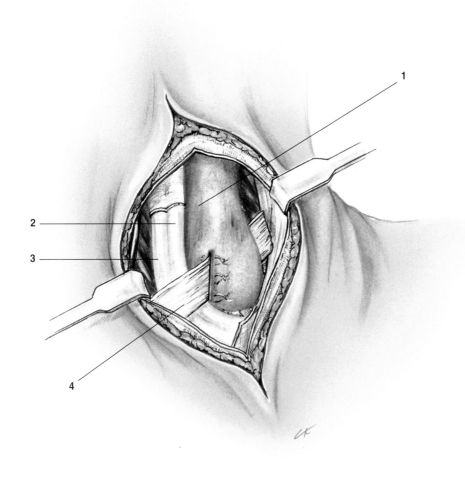

Figure 3

Reefing of the peroneal retinaculum through a sagittal bone slit. Fixation with transosseous sutures

1   Fibula
2   Peroneus longus tendon
3   Peroneus brevis tendon
4   Peroneal retinaculum

expanded to include a posterior bone block procedure (Figure 4). Not only is a slit made into the distal fibula, but a bone block is created and shifted posteriorly to establish the bone ridge which was not present previously. For this purpose, the bone slit is extended distally until it exits the tip of the fibula, and a second cut is made at the proximal end of the slit in a perpendicular orientation, entering from the lateral cortex of the fibula. Again, the use of an oscillating saw is preferable. Once the bone block is fully detached from the remaining fibula, the retinacular flap with the two tag sutures at its corners is pulled anteriorly until sufficient tension is created on the flap. The bone block is then placed back on to the fibula and the flap, displacing it approximately 3–5 mm from its original position in a posterior direction. Alternatively, the bone block may be rotated in a posterior direction. A pointed reduction clamp is used to hold the block in place during fixation with screws. Two small-fragment cancellous screws are generally used. Care must be taken not to enter the ankle joint with the screw tips and ankle joint motion must be checked intraoperatively to ascertain that this is not the case. Once stable bone

fixation is achieved, the retinacular flap is secured by transosseous fixation of the tag sutures.

Deepening of the peroneal groove is an alternative to the bone block procedure. Following displacement of the tendons with a retractor, a rongeur or curette may be used to remove a small amount of bone from the posterior fibular surface to create a concavity. Alternatively, the bone may be impacted to preserve the cartilaginous gliding layer. However, some impairment of tendon gliding will always occur postoperatively. Also, additional reefing of the peroneal retinaculum will be necessary in most cases. Therefore, a fibular grooving procedure is not recommended by the author.

Non-anatomic reconstruction

Procedures that sacrifice normal anatomic relationships at the lateral aspect of the ankle will always compromise function to some degree. Therefore, these procedures should be reserved for special conditions, such as revision cases.

Rerouting of the tendons under the calcaneofibular ligament has been advocated [Steinböck and Pinsger

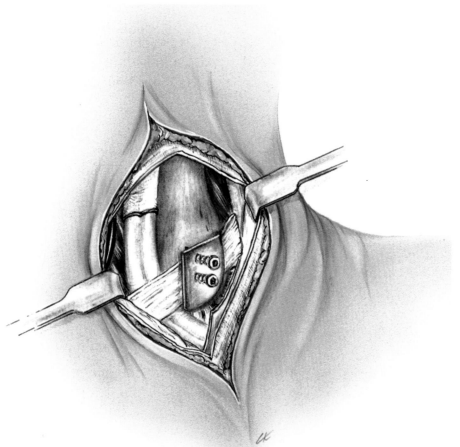

Figure 4

Reefing of the peroneal retinaculum with posterior displacement of a bone block and screw fixation

1994]. The surgical approach described above is extended distally to expose the ligament, which is deep to the peroneal tendons. The calcaneofibular ligament may be divided mid-substance and resutured over the tendons. Alternatively, the distal insertion of the ligament may be detached from the lateral surface of the calcaneus, including a small bone fragment, and the ligament may be pulled out from underneath the tendons. It is then flapped back over the tendons to its distal insertion site and fixed with transosseous sutures or bone anchors. Division of the peroneal tendons and transposition under the intact calcaneofibular ligament has also been used but compromises tendon integrity.

Rerouting of the peroneal tendons through a drill hole in the distal fibula has also been used. Usually only one tendon is rerouted, most commonly the peroneus longus. A 4.5-mm drill hole is made in the sagittal plane through the distal fibula, from posterior superior to anterior inferior, exiting close to the tip of the fibula. The tendon is transected distally, led through the drill hole from posterior to anterior and then sutured to the distal stump. Even though stability of the tendon will be achieved with this technique, it must be questioned whether gliding of the tendon within the cancellous bone canal will occur, or whether a tenodesis effect will result. The latter will compromise hindfoot motion, in particular supination. Therefore, drill hole rerouting of the tendon is not advocated by the author.

Postoperative treatment

With all procedures described above, immobilization is required for 6 weeks after surgery, until soft-tissue and bone healing have occurred. Immobilization in an orthotic device is preferred to a cast. The orthosis must largely eliminate inversion and eversion of the hindfoot and also limit dorsiflexion/plantarflexion of the ankle. A great variety of devices are available. They can usually be worn in a shoe and allow full weightbearing.

At 6 weeks after surgery, aggressive physiotherapy is begun. This includes motion exercises of the ankle and hindfoot, in particular inversion and eversion of the heel. The peroneal muscles are strengthened by exercises, including isokinetic training, if available.

Wobble-board exercises enhance peroneal reflexes and promote stability of the ankle and of the peroneal tendons.

If screws have been used for fixation of a bone block, they should be removed after approximately 1 year. Usually, some tenderness develops over the screw heads because the overlying skin is quite thin.

Bibliography

Beck E (1981) Operative treatment of recurrent dislocation of the peroneal tendons. Arch Orthop Trauma Surg 98: 247–250

Brage ME, Hansen ST Jr (1992) Traumatic subluxation/dislocation of the peroneal tendons. Foot Ankle 13: 423–431

Clanton TO, Schon LC (1993) Athletic injuries to the soft tissues of the foot and ankle. In: Mann R, Coughlin MJ (eds) Surgery of the Foot and Ankle, 6th edn. St Louis, Mosby, pp 1167–1177

Edwards EE (1928) The relation of the peroneal tendons to the fibula, calcaneus and cuboideum. Am J Anat 42: 213–253

Escalas F, Figueras JM, Merino JA (1980) Dislocation of the peroneal tendons. Long-term results of surgical treatment. J Bone Joint Surg 62: 451–453

Karlsson J, Eriksson BI, Sward L (1996) Recurrent dislocation of the peroneal tendons. Scand J Med Sci Sports 6: 242–246

Mabit C, Salanne P, Boncoeur-Martel MP et al. (1996) La gouttière retromalléolaire latérale: étude radio anatomique. Bull Assoc Anat (Nancy) 80: 17–21

Orthner E, Polcik J, Schabus R (1989) Die Luxation der Peroneussehnen. Unfallchirugie 92: 589–594

Platzgummer H (1967) Über ein einfaches Verfahren zur operativen Behandlung der habituellen Peronäussehnenluxation. Arch Orthop Unfallchir 61: 144–150

Radke J, Fink G (1975) Zur Morphologie des Sulcus malleolaris lateralis – ein Beitrag zur Atiologie der Peronaalsehnenluxationen. Z Orthop Ihre Grenzgeb 113: 858–863

Sarmiento A, Wolf M (1975) Subluxation of peroneal tendons. J Bone Joint Surg 52A: 115–116

Steinböck G, Pinsger M (1994) Treatment of peroneal tendon dislocations by transposition under the calcaneofibular ligament. Foot Ankle Int 15: 107–111

Tourne Y, Saragaglia D, Benzakour D, Bezes H (1995) La luxation traumatique des tendons peroniers. A propos de 36 cas. Int Orthop 19: 197–203

Viernstein K, Rosenmeyer B (1972) Ein Operationsverfahren zur Behandlung der rezidierenden Peronealsehnenluxation beim Leistungssportler. Arch Orthop Unfall Chir 74: 175–181

35

Osteochondral lesions of the talus: surgical considerations

Hans Zollinger-Kies

Introduction

Osteochondral lesions of the talus are common articular lesions that are often traumatic in origin. A number of terms are used to describe these lesions: osteochondritis dissecans, transchondral fracture, osteochondral fracture, partial talar necrosis, talar dome fracture and flake fracture. Osteochondritis dissecans is a term reserved for the chronic, non-union stage of an osteochondral fracture of the talus, but may also refer to a loose fragment of cartilage and necrotic subchondral bone resulting from localized vascular ischemia and subsequent fracture.

Etiology and pathogenesis

Supination injuries of the ankle and other biomechanical factors such as ankle ligament laxity appear to have an influence on the development of osteochondritis dissecans, at least if this is located at the medial rim of the talus [Bruns et al. 1992]. In cadaveric experiments [Bruns et al. 1992] the location, size of contact area and the maximum measured pressure at the ankle joint depended on the joint position and on the integrity of the fibular ligaments. However, the peak pressure was located at the medial talar rim even without lateral ligament dissection. This is the area where osteochondral lesions are most commonly observed.

Despite the fact that trauma is recognized as the principal etiological factor, not all patients with osteochondral lesions of the talus have a history of trauma. Osteochondritis may be caused by a pathological fracture through necrotic bone as a consequence of ischemia. The presence of subchondral cysts with overlying chondromalacia, osteochondral fragments and loose bodies may all represent stages in the progression of the disease.

Clinical and radiographic appearance

A flake fracture, which can potentially develop into an osteochondral lesion of the talus, may at times be suspected immediately following an acute ankle injury. More often, patients present with chronic ankle pain, with a history of an inversion episode or with chronic ankle instability. Other symptoms may include chronic ankle swelling, stiffness, weakness and giving way. The differential diagnosis must include soft-tissue ankle impingement, degenerative arthrosis and occult fractures.

Osteochondritis is usually diagnosed by plain radiography [Berndt and Harty 1959]. Magnetic resonance imaging (MRI) has improved the diagnostic accuracy. Computed tomography (CT) is valuable in obtaining detailed information on the extent and the morphology of the bony lesion, once this has been diagnosed radiographically. If the diagnosis is not clear, MRI appears to be more valuable, because it also indicates soft-tissue pathology. In particular, MRI appears to be reliable in detecting the presence and the extent of detachment of an osteochondral fragment at the talus [De Smet et al. 1990], and MRI assessment of osteochondritis dissecans lesions is of comparable value to arthroscopic evaluation [Pritsch et al. 1986, Nelson et al. 1990].

Various classification systems have been developed on the basis of CT findings [Ferkel 1996] and of MRI findings [Anderson et al. 1989].

Indications for surgery

Frequently, osteochondritic talar lesions are not painful, progress slowly and do not impair ankle function. Osteochondritic lesions often represent an incidental finding in an asymptomatic patient. In such cases no treatment is necessary.

The classification of Berndt and Harty [1959] for the assessment and treatment of osteochondral talar lesions has been increasingly replaced by arthroscopic, MRI and/or CT assessment. Treatment criteria are based on the location, size and displacement of the osteochondral fragment [Hepple et al. 1999].

Stage 1 is radiologically a small area of compression of subchondral bone. In arthroscopy an irregularity and softening of the articular cartilage is observed – on MRI a thickening of cartilage with low signal changes. This stage is usually painless at the onset and does not require treatment. However, the lesion may progress to a more advanced stage.

Stage 2 is radiologically a partially detached osteochondral fragment. Arthroscopically the cartilage is breached with a definable but not detached fragment. In MRI the cartilage is breached with a low signal rim behind the fragment, indicating fibrous attachment. In adolescent patients, treatment with cast immobilization for 6–8 weeks may be attempted. If this is unsuccessful and if the patient is sufficiently symptomatic, surgery should be performed. This consists of multiple drilling of the lesion combined with excision of loose fragments and debridement of all diseased articular cartilage. With this technique, over 85% of patients may improve or heal [Angermann and Jensen 1989, Struijs et al. 2001]. However, long-term results are controversial. At follow-up 9–15 years after surgery, more than half of the patients had some degree of pain and swelling of the ankle during activity [Angermann and Jensen 1989]. Other authors reported that, even if surgery were performed for a chronic lesion, the operation gave a high percentage of good results, and the long-term results did not differ appreciably from the results 18 months postoperatively [Alexander and Lichtman 1980].

An alternative treatment in stage II lesions is fixation of the fragment with a screw or a pin. This is indicated only if the fragment is sufficiently large.

Usually, union of the fragment to the talus is achieved only in patients during childhood and adolescence. Bone graft may have to be placed underneath the fragment to bring it to the level of the surrounding articular cartilage. Multiple drilling of the adjacent sclerotic bone should be performed in addition to fixation. Diseased cartilage should be debrided. In very large fragments with a wide area of surrounding sclerosis, retrograde bone grafting through a canal in the talus is possible.

Stage 3 is a completely detached osteochondral fragment that remains in the talar bone defect. Arthroscopically the cartilage is breached, with a definable and detached fragment and some overlying cartilage. In MRI the cartilage is breached with a high signal rim behind the fragment, indicating synovial fluid between the fragment and the surrounding subchondral bone. Fixation of the fragment with drilling of its bed is indicated only in patients under 16 years of age and if the fragment is very large. In all others, the fragment should be removed and the crater at the articular surface of the talus debrided.

Stage 4 is radiologically, arthroscopically and on MRI examination a displaced osteochondral fragment. These fragments are rarely fixed to their beds. Generally, removal of the fragment with drilling and debridement or replacement by cylindrical autologous osteochondral graft of the crater are indicated.

The character of the overlying cartilage, the stability of the fragment, and the subtle differences between stage 2 and stage 3 lesions are best determined arthroscopically or by MRI. Preoperative MRI correlates highly with arthroscopic findings in osteochondral lesions of the talus [Assenmacher et al. 2001]. Arthroscopy is helpful to differentiate between incompletely detached and completely detached but non-displaced fragments, and often permits treatment without open surgery. For experienced arthroscopic surgeons, the indications for open ankle surgery in osteochondritic talar lesions are decreasing. However, with large osteochondritic areas, the need for fixation of a large fragment or autologous osteochondral transplantation techniques and cancellous bone grafting of talar bone cysts may require arthrotomy.

Treatment

Approaches to the talar lesion

Open arthrotomy is used in all patients with osteochondritic lesions that are not suitable for arthroscopic treatment, in particular in large defects and if

a

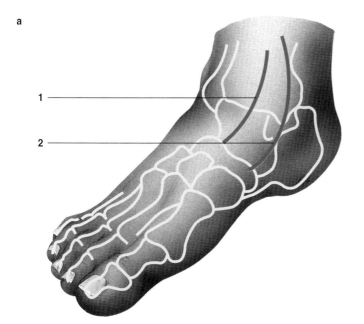

b

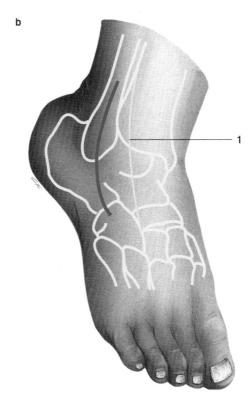

Figure 1

Skin incisions for the treatment of osteochondral lesions of the talus

a. anteromedial approach (1) and medial approach (2);
b. anterolateral approach

1 Superficial peroneal nerve

autologous chondocyte transplantation, mosaicplasty, or a (re-)fixation of the fragment are indicated. The patient is positioned supine. A sandbag should be placed under the ipsilateral hip to internally rotate the leg, if a lateral approach is needed. A tourniquet should be used, which may be placed at the proximal thigh or above the ankle. According to the preference of the patient, arthrotomy may be performed under general anesthesia or under spinal anesthesia.

A number of approaches are available for open surgical treatment of an osteochondral lesion of the talus. The incision has to be placed according to the site of the lesion. The surgical approach must take into account the superficial location of several nerves of the foot, which are particularly at risk owing to their subcutaneous location.

An anteromedial incision is used for lesions of the superomedial aspect of the talus. The skin incision is made over the medial malleolus and extended distally towards the superior medial aspect of the navicular (Figure 1). The anterior part of the deltoid ligament is incised and the ankle joint is inspected (Figure 2). Grooving of the distal tibia in order to improve access to an osteochondritic lesion has also been described, but this is rarely necessary. If adequate exposure of the talar lesion is not possible,

the medial malleolus is osteotomized at its base through a medial approach (Figures 1, 3) to allow full visualization of the talar neck, head and body. A crescentic osteotomy of the medial malleolus may give better exposure of the middle and posterior aspects of the medial margin of the talus [Wallen and Fallat 1989]. As an alternative dorsomedial approach, the deltoid ligament may be incised at its dorsal aspect to the tip of the medial malleolus and the calcaneus dorsalized by means of a distractor to realize a good approach to the dorsomedial aspect of the talus.

A standard anterolateral approach is used for lesions of the talus in an anterolateral location (Figure 1). The incision starts 6 cm above the ankle joint and continues along the anterior border of the fibula to the lateral cuneiform. The dorsal intermediate nerve must be identified and preserved. After transection of the extensor retinaculum and of the anterior talofibular ligament, the capsule of the ankle joint is incised.

Infrequently, a posterolateral incision is used for posterolateral lesions of the talus. This approach may be facilitated by fibular osteotomy. However, dorsiflexion and plantarflexion of the ankle usually expose the lesion adequately, and malleolar osteotomies are only rarely needed.

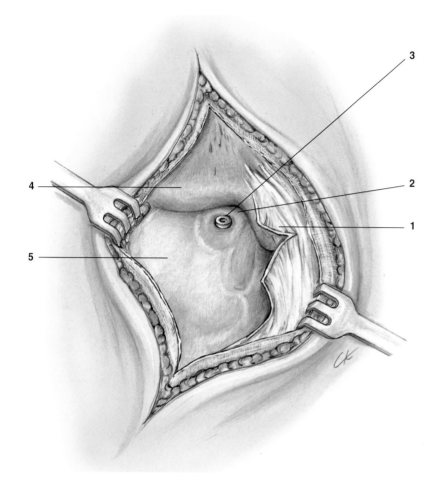

Figure 2

Anteromedial approach to the talus. Forced plantarflexion of the foot may be necessary to bring a dorsally located talar dome lesion into view. Following debridement and drilling a large talar fragment may be fixed with a screw

1 Deltoid ligament
2 Osteochondral lesion
3 Fixation screw
4 Tibia
5 Talus

After the appropriate incision of the skin and subcutaneous tissue, the capsular flaps are retracted to allow visualization of the articular surface around the osteochondritic lesion.

Methods for creating a fibrocartilage repair of the talar lesion

Traditional cartilage repair techniques try to stimulate a revascularization of the lesioned area by breaking up the subchondral bone with drilling, abrasion or microfracturing. The repair tissue will be fibrous cartilage with limited biomechanical proprieties.

Examination with a small probe reveals the presence and extent of attachment of the fragment to the talus, as well as the stage of the osteochondritic lesions. Thorough debridement of all necrotic cartilage and bone is performed. Softened cartilage with an intact surface should be left in place. To increase the vascularity in the area of the lesion, multiple holes through the sclerotic base are made with the 2.0-mm drill, at approximately 3–5-mm intervals and to a depth of 10 mm. If the articular cartilage over the osteochondritic lesion is still intact, drilling

may be performed retrogradely through the lateral or the medial aspect of the talus, and can even be computer-assisted [Fink et al. 2001]. Cystic lesions of the talus are filled with cancellous bone from the distal anterior tibia. If a fragment is large enough, i.e. at least 7 mm in diameter, it is re-attached to the talus with one or two small screws. Care must be taken to place the screw heads underneath the level of the articular surface. Alternatively, steel wires or absorbable pins may be used for fixation. These implants may be inserted retrogradely into the lesion, i.e. through the lateral aspect of the talus in a medial osteochondritic lesion.

The wound is closed in layers over a suction drain. The foot is placed in a well-padded dressing with a dorsal plaster splint. Compression of superficial nerves must be avoided.

Autologous osteochondral transplantation techniques

Poor biomechanical characteristics of the reparative fibrocartilage promoted by these traditional resurfacing techniques provide only moderate clinical

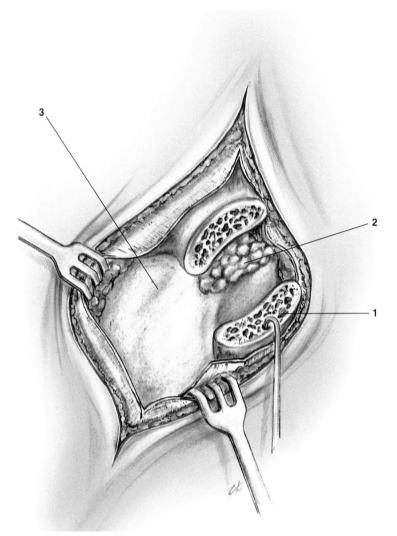

Figure 3

Medial approach to the talus. Temporary osteotomy of the medial malleolus is performed after drill holes for one or two 4.0 mm fixation screws were made

1 Medial malleolus (osteotomized)
2 Osteochondral lesion
3 Talus

outcome in the treatment of such lesions. Newer techniques try to provide a hyaline-like gliding surface for a full-thickness defected area on the weightbearing surface. These favored new methods are autologous osteochondral transplantation techniques, including osteochondral mosaicplasty, chondrocyte transplantation, periosteal and perichondrial resurfacing and allograft transplantation. According to the early and medium-term experiences of these methods it seems that a hyaline or hyaline-like resurfacing of the defect area can provide a more durable gliding surface and a better clinical outcome than the so-called 'traditional resurfacing techniques'.

Autologous osteochondral mosaicplasty

As an easy, one-step procedure providing relatively quick rehabilitation, autologous osteochondral mosaicplasty can be an alternative in the treatment

of small and medium-sized lesions. Excellent clinical outcome, low treatment costs and short rehabilitation time are the main advantages of this method [Hangody et al. 1997 and 1999, Schottle et al. 2001]. Cylindrical osteochondral grafts from the ipsilateral knee are transfered to the area of the lesion in the talar dome with specially designed tube chisels. These grafts taken at the non-weightbearing rim of the medial or lateral condyle of the knee have slightly larger diameters (0.15 mm) than the resected damaged grafts, to allow a good pressfit (Figure 4). The cartilage configuration of the graft should correspond to the anatomy of the talus.

Transplantation of osteochondral allografts

Transplantation of osteochondral allografts can be indicated for massive osteochondral lesions. There is less experience with the clinical use of periosteal

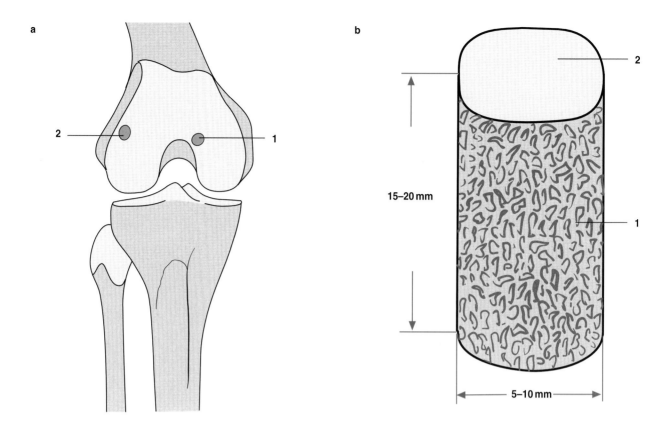

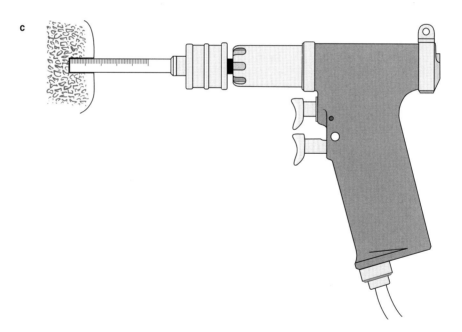

Figure 4

a. Osteochondral cylindrical grafts taken at the non-weightbearing area of the medial (1) or lateral condyle (2) of the knee have slightly larger diameters (0.15 mm) than the resected talar grafts to enable a good press-fit; b. lateral cross-section of an osteochondral cylindrical graft; c. specially designed cylindrical chisels are used to drill the damaged as well as the donor grafts. The diameter

and depth of the grafts are planned on the basis of MRI scans. The height and diameter of the graft have to match the volume and form of the resected graft. Here the normal dimensions are indicated

b
1 Bone
2 Cartilage

and perichondrial resurfacing techniques and biomaterials. Successful treatment of the full-thickness cartilage damage to the weightbearing surfaces depends not only on the method of cartilage repair but also on the treatment of the underlying cause. An effective treatment of full-thickness defects on the weightbearing surfaces requires careful patient selection, a complex operative plan and a well-organized treatment course [Hagody et al. 1999].

Autologous chondrocyte transplantation

Autologous chondrocyte transplantation seems to be a promising option in the treatment of larger full-thickness defects, but requires a relatively expensive two-step procedure and a longer rehabilitation period. Good or excellent long-term outcome results are reported after autologous chondrocyte transplantation of the knee [Peterson et al. 2000], but this does not yet exist for the talus.

Arthroscopy of the ankle joint

Smaller instruments and improved technology have made ankle arthroscopy a valuable technique for the diagnosis and treatment of osteochondral talar lesions, with good or excellent results in the hands of experienced surgeons [Ferkel et al. 1991, Ferkel 1996]. The main advantages of arthroscopy include good visualization, decreased morbidity, short hospitalization and early range of motion. However, the success of ankle arthroscopy depends largely on the expertise of the surgeon. Despite this fact, open surgical approaches are again more popular and used in the treatment of osteochondritic talar lesions for autologous osteochondral transplantation techniques [Seil et al. 2001].

Arthroscopy of the ankle allows direct visualization and palpation of the osteochondritic lesion (see Chapter 39). The base of the lesion can be perforated arthroscopically with a drill. In active individuals with detached lesions, excision, debridement and/or drilling is an effective treatment. The ability to drill arthroscopically significantly reduces the morbidity associated with open procedures. The use of an anterior cruciate ligament guide and the transmalleolar approach has been advocated to drill defects at the posteromedial aspect of the talar dome [Bryant and Siegel 1993].

The anterolateral and anteromedial portals are safe and are used to debride osteochondritic lesions. The posterolateral portal can be used to examine posterior talar lesions and to remove posterior loose bodies. If arthroscopy reveals an osteochondritic lesion which is suitable for arthroscopic screw fixation, this may be done either arthroscopically or by arthrotomy [Ferkel 1996].

Arthroscopy of the ankle joint permits complete examination of the intra-articular structures and may uncover other ankle disorders, such as impingement of soft tissues and of bone and loose bodies [Ferkel 1996]. The use of an ankle joint distractor is not usually necessary.

Surgical technique

The detailed technique is described in Chapter 39. Arthroscopic treatment of osteochondral lesions in particular includes the following:

1. Loose bodies and osteochondral fragments are removed.
2. The extent of cartilaginous softening is assessed by arthroscopic palpation.
3. Debridement is performed with various instruments such as a shaver, a mini-suction punch, curettes, graspers and scalpels.
4. Precise drilling (Figure 5a) and screw fixation of fragments (Figure 5b) can be performed through the standard arthroscopic portals and transmalleolarly.
5. Reversed bone cylinders may be used to fill an osteochondritic bone defect (Figure 6).
6. Autologous osteochondral mosaicplasty and autologous chondrocyte transplantation will be possible by arthroscopy.

Postoperative care

Postoperative treatment depends on the surgical procedure that was used. For patients treated by simple arthrotomy, curettage and drilling, temporary immobilization in a splint is recommended until wound healing occurs. The patient is then started on range-of-motion exercises without weightbearing for 6–8 weeks. The same protocol is used if an osteotomy of the medial malleolus was performed. No prolonged cast immobilization is required.

Following cancellous bone grafting of talar cysts and autologous condrocyte transplantation, weightbearing is not permitted for 3–6 months to allow the cancellous bone and the cartilage to integrate. Following internal fixation of talar dome fragments and after mosaicplasty, no weightbearing is permitted for 12 weeks. Relief of symptoms may take even

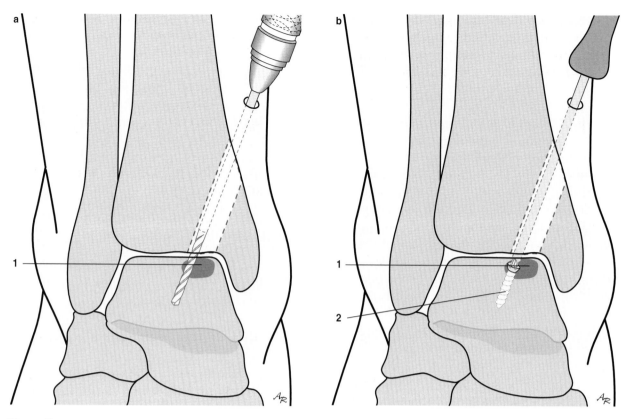

Figure 5

Arthroscopic transmalleolar approach: a. for drilling of a medial osteochondral lesion at the talus; b. for screw fixation of a large osteochondral fragment

a
1   Osteochondral lesion

b
1   Osteochondral lesion
2   Fixation screw

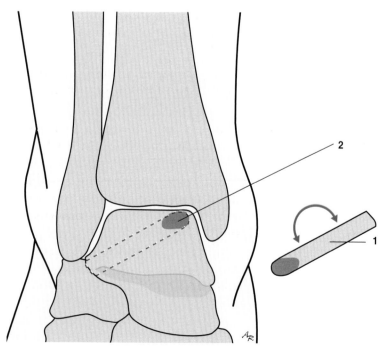

Figure 6

Reversed bone cylinder graft for an osteochondral lesion at the medial talar dome. A bone cylinder is removed from the talus with a cannulated drill and reinserted reversely, transplanting intact cancellous bone into the lesion

1   Reversed bone cylinder
2   Osteochondral lesion

longer, and bony union or fragment revascularization may be demonstrated radiographically only after several months. Fixation screws should be removed arthroscopically after 1–2 years.

Complications

Nerve lesions may result from inadequate handling of the soft tissues. There are multiple variants of nerve anatomy. Therefore, the initial incision must be made only through the skin but not through the subcutaneous tissue, where the nerves are located. Cautery must not be employed indiscriminately and blunt retractors should be used. Nerves may also become entrapped in the subcutaneous or skin sutures. The same diligence must be used when closing the wound as during the incision.

Non-union of the medial malleolus may result from inadequate fixation of the osteotomy. It is recommended to drill two holes prior to the osteotomy and to use two 4.0-mm cancellous screws for fixation.

With autologous osteochondral transplants, problems of transplant stability and congruency may occur.

References

Alexander AH, Lichtman DM (1980) Surgical treatment of transchondral talar-dome fractures (osteochondritis dissecans). Long-term follow-up. J Bone Joint Surg 62A: 646–652

Anderson IF, Crichton KJ, Grattan-Smith T et al. (1989) Osteochondral fractures of the dome of the talus. J Bone Joint Surg 71A: 1143–1152

Angermann P, Jensen P (1989) Osteochondritis dissecans of the talus: long-term results of surgical treatment. Foot Ankle 10: 161–163

Assenmacher JA, Kelikian AS, Gottlob C, Kodros S (2001) Arthroscopically assisted autologous osteochondral transplantation for osteochondral lesions of the talar dome: an MRI and clinical follow-up study. Foot Ankle Int 22: 544–551

Berndt AL, Harty M (1959) Transchondral fractures (osteochondritis dissecans of the talus). J Bone Joint Surg 41A: 988–1020

Bruns J, Rosenbach B, Kahrs J (1992) Etiopathogenetic aspects of medial osteochondrosis dissecans tali. Sportverl Sportschaden 6: 43–49

Bryant DD, Siegel MG (1993) Osteochondritis dissecans of the talus: a new technique for arthroscopic drilling. Arthroscopy 9: 238–241

De Smet AA, Fisher DR, Burnstein MI et al. (1990) Value of MR imaging in staging osteochondral lesions of the talus (osteochondritis dissecans): results in 14 patients. Am J Roentgenol 154: 555–558

Ferkel RD (1996) Arthroscopic Surgery of the Foot and Ankle. Philadelphia, Lippincott Raven

Ferkel RD, Karzel RP, DelPizzo W (1991) Arthroscopic treatment of the anterolateral impingement of the ankle. Am J Sports Med 19: 440

Fink C, Rosenberger RE, Bale RJ et al. (2001) Computer-assisted retrograde drilling of osteochondral lesions of the talus. Orthopäde 30: 59–65

Hangody L, Kish G, Karpati Z et al. (1997) Treatment of osteochondritis dissecans of the talus: use of the mosaicplasty technique – a preliminary report. Foot Ankle Int 18: 628–634

Hangody L, Sukosd L, Szabo Z (1999) Repair of cartilage defects. Technical aspects. Rev Chir Orthop Réparatrice Appar Mot 85: 846–857

Hepple S, Winson IG, Glew D (1999) Osteochondral lesions of the talus: a revised classification. Foot Ankle Int 20: 789–793

Nelson DW, DiPaola J, Colville M, Schmidgall J (1990) Osteochondritis dissecans of the talus and knee: prospective comparison of MR and arthroscopic classifications. J Comput Assist Tomogr 14: 804–808

Peterson L, Minas T, Brittberg M et al. (2000) Two- to 9-year outcome after autologous chondrocyte transplantation of the knee. Clin Orthop Rel Res 374: 212–234

Pritsch M, Horoshovsky H, Farine I (1986) Arthroscopic treatment of osteochondral lesions of the talus. J Bone Joint Surg 68A: 862–865

Schottle PB, Oett GM, Agneskirchner JD, Imhoff AB (2001) Operative therapy of osteochondral lesions of the talus with autologous cartilage–bone transplantation. Orthopäde 30: 53–58

Seil R, Rupp S, Pape D et al. (2001) Approach to open treatment of osteochondral lesions of the talus. Orthopäde 30: 47–52

Struijs PA, Tol JL, Bossuyt PM et al. (2001) Treatment strategies in osteochondral lesions of the talus. Review of the literature. Orthopäde 30: 28–36

Wallen EA, Fallat LM (1989) Crescentic transmalleolar osteotomy for optimal exposure of the medial talar dome. J Foot Surg 28: 389–394

36

Surgical treatment of anterior and posterior impingement of the ankle

Michael M. Stephens

Introduction

Anterior tibiotalar impingement spurs were first described in 1943 [Morris 1943] and the term 'athlete's ankle' was used for this condition. It was also referred to as 'footballer's ankle', and good results from excision of the spurs have been reported [McMurray 1950]. Since then it has been described in many athletes who use repetitive and forceful dorsiflexion movements of the ankle, and is now usually termed 'anterior impingement syndrome' [O'Donoghue 1957, Brodelius 1960, Parkes et al. 1980, Parisien 1991].

The association with narrowing of the anterior joint space and midtarsal changes suggests that anterior spurs may be part of an early degenerative process [McDougall 1955, O'Donoghue 1957, Brodelius 1960].

The clinical features of anterior impingement are pain and limitation of movement when the ankle is dorsiflexed. This is often localized to the anterolateral or anteromedial side of the joint. Lateral weightbearing radiographs in neutral, dorsiflexion and plantarflexion should clearly show a bony spur or osteophyte on the anterior aspect of the tibia, with a corresponding 'kissing' spur on the superior aspect of the talus. These are more likely to arise from the tibia if they are lateral and from the talus if they are medial (Berberian et al. 2001). With the foot in a neutral position the angle between the bevel of the anterior tibia and the neck of the talus should be 60° [Coker 1991]. Anterior impingement of the ankle produces an osteochondral ridge on the anterior tibia, and the bevel is lost. Injection of local anesthetic solution into the area can help to confirm the diagnosis. Rest, physiotherapy, anti-inflammatory medication or local steroid injection, and heel lift should be used initially. When a conservative program fails, surgery is indicated. Posterior impingement, which is also called 'talar compression syndrome', is a painful condition at the back of the ankle. It results from compression of the capsule and synovial membrane between the lower tibia and the upper surface of the calcaneus during repeated and forceful plantarflexion of the foot. The onset is usually gradual. The source of pressure can be a fused posterior tubercle, also called Steida's process when elongated, or an unfused posterior ossicle, known as os trigonum [Marotta and Micheli 1992]. This disorder is often seen in classical ballet dancers [DiRaimondo 1991, Wredmark et al. 1991, Hamilton et al. 1996, Van Dijk and Marti 1999].

The clinical features of posterior impingement are pain and limitation of movement when the ankle is plantarflexed and when jumping in sports or walking downstairs. This impingement can mimic flexor hallucis longus tendinitis, but in the latter symptoms tend to be more medial. However, the two conditions can coexist [Hamilton 1982]. Technetium bone scanning can be useful to confirm the diagnosis. Injection of local anesthetic solution into the posterior ankle capsule can help confirm the diagnosis with complete relief of pain. Initial treatment involves minimizing plantarflexion of the foot. If conservative treatment with rest, physiotherapy, anti-inflammatory medication, low heels and local steroid injection fail, surgery is indicated. Open techniques are safe and useful [Hedrick and McBryde 1994].

Open excision of the anterior tibial and talar spurs was first described in 1950 [McMurray 1950]. Since then, others have also reported good results from open excision [O'Donoghue 1957, Brodelius 1960, Parkes et al. 1980, Hawkins 1988]. Arthroscopic removal of the spurs [Branca et al. 1997, Tol et al. 2001] carries a low risk of infection and faster rehabilitation, but long-term results are the same as with an open technique [Coull et al. 2003].

Infection in ankle portals is higher than in the knee [D'Angelo and Ogilvie-Harris 1988, Ferkel and Fischer 1989, Barber et al. 1990, Ogilvie-Harris et al. 1993]. Prophylactic antibiotics have therefore been recommended [D'Angelo and Ogilvie-Harris 1988].

Anterior ankle impingement may be graded I to IV, according to the size of the spurs and the degree of involvement of the ankle (Figure 1) [Scranton and McDermott 1992]. Grade I is synovial impingement and tibial spurs of less than 3 mm. Grade II is an osteochondral reaction exostosis; radiographs show spurs greater than 3 mm with none on the talus. Grade III is the same as for grade II, with spur formation on the dorsum of the neck of the talus. There is often fragmentation of the osteophytes. Grade IV is pan-talocrural osteoarthritic change: radiographs suggest osteoarthritic changes medially and laterally and posteriorly with narrowing of the whole joint space.

Treatment and recovery were shown to correlate with the grade [Scranton and McDermott 1992]. Grades I, II and III spurs are suitable for resection arthroscopically or by arthrotomy. However, patients who are managed arthroscopically recover in a shorter time than those with an arthrotomy. The range of movement returns earlier after the former, but on long-term follow-up both have the same range. Grade IV disease is not treated by debridement as the whole joint is involved. Arthrodesis is the treatment when all conservative measures fail.

The duration of hospitalization, postoperative recovery and rehabilitation, and the size of the operative scars, are reported to be the only major differences between the arthrotomy and the arthroscopy groups [Scranton and McDermott 1992]. Recent papers suggest that soft-tissue impingement alone can cause anterior impingement symptoms as the synovium is sucked into the joint on dorsiflexion either anterolaterally [Akseki et al. 1999] or anteromedially [Mosier-La Clair et al. 2000]. These could therefore be graded as grade 0, and arthroscopic resection is the treatment of choice. Magnetic resonance imaging (MRI) can confirm this diagnosis [Jordan et al. 2000].

Treatment

Surgical intervention is indicated when conservative measures have failed in the treatment of anterior and posterior impingement syndromes. In cases of anterior impingement, the ankle joint should initially be explored arthroscopically. If the osteophytes are deemed too large to resect arthroscopically, then open arthrotomy is indicated. Initial arthroscopic exploration allows the surgeon to identify on which side of the ankle joint to make the arthrotomy incision. Posterior impingement is best treated safely with open arthrotomy, where assessment of the talar dome can be carried out at the same time.

Arthroscopic technique for anterior impingement

Ankle arthroscopy can be performed as day-case surgery, under regional or general anesthesia. The patient is positioned supine on the operating table with a tourniquet at thigh level. The appropriate leg is prepared and draped. A needle is inserted just lateral to the peroneus tertius tendon and the ankle is inflated with 15–20 ml of saline. A small, longitudinal skin incision is made. Deep dissection prevents soft-tissue damage. Use of a hemostat allows a 4.5-mm, 30° angled arthroscope to be inserted through an anterolateral portal (see Chapter 37). Care is taken to pass the arthroscope across the anterior aspect of the joint and not across the dome of the talus. A separate anteromedial portal is made

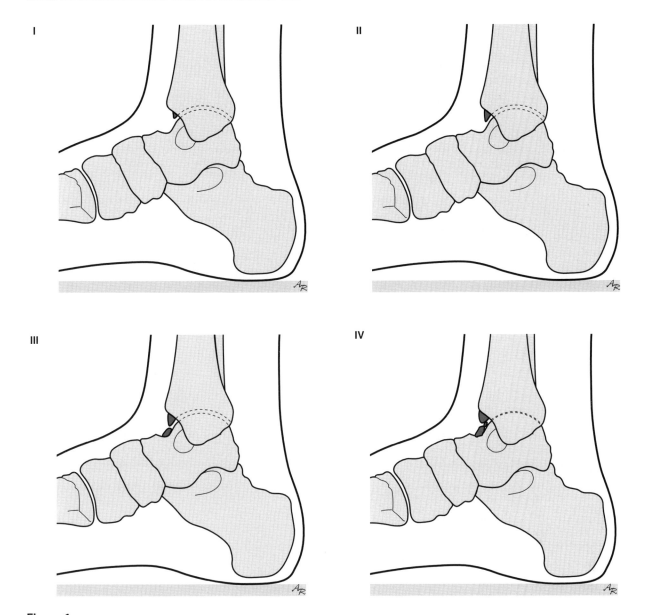

Figure 1

Grading of anterior ankle spurs [Scranton and McDermott 1992]

just medial to the tibialis anterior tendon to allow inflow and outflow of saline (see Chapter 37). Instruments are inserted through the anteromedial portal. A synovator is used to clear the anterior synovium and to define the anterior tibial and superior talar bony spurs. Burrs can then be used to remove the spurs, resecting back until the normal cortical bone of the anterior tibia can be seen. This can be easily distinguished from the soft cancellous bone of the spur, and the tibial surface is smoothed off using the 3.5-mm full radius resector. Resection back to normal-looking articular cartilage produces the 'coconut meat' sign (Figure 2). The osteophyte on the superior neck of the talus is then removed. Finally, the anterior ankle joint is inspected and is

put through its range of motion to confirm complete resection. After the operation and a thorough washout, 10 ml of 0.2% bupivacaine is instilled into the joint and the incisions are sutured. A below-knee cast is usually applied with the foot in plantigrade position, particularly after large resections.

Open technique

The open arthrotomy can be performed under regional or general anesthesia, with a tourniquet. The patient is positioned supine with a sandbag under the ipsilateral buttock. The decision as to whether the approach is anterolateral or anteromedial (Figure 3)

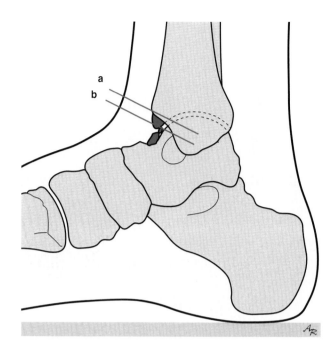

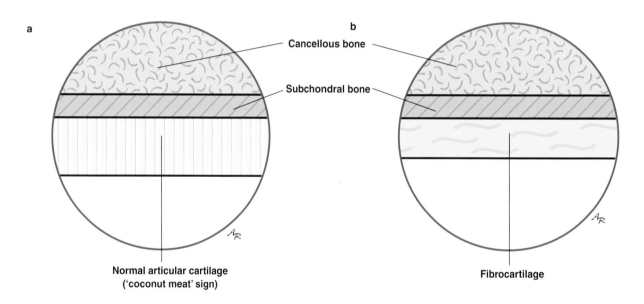

Cancellous bone

Subchondral bone

Normal articular cartilage
('coconut meat' sign)

Fibrocartilage

Figure 2

Tangential transections through anterior impinging spur. a. normal articular cartilage ('coconut meat' sign); b. fibrocartilage

is based on clinical symptoms and signs and radiographs, and on arthroscopic findings. The tourniquet is deflated at the time of closure to allow cautery of bleeding points.

Anterior impingement

The arthrotomy for anterior impingement can be carried out from either the anterolateral approach

between the peroneus tertius and the long extensor tendons (Figure 4), or anteromedially, medial to the tibialis anterior tendon. A 3-cm longitudinal incision is made, avoiding the veins. Anterolaterally the superficial peroneal nerve and anteromedially the saphenous nerve must be avoided. Straight 5-mm and 7-mm osteotomes are used for spur resection. It is important to resect the osteophytes to restore normal anatomy, i.e. the normal anterior tibial bevel and back to normal articular cartilage (coconut

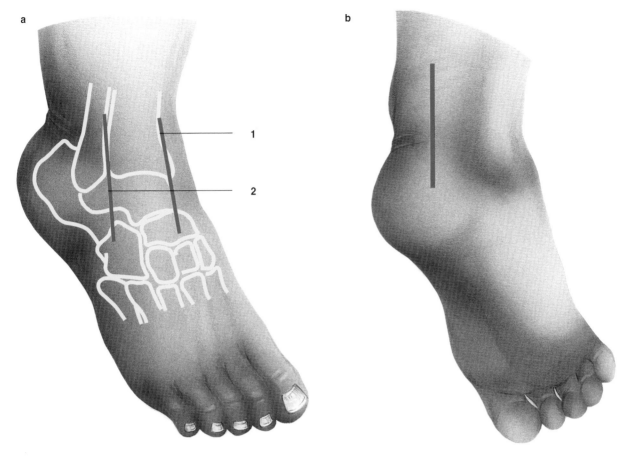

Figure 3

Open spur resection. a. anteromedial and anterolateral incisions; b. posterolateral incision

1 Anteromedial incision
2 Anterolateral incision

meat sign) (Figure 2). Once the impingement is resected, the ankle joint is irrigated and inspected for additional pathology, e.g. osteochondritis dissecans and talar articular damage. Closure is in layers over a drain. A soft dressing is applied, and usually a cast or a walker boot is used for 2 weeks, particularly if the resection was extensive and to lessen the chance of a synovial fistula.

Posterior impingement

The patient is best positioned prone with a jelly roll across the end of the operating table at the level of the ankle so that the toes are allowed to hang free. This facilitates exposure of the ankle joint by ankle dorsiflexion. The arthrotomy for posterior impingement can be carried out either lateral or medial to the Achilles tendon, thus the neurovascular bundle lying medially or the sural nerve lying laterally can be retracted anteriorly (see Figure 3). Deep dissection is through the fat pad to the

posterior joint (Figure 5). The flexor hallucis longus muscle belly is identified and its tendon sheath incised. This allows the tendon to be retracted medially for complete exposure of the posterior tibial and talar margin. The capsule is opened longitudinally and the large posterior process or os trigonum is then excised back to normal talar articular cartilage. Osteotomes and rongeurs are used. The tourniquet is released prior to closure. Closure is in layers using absorbable sutures. A soft dressing is applied, and a cast or a walker boot is used for 2 weeks, with weightbearing as tolerated.

Postoperative care

Patients are allowed to take full weight as tolerated. After 2 weeks the plaster cast is removed and a rigorous rehabilitation program is started which includes ice packs with both active and passive range of motion exercises. A balance (wobble)

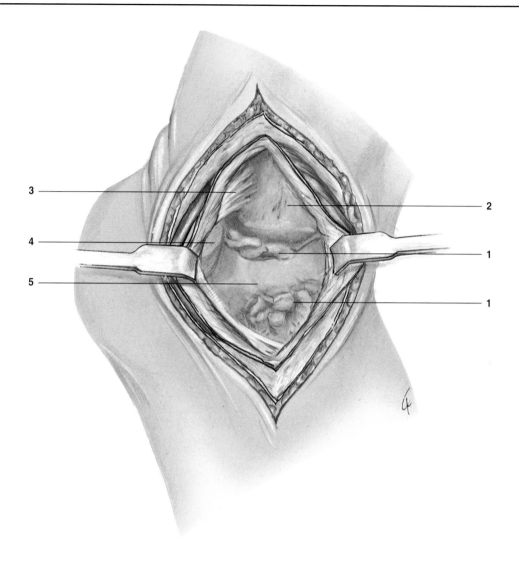

Figure 4

Anterolateral exposure of grade IV anterior impingement of the ankle

1 Spur
2 Tibia
3 Anterior tibiofibular syndesmosis
4 Fibula
5 Talus

board is used for proprioceptive training, and the anterior and posterior muscles of the calf and foot are strengthened. Return to training is encouraged after 6 weeks in a paced accelerated program, with appropriate footwear. High-level competitive contact sports and training can be commenced 3 months from surgery.

Complications

Most arthroscopic complications can be avoided if the surgeon becomes thoroughly familiar with the anatomy of the region [Barber et al. 1990] but the complication rate may be as high as 10% [Ferkel and

Fischer 1989]. However, with careful attention to anatomical structures, this rate can be reduced. The most common complication is neurological, involving the superficial peroneal nerve, the sural nerve or the saphenous nerve [Ogilvie-Harris et al. 1993].

Neurological and arterial damage have also been reported with the use of an anterocentral portal and a posteromedial portal, as well as with the use of distraction pins. This damage can be caused by placement of the pins or instruments through the portal or by powered cutting shavers used during the procedure.

Infection, phlebitis and complex regional pain syndrome can occur postoperatively, as they can after any operative procedure.

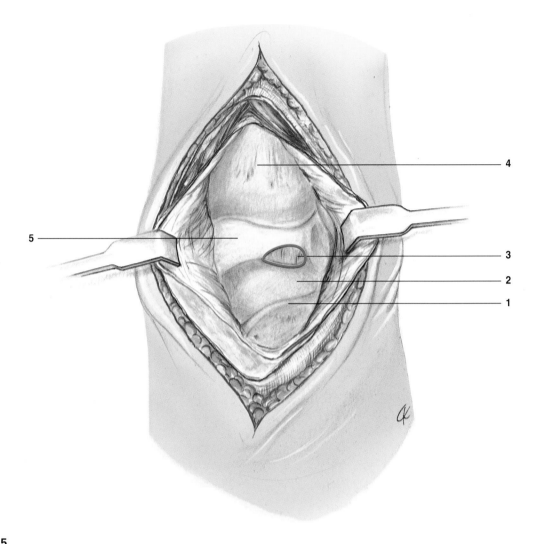

Figure 5

Posterolateral exposure in posterior impingement of the ankle, with the area excised at the site of the os trigonum

1 Subtalar joint
2 Talus
3 Excised area of os trigonum
4 Tibia
5 Talar dome

In open arthrotomy, neurovascular structures can be visualized and protected. However, careful exposure in layers and its repair with 2 weeks of immobilization is advised, to prevent synovial fistula formation.

References

Akseki D, Pinar H, Bozkurt M et al. (1999) The distal fascicle of the anterior inferior tibio-fibular ligament is a cause of anterolateral ankle impingement: results of arthroscopic resection. Acta Orthop Scand 70: 478–482

Barber FA, Click J, Britt BT (1990) Complications of ankle arthroscopy. Foot Ankle 10: 263–266

Berberian WS, Hecht PJ, Wapner KL, DiVerniero R, (2001) Morphology of tibiotalar osteophytes in anterior ankle impingement. Foot Ankle Int 22: 313–317

Branca A, DiPalma L, Bucca C et al. (1997) Arthroscopic treatment of anterior ankle impingement. Foot Ankle Int 18: 418–423

Brodelius A (1960) Osteoarthritis of the talar joints in footballers and ballet dancers. Acta Orthop Scand 30: 309–314

Coker TP (1991) Sports injuries to the foot and ankle. In: Jahss MH (ed) Disorders of the Foot and Ankle: Medical and Surgical Management, 2nd edn. Philadelphia, WB Saunders, pp 2438–2340

Coull R, Raffiy T, James LE, Stephens MM (2003) Open treatment of anterior impingement of the ankle. J Bone Joint Surg 85B: 550–553

D'Angelo GL, Ogilvie-Harris DJ (1988) Septic arthritis following arthroscopy with cost/benefit analysis of antibiotic prophylaxis. Arthroscopy 4: 10–14

DiRaimondo C (1991) Overuse conditions of the foot and ankle. In: Sammarco GJ (ed) Foot and Ankle Manual. Philadelphia, Lea & Febiger, pp 269–270

Ferkel RD, Fischer SP (1989) Progress in ankle arthroscopy. Clin Orthop 240: 210–220

Hamilton WG (1982) Stenosing tenosynovitis of the flexor hallucis longus tendon and posterior impingement upon the os trigonum in ballet dancers. Foot Ankle 3: 74–80

Hamilton WG, Geppert MJ, Thompson FM (1996) Pain in the posterior aspect of the ankle in dancers: different diagnosis and operative treatment. J Bone Joint Surg 78A: 1491–1500

Hawkins RB (1988) Arthroscopic treatment of sports-related anterior osteophytes in the ankle. Foot Ankle 9: 87–90

Hedrick MR, McBryde AM (1994) Posterior ankle impingement. Foot Ankle Int 15: 2–8

Jordan LK 3rd, Helms CA, Cooperman AE, Speer KP (2000) Magnetic resonance imaging findings in anterolateral impingement of the ankle. Skeletal Radiol 29: 34–39

Marotta JJ, Micheli LJ (1992) Os trigonum impingement in dancers. Am J Sports Med 20: 533–536

McDougall A (1955) Footballer's ankle. Lancet 2: 1219–1220

McMurray TP (1950) Footballer's ankle. J Bone Joint Surg 32B: 68–69

Morris LH (1943) Athlete's ankle. J Bone Joint Surg 25: 220

Mosier-La Clair SM, Monroe MT, Manoli A (2000) Medial impingement syndrome of the anterior tibiotalar fascicle of the deltoid ligament of the talus. Foot Ankle Int 21: 385–391

O'Donoghue DH (1957) Impingement exostoses of the talus and tibia. J Bone Joint Surg 39A: 835–852

Ogilvie-Harris DJ, Mahomed N, Demaziere A (1993) Anterior impingement of the ankle treated by arthroscopic removal of bony spurs. J Bone Joint Surg 75B: 437–440

Parisien JS (1991) Arthroscopic surgery in osteocartilaginous lesions of the ankle. In: McGinty JB (ed) Operative Arthroscopy. New York, Raven Press, pp 739–741

Parkes JC, Hamilton WG, Patterson AH, Rawles JG (1980) The anterior impingement syndrome of the ankle. J Trauma 20: 895–898

Scranton PE Jr, McDermott JE (1992) Anterior tibiotalar spurs: a comparison of open versus arthroscopic debridement. Foot Ankle 13: 125–129

Tol JL, Verheyen CP, Van Dijk CN (2001) Arthroscopic treatment of anterior, impingement in the ankle joint. J Bone Joint Surg Br 83: 9–13

Van Dijk CN, Marti RK (1999) Traumatic, post traumatic and over use injuries in ballet: with special emphasis on the foot and ankle. Foot Ankle Surg 5: 1–8

Wredmark T, Carlstedt CA, Bauer H, Saartok T (1991) Os trigonum syndrome: a clinical entity in ballet dancers. Foot Ankle 11: 404–406

37

Ankle arthroscopy

Ian Winson

Introduction

Ankle arthroscopy has progressed from a technique with limited indications and a perception of technical difficulty to the point where it is becoming a required part of the armamentarium to treat foot and ankle conditions. The development of surgical techniques, equipment and clinical understanding has advanced to allow the more widespread use of ankle arthroscopy as a treatment modality. The aim of this chapter is to provide a basic guide to these improved techniques and provide an insight into their use for a variety of conditions.

Ankle arthroscopy as a diagnostic and treatment tool had its origins with Burman in 1931 [Burman 1931]. It progressed slowly, especially compared with knee and shoulder arthroscopy [Small 1986]. This was largely a function of the available equipment and the slow advancement in surgical technique. With an increased appreciation of the requirements of modern ankle arthroscopy and an improved understanding of the pathology accessible, ankle arthroscopy has become an extremely valuable therapeutic tool [Baker and Graham 1993]. With these improvements has come an increasing willingness to utilize arthroscopic techniques for an expanding list of indications. The justification of its continued use in some of these conditions lags behind current usage, owing to a lack of outcome research. Increasing numbers of controlled studies and long-term outcomes being published are addressing this imbalance.

Indications

Arthroscopy has amongst its most common indications the sequelae of the unstable ankle. The assessment and treatment of the unstable ankle in the sporting population and its associated conditions has been measurably improved by the use of ankle arthroscopy [Meislin et al. 1993, Ogilvie-Harris et al. 1997].

Evaluation is aided by a careful examination under anesthesia and diagnostic arthroscopy of the lateral and medial gutter with visualization of the ligamentous insertions. Ligament hypertrophy causing soft-tissue impingement can be treated arthroscopically [Mosier-La Clair et al. 2000]. Injuries to the tibio-fibular syndesmosis can also be adequately assessed and the resultant synovitis and hypertrophy treated [Takao et al. 2001, Pritsch et al. 1993]. Impingement lesions take several forms [Liu and Mirzayan 1993, Pritsch et al. 1993, Mosier-La Clair et al. 2000, Tol et al. 2001], but consist of fibrotic scarring with synovitis. The term 'meniscoid lesion' has been coined for synovial thickening in the lateral gutter. Anterior tibiotalar osteophytic impingement secondary to trauma has been defined and classified. The morphology of these impingement lesions has been further expanded with the identification of reproducible osteophytes on the medial malleolus and anterior fibula [Scranton and McDermott 1992, 2000]. Synovial impingement in the early stages responds well to arthroscopic debridement, with good to excellent results ranging from 70 to 90%. Arthroscopic resection of bony anterior talar or tibial osteophytes has shown sustainable symptomatic benefit and a faster recovery time compared to open techniques, despite some recurrence over time [Tol et al. 2001]. Posterior synovial impingement has also been reported to respond to arthroscopic debridement [Chaytor and Conti 1998, Liu and Mirzayan 1993].

There is considerable radiological and arthroscopic evidence of a high incidence of chondral and osteochondral injury with ankle ligament ruptures [Ogilvie-Harris et al. 1997, Hinterman et al. 2002]. Persistent symptomatology can be accurately diagnosed and treated with arthroscopic intervention.

Osteochondritis desiccans can also be assessed and treated regardless of etiology. Management options depend on site, size and staging. Adjunctive magnetic resonance imaging (MRI) helps elucidate subchondral cysts and gives an indication of stability, but arthroscopic examination is the ultimate way of assessing joint surface integrity [Hepple et al. 1999]. Treatment options include debridement of both cartilage and subchondral bone, fixation, retrograde and antegrade drilling, removal of loose bodies, and more recently bone and osteochondral grafting and chondrocyte transplantation.

Arthroscopy has also been used as an adjunctive tool to assess the accuracy of reduction of intra-articular fractures around the ankle. Chondral and osteochondral damage can be addressed at this time [Thordarson et al. 2001, Loren and Ferkel 2002]. Post-traumatic and idiopathic osteoarthritis presents the options of debridement of both bony and articular abnormalities [van Dijk et al. 1997].

In painful degenerative or inflammatory arthritis, arthroscopic ankle arthrodesis may be indicated. Previously correction of angular or rotational deformity by arthroscopic means was suggested as being minimal, and therefore open techniques have been used. Although caution is advised for deformities with 10° or more of varus or valgus, correction is achievable via the arthroscopic method. Arthroscopic techniques reduce the problems of wound healing which are common after traditional techniques, and the time to union may be faster [Myerson and Quill 1991, O'Brien et al. 1999]. In an area where post-traumatic arthritis predominates, with the implications of extensive soft-tissue damage, the limited incisions of an arthroscopic technique are invaluable.

Pure synovial abnormalities and tumorous conditions can also be addressed arthroscopically. Synovial chondromatosis, pigmented villonodular synovitis, inflammatory arthritides and post-traumatic synovitis can all be treated. Osteoid osteoma and acute pyarthrosis have responded to arthroscopic lavage and synovectomy in addition to antibiotic treatment [Parisien and Schaffer 1992].

Problem areas

Arthroscopy of the ankle has specific problems that are uniquely attributable to its anatomy and the pathology that affects it. The increasing number of indications for its use have brought with it a greater responsibility to investigate fully and appreciate both intra- and extra-articular pathology. A structured approach with careful history taking and examination is advised, to ensure that pathology can be identified and an approach used that facilitates the most appropriate treatment.

Certain types of ankle present a greater challenge to adequate visualization and instrumentation. Post-traumatic scarring and fibrosis can limit distraction and persistent anterior synovitis may obscure view. Again an appreciation of the underlying diagnosis can prepare the surgeon for potential problems that may be encountered.

Anatomically the ankle joint has specific inherent problems. The talar dome is curved and thus special curved instruments or supplementary portals may need to be used. Neurovascular structures pass close to all portals used; therefore anatomical landmarks need to be identified and care taken with the establishment, use and closure of portals [Ferkel et al. 1996].

Contraindications to ankle arthroscopy exist. Overlying soft-tissue infection may introduce infection to a healthy joint. RSD, vascular compromise and significant edema present relative contraindications. Invasive traction is also relatively contraindicated in these groups, as also in high-performance athletes and patients with open physes.

Technique

Power instruments are obligatory to avoid multiple instrument passage, which wastes time and increases the risk of neurovascular complications, but care must be taken in their use. Anterior synovitis is common and a partial anterior synovectomy is often required as it aids view, regardless of pathology. A range of soft-tissue resectors ranging from 2.9 to 4.2 mm in diameter are required. The treatment of chondral lesions, osteophyte resection and arthrodesis requires burrs of sizes varying from 2.9 to 4 mm and shapes from ball tip to barrel. The commonest sizes used for standard arthroscopy are a 3.5-mm soft-tissue resector and a 3.5-mm ball-tipped burr. To accommodate the variety of convex and concave surfaces, some of the available instruments are semi-flexible and in some cases can be pre-bent to aid access to lesions on the convex surface of the talus. Standard smaller arthroscopic instruments can be used in most cases. Instrumentation in the medial and lateral gutter may require the use of small joint instruments, particularly in the younger patient.

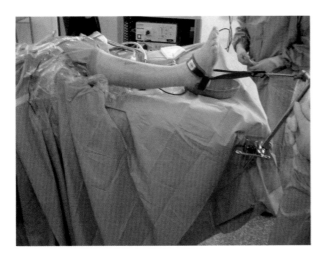

Figure 1

Standard set-up for the supine patient

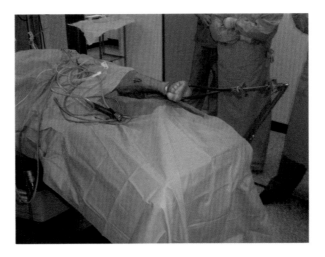

Figure 2

Set-up for patient in lateral decubitus position

Small osteotomes, straight and right-angled small curettes, hooks and angulated awls are particularly helpful in the treatment of osteochondral and chondral abnormalities. Small suckers can be useful in retrieving loose bodies.

Ankle distraction in some form is required in most cases. Non-invasive traction can be applied manually by an assistant or via a sling around the ankle. The surgeon can regulate traction by flexing the knee over the end of the table and applying traction by means of foot pressure through a stirrup attached to a foot sling. Both these methods are unreliable in sustaining traction for longer procedures.

Invasive skeletal distraction can be applied by several methods. The Charnley compression clamp in reverse, other external fixation systems and the AO Femoral distraction require tibial and calcaneal pins. Manderson et al. [1994] and Kumar and Satku [1994] described a technique using the standard fracture table and a calcaneal pin, thereby eliminating the need for a tibial pin. More recently, fine wire, circular frame fixations have been used. These techniques allow the controlled application of distraction force without the risk to skin from a sling, have the potential to overdistract, which may be a disadvantage. Electrophysiological and cadaveric studies have shown ligament injury and reversible disturbances in nerve conduction at forces greater than 135 N for over an hour [Albert et al. 1992, Dowdy et al. 1996]. In addition, neurovascular injury, pin-site infection or fracture and restricted access to portals have been reported subsequent to use of these techniques.

Our preference is the use of a modified clove-hitch sling attached to a distraction device fitted to the table. This enables free access to anterior and posterior portals, applies a constant distraction force that can be altered, and is easily removed for access to the anterior fossa. Using this technique, distraction up to 5 mm can be easily sustained.

Although tourniquet use is not universal it is advisable, particularly during early experience. Several fluid delivery systems are available that are controlled by either pressure or flow. Our preference is for a system that maintains a constant pressure with control over excessive flow. This decreases problems with bleeding and air bubbles. Suction applied via power instrumentation functions best at approximately 50% of normal wall pressure.

Accessory equipment includes an image intensifier, especially in arthrodesis and when contemplating drilling of osteochondral defects with subchondral cysts. Bone biopsy trocars, cannulated drills and drill guides are helpful in bone grafting of such cysts.

Patient preparation and positioning

Preoperative diagnosis may influence patient position. The posterolateral portal is accessible while the patient is supine, but if it is anticipated that there will be significant posterior recess pathology, a lateral decubitus position may be advisable. In a supine position a thigh support large enough to allow suspension of the lower leg is used. The distraction arm is fixed to the side of the table, and the ankle is suspended via a clove-hitch-type sling. Traction is applied by breaking the end of the table. This often necessitates a slightly head-down position (Figure 1). If using the lateral decubitus position a similar technique applies, with the distraction arm on the side facing forward (Figure 2).

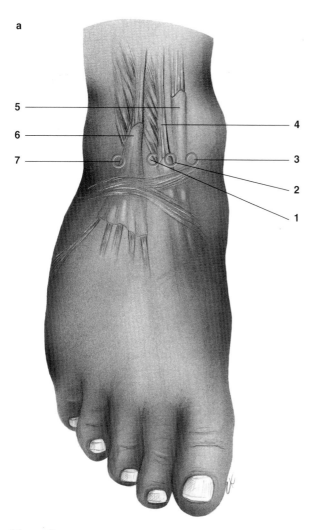

Figure 3

Entry portals for ankle arthroscopy. a. anterior aspect; b. posterior aspect

a
1 Anterior midline portal
2 Additional anterior portal
3 Anterior medial portal
4 Extensor hallucis longus
5 Tibialis anterior
6 Extensor digitorum longus
7 Anterior lateral portal

b
1 Posterior midline portal
2 Sural nerve
3 Lateral malleolus
4 Peroneal tendons
5 Posterolateral portal
6 Achilles tendon
7 Posteromedial portal
8 Flexor tendons
9 Neurovascular bundle

Entry portals

The most commonly used portals are anteromedial/anterolateral and posterolateral. An understanding of anatomy, plus several cadaveric studies, have proved these to be the safest and most amenable for a good visual field and easy access to pathology. The anteromedial portal lies medial to the tibialis anterior and poses the least threat to neurovascular structures. The structures at risk are the saphenous nerve and vein. The anterolateral portal is lateral to the extensor digitorum communis on either side of the peroneus tertius as dictated by the branches of the superficial nerve (Figure 3a). The posterolateral portal is situated posterior to the lateral malleolus and peroneal tendons. An 18-gauge needle directed anterior and medial, aiming to enter the joint medial to the transverse tibiofibular ligament, is useful in establishing the portal. The sural nerve and small saphenous vein are at risk from this approach (Figure 3b). Supplementary anterior portals have also been described. The anterocentral portal has

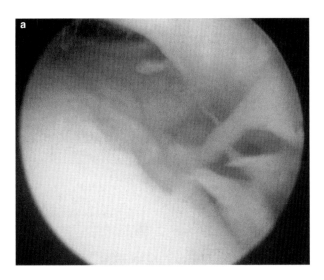

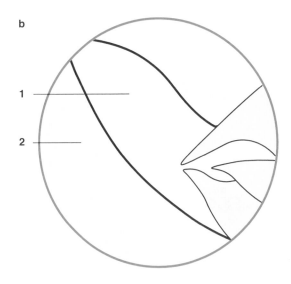

Figure 4

Anterior gutter through anterolateral portal of right ankle. a. arthroscopic view; b. schematic representation

1 Talar neck
2 Talus

traditionally been associated with the potential for damage to the neurovascular bundle [Feiwell and Frey 1993]. Its advantages lie in improved access to both the medial and the lateral gutters and has routinely been described as being lateral to the extensor hallucis longus (EHL) tendon. By moving this portal medially between the EHL tendon and the tibialis anterior, the same benefits of access are imparted with a lower incidence of damage to anterior structures (Figure 3a) [Buckingham et al. 1997].

Further posterior portals, both medial and trans-Achilles, have also been described [Voto et al. 1989]. The posteromedial portal has the disadvantage of its close proximity to the neurovascular bundle and flexor tendon group and is therefore used sparingly. The trans-Achilles portal has the disadvantage of intra-tendinous damage and has limited use (Figure 3b).

Rarely a transmalleolar portal may be advocated for access to osteochondral lesions for therapeutic intervention. In our experience this is unneccessary and carries a risk of subsequent stress fracture.

In establishing all portals, damage to underlying structures is minimized by using a needle to establish position, incising the skin and using a small pair of scissors or hemostat to dissect soft tissue and puncture the capsule and synovium. The initial portal is established after pre-infusion of up to 20 ml of normal saline. Secondary portals can be established by this manner under direct vision. Owing to the increased hydrostatic pressure and limited overlying soft tissue, it is advisable to undertake formal closure of the portals to effect a seal and prevent synovial fistula formation.

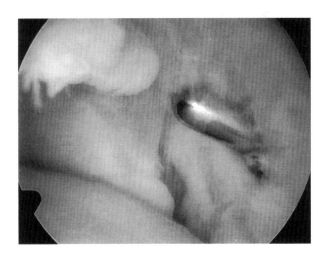

Figure 5

Anterolateral gutter through medial portal showing anterior tibial and lateral malleolus osteophytes; arthroscopic view

Initial survey

In most cases it is best to start with a view through the anterolateral portal. The exception to this is where an extensive lateral osteophyte is blocking access. In this case switching to the medial side (or lowering the entry portal) may improve the ease of access. In many cases a limited anterior synovectomy is needed to allow a thorough view. A systematic nine-point initial survey should include the anterior gutter (Figures 4 and 5), the lateral gutter and talofibular articulation, the lateral ligament and

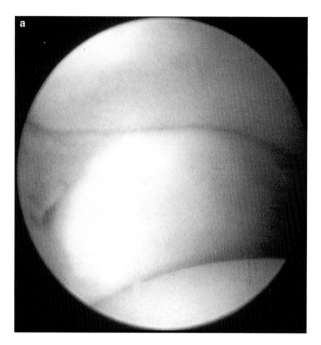

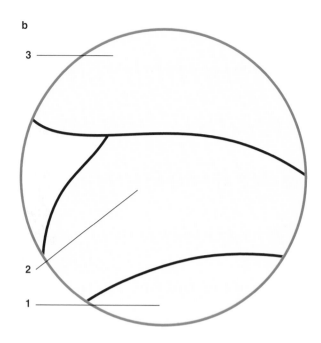

Figure 6

Lateral malleolus, lateral talus, talofibular articulation through anteromedial portal. a. arthroscopic view; b. schematic representation

1 Talus
2 Fibula
3 Tibial plafond

talus (Figures 6, 7, and 8), the central talus and the posterior gutter, including the posterior tibiofibular articulation (Figure 9), and the deltoid ligament, medial gutter and medial talus (Figure 10). A view of the anterior gutter is again helped by synovectomy and releasing the traction. The medial and lateral gutters are better accessed by the more central portals if difficulty is encountered. The posterior gutter and posterocentral talus may be difficult to access from the anterior portals. Options include using a small (3.5 mm or 2.9 mm) scope or a postero-lateral portal.

Specific procedures

Assessment of the unstable ankle

Chondral and osteochondral injury, synovitis, loose bodies and degenerative change have all been reported in ankle arthroscopy prior to lateral ligament reconstruction. Lesions that are seen in distinct postions both medially and laterally have been found in up to 70% of ankles after fracture, and failure to treat these may be a source of ongoing pain [Loren and Ferkel 2002]. Synovial lesions from florid synovitis, fibrous adhesions with overlying mild

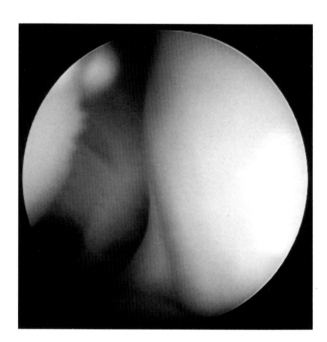

Figure 7

Lateral gutter through anterolateral portal; arthroscopic view

synovitis and synovial impingement can all cause continuing pain following ankle sprain [Ogilvie-Harris et al. 1997].

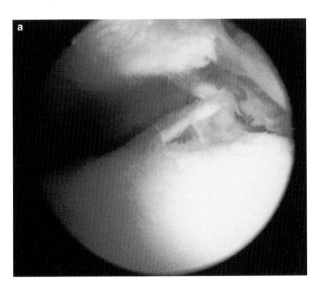

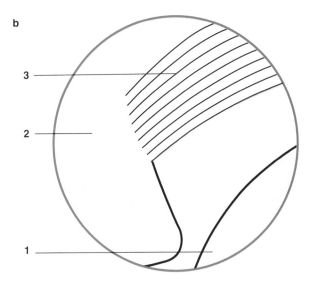

Figure 8

Posterolateral corner of right ankle through anterolateral portal. a. arthroscopic view; b. schematic representation

1 Talus
2 Fibula
3 Posterior tibiofibular ligament

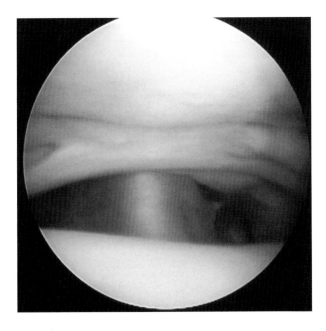

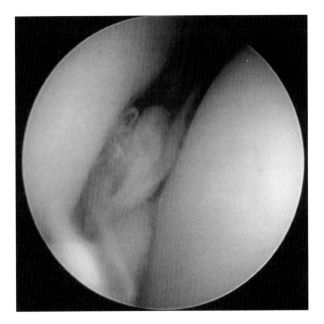

Figure 9

Central talus, posterior gutter; arthroscopic view

Figure 10

Medial gutter including deltoid ligament through antero-medial portal; arthroscopic view

An examination under anesthetic prior to ligament reconstruction is routinely undertaken by most surgeons but we believe that a routine arthroscopy should also be performed. Talar tilt of more than 15° and a forward translation of the talus of more than 10 mm, along with a direct observation of the anterior talofibular and calcaneofibular ligament in the lateral gutter, may aid in assessment and choice of stabilization procedure (Figure 11) [Hinterman et al. 2002].

Anterior chielectomy

Osseous and synovial impingement in dorsiflexion is a significant cause of anterior pain in the ankle following acute or chronic trauma. Large osteophytes

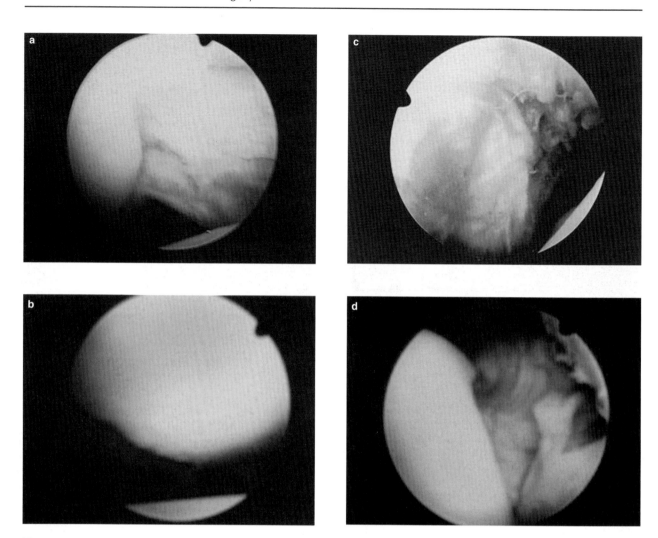

Figure 11

Severe case of instability where, with traction, both malleolar tips (a and b) and extensive scarring of the ligaments (c and d) can be seen

are often the sequelae of continued instability, malalignment and more extensive degenerative change. In the presence of established osteoarthritis or malalignment, results of debridement of these lesions fall to approximately 50% [van Dijk et al. 1997]. In the absence of generalized changes, debridement of both osseous and synovial impingement lesions yields good to excellent results in up to 90% of patients.

It is important to appreciate the extent of both tibial and talar osteophytes. These generally have a distinct morphology consisting of a large lateral tibial osteophyte, which may impede access, and accompanying osteophytes on the anterior surfaces of the medial and lateral malleolus. Talar osteophytes are variable in their morphology, but commonly lie more medially on the talar neck.

For accurate assessment it is necessary to identify the recess immediately above the bony ledge which may require anterior synovectomy (Figure 12). Once

identified it is best dealt with systematically, working from medial to lateral to reconstitute the natural 30° bevel of the tibia. Resection should continue to a point where normal cartilage is reached ('cliffs of Dover' appearance), and is aided by the release of traction (Figure 13). The talar osteophyte is more difficult to access and care must be taken to protect the neurovascular bundle. An assessment of the extent of resection can be made by viewing the anterior recess arthroscopically in maximal dorsiflexion [Ogilvie-Harris 1993a].

Treatment of osteochondral lesions and subchondral cysts

The treatment of chondral flaps and osteochondral lesions remains controversial. Small chondral flaps are resected, and loose bodies are removed. The question remains as to what treatment may yield the best results in those lesions up to 1 cm in size, with

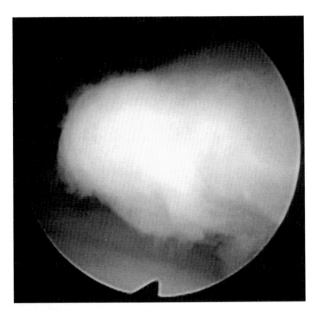

Figure 12

Pre-resection view showing the recess above the bony ledge

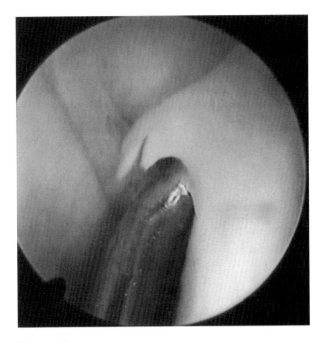

Figure 14

Chondral flap through anterolateral portal; arthroscopic view

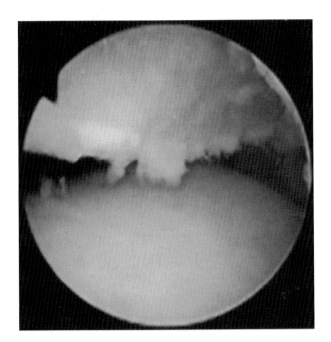

Figure 13

Post-resection view showing reconstitution of the anterior tibial bevel

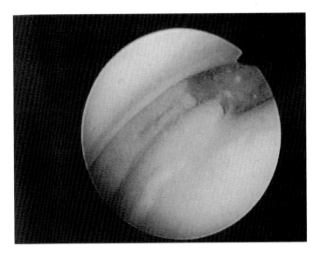

Figure 15

Osteochondral lesion of the anterolateral talus; arthroscopic view

either a partially free or an intact cartilage layer and evidence of subchondral erosion. There is some disparity in outcome between medial and lateral lesions, perhaps due to their different morphologies and theoretically different etiologies (Figures 14 and 15).

The treatment options include transarticular drilling, abrasion of subchondral bone, subchondral drilling, either bone or osteochondral grafting and potentially chondral transplantation. Flaps and loose osteochondral fragments can be removed and treated by debridement of the underlying

bony surface. The author's preference is to debride cysts with a mobile cartilage cap back to bleeding cancellous bone. If the cartilage is intact and a subchondral cyst is evident, subchondral drilling is undertaken using a drill guide and entry through the sinus tarsi. This should be augmented with bone graft, especially in the younger patient. The larger medial lesions present a greater dilemma; access is often difficult, being frequently posteromedial. Transmalleolar drilling is not favored, owing to the inherent risk of stress risers and fractures in

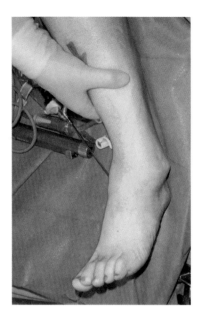 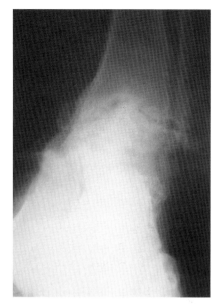 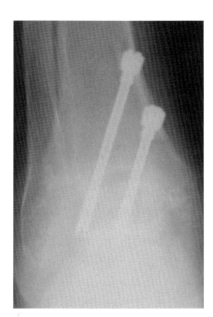

Figure 16

Varus deformity of the ankle corrected by arthroscopic means and arthrodesed

the malleolus itself. Chondral grafting may be a treatment option in specific cases, but is largely experimental at present.

Arthroscopic ankle arthrodesis

Arthroscopic ankle arthrodesis is protective of the overlying soft tissue, which potentially reduces infection rates, preserves overall joint anatomy and decreases complication rates while achieving fusion rates comparable to those of open techniques [Ogilvie-Harris 1993a, Tasto et al. 2000]. Deformities of increasing size can be corrected by addressing predominantly the tibial and, to a lesser degree, the talar surfaces during debridement (Figure 16). Care should be taken to decompress the lateral gutter to prevent lateral impingement.

A standard set-up is used and minimal synovial debridement required. Opposing cancellous surfaces are achieved by a combination of power burrs of both barrel and ball-tipped shape and occasional use of hand-held curettes. Debridement to bleeding cancellous bone is mandatory and attention should be paid to ensuring a uniform surface, addressing the potential for 'shoulders' to form on either side of the talar dome. Correction is achieved by assessing and compensating for tibial bone loss during debridement (Figure 17). Fixation of the arthrodesis is achieved with two cannulated titanium screws inserted from proximal–medial to distal–anterior and lateral. Compression of these screws will also

aid in clearing the lateral gutter as the talus is drawn medially. Image intensification is required.

Postoperative care

Routine arthroscopic examination

In all cases portals are closed with non-absorbable sutures to decrease the risk of synovial fistula. A simple wool and crêpe compression bandage is applied. Routine use of bupivacaine local anesthetic infiltration into portal sites and intra-articularly provides good analgesia for several hours.

Provided minimal soft-tissue trauma has occurred, within a few hours patients can walk short distances with the aid of a single stick or crutch. Domestic mobility is allowable and achievable by day 1 and return to sedentary work by day 4. Driving is allowed after 1 week.

Physiotherapy is instigated early in the postoperative phase and compression bandaging continued for at least 2 weeks. Continued elevation and icing should also be encouraged in the first 2 weeks. Regardless of pathological findings a progressive program of movement, proprioception and strengthening exercises is given.

Arthroscopic ankle arthrodesis

Patients are placed into a below-knee cast for a minimum of 12 weeks. They remain non-weightbearing

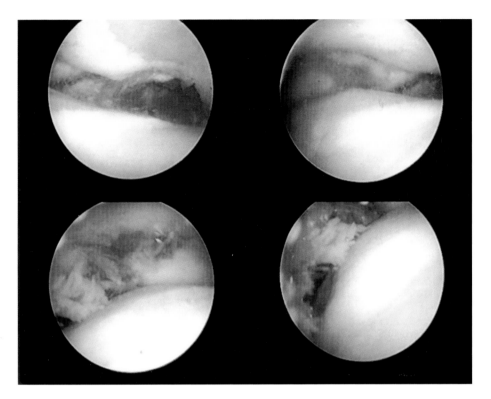

Figure 17

Arthroscopic view of cartilage loss pattern and ridge formation in the tibia caused by progressive deformity

for the initial 6 weeks and are allowed partial weightbearing for the remainder, depending on radiographic appearances at the 6-week review. If necessary, patients are then transferred to a rigid removable walking brace or ankle–foot orthosis until radiological fusion has occurred.

Drilling and grafting procedures

Following the treatment of chondral or osteochondral problems, an effort is made to protect the joint surface. If simple chondral flaps are removed and the joint surface abraded, the standard progressive mobilization regimen is slowed and altered to avoid activity for 6 weeks. More extensive treatment, such as bone grafting, and larger lesions are followed by protected weightbearing on crutches for 6 weeks.

References

Albert J, Reiman P, Njus G et al. (1992) Ligament strain and ankle joint opening during ankle distraction. Arthroscopy 8: 469–473

Baker CL, Graham JM Jr (1993) Current concepts in ankle arthroscopy. Orthopedics 16: 1027–1035

Buckingham RA, Winson IG, Kelly AJ (1997) An anatomical study of a new portal for ankle arthroscopy. J Bone Joint Surg 79B: 650–652

Burman MS (1931) Arthroscopy of direct visualisation of joints: an experimental cadaver study. J Bone Joint Surg 13: 669

Chaytor ER, Conti SF (1998) Arthroscopy of the foot and ankle: current concepts review. Foot Ankle Int 19: 184–192

Dowdy PA, Watson BV, Amendola A, Brown JD (1996) Noninvasive ankle distraction: relationship between force, magnitude of distraction, and nerve conduction abnormalities. Arthroscopy 12: 64–69

Feiwell LA, Frey C (1993) Anatomic study of arthroscopic portal sites of the ankle. Foot Ankle 14: 142–147

Ferkel RD, Heath DD, Guhl JF (1996) Neurological complications of ankle arthroscopy. Arthroscopy 12: 200–208

Hepple S, Winson IG, Glew D (1999) Osteochondral lesions of the talus: a revised classification. Foot Ankle Int 20: 789–793

Hintermann B, Boss A, Schafer D (2002) Arthroscopic findings in patients with chronic ankle instability. Am J Sports Med 30: 402–409

Kumar VP, Satku K (1994) The AO femoral distractor for ankle arthroscopy. Arthroscopy 10: 118–119

Liu SH, Mirzayan R (1993) Posteromedial ankle impingement. Arthroscopy 9: 709–711

Loren GJ, Ferkel RD (2002) Arthroscopic assessment of occult intra-articular injury in acute ankle fractures. Arthroscopy 18: 412–421

Manderson EL, Nwaneri UR, Amin KB (1994) The fracture table as a distraction mode in ankle arthroscopy. Foot Ankle Int 15: 444–445

Meislin RJ, Rose DJ, Parisien JS, Springer S (1993) Arthroscopic treatment of synovial impingement of the ankle. Am J Sports Med 21: 186–189

Mosier-La Clair SM, Monroe MT, Manoli A (2000) Medial impingement syndrome of the anterior tibiotalar fascicle of the deltoid ligament on the talus. Foot Ankle Int 21: 385–391

Myerson MS, Quill G (1991) Ankle arthrodesis. A comparison of an arthroscopic and an open method of treatment. Clin Orthop 268: 84–95

O'Brien TS, Hart TS, Shereff MJ et al. (1999) Open versus arthroscopic ankle arthrodesis: a comparative study. Foot Ankle Int 20: 368–374

Ogilvie-Harris DJ, Mahomed N, Demaziere A (1993a) Anterior impingement of the ankle treated by arthroscopic removal of bony spurs. J Bone Joint Surg 75B: 437–440

Ogilvie-Harris DJ, Lieberman I, Fitsialos D (1993b) Arthroscopically assisted arthrodesis for osteoarthritic ankles. J Bone Joint Surg 75A: 1167–1174

Ogilvie-Harris DJ, Gilbart MK, Chorney K (1997) Chronic pain following ankle sprains in athletes: the role of arthroscopic surgery. Arthroscopy 13: 564–574

Parisien JS, Shaffer B (1992) Arthroscopic management of pyarthrosis. Clin Orthop 275: 243–247

Pritsch M, Lokiec F, Sali M, Velkes S (1993) Adhesions of distal tibiofibular syndesmosis. A cause of chronic ankle pain after fracture. Clin Orthop 289: 220–222

Schimmer RC, Dick W, Hintermann B (2001) The role of ankle arthroscopy in the treatment strategies of osteochondritis dissecans lesions of the talus. Foot Ankle Int 22: 895–900

Scranton PE Jr, McDermott JE (1992) Anterior tibiotalar spurs: a comparison of open versus arthroscopic debridement. Foot Ankle 13: 125–129

Scranton PE Jr, McDermott JE, Rogers JV (2000) The relationship between chronic ankle instability and variations in mortise anatomy and impingement spurs. Foot Ankle Int 21: 657–664

Small NC (1986) Complications in arthroscopy: the knee and other joints. Arthroscopy 2: 253–258

Takao M, Ochi M, Naito K et al. (2001) Arthroscopic diagnosis of tibiofibular syndesmosis disruption. Arthroscopy 17: 836–843

Tasto JP, Frey C, Laimans P et al. (2000) Arthroscopic ankle arthrodesis. Instr Course Lect 49: 259–280

Thordarson DB, Bains R, Shepherd LE (2001) The role of ankle arthroscopy on the surgical management of ankle fractures. Foot Ankle Int 22: 123–125

Tol JL, Verheyen CP, van Dijk CN (2001) Arthroscopic treatment of anterior impingement in the ankle. J Bone Joint Surg 83B: 9–13

van Dijk CN, Tol JL, Verheyen CC (1997) A prospective study of prognostic factors concerning the outcome of arthroscopic surgery for anterior ankle impingement. Am J Sports Med 25: 737–745

Voto SJ, Ewing JW, Fleissner PR Jr et al. (1989) Ankle arthroscopy: neurovascular and arthroscopic anatomy of standard and trans-achilles tendon portal placement. Arthroscopy 5: 41–46

Yates CK, Grana WA (1988) A simple distraction technique for ankle arthroscopy. Arthroscopy 4: 103–105

38

Ankle fractures: open reduction and internal fixation

Hajo Thermann
Harald Tscherne

Introduction

Ankle fractures are the most common type of lower limb fracture. About 87% occur during walking, running or falling. In 13% the injury is caused by direct force, for example in contact sports or accidents [Browner et al. 1992, Zwipp 1994].

Biomechanics and anatomy

The anterior part of the trochlea tali is approximately 5 mm wider than the posterior part. In dorsiflexion of the ankle, the lateral malleolus displaces laterally and away from the tibia. It also moves proximally and into internal rotation. In plantarflexion the lateral malleolus moves toward the tibia, moves distally and rotates externally. In the stance phase, a lateral thrust occurs from the talus to the lateral malleolus. This force is transferred back to the tibia. Thus, the lateral malleolus is a weightbearing structure, maintaining approximately one-sixth of body weight [Schatzker and Tile 1994].

The ankle joint is fully congruent in all positions. Talar tilt of 2–4° in the frontal plane, lateral displacement of the talus and shortening of the lateral malleolus by more than 2 mm result in a reduction of contact area of about 40%. Minor displacement of the ankle mortise may compromise the long-term prognosis [Weber 1966, Schatzker and Tile 1994]. Therefore, the ultimate goal of fracture treatment is the anatomic and stable restoration of ankle joint congruity.

The sural nerve is located 10 cm above the tip of the fibula at the lateral border of the Achilles tendon. It lies anterolateral to the short saphenous vein, turns around the posterior border of the lateral malleolus and passes forward 1–1.5 cm from the tip of the lateral malleolus. The superficial peroneal nerve is at higher risk for iatrogenic injury, owing to its anatomic variety. In general, the superficial peroneal nerve pierces the crural fascia about 12 cm proximal to the ankle joint. In most cases, the nerve divides at a mean distance of just over 4 cm into the medial cutaneous and the intermediate dorsal nerves. In some cases the two branches originate independently and the intermediate cutaneous nerve penetrates the crural fascia posterior to the fibula 5.5 cm proximal to the ankle joint, and courses medially to cross the lateral aspect of the fibula, proximal to the ankle joint. The intermediate dorsal cutaneous nerve may also penetrate the fascia anterior to the fibula approximately 5 cm above the ankle and travel adjacent to the anterior border of the fibula.

Mechanism of injury

When the foot is fixed on the ground by the body weight, the talus produces bending or shearing forces to the malleoli. The variety of different fracture patterns results from bending moments produced with rotation, either in the coronal plane, i.e. adduction or abduction of the talus relative to the tibia, or in the transverse plane, i.e. internal or external rotation. In severe cases, there is more than a single force vector during the injury, causing variable impaction of the tibial plafond. Axial loading of the ankle joint results in posterior and anterior lip fractures at the plafond and in malleolus fractures with metaphyseal components.

Classification

Ankle fractures may be classified according to the mechanism of injury [Lauge-Hansen 1948] and according to practical therapeutic considerations [Weber 1966].

Lauge-Hansen classification

In the Lauge-Hansen system, supination–adduction fractures account for 10–18% of malleolar fractures. There is a distal transverse fracture of the fibula in the first stage, and a vertical fracture line of the medial malleolus in the second stage.

Supination–eversion (external rotation) is the most common mechanism of ankle fracture, accounting for 40–70% of cases. This injury starts with a rupture of the anterior tibiofibular syndesmosis or a corresponding bone avulsion. Subsequently, an oblique spiral fracture of the lateral malleolus develops. This runs from anterior–distal to posterior–proximal, beginning at the level of the tibial plafond. The posterior tibiofibular syndesmosis fails in substance or by avulsion of its tibial attachment as an intra-articular fragment of different size. This is also referred to as the posterior malleolar or Volkmann's fragment. The fourth stage is medial failure of either the malleolus or the deltoid ligament.

Pronation–abduction trauma accounts for 5–15% of fractures and starts with a failure of the deltoid ligament or a transverse medial malleolus fracture. The second stage is a rupture of the anterior or posterior syndesmosis. The bending mechanism results in a laterally comminuted transverse fibular fracture.

In pronation–eversion (external rotation) injuries, the external rotation produces an initial failure of the deltoid ligament or an avulsion of the medial malleolus. The anterior syndesmosis then fails. The third stage is a spiral or oblique fracture of the fibula, which runs from anterior–proximal to posterior–distal. The level of the fibular fracture is characteristically above the level of the ankle joint. In the fourth stage, a rupture or an avulsion of the posterior syndesmosis occurs. Pronation–eversion fractures account for 8–14% of all ankle fractures.

Danis–weber classification

In the Danis–Weber classification, type A injuries have a transverse fibular fracture below the syndesmosis. They are caused by a supination–adduction mechanism. On the medial side, a more or less displaced oblique fracture may occur. Type B injuries have a fibular fracture at the level of the syndesmosis. They are biomechanically pronation–abduction or supination–external rotation injuries. Disruption of the syndesmosis is optional. The lateral malleolus fracture pattern depends on the mechanism of injury. The supination–external rotation injuries have an oblique spiral fracture. This runs from anterior–distal to posterior–proximal and begins at the level of the tibial plafond. Avulsion of the anterior syndesmosis is common. This fracture is well differentiated from the transverse, lateral comminuted fracture in pronation–abduction trauma, which is located at or just above the level of the tibial plafond. The medial side suffers a deltoid ligament rupture or an avulsion fracture of the medial malleolus. Stability depends on the extent of syndesmosis rupture, on posterior or anterior lip fractures and on impaction of the tibial plafond. In type C injuries, the fibular fracture is located at a variable distance proximal to the tibial plafond and to the syndesmosis. The trauma mechanism is pronation–external rotation. Typically, an oblique or spiral fracture is found, which runs from anterior–proximal to posterior–distal. Instability is increased with disruption of the syndesmosis. Significantly more proximal fractures involve the interosseous membrane and are referred to as Maisonneuve fractures.

Soft-tissue trauma

The evaluation of soft-tissue trauma is important for its acute management and the timing of surgery. Soft-tissue damage may be difficult to assess, especially within the first few hours, or if the patient is in shock. Significant fracture–dislocation jeopardizes local perfusion, stretches neurovascular structures, interferes with distal blood circulation and promotes swelling. Early reduction and the application of a well-padded below-knee plaster splint are mandatory until operative treatment is performed.

Treatment

Indications for surgery

The decision about surgical fixation of ankle fractures depends on the stability of the fracture, its displacement, the age of the patient and contraindications to surgery. Further considerations are the extent of soft-tissue trauma and concomitant injuries, which may influence the timing of surgery and the choice of the surgical technique.

The stability of the fracture is assessed by translating the talus medially and laterally. A noticeable impact may be present against the medial malleolus and a minor resistance against the fibula. Displaced and unstable fractures are treated operatively. Undisplaced and stable fractures are treated non-operatively [Hamilton 1984]. Stable fibular fractures with minimal displacement and with no more than 2 mm of shortening are reported to have good results at long-term follow-up if treated non-operatively [Bauer et al. 1985a, Browner et al. 1992, Schatzker and Tile 1994]. For patient comfort, an ankle–foot orthosis or walking boot may be applied instead of a plaster cast. However, internal fixation of these fractures allows full weightbearing in an ankle orthosis postoperatively, which may be preferable in younger patients with high professional or athletic ambitions [Segal et al. 1985]. Surgical complications are uncommon in the hands of an experienced surgeon.

A short interval between trauma and surgery is the best assurance of uncomplicated healing, especially in open fractures or if skin abrasions are present [Fogel and Morrey 1987, Carragee and Csongradi 1991]. In significant soft tissue trauma with blisters and marked swelling, delayed open reduction and internal fixation are recommended, until the local soft tissue has recovered and edema has subsided. In fractures with severe soft-tissue contusion, the choice of approach and surgical technique is of particular importance. A dorsolateral approach and dorsal plating are more appropriate in anterolateral soft-tissue problems. Percutaneous insertion of a 3.5-mm cannulated screw through a stab incision should be considered as an alternative procedure.

In elderly patients osteoporotic bone, vulnerable soft-tissue coverage and concomitant diseases may pose problems [Beauchamp et al. 1983]. Minor displacement of the malleoli is less important than in younger patients. On the other hand, ankle fractures in older patients are often very unstable and cause considerable difficulty with conservative treatment.

In patients with multiple injuries, displaced malleolar fractures require fast and stable fixation. This is best accomplished by tarsotibial transfixation with an external fixator, in some cases with additional Kirschner wires for correction and stabilization of the anatomic alignment. Compared with plaster immobilization, this facilitates soft-tissue management

and care. In multiple lower extremity fractures the ankle fracture has a lower priority, except in cases with skin abrasion or in open fractures.

Surgical technique

The patient is placed supine with a cushion under the ipsilateral pelvis to rotate the trunk and lower leg internally, because the fibula is located posteriorly. A safety support or strap at the contralateral pelvis allows the table to be tilted further, if needed. A pneumatic tourniquet is not recommended in compromised soft tissues or with impaired perfusion.

Incision

The surgical landmarks for the incision (Figure 1) are the tip and the anterior and posterior borders of the fibula, and the base of the fifth metatarsal bone. For the posterolateral approach, the Achilles tendon serves as a landmark. On the medial side, the tip and the width of the medial malleolus and the fracture are palpated.

The placement of the incisions depends on the location of the injury relative to the tibiofibular ligament complex. A longitudinal lateral incision provides sufficient access to the fibula. The incision should be sufficiently long to avoid tension on the soft-tissue flap. Distally, the incision is angled slightly anteriorly, to permit arthrotomy, inspection and irrigation of the ankle joint surfaces. The proximal extension of the incision is determined by the location of the fracture. In compromised soft tissues, the skin flap should be retracted by subcutaneous sutures instead of retractors. The fracture is exposed minimally to evaluate the restoration of anatomy on the lateral side, at the dorsal spike and at the anterior syndesmosis. For anatomic reduction, the periosteum is reflected 1–2 mm at the fracture, small fragments and comminuted areas are kept in their soft-tissue envelope and are aligned anatomically. At the medial side, the incision is placed more anteriorly to facilitate the reduction at the anteromedial corner of the ankle joint.

Reduction and internal fixation

In *type A fractures*, the bone avulsion is retracted with a small forceps or a sharp dental probe, the clots are removed and anatomic reduction is secured with two parallel 1.6-mm Kirschner wires. A 1.25-mm tension-band wire provides compression at the fracture site (Figure 2a). This is anchored proximally through a 2.5-mm drill hole, with a bony bridge in

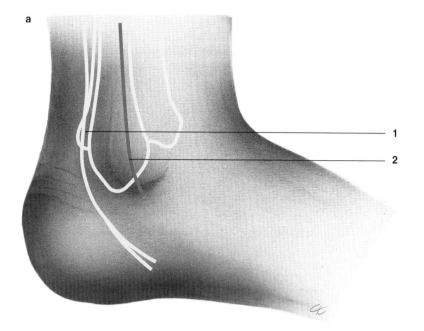

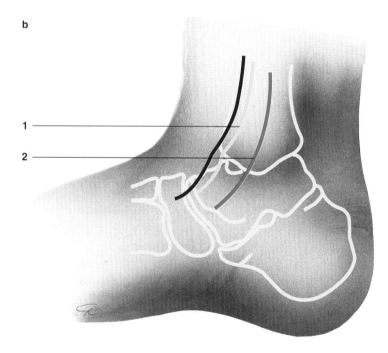

Figure 1

Skin incision for fixation of malleolar fractures.
a. approach to the lateral malleolus; b. approach
to the medial malleolus

a
1 Sural nerve
2 Incision

b
1 Saphenous nerve and vein
2 Incision

the fibula of at least 3 mm. The tension band must be directed perpendicularly to the fracture line, i.e. the drill hole must be more medial in slightly oblique fractures. The Kirschner wires are cut and the distal ends are bent proximally. Alternatively, one or both Kirschner wires are replaced by a 3.5-mm oblique lag screw (Figure 2b), which should penetrate the medial cortex with one or two threads. In atypical, very low, comminuted lateral malleolar fractures, the use of multiple Kirschner wires [Bauer et al. 1985b], in the same way as intramedullary rodding, with a tension wire for lateral support and rotational control, is a possible solution.

In *supination–adduction injuries*, the vertical shear fracture of the medial malleolus with medial

impaction of two or three small fragments is technically difficult to reduce. One of these fragments may be from the tibial plafond and commonly has a width of 2–4 mm. Removal of this fragment may result in internal rotation and in malunion of the medial malleolus. Therefore, anteromedial impaction of the tibial plafond must be elevated and reduced anatomically with a 5–10-mm osteotome (Figure 3a). The bone bridge between the medial malleolus and the tibia must be at least 8–10 mm wide to prevent displacement. Small defects may be filled with autogenous bone graft from the adjacent tibial plafond. The fracture is then stabilized with two horizontal screws (Figure 3b).

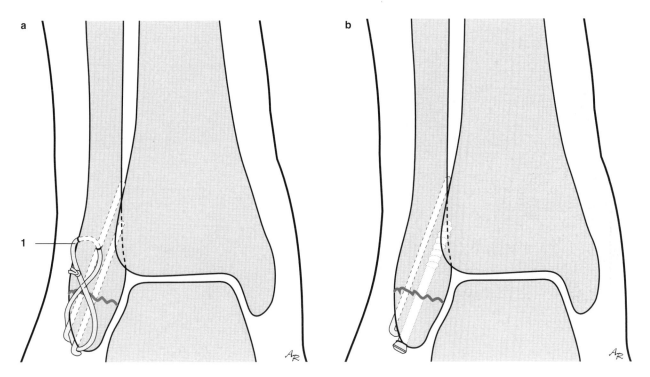

Figure 2

Fixation of type A fractures. a. tension-band fixation; b. alternatively, one or both Kirschner wires may be replaced with an oblique lag screw

a
1 Tension band wire

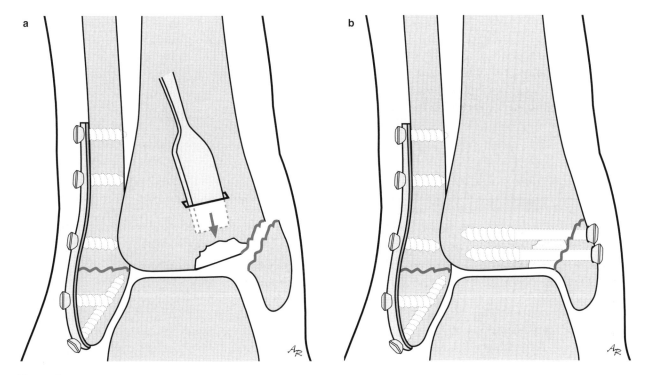

Figure 3

Shear fracture of the medial malleolus. a. anteromedial impaction of the tibial plafond is elevated anatomically; small defects are filled with autogenous bone graft; b. the medial malleolus fracture is fixed with screws

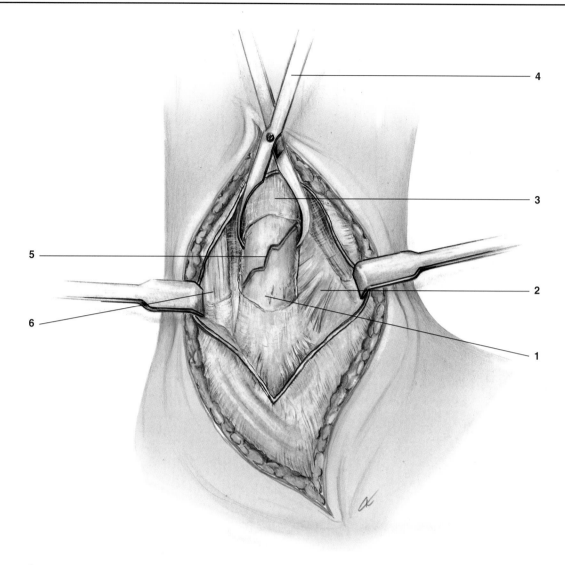

Figure 4

Supination–external rotation type B injuries are the most common ankle fractures. For reduction of the lateral malleolus, the distal fragment is grasped with a pointed forceps or towel clip and brought into anatomic position with the proximal fragment. A reduction clamp is then tightened across the fracture plane

1 Distal fibular fragment
2 Anterior tibiofibular syndesmosis
3 Proximal fibular fragment
4 Reduction clamp
5 Fracture line
6 Peroneal tendons

In *supination–external rotation type B fractures*, anatomic reduction of the posterior spike is the clue for restoration of length and rotation of the fibula (Figure 4). This is accomplished by inversion of the hindfoot. The distal fragment is grasped with a pointed forceps or a towel clip and brought into anatomic alignment with the proximal fragment. A reduction clamp is tightened perpendicularly to the fracture plane. The fracture is fixed with a 3.5-mm lag screw from anterior to posterior and parallel to the reduction clamp. A five- or six-hole, one-third tubular plate is contoured anatomically to the distal

fibula. In most cases, the distal fragment has room for only two screws. The screw in the proximal hole is drilled slightly anteriorly. The most distal screw is directed proximally and posteriorly, to obtain purchase in the two cortices without interfering with the tibiofibular joint (Figure 5). In osteoporotic bone, the use of a pointed forceps for reduction is hazardous because it may further damage the distal fragment. An indirect reduction technique may have to be used (see below) (Figure 6). Ruptures of the anterior syndesmosis are sutured with absorbable material. Avulsion fractures of the

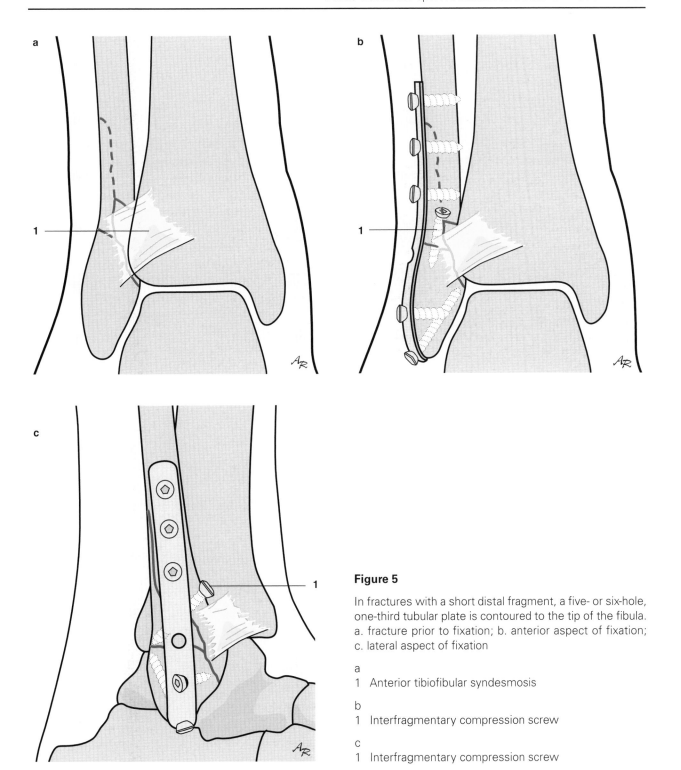

Figure 5

In fractures with a short distal fragment, a five- or six-hole, one-third tubular plate is contoured to the tip of the fibula. a. fracture prior to fixation; b. anterior aspect of fixation; c. lateral aspect of fixation

a
1   Anterior tibiofibular syndesmosis

b
1   Interfragmentary compression screw

c
1   Interfragmentary compression screw

posterior syndesmosis complex are reduced with a clamp, which is placed anterior–posterior into the tibia through stab incisions. A 3.5-mm or 4.0-mm cannulated cancellous bone screw is drilled slightly obliquely from medial–anterior to the posterolateral fragment, under radiographic control. Supination–eversion injuries with a large posterior malleolar fragment are better addressed through a postero-lateral approach, to facilitate anatomic reduction

(Figure 7). In this case, screws and an anti-glide plate are placed on the lateral malleolus from posterior.

In *pronation–abduction type B fractures*, exten-sive comminution and anterolateral impaction complicate the reduction. Landmarks for precise reduction are the fibular groove, the medial subchondral surface and the tip of the fibula. Exposure of the comminuted fragments must be minimal. The contoured plate is clamped proximal

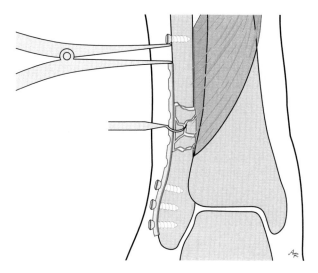

Figure 6

Indirect reduction technique: the contoured plate is fixed distally and the length is restored with a bone spreader against a more proximal screw

to the fracture. With a pointed clamp, the major distal fragment is distracted by an assistant. Usually, congruent fragments can be found to restore the length of the fibula. The surgeon carefully holds the plate to the fibula with one hand. With a dental probe, the other fragments are aligned and the plate is fixed by placing a screw in the distal fragment. This screw hole is drilled slightly eccentric to achieve minimal compression. A second distal or proximal screw is placed, providing rotational stability of the plate. The fibular groove is exposed, if present, and an intraoperative radiograph is taken to ascertain the reduction, including a comparison with the opposite ankle. If the area of the comminution is very large and the patient is big, a stiffer 3.5-mm low-contact dynamic compression plate or reconstruction plate should be used. Anterolateral impaction may lead to talar tilt with significant ankle joint incongruence and must be corrected.

Avulsion of the anterior syndesmosis with a bone fragment is repaired with a 3.5-mm cancellous screw and a plastic ligament washer. Treatment of damage to the posterior syndesmosis depends on the stability of the ankle joint. Ruptures or small avulsion fragments are often visible after anatomic fixation of the lateral malleolus. If instability of the posterior syndesmosis can be demonstrated, fixation is mandatory. The stability of the syndesmosis is assessed clinically and radiographically by external rotation and valgus stress to the hindfoot. A demonstrable laxity of the anterolateral corner of the fibula of more than 3–4 mm is an indication

for a syndesmosis transfixation screw (Figure 8) [Parfenchuck et al. 1994].

In *pronation–external rotation type C injuries*, the reduction is performed by distraction of the distal fragment with a pointed clamp. A four-hole, one-third tubular plate and an interfragmentary screw suffice for fixation in most cases. In cases of gross comminution, the fracture is reduced indirectly with a bone spreader (see Figure 6). Instability of the syndesmosis after fixation of the lateral malleolus fracture requires syndesmosis transfixation (Figure 8). A 3.5-mm cortical screw is placed from posterolateral in the fibula to anteromedial in the tibia, about 2–3 cm above the tibial plafond, at an angle of 25–30° to the frontal plane. The ankle has to be in neutral position during this maneuver. The screw penetrates only the lateral cortex of the tibia and is gently tightened [Lauge-Hansen 1948]. The anterolateral corner of the ankle joint is evaluated for anatomic reduction of the fracture. In very proximal fibula fractures, i.e. Maisonneuve fractures with ankle instability, only the ankle mortise is reduced and syndesmosis transfixation is carried out.

Closure

Insertion of a small suction drain is optional. The subcutaneous tissue is closed with interrupted absorbable sutures to cover the plate. Interrupted non-absorbable sutures are used for skin closure. The lower leg is placed in a soft splint with the ankle in neutral position. In very unstable fractures with poor bone stock, a bivalved, well-padded below-knee plaster cast is used.

Special considerations

In osteopenic bone, it is risky to reduce the fracture with a pointed clamp. In this circumstance, an indirect reduction technique has to be applied (see Figure 6). In supination–adduction/eversion injuries, the assistant first distracts the fracture by maximum supination and adduction of the foot. With a sharp dental probe, the posterior spike is reduced anatomically to the proximal fragment by gentle abduction. Instead of a reduction clamp, a 1.4–1.6-mm Kirschner wire is advanced through the fragments, perpendicular to the fracture plane, to secure the reduction until the plate is applied. In pronation–abduction/eversion fractures with a transverse fracture and often with comminution, the contoured plate is fixed distally with one screw. Reduction is achieved by initial pronation and

a

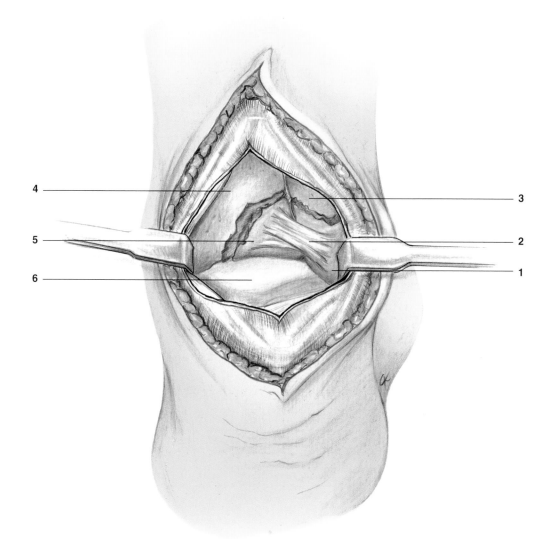

b

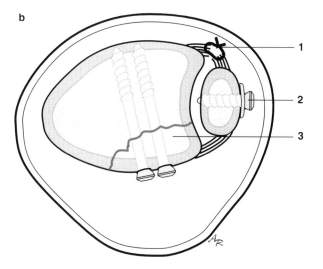

Figure 7

Large posterior malleolar fragments are reduced through a posterolateral approach. a. intraoperative aspect from posterior; b. fixation technique

a
1 Distal fibular fragment
2 Posterior tibiofibular syndesmosis
3 Fibula
4 Tibia
5 Posterior malleolar fragment
6 Talus

b
1 Suture of anterior tibiofibular syndesmosis
2 Fixation of fibular fracture
3 Posterior malleolar fragment

abduction. The small fragments are aligned beneath the plate and fixed with a second proximal screw. While tightening the screws, the reduction of the small fragments is ascertained with a dental probe or a small curette.

Displaced ankle fractures, which cannot be reduced by closed techniques and have very poor soft-tissue conditions, are difficult to manage. Open reduction and internal fixation is contraindicated. These injuries may be a rare indication for

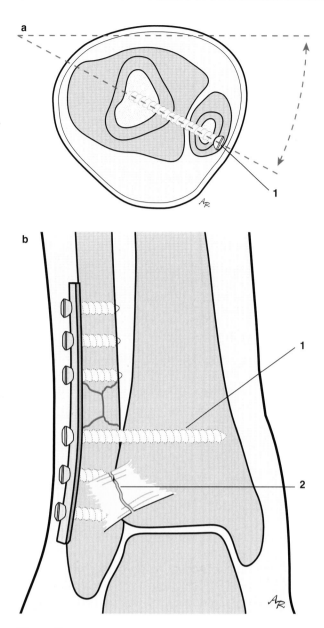

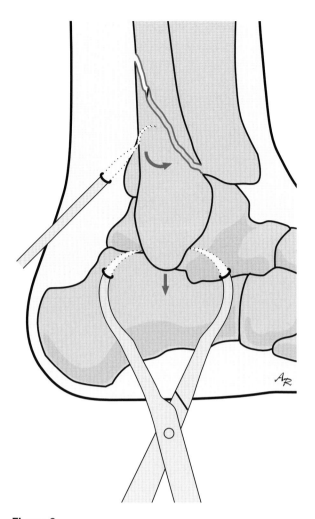

Figure 9

Technique of percutaneous reduction and screw fixation

Figure 8

Transfixation of the syndesmosis with a 3.5 mm cortical screw, which is placed from posterolateral in the fibula to anteromedial in the tibia about 2–3 cm above the plafond in an angle of 25–30° to the frontal plane. a. transverse section; b. anterior aspect

a
1 Syndesmosis transfixation screw

b
1 Syndesmosis transfixation screw
2 Anterior tibiofibular syndesmosis (ruptured)

percutaneous screw fixation (Figure 9). A stab incision is placed at the tip of the fibula. With a sharp clamp, the soft tissues posterior to the distal fragment are gently undermined. With a pointed clamp, the distal fragment is grasped percutaneously and manipulated. The dental probe is inserted posteriorly to finish the reduction. The fracture is stabilized with two Kirschner wires, which are subsequently replaced by cannulated screws. This is a difficult technique, which requires an experienced surgeon.

Postoperative care

The dressing is removed on the first or second day after surgery, cold packs are applied and the patient is started on careful dorsiflexion and plantarflexion exercises for relief of pain and edema. The extrinsic and intrinsic foot muscles are trained by pushing the foot in the neutral position against a foot board.

Bimalleolar fractures treated with stable open reduction and internal fixation are allowed full weightbearing, depending on soft-tissue healing, on the patient's complaints and walking capacity. In uncomplicated cases, the patient starts walking on crutches on the third or fourth day, with 30-kg weightbearing. This is increased to full weightbearing, according to the patient's complaints. A therapy boot with a long shaft and medial and lateral stabilizers, or a walking boot with an unfixed hinge, may be used instead of a below-knee walking cast, to improve the range of motion. Protection is continued for 6 weeks postoperatively. In more complex cases, such as unstable fractures with combined anterior and posterior syndesmosis reconstruction, a walking cast with 15-kg weightbearing is applied for 6 weeks. Full weightbearing is permitted after 8 weeks. In cases with bone grafting, e.g. in anterior lip fractures, partial weightbearing for 3 months is recommended.

Complications

Postoperative soft-tissue problems have to be treated aggressively. Hematoma compromising the skin and possibly leading to necrosis has to be evacuated without delay, accompanied by meticulous hemostasis. Superficial infection is treated initially with rest, cold packs and antibiotics. In cases of persisting local or systemic evidence of infection, debridement with jet lavage cleansing is mandatory. Delayed skin closure may be necessary. If infection persists, a second debridement is performed and the plate is removed. The fracture is fixed with Kirschner wires to maintain gross alignment.

Postoperative loss of reduction requires reosteosynthesis with a stiffer 3.5-mm plate. In osteopenic bone, fully threaded cancellous screws may be used.

Inadequate handling of the soft tissue, such as the use of forced retraction to expose the most proximal screw hole in too short an incision, may lead to skin sloughing, necrosis and infection. The skin may suffer from contact with the drill during placement of the interfragmentary screw in oblique or spiral fractures. In bimalleolar fractures with massive swelling, primary skin closure may be difficult. In order to avoid undue tension, only the lateral or medial side may be sutured, the other side covered with skin substitute and closure delayed for 2 days.

Delayed bone healing may be caused by soft-tissue trauma, by stripping of the periosteum and soft-tissue envelope during surgery, by poor bone stock and by prolonged delay in weightbearing. Postoperative physiotherapy must aim to improve regional perfusion, to increase weightbearing, especially in patients with low pain resistance, and to improve the range of ankle motion with appropriate exercises.

References

Bauer M, Bergström B, Hemborg A, Sandegaard J (1985a) Malleolar fractures: nonoperative versus operative treatment: a controlled study. Clin Orthop 199: 17–27

Bauer M, Johnsson K, Nilsson B (1985b) Thirty-year follow-up of ankle fractures. Acta Orthop Scand 5: 103–106

Beauchamp CG, Clay NR, Thexton PW (1983) Displaced ankle fractures in patients over 50 years. J Bone Joint Surg 63B: 329–332

Browner BD, Jupiter JB, Levine AM, Trafton PG (1992) Fractures and soft tissue injuries of the ankle. Skel Trauma 2: 1887–1957

Carragee EJ, Csongradi JJ (1991) Early complications in the operative treatment of ankle fractures. Influence of delay before operation. J Bone Joint Surg 73B: 79–82

Fogel GR, Morrey BF (1987) Delayed open reduction and fixation of ankle fractures. Clin Orthop 215: 187–195

Hamilton WC (1984) Traumatic Disorders of the Ankle. Berlin, Springer

Lauge-Hansen N (1948) Analytic historic survey as basis of new experimental roentgenologic investigation. Arch Surg 60: 259–317

Parfenchuck TA, Frix JM, Bertrand SL, Corpe RS (1994) Clinical use of a syndesmosis screw in stage IV pronation–external rotation ankle fractures. Orthop Rev (Suppl) 23–28

Schatzker J, Tile M (1994) The Rationale of Operative Fracture Care. Berlin, Springer, pp 371–405

Segal D, Wiss DA, Whitelaw GP (1985) Functional bracing and rehabilitation of ankle fractures. Clin Orthop 199: 39–45

Weber BG (1966) Die Verletzungen des oberen Sprunggelenkes. Bern, Hans Huber

Zwipp H (1994) Chirurgie des Fusses, OSG-Frakturen. Berlin, Springer

39

Ankle arthrodesis

Andrea Cracchiolo III

Introduction

Arthrodesis of the ankle is still the standard salvage operation to treat the painful, arthritic ankle joint which has been unresponsive to non-operative care. Occasionally, arthroscopic debridement of an arthritic ankle, depending on the degree of arthritis, may give some relief of pain. However, with progressive arthritic changes, particularly in a patient with a systemic arthritis, the positive results of arthroscopic debridement diminish with time.

The ankle presents certain difficulties when an arthrodesis is attempted. These problems are: the surfaces for fusion are small; the leg is a long lever arm which is to be attached and eventually fused to a much smaller distal part, i.e. the foot and ankle; and the blood supply to the talus may have been impaired by previous injury, surgery or disease.

Historically, a wide variety of techniques for ankle fusion have been reported [Cracchiolo 1991]. It was found that compression across the arthrodesis site reduced the risk of complication, especially pseudarthrosis, and became the treatment of choice for performing an ankle fusion.

External fixators were developed to produce compression across the arthrodesis; they were initially proposed by Charnley, and later popularized by Calandruccio. More recently, arthroscopically assisted techniques to gain ankle arthrodesis have become popular among clinicians who routinely perform arthroscopy of the ankle. The success of these techniques depends on the operator's skill, and sometimes lengthy operating times are needed. Using an arthroscopic technique for ankle arthrodesis may result in an ankle fusion which is said to

occur sooner than if an open operative technique is used [Dent et al. 1993, Ogilvie-Harris et al. 1993]. The reports of this technique mention a significant number of non-unions and other complications [Crosby et al. 1996]. O'Brien et al. [1999] reported equal success following open versus arthroscopic ankle arthrodesis. However, only patients with limited angular deformities were suitable candidates for arthroscopic ankle arthrodesis.

Ankle arthrodesis techniques can be divided into two categories according to the condition of the ankle. Deformed ankles requiring re-alignment are suitably treated by open techniques and a wide surgical exposure. Arthritic ankle joints which are in relatively good alignment and have only loss of the joint surface may simply require fusion in situ; these ankles can be approached using a more limited exposure, an arthroscopically assisted technique or a mini-arthrotomy technique [Paremain et al. 1996].

Treatment

Surgical technique

Ankle arthrodesis is usually performed under thigh-high tourniquet control. However, this is mainly for the surgeon's convenience, as the operation does not usually result in excessive blood loss. Therefore, if there are any contraindications to the use of a tourniquet, the procedure can still be performed. Keeping the operating table in the Trendelenburg position may minimize bleeding. If a tourniquet is used it can be deflated after fixation of the joint surfaces and hemostasis performed prior to closure.

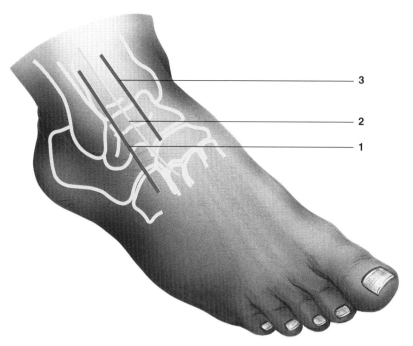

Figure 1

The anterolateral incision to the ankle joint is placed about 1–2 cm anterior to the edge of the fibula. This incision can be extended proximally and distally if greater exposure is required. The anterior incision begins about 5 cm superior to the ankle joint and extends distally in a straight line, almost to the talonavicular joint

1 Anterolateral incision
2 Superficial peroneal nerve
3 Anterior incision

Most surgical approaches to the ankle involve an incision on the lateral or anterolateral side of the ankle joint. Placing a towel roll under the ipsilateral buttock will provide internal rotation to the hip joint and keep the foot in neutral or possibly slight internal rotation. This is useful in the exposure and allows access to both sides of the ankle joint.

It is helpful to prepare and drape the entire lower extremity into the operative field so that the knee joint can be used as a reference point for the final position of the ankle fusion.

Incisions

Anterolateral approach

The anterolateral approach is the most versatile for exposure of the ankle joint. The subtalar joint and calcaneocuboid joint can also be exposed if necessary. The length of the incision depends upon the arthrodesis technique that has been planned. For arthrodesis in situ, the incision begins about 2 cm anterior to the anterior border of the fibula and approximately 3 cm above the ankle joint. The incision then curves inferiorly and slightly anteriorly, ending just below the sinus tarsi (Figure 1). Deep dissection then exposes the tibiotalar joint and clears the undersurface of the talus at the sinus tarsi. The deep subcutaneous tissues should be preserved as this aids in wound closure and healing. Through this incision most of the ankle joint can be exposed, particularly if the ankle

is not overly stiff. Right-angled Hohmann retractors are helpful. They are placed between the fibula and tibia after release of the interosseous ligament, and over the tibia at the medial side of the joint surface. A small lamina spreader is useful in distracting the joint surfaces. The anterior talofibular ligament, if present, can also be released from the fibula.

In a complex ankle arthrodesis, which may also require arthrodesis of the subtalar joint, a longer anterolateral incision is usually needed. This is the best approach to use if there is a moderate to severe ankle/hindfoot deformity which must be corrected. The incision should extend approximately 5–6 cm above the ankle joint and then inferiorly and anteriorly to the anterior process of the calcaneus and over the dorsal portion of the calcaneocuboid joint (Figure 1). Care should be taken to avoid injury to the superficial peroneal nerve. Sharp dissection is carried down, freeing the intraosseous ligament between the tibia and fibula, and then a subperiosteal dissection begins at the joint line to expose the anterior distal tibia. The sinus tarsi is exposed and the exposure can be carried more distally if significant hindfoot surgery is to be included (Figure 2). If the fibula is to be osteotomized, then an incision is made along its anterolateral border and the periosteum is reflected from the anterior and lateral half of the fibula. The periosteum and soft tissues on the posterior side of the fibula should remain intact, as they may aid in stability and blood supply to the bone, if it is to be used as a

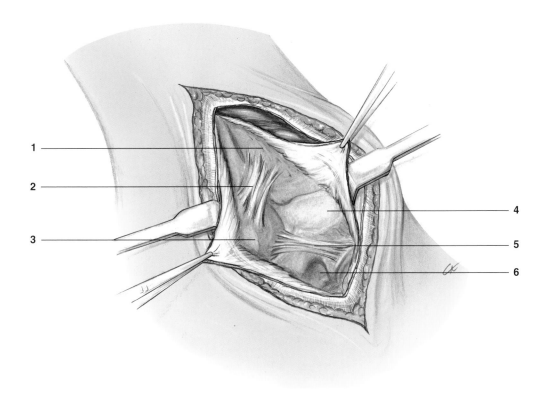

Figure 2

Anterolateral approach: sharp dissection is carried down to the periosteum of the tibia and along the anterior border of the fibula, if a fibular strut graft is to be used. The ankle joint is exposed and subperiosteal dissection across the anterior rim of the tibia allows for good visualization

1   Tibia
2   Anterior tibiofibular ligament
3   Fibula
4   Talar dome
5   Anterior talofibular ligament
6   Sinus tarsi

graft. The fibula can be osteotomized at any level, but if it is to be used as a strut graft the osteotomy is usually made about 6–7 cm above the tip of the lateral malleolus. An oblique osteotomy is preferred and the inner third of the fibula can be divided longitudinally and removed from the ankle. The remaining lateral two-thirds of the fibula can then be used as a strut graft. The resected portion of fibula, in some cases, can also be used as supplemental bone graft. Depending upon the type of fixation and the degree of deformity, it may be necessary to add a short supplemental medial incision. This incision begins about 3 cm superior to the tibial plafond and courses inferiorly and slightly anteriorly along the anterior edge of the medial malleolus. Subperiosteal dissection clears the medial side of the tibia just above the joint line. This incision can also be used to expose the anterior third of the medial malleolus should it require resection (see below).

Short medial and lateral incisions

In patients having an arthrodesis in situ, short medial and lateral incisions are helpful in gaining exposure. These shorter incisions are made in the same sites that would be used for portals for ankle arthroscopy. On the medial side it is important to remember the location of the saphenous nerve, although it is rarely seen. On the lateral side, care is needed to avoid the superficial peroneal nerve. This type of exposure only permits access to the tibiotalar joint. Usually some type of high-speed power burr is required for joint preparation. Distraction of the ankle joint can be done manually or with a mechanical ankle distractor.

Arthroscopic portals

The standard anteromedial and anterolateral arthroscopic portals are used if an ankle arthrodesis is to be performed using arthroscopic techniques to prepare the joint surfaces. Ankle distraction is most helpful. Small supplemental incisions will be necessary, depending on the type of fixation that is selected.

Anterior approach

An anterior approach to the ankle joint can be used if an arthrodesis in situ is planned, or in patients with only mild deformity where an external fixator is going to be used. The anterior incision begins about 4–5 cm superior to the ankle joint and extends inferiorly almost to the talonavicular joint (see Figure 1). The interval between the anterior tibial tendon and the extensor hallucis longus is a safe one to use, as the deep peroneal neurovascular bundle remains lateral to the approach. Alternatively, some prefer to enter the ankle through the sheath of the anterior tibial tendon. This may be important if there has been a previous incision or extensive scarring anteriorly. Dissection is carried down to the ankle joint, which is exposed by subperiosteal elevation at the tibial side of the joint. This incision gives satisfactory exposure, particularly if the joint surfaces are to be resected with a power oscillating saw. Otherwise, there may be some limitation in clearing the posterior malleolus of its articular surface, if that is necessary.

Posterior approach

The posterior approach is reserved for complicated ankle arthrodesis, usually a revision procedure, or when there is extensive scarring or poor skin anterolaterally. However, it may be difficult using this approach to correct severe ankle and hindfoot deformities, so it is best to use this when one is performing a tibeotalocalcaneal arthrodesis, where there is mild to moderate deformity and extensive bone grafting is necessary. The patient is in a prone position. The incision is approximately 10–12 cm long and begins at the tip of the calcaneus, extending proximally just along the medial border of the Achilles tendon. Depending on the pathology, the Achilles tendon can either be divided in a Z-fashion for exposure, or be detached with a small piece of bone from its insertion on the calcaneus. If the latter method is selected, the tendon with its fragment of bone can be placed superiorly under the subcutaneous tissues for protection. Dissection is carried down in the midline, finding the tendon of the flexor hallucis longus and incising the periosteum just lateral to that tendon, reflecting the flexor hallucis longus and its muscle belly medially, and the other

soft tissues laterally. A wide exposure of the posterior portion of the ankle joint is possible. The subtalar joint is usually found first in the subperiosteal dissection. This exposure is excellent if a blade plate or an intramedullary rod is to be used for fixation. This approach can also be used if extensive bone grafting is necessary to obtain an arthrodesis.

Joint preparation

Debridement of joint surfaces

A sharp periosteal elevator is best used to remove whatever joint surface remains in the arthritic ankle. A 4–5-mm oval power burr is helpful as long as a smooth surface is maintained. At times it is necessary to osteotomize the posterior malleolus in order to obtain proper alignment of the ankle arthrodesis, and this can be done with a power oscillating saw. Surface debridement is performed using arthroscopic equipment if that technique has been selected.

Resection of joint surfaces

The dome of the talus and the articular surface of the tibia can be resected with an oscillating power saw. As little subchondral bone as possible should be removed. Resection of large amounts of bone reduces the height of the dome of the talus and may cause significant impingement of the malleoli on the counter of the shoe, if they are not resected.

Malleolar resection

Generally, the medial malleolus can be retained when an ankle arthrodesis is performed. It may provide some increased stability to the fusion construct. When bone is deficient, as in severe arthritis, previous trauma, sepsis or a failed implant, the malleoli prevent the remaining bony surfaces from coming into contact. In severe cases, such as a failed ankle replacement, the gap is so large that an interpositional bone graft is needed. In others, simply removing a portion of each malleolus will allow good bony contact between the tibia and the talus. Even after a successful ankle arthrodesis, the malleoli may be excessively prominent medially and laterally and may impinge on the counter of the patient's shoe, causing pain. Partial resection of the malleoli is preferable. The lateral malleolus is prepared as it would be for a strut graft (see above). The anterior two-thirds of the medial malleolus is resected using the short medial incision (see above).

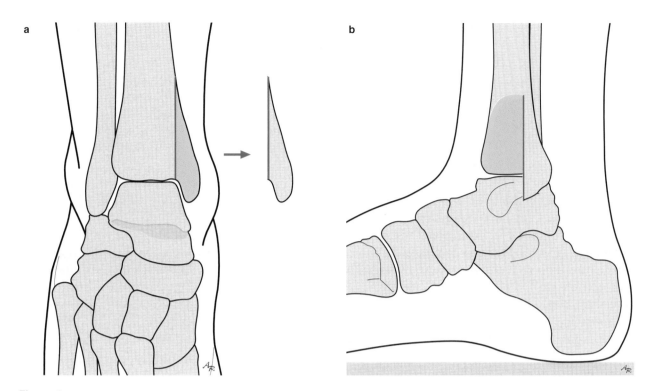

Figure 3

The anterior two-thirds of the medial malleolus can be resected if necessary. a. anterior aspect; b. medial aspect

Using a small oscillating saw and an osteotome, the malleolus is first cut on the medial side longitudinally at the junction between the anterior two-thirds and posterior one-third. A short cut is then made from anterior to posterior at a 90° angle to the first cut to remove the anterior two-thirds of the medial malleolus (Figure 3). This usually removes the prominent inferior tip of the malleolus. Retaining the posterior third protects the tendons and the neurovascular bundle.

Foot position in an arthrodesis

As important as obtaining an arthrodesis is positioning the foot in the optimum position to improve the patient's gait. Fusing the ankle in a neutral position allows the use of any remaining midfoot motion, which simulates some ankle joint motion and gives a better functional result [King et al. 1980]. At the transverse tarsal joints, the midfoot moves approximately 15–20° in a dorsal–plantar direction. If an ankle is fused in plantarflexion it cannot utilize this motion. Thus, positioning the tibiotalar surfaces so the foot and ankle are in a neutral position is important. If the hindfoot is stiff or has been previously fused, positioning the foot and ankle

in about 10° of dorsiflexion may be helpful. This position allows the patient to rise more easily from a chair. The hindfoot alignment is also important, and the heel should be in 5–10° of valgus. A heel in varus will lock the transverse tarsal joints, limiting any compensatory tarsal motion. External rotation should approximate the contralateral normal ankle and is usually about 10°. This degree of external rotation is achieved when the anteromedial crest of the tibia is parallel to the second ray. The foot should be positioned directly under the tibia. Therefore, the anterior edge of the talar dome should be directly under the anterior cortex of the tibia. If the foot remains too anterior to the tibia, gait will be impaired and the patient will need to vault over an overly long foot.

At times it is impossible to achieve the perfect position for ankle arthrodesis. This is usually due to the ankle deformity or malalignment of the tibia, which may distort the anatomy. Likewise, deformities of the adjacent joints, i.e. the subtalar and transverse tarsal joints, may have a limiting effect on gait following an ankle arthrodesis. These factors should be carefully explained to the patient preoperatively. The main indication to perform an ankle arthrodesis is to relieve pain caused by the arthritic ankle.

Fixation for ankle arthrodeses

The optimum type of fixation should be used in ankle arthrodesis. Good bone quality, such as is seen in patients with traumatic arthritis or osteoarthritis, allows the most rigid type of fixation. At least two 6.5-mm cancellous bone screws give satisfactory stability to an arthrodesis construct [Thordarson et al. 1990]. The addition of a fibular strut graft provides additional stability in ankles with good bone quality. However, a strut graft appears to contribute more stability when the bone quality is poor, and is an excellent addition when performing an ankle fusion in patients with osteoporosis [Thordarson et al. 1990]. The screws should be tested after insertion to determine whether they provide enough stability across the arthrodesis site. If mild torque is applied manually to the foot there should be no visible motion at the site of the arthrodesis, indicating satisfactory fixation is provided by the screws. If the quality of the bone is questionable and suboptimal purchase of the screws results in obvious torsional motion at the site of the arthrodesis, the graft technique should be considered. Alternatively, it may be possible to add an external fixator, depending on the screw placement. Colgrove and Bruffey [2001] reported 100% fusion in 26 consecutive ankles using two screws and an external fixator. If, however, the screws are giving no fixation they should be removed and an external fixator utilized (this is indeed a rare situation). The external fixator has been shown to improve the control of tibial rotation, a motion that is probably not well controlled by a below-knee cast [Thordarson et al. 1992]. However, screw fixation, even in poor-quality bone, was found to be superior to the use of an external fixator for plantarflexion and dorsiflexion loading [Thordarson et al. 1992]. This motion can be controlled, in part, by a below-knee cast.

Patients with rheumatoid arthritis frequently have osteoporotic bone, and fixation may be difficult. Fusion rates seemed to be equal in a group of rheumatoid patients who underwent ankle arthrodesis using either an external fixator or cancellous bone screws [Cracchiolo et al. 1992].

Cancellous bone screws

Internal fixation using cancellous bone screws has now gained wide acceptance. This method avoids most of the pitfalls and postoperative care required when using an external fixator. Thus, the advantages of internal fixation may be:

- Better acceptance by the patient
- Less frequent medical care because pin care is unnecessary, as it is when an external fixator is used; also, all external fixation devices require removal at some point, and this usually means performing another (although relatively minor) operation
- A below-knee cast can be used to give additional stability to the arthrodesis site
- There may be decreased rates of infection
- There may be higher rates of fusion.

Cannulated screws placed over a guide wire, and self-reaming and self-tapping screws have been developed which are very helpful in ankle arthrodesis procedures. The screw diameter most commonly used is 6.5 mm. However, diameters vary between 5.5 and 7.0 mm.

Using cannulated screws, two guide wires are placed across the ankle and the position checked with an image intensifier. When the position is optimal, screws are placed over the wires.

Placement of screws can be in any direction. They can go from the tibia both anteromedial and anterolateral into the talus (Figure 4). These screws cross each other, and the drill holes should therefore be placed far enough apart so that the screws do not impinge on each other. A screw may also be placed from the posterior malleolus into the neck of the talus (Figure 5). This gives excellent fixation and positions the foot properly under the tibia. Exposure to place this screw and the technique of placing can be difficult. A medial and/or lateral screw can be used to augment the fixation site. Another good method is to place the screws from the lateral aspect of the talus, directing them superiorly and medially into the tibia (Figure 6) [Mann et al. 1991]. The entry points are at the junction between the neck and body of the talus and the second screw enters the lateral process of the talus. This method is made easier if there is some remaining motion in the subtalar joint.

Guide wires are directed superiorly, slightly posteriorly, medially and across the medial cortex of the tibia. Radiographs can then be used to check the position of the fusion. Appropriate-length (6.5 mm) cannulated self-tapping and self-reaming screws are then placed over the guide wires. A biomechanical analysis using cadaver specimens indicated that a crossed-screw technique was more rigid than the parallel-screw technique [Friedman et al. 1994]. The crossed-screw construct was more effective in controlling torsional motion, which is not controlled by a short leg cast frequently used postoperatively. Whenever cancellous bone screws

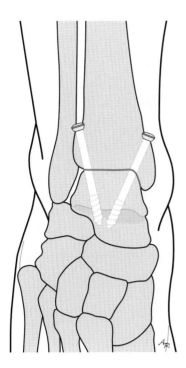

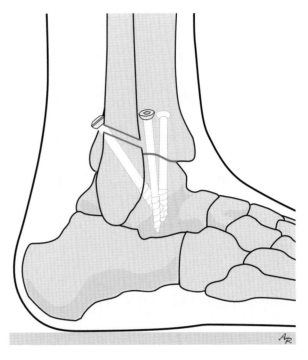

Figure 4

The use of cancellous bone screws has become popular in ankle arthrodesis procedures. Originally, screw placement was described from the tibia into the talus using one screw medially and one screw laterally

Figure 5

If a lateral approach is used, a screw may be placed from the posterior malleolus into the neck of the talus

are used, no threads should cross the arthrodesis site. If this is not possible, then a 6.5-mm drill is used to overdrill from the entry drill hole across the joint. However, this is rarely necessary. Metal washers are helpful in osteoporotic bone. Regardless of the method of fusion, cancellous bone grafts should be used to augment any ankle arthrodesis.

Fibular strut graft

The fibula is cut about 7 cm superior to the tibiotalar joint line (Figure 7). The medial third of the fibula is then transected longitudinally to decrease the width of the graft. This resected portion of the fibula can be used as a supplemental bone graft if necessary. The lateral edge of the tibia at the joint line must also be shaved so that there is a flat surface against which the fibula can be placed. It is then possible to place the narrowed lateral malleolus against the lateral side of the dome of the talus, and fixation is achieved with a short (3.5–4.0 mm) cancellous bone screw. If necessary, a 4.5-mm cortical screw can also be placed across the superior portion of the strut graft across all cortices, including the medial cortex of the tibia.

Morgan et al. [1999] have described salvage of tibial pilon fractures by fusing the ankle using a 90° cannulated blade-plate for fixation (90° cannulated LC-angled blade plate, Synthes, Paoli, PA, USA). These patients have severe destruction of the ankle and the distal metaphysis of the tibia. By use of the blade-plate, rigid internal fixation is achieved not only of the ankle but also of the distal tibial deformities, while avoiding fusion of the subtalar joint. However, these patients must have a talus which is large enough to accommodate the blade of this device. A posterior approach is used through a Z-plasty of the Achilles tendon. The posterior capsule of the ankle is resected, protecting the subtalar joint. Any remaining cartilage is removed from major tibial fragments and the dome of the talus. Metaphyseal defects are prepared for bone grafting. Under fluoroscopic control a guide wire is placed from the posterior talus into the center of the head parallel to the plantar aspect of the foot. An appropriate length blade-plate is driven over the guide wire and impacted flush with the posterior talus. The metaphyseal defects and ankle joint are packed with graft. The plate is provisionally fixed to the proximal tibia (usually intact). The alignment is checked with the fluoroscope and adjusted if needed. The plate is then secured to the tibia. Choi et al. [2001] also reported using the 90° angled blade-plate inserted laterally in a patient requiring revision arthrodesis of the tibiotalar joint.

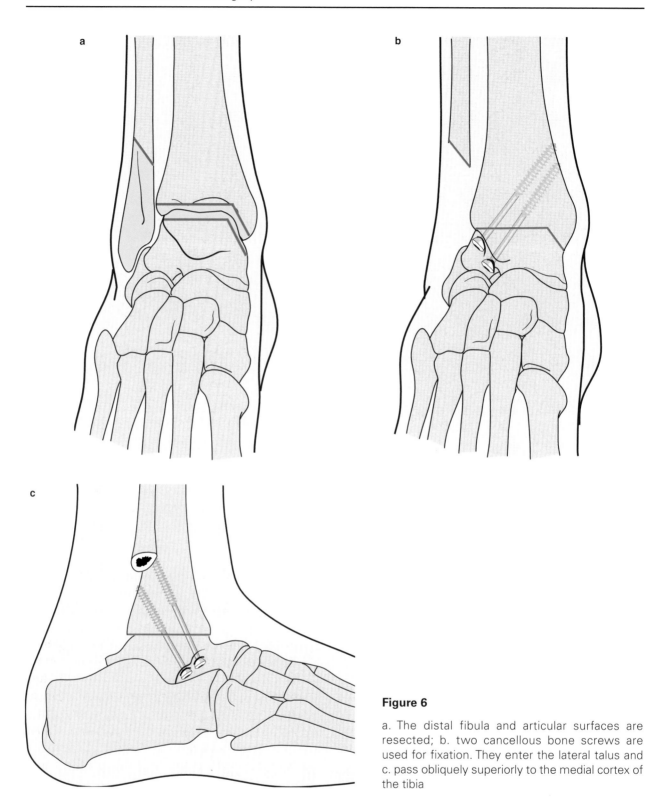

Figure 6

a. The distal fibula and articular surfaces are resected; b. two cancellous bone screws are used for fixation. They enter the lateral talus and c. pass obliquely superiorly to the medial cortex of the tibia

The use of implantable electrical stimulators

Implantable electrical stimulators are available and have been utilized to promote arthrodesis. The stimulator can be placed through a separate skin incision in the distal posterior lateral portion of the calf. The electrodes are tunneled distally and placed into the fusion site, with care being taken to avoid contact between the titanium leads and the internal fixation devices. They should be considered in patients with known risk factors for non-union, such as active smoking, infection, osteonecrosis and failed arthrodesis, as they are expensive.

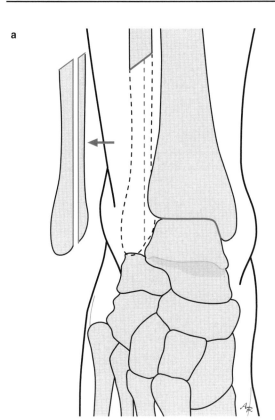
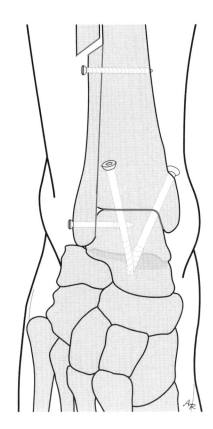

Figure 7

The fibula can be utilized as a strut graft to provide increased fixation for an ankle arthrodesis. a. preparation of graft; b. fixation of graft and arthrodesis

Although the controlled study has not yet been published, there is evidence that implantable electrical stimulators aid in achieving an arthrodesis.

External fixation

External fixators are now rarely used for ankle arthrodesis. However, the use of an external fixator may be indicated for arthrodesis in the presence of a suspected infection or severe osteoporosis; and arthrodesis in ankles that have marked loss of bone – from a previous fracture, a failed ankle replacement or a failed ankle fusion. In such patients, a tibiotalocalcaneal arthrodesis is performed. Some of these indications also require the use of extensive bone grafting to obtain a solid fusion. It is important to use an external fixator that provides relatively rigid fixation, with no plantarflexion or dorsiflexion movement. It is usually not possible to supplement the arthrodesis site with a below-knee cast.

Two types of external fixator are available for ankle arthrodesis. The first uses pins which pass across both the medial and the lateral sides of the tibia, and either the talus or the calcaneus.

Usually, 4-mm or 5-mm centrally threaded pins are used. The second method uses a unilateral frame [Thordarson et al. 1994]. This device is placed on the medial side of the ankle, using two cortical pins in the tibia and two cancellous pins in the body of the talus or in the calcaneus. Pins tapering from 6 mm to 5 mm in diameter are most frequently used. When using external fixation it is important to make a small transverse incision medially, just posterior to the medial malleolus, to avoid injury to the neurovascular bundle. Through this incision it is possible to expose a portion of the talus by blunt dissection. At times, it is necessary to identify the neurovascular bundle. Occasionally, a small amount of the posterior part of the medial malleolus needs to be removed, so that the posterior pin will not impinge on the malleolus. This is most often necessary if the pins traverse the talus. At times, little talar bone remains and it is necessary to place the pins in the calcaneus (Figure 8). Again, care should be taken not to injure the neurovascular bundle, which can be protected further by the use of a drill sleeve. With the foot and leg held in the proper position for fusion, a power drill is used to drive the pins from medial to lateral across the talus or calcaneus,

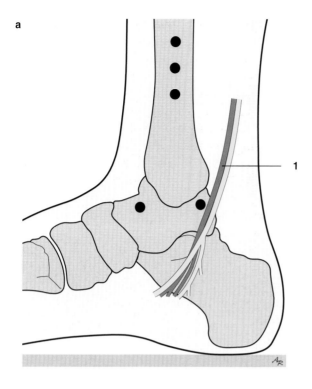

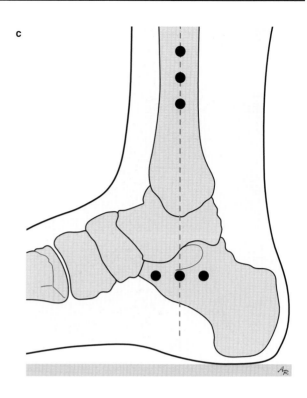

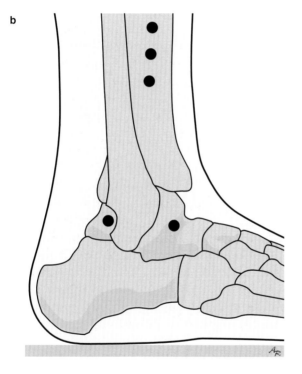

Figure 8

Pin placement in external fixation of ankle arthrodesis. a. medial aspect; b. lateral aspect; c. if the talus is deficient, the pins are placed in the calcaneus

a

1 Tibial nerve and posterior tibial artery

should the fixator be one having a medial and a lateral frame. If sufficient bone is present, three pins can be used when placing an external fixator in the talus or the calcaneus. Sometimes it is only possible to place two pins. The pins in the talus should be about 2 cm distal to the arthrodesis site. Since the fibula is a posterior structure, the posterior transfixion pin will usually impinge on the fibula. That portion of the fibula should be exposed

and removed so that the pin will not touch the fibula, particularly after compression has been placed (Figure 8b). Appropriate drill guides and the distal portion of the fixator can then be used to aid in positioning the additional pins in the talus or calcaneus. In the tibia the pins are placed across the midsagittal portion of the bone. Although three pins may not be necessary, it is helpful to have them in place, because occasionally one has to be removed if a superficial infection develops around it. In placing the pins in the tibia it is important to use the center of the tibia and not place the pins into the anterior cortex. Pins placed just under the subcutaneous anterior cortex of the tibia can cause drainage or pin tract infection. It may be necessary to pre-drill the tibial holes if dense cortical bone is present. Following placement of the pins, the external fixator is attached and the position of arthrodesis is usually checked visually. It may be difficult to see the tibiotalar arthrodesis site on the lateral radiograph with the fixator in place. Sufficient compression is used to hold the ankle arthrodesis construct as stable as possible, until the transfixion pins just begin to bend. The use of fixation pins requires daily care to avoid the occurrence of sepsis, which might require premature removal of one of the pins.

Ankle and pantalar fusions can also be accomplished using the Ilizarov fixation method (Khodadadyan-Klostermann et al. 2001). This method is somewhat complex and should be used only by surgeons who use it regularly. Its main use is in patients with failed fusion, in patients with sepsis after failed fusion, and in patients with severe anatomic deformity who may have substantial bone loss and who may also have poor skin.

Postoperative care

Following the use of internal fixation, the ankle should be placed in a short leg cast. The cast is initially split to allow for swelling. The patient should use crutches or a walker and should not bear weight on the ankle arthrodesis side for approximately 6 weeks. Sutures are removed about 2 weeks postoperatively. At about 6 weeks postoperatively the cast is removed and non-weightbearing anteroposterior and lateral radiographs are obtained. If the ankle arthrodesis appears stable, weightbearing is permitted after a walking cast has been applied. The patient can place more weight on the cast on a weekly basis. Four to six weeks later, if the patient is asymptomatic while putting full weight on the cast, the cast is removed and new weightbearing radiographs are taken. If there is evidence of bone union both clinically and radiographically, a cast is no longer needed. An inexpensive athletic shoe can be worn while the patient continues to use crutches or a walker for several days until the gait pattern has adjusted. An oversized shoe is usually selected as there will be postoperative swelling, which can be controlled using elastic stockings. The patient must

be warned that should the ankle become painful it may indicate that insufficient fusion is present despite the clinical and radiographic evaluation. They must return immediately and can be fitted with a postoperative boot to be worn for a few weeks. Some patients require physical therapy for gait training. The patient should be evaluated about 4–6 weeks later. If they have difficulty with gait the shoe can be adapted using a modified solid ankle cushion heel and a rocker-bottom sole. Leg length inequality can be checked at that time, and if significant shortening is present on the operative side, a lift can be added to the outside of the shoe. Usually, 1 cm of shortening is acceptable, but anything greater may require a lift. At about 1 year, when the patient returns for routine follow-up, they are usually wearing ordinary shoes.

Complications

The major complications following an ankle arthrodesis are sepsis, non-union, delayed union, wound healing problems, peripheral neurovascular complications and stress fractures of the tibia. Many of these complications may be minimized by carefully ascertaining the medications that the patient is taking before the arthrodesis procedure. It may be possible to discontinue many of these drugs, which may interfere with a successful outcome. Thus, non-steroidal anti-inflammatory medications should be discontinued approximately 10 days before surgery, and preferably not restarted for as many weeks as the patient can tolerate following the operation, as they are known to interfere with bone healing. Patients taking oral corticosteroids, especially those taking more than 7.5 mg of prednisone per day, also run a much higher risk of delayed union or non-union [Cracchiolo et al. 1992]. Patients with rheumatoid arthritis taking methotrexate may also have a higher incidence of delayed wound healing; it is appropriate to discontinue methotrexate about a week before the operation and for about 2 weeks afterwards.

Tibiotalocalcaneal arthrodesis

At times it is necessary to include the subtalar joint and the calcaneus in the fusion construct. This is usually seen when there is subtalar arthritis or when a severe varus or valgus deformity of the hindfoot; or when there is a loss of the dome of the talus (trauma, necrosis, sepsis, prior operations, failed total ankle implant). Such an arthrodesis requires

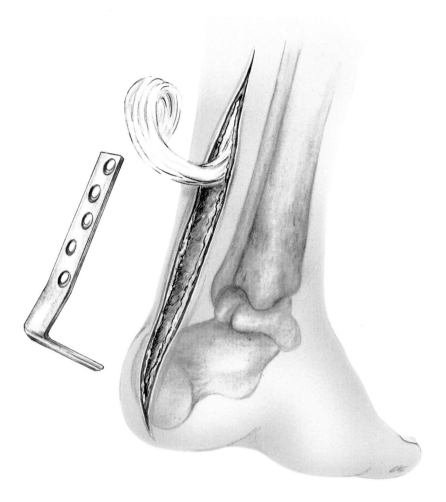

Figure 9

A 95° blade-plate is used to secure the tibiotalocalcaneal arthrodesis through a posterior approach

bone grafting, usually posteriorly so that the tibia fuses to the calcaneus across the posterior portion of what was the tibiotalar joint; rigid internal fixation if possible (blade-plate or intramedullary rod); and an external fixator (this is less desirable as time to even early evidence of fusion is prolonged, and the fixator may need to be removed if there are pin problems). Prolonged use of external fixators such as the Ilizarov device may be poorly tolerated by patients. Although screw fixation can be used (Acosta et al. 2000), especially in thin patients with small stature, they do not give sufficient fixation in large patients, patients with deformity and where there is bone loss. An intramedullary rod, even one placed without compression, has been shown to be superior to crossed lag screws as a method of internal fixation (Berend et al. 1997).

Blade-plate fixation

Posterior approach

The posterior approach and use of a standard 95° angled blade-plate with extensive bone grafting is an excellent method of securing a solid tibiotalocalcaneal arthrodesis [Gruen and Mears 1991]. The patient is in the prone position and the posterior iliac crests are available for autogenous bone grafts. This method is best used in patients with mild to moderate deformity and when the transverse tarsal joints are spared. Gross, severe deformity may be difficult to correct with the patient prone. It is not absolutely necessary to completely denude the surfaces of the ankle and subtalar joint; the former is usually destroyed and the latter frequently arthritic. However, the use of sharp Cobb periosteal elevators assists in clearing the joint surfaces. The fibula is separated from the tibia by sharp dissection. It may be necessary to osteotomize the fibula to correct a mild to moderate varus/valgus deformity.

Alignment can be maintained manually and the blade inserted into the calcaneus, usually into a prepared trough (Figure 9). Using a single screw under compression the plate is then secured to the posterior tibia; the flexor hallucis muscle must be swept aside medially using a periosteal elevator but must not be damaged. An image intensifier is used to check the position of the blade-plate and the angle of arthrodesis. If satisfactory, the remaining screws are placed. Autogenous bone graft is placed along the posterior of the tibia just above the ankle

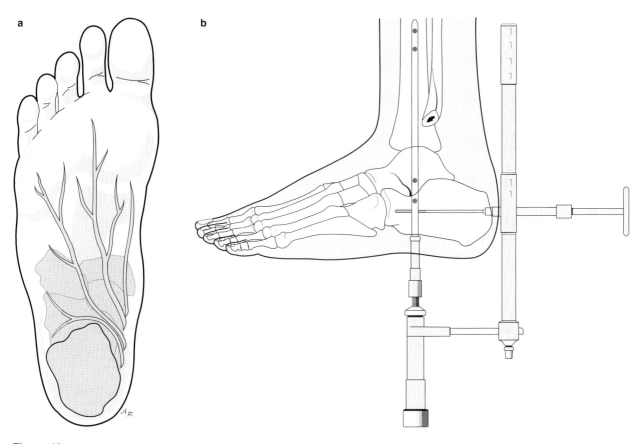

a   b

Figure 10

a. Site of the Steinman pin placement through the body of the calcaneus. b. the tibial interlocking screws are placed from lateral to medial. With this particular intramedullary nail, compression can be placed distal and plantar on the calcaneus and after compression is secured the calcaneal and talar screws are placed from lateral to medial. A posterior to anterior screw can be used with selected intramedullary nails and such a screw is essential when there is insufficient talus, as occurs in severe erosive arthritis, osteonecrosis, or previous failed arthrodesis or failed ankle replacement

joint and inferiorly to the calcaneus. Voids are also filled with cancellous graft. The muscle is repositioned and the Achilles tendon can be re-attached to the calcaneus using either a 4.5-mm screw through a bone fragment in the tendon or bone anchors with 2-0 sutures. Closure must be meticulous and without undue tension, as wound healing is always a concern.

Anterolateral approach

Patients with moderate to severe ankle and/or hindfoot deformities or who may also require arthrodesis of the transverse tarsal joints (pantalar fusion) are operated upon using the anterolateral approach and an ancillary medial incision. The fibula can be used for a bone graft; it can be morcellized using a 43-mm sharp acetabular reamer [Raikin and Myerson, 2000], or it can be excised and later broken into pieces or placed in a bone mill to be used as graft. It is usually necessary to excise the distal 12–15 mm of fibula. This gives excellent exposure to the ankle and subtalar joints. The medial

incision is used to excise the anterior two-thirds of the malleolus, which is usually necessary, and to expose the talonavicular joint if needed. After the joints are prepared (see Joint preparation) the blade-plate drill guide is used to place a 2-mm guide wire from the lateral side of the calcaneus medially to exit just under the sustentaculum tali about 1.5 cm inferior to the subtalar joint. This orients the blade at 90° to the shaft of the tibia. The depth of the guide wire determines the length of the blade: usually 40–50 mm. The 90° angle blade-plate is selected, usually a 5–8-hole plate, attached to the inserter/extractor handle and driven over the guide wire, which is then removed. Using an impactor the blade can be driven a few millimeters further into the calcaneus, which may improve the position of the plate against the lateral tibia.

The position of the arthrodesis and the blade-plate should be checked with the image intensifier; if satisfactory the screws are placed, compressing the arthrodesis site. Bone grafts are placed, mostly posteriorly and within all voids at the joint lines.

Meticulous skin closure is necessary to avoid delayed wound healing.

Intramedullary nail fixation

Intramedullary fixation has also been utilized for tibiotalocalcaneal arthrodesis. Initially a Trifin nail was used [Stone and Helal 1991]. More recently interlocking screws have been used to secure the nail proximally through the tibia and distally through the calcaneus. To date, the choice of a nail versus blade-plate fixation seems more dependent on the surgeon's choice and experience with the devices than on specific preoperative indications. Both the posterior and anterolateral approaches can be used; again the degree of deformity and surgeon's preference seem to determine the surgical procedure. The approaches, bone preparations and the use of bone grafts have been previously described.

Using the posterior approach, Kile et al. [1994] described making a trough through the posterior cortex of the tibia just above the ankle joint and extending the trough inferiorly across what remained of the posterior talus and the superior cortex of the calcaneus. This would be the recipient site for the extra-articular portion of the bone graft. Placement of the nail is similar, regardless of the approach. McGarvey et al. [1998] determined that it was important to remove both malleoli in order to avoid damage to the neurovascular structures – especially the lateral plantar nerve and the flexor hallucis longus – when the nail was introduced through the body of the calcaneus. Following malleolar resection, the talus (foot) can be medially displaced 7–11 mm, which protects the structures and allows the nail to pass through the body of the calcaneus rather than the sustentaculum tali, thus enhancing purchase within the calcaneus (Figure 10). Following bony preparation a 3-cm longitudinal incision is made anterior to the fat pad of the heel (Figure 10a). Blunt dissection is carried through the plantar fascia, and if possible the intrinsic muscles are moved as medial as possible. A Steinmann pin is passed through the calcaneus and talus into the distal tibia. This is checked with an image intensifier. An appropriate-sized cannulated reamer, depending on which nail is used, is then passed over the pin. The pin is removed and under image control a ball-tipped guide wire is passed up the center of the tibia for a distance that corresponds to the length of nail selected for the fixation (Figure 10b). Flexible reamers in 0.5-mm increments are passed over the guide wire to open the distal tibia. The tibia is usually reamed 0.5 mm more than the diameter of the nail. The nail is then attached to its specific drill guide and impacted. Bone cuts, usually on the tibial side, may need to be adjusted so that good bony opposition is achieved between tibia and talus. Interlocking screws are then placed from lateral to medial avoiding the fibula superiorly. Whether to place the tibial or calcaneal interlocking screws first depends on the specific nail. In patients with loss or absence of the talus one nail allows the calcaneal interlocking screw from posterior to anterior of ensuring purchase distally and resulting in a stiffer construct [Mann et al. 2001]. Depending on the nail selected, up to 15 mm of compression of the fusion site is possible. Bone grafting is essential, as is careful wound closure.

Stress risers occur in the tibial diaphysis around the proximal interlocking screws of intramedullary nails used for tibiotalocalcaneal fusions. Stress fractures may also occur in this area. It may be prudent to remove the proximal screws once a solid fusion has occurred.

Postoperative care

Postoperative care is similar to that used following ankle arthrodesis (see above). However, some time may be required, depending on the bone quality and security of internal fixation. Thus, time in the non-weightbearing cast might be extended to 8 weeks. The weightbearing cast should be continued until the patient is completely pain free when walking and the radiograph shows some early evidence of fusion. A walking boot should be used for 3–4 weeks after the cast has been discontinued.

References

Acosta R, Ushiba J, Cracchiolo A III (2000) The results of a primary and staged pantalar arthrodesis and tibiotalocalcaneal arthrodesis in adult patients. Foot Ankle Int 21: 182–194

Berend ME, Glisson RR, Nunley JA (1997) A biomechanical comparison of intramedullary nail and crossed lag screw fixation for tibiotalocalcaneal arthrodesis. Foot Ankle Int 18: 639–643

Choi G, Ghalambor N, Nihal A, Trepman E (2001) Revision ankle arthrodesis with lateral cannulated angled blade plate fixation. Foot Ankle Surg 7: 187–191

Colgrove RC, Bruffey JD (2001) Ankle arthrodesis: combined internal–external fixation. Foot Ankle Int 20: 92–97

Cracchiolo A (1991) Methods and follow-up statistics on ankle arthrodesis. Clin Orthop 268: 2–111

Cracchiolo A, Cimino W, Lian G (1992) Arthrodesis of the ankle in patients who have rheumatoid arthritis. J Bone Joint Surg 74A: 903–909

Crosby LA, Yee TC, Formanek TS, Fitzgibbons TC (1996) Complications following arthroscopic ankle arthrodesis. Foot Ankle 17: 340–342

Dent CM, Patil M, Fairclough JA (1993) Arthroscopic ankle arthrodesis. J Bone Joint Surg 75B: 830–832

Friedman RL, Glisson RR, Nunley JA (1994) A biochemical comparative analysis of two techniques for tibiotalar arthrodesis. Foot Ankle 15: 301–305

Gruen GS, Mears DC (1991) Arthrodesis of the ankle and subtalar joints. Clin Orthop 268: 15–20

Khodadadyan-Klostermann C, Raschke M, Mittlemeier T et al. (2001) Ankle and pan-talar arthrodesis with Ilizarov composite hybrid fixation: operative technique and review of 21 cases. Foot Ankle Surg 7: 149–156

Kile TA, Donnelly RE, Gehrke JC et al. (1994) Tibiotalocalcaneal arthrodesis with an intramedullary device. Foot Ankle 15: 669–673

King HA, Watkins TB, Samuelson KM (1980) Analysis of foot position in ankle arthrodesis and its influence on gait. Foot Ankle 1: 44–49

Mann RA, Van Manen JW, Wapner K, Martin J (1991) Ankle fusion. Clin Orthop 268: 49–55

Mann MR, Parks BG, Pak SS, Miller SD (2001) Tibiotalocalcaneal arthrodesis: a biomechanical analysis of the rotational stability of the Biomet ankle arthrodesis nail. Foot Ankle Int 22: 731–733

McGarvey WC, Trevino SG, Baxter DE et al. (1998) Tibiotalocalcaneal arthrodesis: anatomic and technical considerations. Foot Ankle Int 19: 363–369

Morgan SJ, Thordarson DB, Shepherd LE (1999) Salvage of tibial pilon fractures using fusion of the ankle with a 90° cannulated blade-plate: a preliminary report. Foot Ankle Int 20: 375–383

O'Brien TS, Hart TS, Shereff MJ et al. (1999) Open versus arthroscopic ankle arthrodesis: a comparative study. Foot Ankle Int 20: 368–374

Ogilvie-Harris DJ, Lieberman I, Fitsialos D (1993) Arthroscopically assisted arthrodesis for osteoarthrotic ankles. J Bone Joint Surg 75A: 1167–1174

Paremain GD, Miller SD, Myerson MS (1996) Ankle arthrodesis: results after the miniarthrotomy technique. Foot Ankle 17: 247–252

Stone KH, Helal B (1991) A method of ankle stabilization. Clin Orthop 268: 102–106

Raikin SM, Myerson MS (2000) A technique for harvesting bone graft for arthrodeses around the ankle. Foot Ankle Int 21: 778–779

Thordarson DB, Markolf KL, Cracchiolo A (1990) Biomechanical analysis of ankle arthrodesis using cancellous screws and fibular strut graft. J Bone Joint Surg 72A: 1359–1363

Thordarson DB, Markolf K, Cracchiolo A (1992) Stability of the ankle arthrodesis fixed by cancellous bone screws compared with that fixed by an external fixator. A biomechanical study. J Bone Joint Surg 74A: 1050–1055

Thordarson DB, Markolf K, Cracchiolo A (1994) External fixation in arthrodesis of the ankle. J Bone Joint Surg 76A: 1541–1544

40

Ankle joint replacement

Beat Hintermann
Victor Valderrabano

Introduction

Arthritis of the ankle joint can be very painful and can substantially affect normal locomotion. Ankle arthrodesis is a surgical intervention recommended for end-stage ankle arthritis that typically relieves pain in the short term. The results of long-term follow-up studies (at an average of 7–10 years after surgery) are not consistent. There are reports with very positive outcomes of ankle arthrodesis [Lynch et al. 1988, Glick et al. 1996]. However, many reports describe short-term and long-term problems with ankle arthrodesis [Kofoed and Stürup 1994, Pyevich et al. 1998], including problems when climbing stairs, getting up from a chair, walking on uneven surfaces and running. Additionally, the patient's level of satisfaction is often reported as being unsatisfactory, as the decreased functional ability often causes a need for ambulatory aids and/or permanent shoe modifications [Mazur et al. 1979, Boobbyer 1981]. A 16% decrease in gait velocity, a 3% increase in oxygen consumption and an overall decrease of 10% in gait efficiency was found [Waters et al. 1988].

Theoretically, an ankle arthrodesis would naturally cause increased stress in contiguous joints, forced to perform motions the fused ankle is unable to perform. Because increased contact stress and shear forces are primary causal factors for joint degeneration, the widespread advocacy of arthrodesis as the final treatment for ankle arthritis seems imprudent. These concerns have led several investigators to continue to search for a workable joint replacement that would allow the normal functional range of motion of the joint, reduce the pain and disability resulting from arthritis and preserve the integrity of adjacent articulations.

However, the biomechanics of the ankle present a unique set of challenges for arthroplasty surgery [Deland et al. 2000]. Despite a relative congruency of this joint, the axis of rotation does not stay constant during range of motion [Lundberg et al. 1989], therefore rotational forces must be taken into account [Hintermann et al. 1994]. The success of arthroplasty depends on how well a design can dissipate these rotational forces while maintaining the stability of the joint. It is not yet clear whether this dissipation of forces has been accomplished successfully with modern implants, although early reults in the semi-constrained designs with two components [Pyevich et al. 1998] or three components [Hintermann 1999, Kofoed and Lundberg-Jensen 1999, Hintermann and Valderrabano 2001] are encouraging.

Ankle replacement design

The differences between current ankle prostheses are striking, and many questions still remain regarding their design. In recent years, however, two different generic approaches to total ankle replacement design have emerged to permit semi-constrained motion:

1. Two-component design, incorporating a tibial and a talar component with some congruency mismatch (Agility™ Total Ankle System; DePuy Inc, Warsaw, IN, USA) or a ball-and-socket configuration (Ramses), allowing little sliding and/or rotational motion.

2. Three-component design, incorporating a flat metal tibial plate, a metal talar resurfacing component, and a mobile polyethylene bearing between

the two metal components, allowing flexion and extension at the talopolyethylene prosthetic interface and internal and external rotation and translation in the frontal and sagittal planes at the tibiopolyethylene prosthetic interface (Buechel-Pappas Ultra total ankle, Endotec, Inc, S. Orange, NJ; Hintegra® Total Ankle, NewDeal SA, Vienne, France (Figure 1); Salto; Link® STAR Scandinavian Total Ankle Replacement; Waldemar Link, Hamburg, Germany).

Fixation

All current ankle arthroplasty designs rely on bone ingrowth for implant stability. There are several major advantages to bone ingrowth [Kofoed and Danborg 1995, Saltzman 2000]:

- Less bone resection is required because no space between bone and implant is necessary for fixation
- Inadvertent cement displacement or spillage is avoided
- Because acrylic cement curing is an exothermic process, damage to local soft tissues and bony surfaces from the heat is avoided
- Loosening and fragmentation of cement probably cause accelerated third-body wear.

Ingrowth prostheses incorporate:

- Porous surfaces along the interface with bone (allow bone ingrowth, usually take 6–12 weeks, result in long-term stability of the implant–bone interface)
- A hydroxyapatite layer covering (encourages molecular bonding between the crystals of the calcium hydroxyapatite and the bone bed, takes 3–6 weeks, is totally resorbed with time, thus leaving concerns regarding long-term component fixation)
- A combination of porous and hydroxyapatite coating (theoretically allows early fixation of the implant through hydroxyapatite bonding and the later secure ingrowth of bone within the porous interstices).

Indications and contraindications

No consensus exists regarding the indications for ankle arthroplasty. The ideal patient is an elderly person with low physical demands. The patient with bilateral ankle arthritis or ipsilateral hindfoot arthritis who has had or will require a triple arthrodesis is particularly appropriate to consider as a candidate

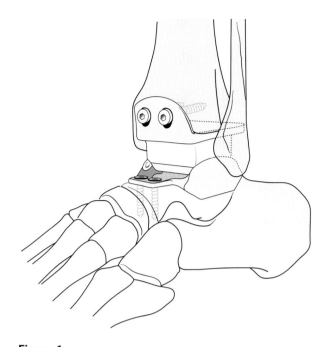

Figure 1

Three component ankle prosthesis

for ankle arthroplasty because bilateral ankle fusions and pantalar (ankle and triple) arthrodeses function poorly.

Indications

- Good bone stock
- Normal vascular status
- No immunosuppression
- Correct hindfoot–ankle alignment
- Well-preserved ankle joint motion
- Sufficient medial and lateral ankle stability.

Contraindications

- Neuroarthropathic degenerative disease (Charcot's ankle)
- Active or recent infection
- Avascular necrosis of the talus (of more than two-thirds of the talar body)
- Severe benign joint hypermobility syndrome
- Non-reconstructible malalignment
- Severe soft-tissue problems around the ankle
- Sensory or motor dysfunction of the foot or leg.

Surgical procedure

Preoperative planning

Anteroposterior and lateral weightbearing radiographs are necessary for planning of the procedure,

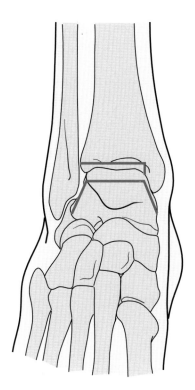
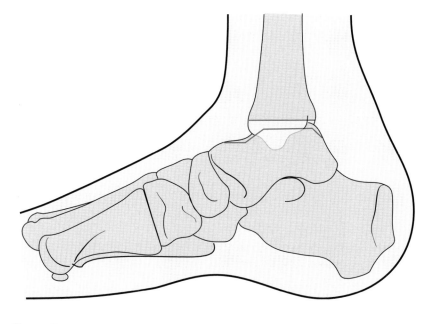

Figure 2

Bone resection for the tibial and the talar components of an ankle prosthesis, viewed from anterior and from medial

such as bony resection of tibia and talus, correction of malalignment and size of the components. In most ankle prostheses, templates are available to plan and to assess the most appropriate size of the tibial and talar components (Figure 2).

Anesthesia

General or regional anesthesia is used, depending on the anesthesiologist's and the patient's preference.

Positioning and preoperative preparation of the patient

The patient is positioned supine with the feet just on the distal border of the table, allowing the surgeon optimal access to the anterior side of the ankle. A support beneath the ipsilateral pelvis allows a correct anteroposterior position of the foot to be obtained. The patient's position should take into account the need for intraoperative image intensification, with the ability to obtain anteroposterior and lateral views. The leg is draped, maintaining the whole shank free (the tibial tuberosity must be visible, the ankle and knee mobile). A tourniquet is placed at the thigh.

Surgical approach and technique

Various approaches to the ankle have been recommended:

- Lateral transfibular approach [Buchholz et al. 1973]
- Anterolateral approach between the peroneal tertius and extensor digitorum longus tendons [Dini and Bassett 1980, Buechel et al. 1988]
- Anterior approach between extensor hallucis longus and anterior tibial tendons [Takakura et al. 1990, Kofoed and Stürup 1994, Hintermann 1999].

The authors' preferred surgical technique

Based on a three-component total ankle replacement design, the technique is as follows:

- Anterior longitudinal incision between extensor hallucis longus and anterior tibial tendons, paying attention to the neurovascular bundle that is on the lateral side covered by the extensor tendons (Figure 3)
- Longitudinal arthrotomy and capsulectomy
- Positioning of a self-retaining wound-spreader (hooks should be avoided)
- Removal of anterior osteophytes on tibia and talus
- Positioning of a special distractor, usually on the medial side, in the case of valgus malalignment on the lateral side, in order to provide optimal ankle joint exposure
- Positioning and alignment of the tibial cutting block, using the anteromedial corner of the ankle as a reference for implantation of the prosthesis (*)

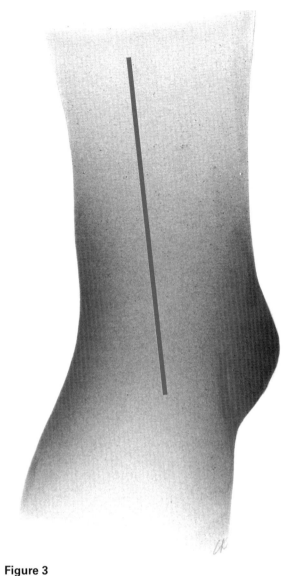

Figure 3

Anterior longitudinal incision between extensor hallucis longus and anterior tibial tendons

- Tibial cut, removal of the distal tibia and the posterior capsule (*)
- Positioning of the talar cutting block while the foot is held strictly in neutral position (*)
- Talar cut and removal of the superior talar surface (*)
- Insertion of the spacer into the created joint space in order to check hindfoot alignment and ligamentous stability of the ankle (*)
- Talar cut step by step on cranial, then posterior, medial and lateral aspects (*)
- Insertion of the trials and check of achieved alignment, stability and joint motion (*)
- Check of the component position by image intensification
- Insertion and fixation of the selected implants (Figure 4) (*)

- Insertion of one suction drain
- Closure of the extensorum retinaculum using non-interrupted resorbable sutures
- Wound closure using interrupted sutures
- Compressive dressing
- Well-padded short leg splint to keep the foot in neutral position.

The steps marked by (*) should be performed following the instructions of the prosthesis producer. In the case of malalignment, ligamentous instability and concomitant arthritis of the distal joints, additional operations might be considered prior to prosthetic implantation.

Postoperative protocol

When the wound condition is favorable, typically 2–4 days after surgery, the foot is placed in a brace (e.g. Vacuped®) that protects the ankle against eversion, inversion and plantarflexion movements for 6 weeks, allowing weightbearing immediately as tolerated. A program is started immediately for rehabilitation of the foot and ankle, including stretching of the triceps surae. In the case of poor bone quality, with additional operations such as re-alignment, ligament reconstruction and/or joint fusions, a short leg weightbearing cast is used for 6 weeks and a brace for an additional 4–6 weeks. After the cast is removed, the rehabilitation program is started, with gradual return to full activities as tolerated.

The authors have not seen any complications regarding wound healing and bone ingrowth with this postoperative protocol in 200 consecutive ankle arthroplasties using a three-component design with double-coated (hydroxyapatite and metal porous-coated) surface. However, it has to be emphasized that many authors suggest an immobilization restriction and do not allow full weightbearing until ingrowth of bone into the prosthetic components has been confirmed radiographically. Whether early postoperative motion has beneficial effects (greater final range of motion) or detrimental effects (less solid implant fixation) remains a matter of controversy and requires further controlled trials.

Radiographic follow-up images, including non-weightbearing anteroposterior and lateral radiographs of the ankle, are made intraoperatively, at 6 weeks, at 6 months, at 1 year, and then depending on the patient's complaint. Image intensification is used to obtain straight anteroposterior and lateral views of the tibial component, which allows reliable recognition of any component migration.

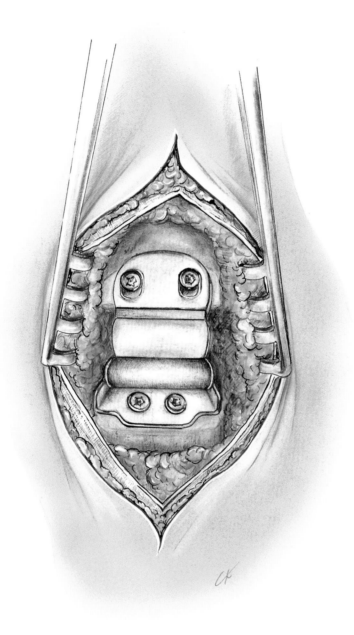

Figure 4

Intraoperative view of ankle prosthesis: a polyethylene bearing is inserted between the tibial and talar components

Hazards, complications and design problems

Wound problems

Total ankle arthroplasty has been plagued with an unusually high incidence of wound problems. Soft tissues around the ankle, especially in elderly patients and patients with rheumatoid arthritis, provide a relatively thin envelope for arthroplasty containment. In the authors' experience, meticulous handling of the soft tissues during surgery, compressive dressing and initial use of a well-padded short leg splint until the wound is healed are some effective measures to avoid skin necrosis, and superficial and deep wound infection.

Bone fracture

A fracture of the medial malleolus or, more seldom, of the fibula may occur while using an inappropriate saw blade. Some instrumentations therefore offer a protection device. If the bone is weakened too much, a fatigue fracture of the medial malleolus may occur. A vertical cut with the osteotome prior to the tibial cut with the saw might prevent this complication.

Poor range of motion

If the posterior capsule is not totally removed, the residual scar tissue may limit dorsiflexion. This may be especially true for the posteromedial corner, including the posterior tibiotalar bundle of the deltoid ligament. Accurate resection and early postoperative mobilization might help to prevent this problem, which may be more common in post-traumatic ankles.

Poor bone quality

A poor bone quality may result in breakage of the bone in contact with the implant, which is probably more the case for the tibial than the talar side. The use of larger implants may increase this potential complication, as the created moments at the interface between implant and bone increase with increasing size of the implants. Therefore, smaller implants should be considered in patients with poor bone quality, especially with respect to the medial–lateral and anterior–posterior dimension.

Proper bone resection

Another concern is the amount of bone resection. The more bone has to be removed, the more difficult is the salvage by revision arthroplasty or secondary fusion. Therefore, ankle replacement designs with minimal bone resection should be considered for primary implantation.

Instability of the polyethylene-bearing insert

One of the potential disadvantages of any mobile bearing design is the risk that a polyethylene-bearing insert will dislocate, when the capture mechanism is not able to withstand loads and wear, or if the ligament stability is insufficient. Therefore, meticulous care must be taken during prosthesis implantation with respect to restoring ligament tension and hindfoot alignment. A major concern with this approach, however, is that the periankle ligaments can become so taut that they decrease the mobility of the bearing construct, causing increased implant stresses and decreased range of motion.

Non-anatomically shaped prosthesis design

Finally, most current designs for the talar component are cylindrical, thus restricting flexion and extension about a single axis of rotation relative to the talus. If the mobile bearings are inserted in a tight-fit fashion, the axis of rotation must become the axis of rotation of the talar component, which might be substantially different from that of the normal ankle. Both the cylindrical talar design and the deviation to the intact ankle might increase ligament stress on the medial ankle, thus causing posteromedial ankle pain, restriction of motion and polyethylene wear.

References

Boobbyer GN (1981) The long-term results of ankle arthrodesis. Acta Orthop Scand 52: 107–110

Buchholz HW, Engelbrecht E, Siegel A (1973) Totale Sprunggelenkendoprothese Modell 'St. Georg'. Chirurgie 44: 241–244

Buechel FF, Pappas MJ, Iorio LJ (1988) New Jersey low contact stress total ankle replacement: biomechanical rationale and review of 23 cementless cases. Foot Ankle 8: 279–290

Deland JT, Morris GD, Sung IH (2000) Biomechanics of the ankle joint. A perspective on total ankle replacement. Foot Ankle Clin 5: 747–759

Dini A, Bassett FH III (1980) Evaluation of the early result of Smith total ankle replacement. Clin Orthop 146: 228–230

Glick JM, Morgan CD, Myerson MS et al. (1996) Ankle arthrodesis using an arthroscopic method: long-term follow-up of 34 cases. Arthroscopy 12: 428–434

Hintermann B (1999) The S.T.A.R. total ankle replacement. Short- and mid-term results. Orthopaede 28: 792–803

Hintermann B, Nigg BM, Cole GK (1994) Influence of selective arthrodesis on the movement transfer between calcaneus and tibia in vitro. Clin Biomech 9: 356–361

Hintermann B, Valderrabano V (2001) Total joint replacement of the ankle. Z Aerztl Fortbild Qualitätssich 95: 187–194

Kofoed H, Danborg L (1995) Biological fixation of ankle arthroplasty. Foot 5: 27–31

Kofoed H, Lundberg-Jensen A (1999) Ankle arthroplasty in patients younger and older than 50 years: a prospective series with long-term follow-up. Foot Ankle Int 20: 501–506

Kofoed H, Stürup J (1994) Comparison of ankle arthroplasty and arthrodesis. A prospective series with long-term follow-up. Foot 4: 6–9

Lundberg A, Svennson OK, Nemeth G, Selvik G (1989) The axis of rotation of the ankle joint. J Bone Joint Surg 71B: 94–99

Lynch AF, Bourne RB, Rorabeck CH (1988) The long-term results of ankle arthrodesis. J Bone Joint Surg 70B: 113–116

Mazur J, Schartz E, Simon S (1979) Ankle arthrodesis. Long-term follow-up with gait analysis. J Bone Joint Surg 61A: 964–975

Pyevich MT, Saltzman CL, Callaghan JJ, Alvine FG (1998) Total ankle arthroplasty: a unique design. Two to twelve-year follow-up. J Bone Joint Surg 80A: 1410–1420

Saltzman CL (2000) Perspective on total ankle replacement. Foot Ankle Clin 5: 761–775

Takakura Y, Yanaka Y, Sugimoto K et al. (1990) Ankle arthroplasty. A comparative study of cemented metal an uncemented ceramic prostheses. Clin Orthop 252: 209–216

Waters RL, Barnes G, Husserl T et al. (1988) Comparable energy expenditure after arthrodesis of the hip and ankle. J Bone Joint Surg 70A: 1032–1037

41

Surgical treatment of superior heel pain

Michael M. Stephens

Introduction

Superior heel pain is a challenging clinical problem, as many conditions can cause this symptom. The most common observed conditions are Haglund's syndrome, superficial Achilles bursitis, retrocalcaneal bursitis and insertional Achilles tendinitis [Dickinson et al. 1966].

Anatomy

To make an accurate diagnosis and render effective treatment, a surgeon must understand the pertinent heel anatomy (Figure 1). The posterior lip of the talar articulation is an important anatomical landmark at the upper surface of the calcaneus. The medial calcaneal tuberosity is the most distal portion and relates to the part of the calcaneus that bears weight, and is the attachment of the long plantar ligaments. The posterior calcaneal tuberosity is easily palpable in the normal heel and is the area of attachment of the Achilles tendon. Above this is a smooth area without tendinous attachment, and uppermost is the postero-superior tuberosity of the calcaneus or bursal projection. The retrocalcaneal bursa is lined with synovium except for the anterior bursal wall, which is composed of fibrocartilage on the calcaneus. Proximally, the bursa lies against the Achilles fat pad. The normal retrocalcaneal bursa contains 1–1.5 ml of fluid.

The Achilles tendon inserts into the inferior two-thirds of the posterior surface of the calcaneus.

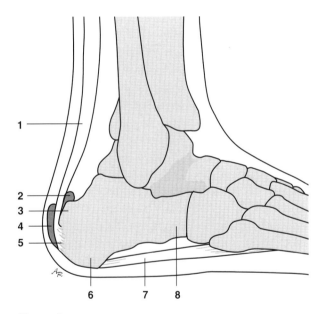

Figure 1

Normal heel anatomy

1 Achilles tendon
2 Retrocalcaneal bursa
3 Bursal projection
4 Superficial bursa
5 Posterior calcaneal tuberosity
6 Medial calcaneal tuberosity
7 Long plantar ligament
8 Anterior calcaneal tuberosity

Medial and lateral expansions of the tendon continue plantarly and are continuous with the long plantar ligament or the plantar fascia. Superficial and posterior to the Achilles tendon, at approximately the level of the postero-superior tuberosity, an adventitious bursa can often be found.

Etiology and clinical evaluation

Superior heel pain is seen commonly in adolescent females, particularly when they start wearing high-heeled shoes with restrictive heel counters. In Haglund's syndrome [Haglund 1928] there is an excessive prominence of the bursal projection, easily seen when viewed from behind. The swelling is located laterally, anterior to the distal portion of the Achilles tendon. Local pain and swelling indicate retrocalcaneal bursitis palpable behind the Achilles tendon on the bursal projection. The most common cause of retrocalcaneal bursitis is overuse, with the bursa compressed between the bursal projection, the Achilles tendon and the heel counter during dorsiflexion of the foot, which causes maximal symptoms in athletes running uphill.

A varus hindfoot is often associated with this deformity because, in such a position, the bursal projection is more prominent laterally. In the cavus foot, the calcaneus is not only in varus but is also more vertical, making the bursal projection even more prominent. A rigid plantarflexed first ray can be another cause of retrocalcaneal bursitis, because indirectly it will cause hindfoot varus. It can be seen as a manifestation of rheumatoid arthritis or indeed other arthropathies, such as gout and Reiter's syndrome.

The Achilles tendon itself may be tender and thickened, indicative of peritendinitis or tendinitis. Swelling may be palpable superficial to the Achilles tendon, which indicates inflammation of the subcutaneous Achilles tendon bursa. Degenerative processes of the Achilles tendon may cause superior heel pain, such as degenerative nodules, ossification within the tendon [Lotke 1970] and Achilles tendon insufficiency from lengthening, secondary to microtears. Overuse injuries can cause tendinosis, which is tendon degeneration without associated inflammation.

Partial tears may develop from overload injuries which occur in the hypovascular area 2–6 cm above the tendon insertion, where a fusiform swelling is found. Eccentric loading of a fatigued muscle–tendon unit from overtraining, hill running, poor-quality running shoes and insufficient gastrosoleus strength have all been associated with the onset of tendinitis. Achilles tendinitis has been demonstrated in hyperpronation of the foot, causing a whipping action on the Achilles tendon as the heel goes from varus to valgus after heel strike.

Radiographic findings

Haglund's deformity can be measured by assessing the superior calcaneal angle on lateral weightbearing radiographs [Fowler and Phillips 1945] (Figure 2). A normal angle is less than 75°. Taking into account the relationship between the calcaneus and the sole of the foot, the angle X + Y (Figure 2) should normally measure less than 90°.

Parallel pitch lines are another radiographic measurement to assess bursal projection [Pavlov et al. 1982]. They are drawn by dropping a perpendicular line from the posterior lip of the talar articulation on to a line that joins the medial and anterior calcaneal tuberosities. A parallel line is drawn from the posterior lip. The portion of bone lying above this line constitutes the 'bursal projection' (Figure 3). This latter measurement correlates best with clinical symptoms.

Lateral radiographs will also reveal calcification within the substance of the Achilles tendon. Erosions of the posterior calcaneus are seen in chronic bursitis, e.g. rheumatoid arthritis. Bursography normally demonstrates well-defined borders, but in bursitis a decreased filling volume with an irregular bursal outline may be observed. Magnetic resonance imaging is useful in the assessment of Achilles tendon degeneration.

Treatment

Conservative treatment is always undertaken initially and consists of reducing the inflammation by rest, ice, massage and anti-inflammatory medication, and physiotherapy in the form of Achilles tendon stretching exercises. The heel counter may be modified, and a heel insert effectively lifts the heel and decreases the calcaneal inclination. Custom-made orthoses to alleviate hyperpronation caused by tibia varum or by subtalar or forefoot varus may also be of benefit. Failure of these regimens is the indication for surgical intervention, although patients must be counseled that surgery has a guarded prognosis [Taylor 1986, Nesse and Finsen 1994].

Surgical technique

Surgical techniques for the treatment of superior heel pain can be generally divided into those related to the bursal projection and retrocalcaneal bursitis, and those that relate to the Achilles tendon itself.

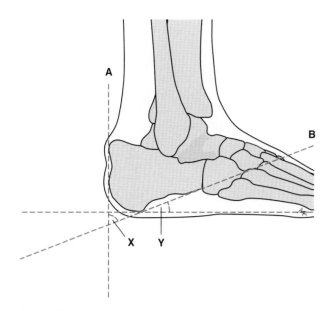

Figure 2

Superior calcaneal angle (X) and calcaneal pitch (Y). Line A is drawn from the bursal projection to the posterior tuberosity and line B joins the medial and anterior calcaneal tuberosities

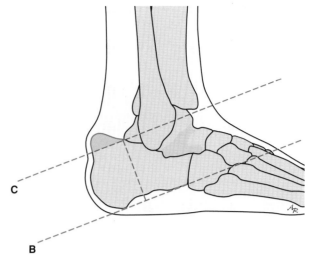

Figure 3

Parallel pitch lines. Line B is drawn between the medial and anterior calcaneal tuberosities. A parallel line C is drawn from the posterior lip of the talar articulation, and the bone above this line is a pathological bursal projection

Bursal projection and retrocalcaneal bursitis

Surgical options for this group of conditions are excision of the prominent posterosuperior tuberosity and the adjoining portion of the calcaneus, or a calcaneal osteotomy.

Excision of calcaneal tuberosity

Under spinal or general anesthesia, the patient is placed in the prone position with a thigh tourniquet. Bolsters are positioned under the patient's distal tibia.

A medial paratendinous incision is performed from the level of the Achilles tendon insertion proximally for 7 cm (Figure 4) [Stephens 1994]. Full-thickness skin flaps are fashioned and branches of the saphenous and medial calcaneal nerves are retracted anteriorly. The deep fascia is incised anterior to the Achilles tendon. The retrocalcaneal bursa is excised and the medial portion of the insertion of the Achilles tendon identified. Plantarflexion of the ankle allows easy retraction of the Achilles tendon posteriorly. The fat pad is retained.

With an oscillating saw or a 15-mm osteotome, the bursal projection can be excised by directing the blade obliquely from the posterior aspect of the talar articulation to the posterior calcaneal tuberosity. The blade must also be inclined laterally and in the plantar direction, which allows the superior and superolateral aspects of the bursal projection and adjoining calcaneus to be excised (Figure 5).

Once the osteotomy is complete, the bone is easily enucleated from the surrounding soft-tissue envelope. Any sharp bony ridges are smoothed near the Achilles tendon insertion. The wound is closed over a suction drain which is removed after 24 h, and the foot is immobilized in a below-knee cast for 2–6 weeks. This can also be performed endoscopically [van Dijk et al. 2001].

Calcaneal osteotomy

The patient is positioned prone and a medial paratendinous incision, 10 cm in length, is used to expose the posterosuperior aspect of the calcaneus. Excision of a dorsally based wedge from between the posterior lip of the talar articulation and the posterosuperior tuberosity is performed [Keck and Kelly 1965] (Figure 6). The base of the wedge varies from 0.6 to 1.5 cm and is determined on preoperative radiographs. This procedure rotates the posterior portion of the calcaneus forward and the calcaneal tuberosity is brought anteriorly away from the Achilles tendon and the retrocalcaneal bursa. Care should be taken not to disturb the periosteum on the inferior aspect of the calcaneus, as this hinge adds significant stability to the osteotomy. The osteotomy is compressed and fixed with one staple or a 4.5-mm cancellous screw perpendicular to the osteotomy. Such a procedure is

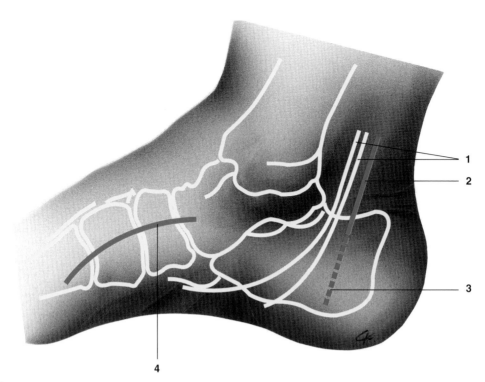

Figure 4

Surgical approaches to excision of calcaneal tuberosity; medial aspect of the foot

1 Neurovascular bundle
2 Incision for excision of bursal projection and bursa
3 Extension for calcaneal osteotomy
4 Incision for harvesting flexor hallucis longus tendon for Achilles tendon augmentation

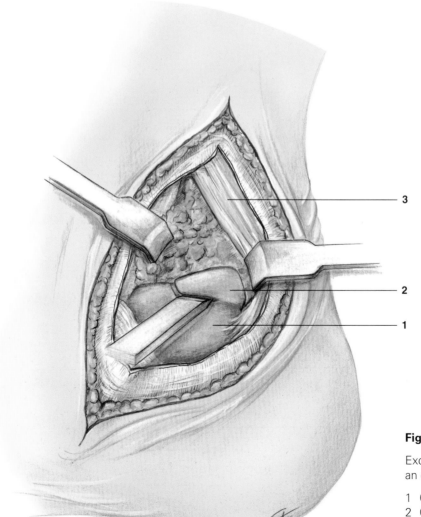

Figure 5

Excision of calcaneal tuberosity with an osteotome

1 Calcaneus
2 Calcaneal tuberosity
3 Achilles tendon

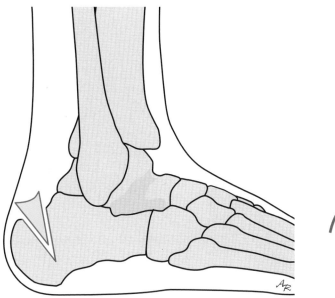
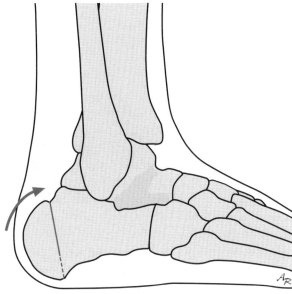

Figure 6

Calcaneal wedge osteotomy

extensive and requires a prolonged period of casting as the osteotomy unites. Therefore, excision of the bursal projection is the procedure of choice in primary cases.

Surgery for the Achilles tendon

Achilles tendinitis

The patient is positioned prone with a thigh tourniquet. A 7-cm longitudinal incision is performed 1 cm medial and parallel to the Achilles tendon. If further exposure is required, the incision may be extended from medial to lateral at the tendon insertion. Full-thickness skin flaps are developed, dissecting between the Achilles tendon and the subcutaneous tissue to preserve the blood supply to the flap.

If the tendon sheath is hyperemic, thickened, fibrotic and adherent to the underlying tendon, as it is in a peritendinitis, sharp dissection is undertaken to free the sheath from the tendon and to excise it. The mesotenon and the anterior fatty tissue must not be disturbed. The tendon is inspected and palpated for thickening, defects or softening. If pathological changes are identified, a longitudinal splitting incision is made to curette the foci of degeneration, to excise ossification and bony spurs, and to stimulate a local inflammatory response [Leach et al. 1992]. The edges are approximated with 3-0 Maxon (glycolide trimethylene carbonate) or PDS (polydioxanone) sutures after debridement

or, if necessary, the tendon is augmented with flexor hallucis longus tendon, as described below.

Augmentation of the Achilles tendon

After debridement the Achilles tendon is occasionally weakened sufficiently to require augmentation using a tendon graft (see Chapter 26). The indication for augmentation is a clinical decision. If, after excision of the degeneration and of bony fragments, the tendon is judged to be insufficient, augmentation should be performed. Tendon transfer is used to augment and increase the vascularity of the weakened tendon [Wapner et al. 1993]. This is also useful to augment the power of plantarflexion if there is triceps weakness or after an untreated rupture, as this muscular tendinous unit is in phase for the gait cycle.

The patient is positioned supine following induction of spinal or general anesthesia using a thigh tourniquet. The foot and knee are disinfected and draped free. Two incisions are required. First, a 10-cm linear incision is made along the medial border of the foot just above the level of the abductor hallucis, from the first metatarsal head to the navicular. The skin and subcutaneous tissue are incised sharply down to the fascia. The abductor hallucis and flexor hallucis brevis are retracted in a plantar direction, allowing identification of the flexor hallucis longus and flexor digitorum longus. The flexor hallucis longus is divided as far distally as possible and the distal stump is inserted into the flexor digitorum slip to the second toe, with all five toes in the neutral position. The proximal portion is tagged with a suture. A second longitudinal incision is made posteriorly along the medial aspect of the Achilles tendon, from the musculotendinous junction to 1 cm below the tendinous insertion, maintaining full-thickness skin flaps. The fascia overlying the posterior compartment of the leg is then incised longitudinally and the flexor hallucis longus is identified. The tendon is retracted from the midfoot into the posterior incision. A drill hole is placed just distal to the Achilles tendon insertion halfway through the bone, from medial to lateral. A second drill hole is placed vertically just deep to the insertion of the tendon to join the first hole. A curved awl is used to augment the tunnel created. The tendon is then passed through the tunnel using the tag suture from proximal to distal. The tendon is woven from distal to proximal through the Achilles tendon using a tendon weaver [Wapner et al. 1993] (Figure 7). The distal stump of the tendon is sutured to the Achilles tendon proximal to the weakened area. The paratenon is repaired and the subcutaneous tissue and skin are closed.

The plantaris, peroneus brevis and the median raphe of the gastrocnemius have all been used in augmentation of the Achilles tendon with good effect, but the strength, axis of contractility, excursion and phasic relationship with the gastrocnemius–soleus complex make the flexor hallucis longus most suitable.

Postoperative care

A short leg cast with the ankle in slight equinus is applied. Indomethacin may prevent recurrent calcification. The cast is worn for 2–6 weeks, depending on the surgical integrity of the Achilles tendon complex and whether a tendon transfer has been performed. Passive motion exercises are begun, emphasizing dorsiflexion. A progressive exercise program is instituted with particular attention to Achilles tendon stretching. A small heel raise for 4 weeks is sometimes necessary for comfort. Jogging is allowed at 8–12 weeks. Full return to competitive athletic activity is usually possible at 5–6 months.

Complications

Knowledge of the surgical anatomy is essential to avoid damage to branches of the saphenous nerve and the medial calcaneal nerves, or the sural

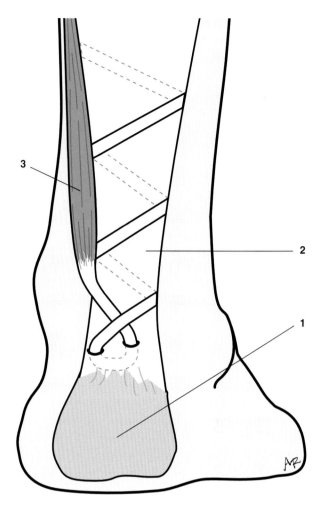

Figure 7

Augmentation of Achilles tendon with flexor hallucis longus

1   Calcaneus
2   Achilles tendon
3   Flexor hallucis longus

nerve if a lateral approach is chosen. Sensitive wounds and neuromas will inevitably cause great discomfort and an unhappy outcome. Occasionally, re-exploration and resection of a neuroma may need to be undertaken.

Iatrogenic damage at the time of surgery may weaken an already susceptible Achilles tendon and postoperative rupture has been documented. Surgical care and protection of the tendon at the time of an ostectomy will avoid this complication.

The incidence of wound hematoma and infection may be decreased by the insertion of a surgical drain and careful handling of the soft tissues and hemostasis prior to wound closure. Women commonly complain about an unsightly lateral scar. A medial scar is less likely to result in such complaints [Stephens 1994].

The optimal size of the excised piece of bone has been disputed, and some authors [Nesse and Finsen 1994] have not correlated the size of the resection with the clinical outcome. Other authors [Huber 1992, Stephens 1994] feel that a good result is dependent on the adequacy of resection. Although good results have been reported [Sammarco and Taylor 1998] patients must be advised that this surgery does have failures [Schneider et al. 2000].

The poor results reported may in part be due to inadequate resection and to inadequate preoperative screening to diagnose the various forms of arthropathies in which this condition is prevalent. The results of excision of the bursal projection are better than those for excision of insertional spurs [Watson et al. 2000].

Careful selection of patients is essential, as is preoperative clarification of these possible complications, because the incidence of complications in some reports is as high as 50% [Nesse and Finsen 1994].

References

Dickinson P, Coutts M, Woodward P et al. (1966) Tendo-Achilles bursitis. J Bone Joint Surg 48A: 77–81

Fowler A, Phillip JF (1945) Abnormality of the calcaneus as a cause of painful heel. Br J Surg 32: 494–498

Haglund P (1928) Beitrag zur Klinik der Achillessehne. Arch Orthop Chir 49: 49–58

Huber HM (1992) Prominence of the calcaneus: late results of bone resection. J Bone Joint Surg 74B: 315–316

Keck S, Kelly P (1965) Bursitis of the posterior part of the heel. J Bone Joint Surg 47A: 267–273

Leach RE, Schepsis AA, Takai H (1992) Long-term results of surgical management of Achilles tendinitis in runners. Clin Orthop 282: 208–212

Lotke PE (1970) Ossification of the Achilles tendon. J Bone Joint Surg 52A: 157–160

Nesse E, Finsen V (1994) Poor results after resection for Haglund's heel. Acta Orthop Scand 65: 107–109

Pavlov H, Heneghan MA, Hersh A (1982) The Haglund syndrome: initial and differential diagnosis. Diagn Radiol 144: 83–88

Sammarco GJ, Taylor AL (1998) Operative management of Haglund's deformity in the non-athletic. Foot Ankle Int 19: 724–729

Schneider W, Niehus W, Knahr K (2000) Haglund's syndrome: disappointing results following surgery – a clinical and radiographic analysis. Foot Ankle Int 21: 26–30

Stephens MM (1994) Haglund's deformity and retrocalcaneal bursitis. Orthop Clin North Am 25: 41–46

Taylor GJ (1986) Prominence of the calcaneus: is operation justified? J Bone Joint Surg 68B: 467–470

van Dijk CN, van Dijk GE, Scholten PE, Kort NP (2001) Endoscopic calcaneoplasty. Am J Sports Med 29: 185–189

Wapner KL, Pavlock GS, Hecht PJ et al. (1993) Repair of chronic Achilles tendon rupture with flexor hallucis longus tendon transfer. Foot Ankle 14: 443–449

Watson AD, Anderson RB, Davis WH (2000) Comparison of results of retrocalcaneal decompression for retrocalcaneal bursitis and insertional Achilles tendinitis with calcific spur. Foot Ankle Int 21: 638–642

42

Repair of acute Achilles tendon rupture

Sandro Giannini
Francesco Ceccarelli

Introduction

The Achilles tendon is the thickest and most powerful tendinous structure below the knee and its subcutaneous rupture accounts for about 35% of all tendon ruptures in the body [Rooks 1994]. This injury is most common in men aged 30–50 years who continue to practice amateur sports. Conditions that favor the rupture are degeneration or inflammation of the tendon or peritendinous structures, hyperuricemia, hyperthyroidism, renal insufficency and arteriosclerosis [Myerson 1999], general cortisone treatment and previous local infiltration therapy with corticosteroids [Maffulli 1999].

Pathogenesis

There is still much controversy in the literature regarding the pathogenic mechanism of the injury. The two main theories are the degeneration theory [Puddu et al. 1976], and the mechanical theory [Barfred 1973, Popovic and Lemaire 1999]. The mechanical theory, which is less supported, explains the rupture as arising from different types of indirect tensional injury to the tendon [Armer and Lindholm 1959]. According to the degeneration theory, however, subcutaneous rupture of the Achilles tendon is secondary to a degenerative process of the tendon and peritendinous structures. The rupture usually occurs about 2–6 cm from the insertion at the calcaneus in an area known to have poor vascularization. Thus, local hypoperfusion may play a role in the etiology of acute Achilles tendon rupture [Leppilahti and Orawa 1998].

Clinical appearance

Patients often recall hearing a 'snap' at the time of sprinting and may think that they have been kicked in the area of the involved tendon. This is immediately followed by pain, not always severe, and difficulty in walking. Generally edema is present, mainly behind the ankle, and there may be marked ecchymosis. The patient cannot stand on tiptoe.

On palpation, the rupture can be felt as a defect in the tendon, but sometimes it cannot be palpated owing to the edema and the hematoma inside the tendon sheath. Some patients are able to flex their foot plantarwards against some resistance by vicarious action of the posterior tibialis and the long flexor muscles to the toes. Popovic and Lemaire [1999] reported the tendon rupture being missed on the first consultation in 25% of cases. The Thompson and Doherty test [1962], also known as the 'squeeze' test, is helpful in making the diagnosis. The calf is squeezed with one hand while the patient is in a prone position. If the tendon is in continuity, there will be slight plantarflexion of the foot. This does not occur if the tendon is completely ruptured. In case of doubt, the O'Brien test [1984] can also be performed. A syringe needle is inserted at a right angle to the Achilles tendon, about 10 cm above the top edge of the calcaneus, with the patient prone. When the foot is moved plantarly or dorsally, there will be pendular movement of the needle if the tendon is in continuity. If the tendon is ruptured, there will be little or no pendular movement.

Standard radiographs can be taken to exclude bony injury to the calcaneus. Ultrasonography and a magnetic resonance imaging (MRI) scan are rarely essential for the diagnosis, which is predominantly clinical in nature. These imaging techniques can be utilized to evaluate the severity of degenerative changes of the tendon.

Treatment

There is controversy concerning the type of treatment of acute Achilles tendon rupture. Some authors support conservative treatment, whereas others advocate surgical treatment (open or minimally invasive).

The re-rupture rate may be as high as 10–30% with conservative traditional treatment [Carden et al. 1987, Cetti et al. 1993, Popovic and Lemaire 1999]. This rate may be considerably reduced if treatment is initiated within the first 48 h [Carden et al. 1987, Roberts et al. 2001, Wallace et al. 2004], but it is still considerably higher than the 0.4–5% re-rupture rate following open surgical treatment [Carden et al. 1987, Zwipp et al. 1989, Cetti et al. 1993, Winter et al. 1998, Mellor and Patterson 2000]. With open surgery, however, complications may occur in 4–20%; these include skin or tendon necrosis, nerve damage or infection [Carden et al. 1987, Zwipp et al. 1989, Cetti et al. 1993, Myerson 1999, Mellor and Patterson 2000]. Regarding open surgery, there is still also controversy concerning the technique utilized: in particular some authors advise the use of biological augmentation such as gastrocnemius–soleus fascia [Winter et al. 1998, Zell and Santoro 2000], plantaris tendon [Lynn 1966], fascia lata [Bug and Boyd 1968], peroneus brevis [Turco and Spinella 1987], flexor digitorum longus [Mann et al. 1991] and flexor hallucis longus [Wapner et al. 1995]. Other authors state that these augmentation techniques are not necessary in the treatment of acute ruptures [Myerson 1999, Popovic and Lemaire 1999].

Regarding minimally invasive surgery, the percutaneous suture [Ma and Griffith 1977] avoids the disadvantages of open surgical treatment and improves the quality of the scar tissue, preserving the blood supply and the paratenon. Stabilizing the tendon stumps, on the other hand, avoids the most important complications of conservative treatment such as elongation of the tendon.

The overall re-rupture rate reported in the literature is 6.4% [Bradley and Tibone 1990]. Other problems may arise, such as malaligned stumps, skin retraction, nodules at the site of the suture and, in particular, trapping of the sural nerve in 13% of cases [Klein et al. 1991]. To reduce these drawbacks some authors have proposed modifications of the original

technique [Gorschewsky et al. 1999, Mertl et al. 1999, Webb and Bannister 1999, Martinelli 2000].

Majewski et al. [2000] reported 88% good or excellent results with percutaneous suture compared to 77.3% with open surgery and 75% with conservative treatment. To reduce entrapment of the sural nerve and to obtain a suture inside the paratenon and consequently a minor tendency to hypertrophic scarring, other authors have developed the use of metal wires [Nasaaki Kakiuchi 1995] or particular instrumentation such as the Achillon System™ (Newdeal, Geneva, Switzerland) (M. Assal, personal communication, ESSKA, Nice, April 1998).

Considering the literature of the past 10 years, the better clinical results are probably determined not only by the methods of repair, but also and perhaps more importantly by the functional rehabilitation [Popovic and Lemaire 1999]. Many authors report improved results in terms of functionality of the tendon and the ankle, quality of the scar and return to previous activities with open surgery [Aoki et al. 1998, Speck and Klaue 1998, Mortensen et al. 1999, Pneumaticos et al. 2000] or minimally invasive surgery [Buchgraber and Passler 1997] and even with conservative treatment [Rickter et al. 1997, Thermann et al. 2000, Roberts et al. 2001].

The conservative functional treatment must be sonographically monitored in order to assess the position of the tendon stumps in plantarflexion of the foot.

Many protocols are reported, characterized by functional rehabilitation with aggressive early motion and weightbearing, in many cases using a removable ankle–foot orthosis with rocking sole to minimize the lever effort of the foot and joints to permit passive range of motion exercises.

In the authors' experience, when prolonged cast immobilization was used to treat the rupture, either surgically or non-surgically, open surgery guaranteed a higher percentage of good results and a shorter postoperative period of immobilization than conservative treatment. The techniques utilized were the open end-to-end suture in cases without excessive degeneration, and end-to-end suture augmented with plantaris tendon, gastrosoleus fascia or peroneus brevis or with polypropylene braid in cases of severe degenerative changes [Giannini et al. 1986, 1994].

The authors' choice in the treatment of acute Achilles tendon rupture is a minimally invasive technique such as modified percutaneous suture according to Ma and Griffith [1977], or the Achillon System [Assal et al. 2002] with lesions up to 6 days

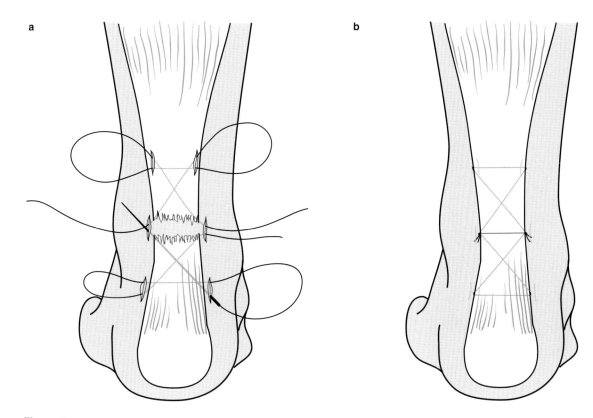

Figure 1

Percutaneous suture. a. method used to pass the suture threads in the two stumps; b. after knotting of the threads

old and 2–8 cm from the calcaneal insertion. The percutaneous technique offers two main advantages: the minimal incision permits control of the site of the lesion and the stumps; and the stitches pass inside the paratenon, reducing the risk of its entrapment and damage to the sural nerve. If the higher risk of re-rupture is accepted, owing to severe degenerative modifications of the tendon (such as renal insufficiency or rheumatoid arthritis), open augmented surgery is utilized.

Non-surgical functional treatment, sonographically monitored, can be indicated for elderly patients who have lower functional requirements, or for patients with an increased risk of poor surgical wound healing, such as insulin-dependent diabetic patients, heavy smokers, patients under heavy immunosuppressive therapy or those with circulatory disorders.

Operative technique

Percutaneous suture

The patient, under general spinal or block anesthesia, is placed in a prone position with the knee flexed at 15°. Both feet are prepared in the surgical field in order to adapt the tension of the suture to the physiological equinus of the uninvolved side. The pneumatic tourniquet is an option.

The tendon defect is identified on palpation and three pairs of 5-mm skin incisions are made medial and lateral to the tendon edge: one pair at the lesion site, one pair 3–4 cm distally at the distal stump site and one pair 3–4 cm proximally at the proximal stump site (Figure 1). At this level, to minimize the risk of trapping the sural nerve the two skin incisions are made more medially than the lateral and medial border of the tendon. The sural nerve crosses the lateral edge of the tendon approximately 9.83 cm proximal to the calcaneal insertion of the tendon [Webb et al. 2000].

With a small forceps the paratenon is opened at each incision level. Two no. 2 Bunnell-type bioresorbable stitches are passed on each stump with a large needle, starting transversely from the proximal and distal pairs of incisions. The stitches are tightened and knotted until the foot reaches the same equinus position as the uninvolved foot. The skin is sutured.

Minimally invasive suture

With the patient in the same position and using a tourniquet at thigh level, a longitudinal 2–3 cm

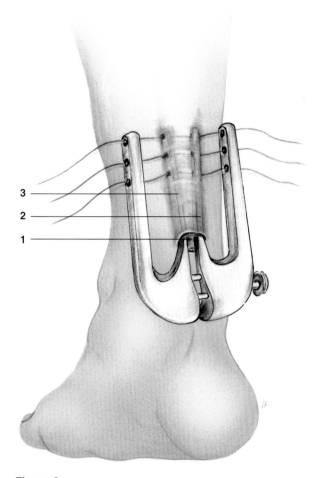

Figure 2

The minimally invasive suture using the Achillon System™. The skin incision is shown (1); after the paratenon is divided with a forceps, the proximal stump is identified and pulled down (2); the system is introduced and progressively widened under the fascia with the stump coming between the two internal branches (3). Three no. 1 absorbable suture threads are passed through the system holes and the tendon stump; the same procedure is repeated for the distal stump

paratendinous medial incision is made at the level of the lesion. The paratenon is incised and the proximal stump identified. Pulling the proximal tendon stump with forceps, the Achillon System is introduced under the fascia with the stump coming between the two internal branches. When the Achillon System is introduced, it is gradually widened to follow the progressive proximal enlargement of the tendon (Figure 2). Three no. 1 absorbable threads are then passed through the Achillon holes and the tendon with a straight needle. The System is then slowly withdrawn by progressive closure [Assal et al. 2002].

The same maneuvers are performed in the distal stump. The six threads are knotted with the foot in the same equinus position as the uninvolved side. The same technique can be used with

prepared metal wires. The fascia and the skin are then sutured.

Open surgery

The anesthesia and the patient position are the same as in minimally invasive surgery; in open surgery a pneumatic tourniquet is used.

Surgical approach

A 10–12 cm posteromedial S-shaped incision is made 0.5 cm from the medial edge of the tendon (Figure 3). This reduces postoperative scar retraction. The posteromedial approach is preferred to the posterolateral approach, to avoid damage to the sural nerve and to the short saphenous vein, and because the cosmetic appearance of the scar is thinner and less visible with time. Following the incision of the skin and the subcutaneous tissue, the tendon sheath is reached. This must be divided without its being dissected from the subcutaneous tissue, in order to avoid compromising skin vascularization and to avoid postoperative adhesions. The two stumps of the tendon are identified and the hematoma is removed by repeated irrigation (Figure 4).

Tendon repair

The tendon stumps are joined with the knee flexed 15° and the foot in 5° of equinus. The tendon is sutured end-to-end with two absorbable no. 2 Kessler stitches, which are placed in healthy tissue, usually 3–4 cm from the tendon tear (Figure 5). The two stumps must be joined as accurately as possible, in order to avoid loss of tension of the tendon, or shortening, which could result in painful nodules in the scar tissue. The sutures must be strong and the stitches must be placed far enough from the injury.

The plantaris longus tendon is harvested with a stripper and then looped once through the two stumps and sutured to them. The remaining plantaris longus tendon is fanned out and sutured to cover the repaired Achilles tendon injury. This maneuver avoids adhesions between the tendon and the sheath, and prevents an excessive increase in volume of the repaired tendon. When the plantaris tendon is not present, a turned-out flap of aponeurosis from the calf muscle may be used to reinforce the repair, after one Kessler stitch (Figure 6) [Giannini et al. 1986]. The flap is reflected

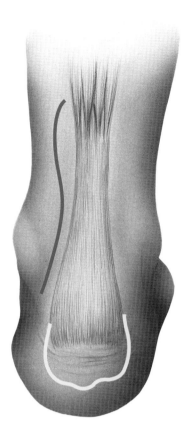

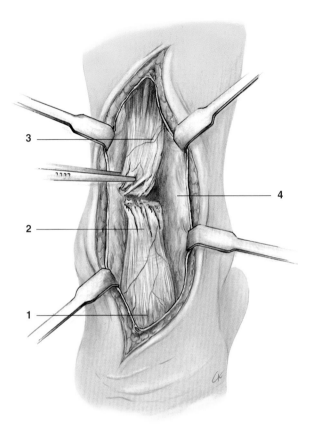

Figure 3

The 'open' approach to the Achilles tendon rupture is through an S-shaped incision medial to the tendon

Figure 4

Intraoperative aspect of the ruptured tendon following division of the tendon sheath

1 Calcaneus
2 Distal tendon stump
3 Proximal tendon stump
4 Achilles tendon sheath

on to the area of the repair and twisted into the sagittal plane. A groove is made in both the distal and the proximal Achilles tendon stumps, and the stumps are sutured to the flap with two or three U-shaped stitches on each side, which are oriented in the frontal plane and perpendicular to the tendon. Subsequently, the ends of the stumps are sutured together, closing the fibers of the tendon to cover the turned-out flap. This restricts the thickness of the repaired tendon. The peroneus brevis tendon [Turco and Spinella 1987] or flexor hallucis longus [Wapner et al. 1995] can also be used to reinforce the Achilles tendon repair.

Following suture of the tendon and augmentation, the tendon sheath is closed with 2–0 absorbable sutures and the skin is closed with 3–0 absorbable sutures.

Postoperative care

The patient leaves the operating theater with a dressing and an ankle–foot orthosis, which is maintained for 8 weeks. In case of minimally

invasive techniques, passive motion is permitted from the first day after operation from 10 to 25° of plantar-flexion associated with 15 kg partial load assisted by two sticks. After 3 weeks the passive motion is increased from 0 to 30° of plantarflexion. After 6 weeks the partial load is permitted up to 25 kg associated with passive motion and dorsiflexion. After 8 weeks progressive full load is allowed and the orthosis is abandoned. Then, physical therapy such as hydrotherapy, stretching, isometric and propioceptive rehabilitation begins. Return to normal activity is permitted after 3 months, and to sports activity after 5 months.

In case of open augmented surgery the partial load from the first day after operation is 25 kg and the passive motion is permitted from 0 to 25° of plantarflexion. After 4 weeks full loading is permitted with an orthosis. After 8 weeks, without orthosis, the physical therapy protocol is the same as for minimally invasive surgery.

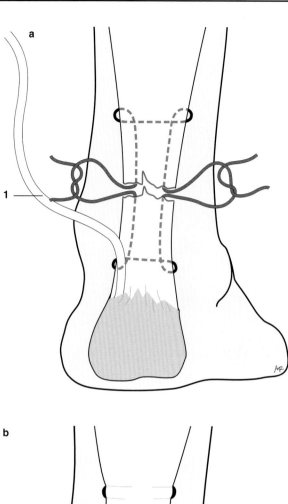

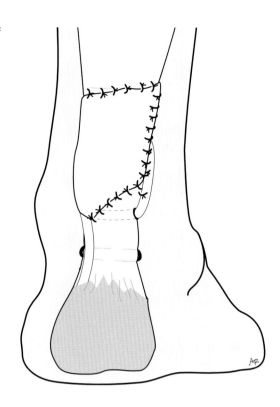

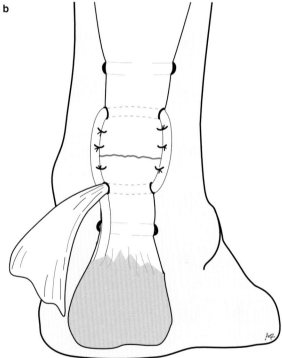

Figure 5

The plantaris longus tendon augmentation technique

a. insertion of sutures; b. weaving of the plantaris longus tendon through the Achilles tendon; c. the remaining plantaris longus tendon is fanned out and sutured around the repair.

1 Plantaris longus tendon

Complications

The complications that can arise from minimally invasive surgery are skin retraction, nodules, and above all the trapping of the sural nerve and tendon

lengthening with insufficient plantarflexion force. Complications with the open surgical techniques are dehiscence of the wound, superficial infection, hypertrophic scarring and restriction of dorsiflexion of the ankle. Undue thickness of the repair may lead

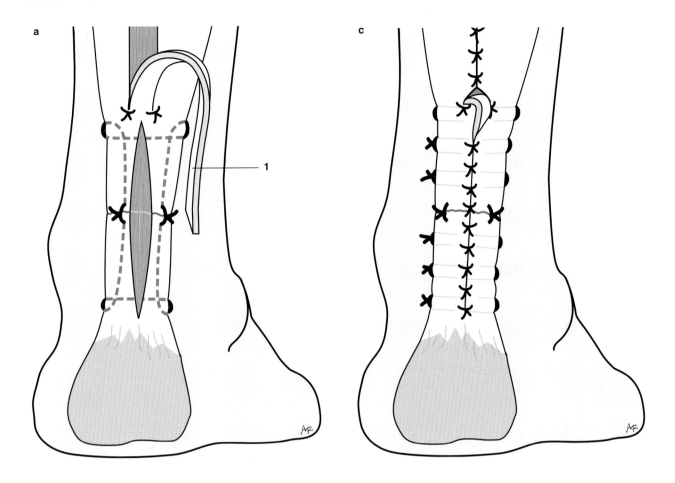

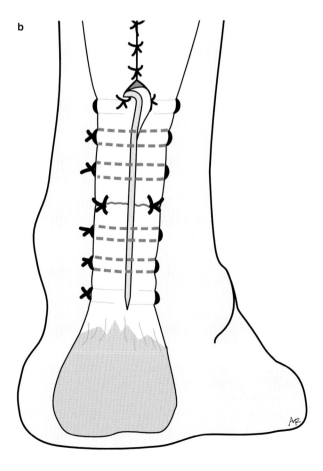

Figure 6

Augmentation with calf muscle aponeurosis. a. the flap is obtained from the gastrosoleus fascia; b. the flap is inserted into the repair; c. the flap is fixed into the tendon after end-to-end suture, being twisted in the frontal plane

1 Gastrosoleus fascia flap

to excessive tension in the sheath and in the skin, with subsequent wound dehiscence and possibly infection.

References

Aoki M, Ogiwara N, Ohta T, Nabeta Y (1998) Early active motion and weightbearing after cross-stitch Achilles tendon repair. Am J Sports Med 26: 794–780

Armer O, Lindholm A (1959) Subcutaneous rupture of the Achilles tendon: a study of 92 cases. Acta Chir Scand 239 (Suppl): 1–51

Assal M, Jung M, Stern R et al. (2002) Limited open repair of Achilles tendon ruptures. J Bone Joint Surg 84A: 161–170

Barfred T (1973) Achilles tendon rupture. Acta Orthop Scand 152 (Suppl): 12–125

Bradley JP, Tibone JE (1990) Percutaneous and open surgical repairs of Achilles tendon ruptures. A comparative study. Am J Sports Med 18: 188–195

Buchgraber A, Passler HH (1997) Percutaneous repair of Achilles tendon rupture. Immobilization versus functional postoperative treatment. Clin Orthop 341: 113–122

Bug EL Jr, Boyd BM (1968) Repair of neglected rupture or laceration of the Achilles tendon. Clin Orthop 56: 73–75

Carden DG, Noble J, Chalmers J et al. (1987) Rupture of the calcaneal tendon. The early and late management. J Bone Joint Surg 69B: 416–420

Cetti R, Christensen SE, Ejsted R et al. (1993) Operative versus nonoperative treatment of Achilles tendon rupture. A prospective randomized study and review of the literature. Am J Sports Med 21: 791–799

Giannini S, DiSilvestre M, Ceccarelli F et al. (1986) Le suture con plastica nel trattamento delle rotture sottocutanee del tendine di Achille. Chir Piede 10: 273–277

Giannini S, Girolami M, Ceccarelli F et al. (1994) Surgical repair of Achilles tendon ruptures using polypropylene braid augmentation. Foot Ankle Int 15: 372–375

Gorschewsky O, Vogel V, Schweizer A, Van Laar B (1999) Percutaneous tenodesis of the Achilles tendon. A new surgical method for the treatment of acute Achilles tendon rupture through percutaneous tenodesis. Injury 30: 315–321

Klein W, Lang DM, Soleh M (1991) The use of the Ma–Griffith technique for percutaneous repair of fresh ruptured tendo Achillis. Chir Org Mov 76: 223–228

Leppilahti J, Orawa S (1998) Total Achilles tendon rupture. J Sports Med 2: 79–100

Lynn TA (1966) Repair of torn Achilles tendon using the plantaris tendon as a reinforcing membrane. J Bone Joint Surg 48A: 268–272

Ma GWC, Griffith TG (1977) Percutaneous repair of acute closed ruptured Achilles tendon. A new technique. Clin Orthop 128: 247–255

Maffulli N (1999) Rupture of the Achilles tendon. J Bone Joint Surg 81A: 1019–1036

Majewski M, Rickert M, Steinbruck K (2000) Achilles tendon rupture. A prospective study assessing various treatment possibilities. Orthopäde 29: 670–676

Mann RA, Holmes GB, Seale KS, Collins DN (1991) Chronic ruptures of the Achilles tendon: a new technique of repair. J Bone Joint Surg 73A: 214–219

Martinelli B (2000) Percutaneous repair of the Achilles tendon in athletes. Bull Osp Joint Dis 59: 149–152

Mellor SJ, Patterson MH (2000) Tendo Achillis rupture, surgical repair is a safe option. Injury 31: 489–491

Mertl P, Jarde O, Van FT et al. (1999) Percutaneous tenorraphy for Achilles tendon rupture. Study of 29 cases. Rev Chir Orthop Reparatrice Appar Mot 85: 277–285

Mortensen HM, Skov O, Jensen PE (1999) Early motion of the ankle after operative treatment of a rupture of the Achilles tendon. A prospective randomized clinical and radiographic study. J Bone Joint Surg 81A: 983–990

Myerson M (1999) Achilles tendon ruptures. Instr Course Lectures 48: 219–230

Nasaaki Kakiuchi (1995) A combined open and percutaneous technique for repair of tendo Achillis. J Bone Joint Surg 77B: 60–63

O'Brien T (1984) The needle test for complete rupture of the Achilles tendon. J Bone Joint Surg 66A: 1099–1101

Pneumaticos SG, Noble PC, McGarvey WC et al. (2000) The effect of early mobilization in the healing of Achilles tendon repair. Foot Ankle Int 21: 551–557

Popovic N, Lemaire R (1999) Diagnosis and treatment of acute ruptures of the Achille tendon: current concepts review. Acta Othop Belg 65: 458–471

Puddu G, Ippolito E, Postacchini F (1976) A classification of Achilles tendon diseases. Am J Sports Med 4: 145

Rickter J, Pommer A, Hahn M et al. (1997) Possibilities and limits of functional conservative therapy of acute Achilles tendon ruptures. Chirurgie 68: 517–524

Roberts CP, Palmer S, Vince A, Delisse LJ (2001) Dinamized cast management of Achilles tendon rupture. Injury 32: 423–426

Rooks MD (1994) Tendon vascular nerve and skin injuries. In: Gould JS (ed) Operative Foot Surgery. Philadelphia, WB Saunders, pp 522–526

Speck M, Klaue K (1998) Early full weightbearing and functional treatment after surgical repair of acute Achilles tendon rupture. Am J Sports Med 26: 789–793

Thermann H, Hufner T, Tscherne H (2000) Achilles tendon rupture. Orthopäde 29: 235–250

Thompson TC, Doherty JH (1962) Spontaneous rupture of tendon of Achilles. A new clinical diagnostic test. J Trauma 2: 126–129

Turco VJ, Spinella AJ (1987) Achilles tendon ruptures – peroneus brevis transfer. Foot Ankle 7: 253–259

Wallace RG, Traynor IE, Kernohan WG, Eames MH (2004) Combined conservative and orthotic management of acute ruptures of the Achilles tendon. J Bone Joint Surg 86A: 1198–1202

Wapner KL, Hecht PJ, Mills RH (1995) Reconstruction of neglected Achilles tendon injury. Orthop Clin North Am 26: 249–263

Webb JM, Bannister GC (1999) Percutaneous repair of the ruptured tendo Achillis. J Bone Joint Surg 81B: 877–880

Webb J, Moorjani M, Radford M (2000) Anatomy of the sural nerve and its relation to the Achilles tendon. Foot Ankle Int 21: 475–477

Winter E, Weise K, Weller S, Ambacher T (1998) Surgical repair of Achilles tendon rupture. Comparison of surgical with conservative treatment. Arch Orthop Trauma Surg 117: 364–367

Zell RA, Santoro VM (2000) Augmented repair of acute Achilles tendon ruptures. Foot Ankle Int 21: 469–474

Zwipp H, Sudkamp N, Therman H, Samek N (1989) Rupture of the Achilles tendon. Results of 10 years' follow-up after surgical treatment. A retrospective study. Unfallchirurgie 92: 554–559

43

Surgical management of rigid congenital talipes equino-varus (clubfoot)

Alvin H. Crawford
Abubakar A. Durrani

Introduction

Congenital talipes equinovarus (CTEV) is a syndrome comprising an in utero malalignment of the talocalcaneonavicular and calcaneocuboid axes of the child's foot, atrophy of the calf and a concomitant variable decrease in foot size and tibial length. It is one of the most common birth defects (1 in 1000 live births). Lochmiller et al. [1998] reported a male to female preponderance of 2.5:1 and a family history in 24.4%, while Palmer et al. [1974] found that 37.3% had at least one other family member affected. An affected male's male offspring has a 1 in 42 chance although there is no additional risk for a female, but an affected female's child has a 1:16 risk for males and 1:40 risk for females. With an affected parent and child in a family, the risk in subsequent siblings increases to 1:4. Ching et al. [1969], while analyzing the incidence of CTEV in different racial groups, reported the highest incidence when both parents were of Hawaiian origin and the lowest in Chinese, whereas Lochmiller et al. [1998] noted no racial predilection.

A deformed talus with a plantarflexed and medially deviated anterior part leads to contracture of the posterior ankle structures, including the posterior ankle capsule, and a talonavicular subluxation, with the navicular often articulating with the medial malleolus

(medial column shortening). The plantarflexed talus forces the calcaneus into plantarflexion, leading to contracture of the Achilles tendon. The calcaneus in turn rotates in the horizontal plane, pivoting on the interosseous ligament, and slips under the head and neck of the talus anteriorly. The calcaneal tuberosity moves towards the fibular malleolus. The posterolateral structures become shortened and a varus heel develops from calcaneal internal rotation. This leads to medial displacement of the cuboid on the long axis of the os calcis, and the medially displaced navicular leads to adduction of the midfoot, varus and adduction deformity of the heel and midfoot. The forefoot supinates, known radiographically by 'stacking' of the cuneiforms and metatarsal bases.

Cahuzac et al. [1999], using a three-dimensional magnetic resonance imaging (MRI) scan, concurred with the findings of Carroll [1997] that there is external rotation of the talus in the mortice, suggesting that the talus must be derotated medially by surgery. However, Johnston et al. [1995], in their three-dimensional analysis of CTEV deformities, described the talus as being in pronation. Cuevas et al. [1998] recently discussed the issue of tibial torsional deformities in CTEV by computed tomography (CT) scans and found no appreciable difference in the amount of femoral or tibial torsion in limbs with or without CTEV.

Neonatal diagnosis

In CTEV the foot plantiflexes with the small calcaneus drawn up and rolled in under the talus in an inverted position, leaving the heel pad empty. There is a deep crease at the posterior aspect of the ankle which, in combination with the empty heel pad, gives rise to the so-called 'keel-shaped heel'. The mid- and forefoot are adducted and supinated. The anterior end of the talus is prominent on the dorsolateral aspect of the foot. The skin creases are deeply furrowed on the concave medial and plantar aspects of the foot. The navicular abuts the anterior aspect of the medial malleolus with a varying degree of calf atrophy and shortening of the affected leg and foot. CTEV must be differentiated from a postural deformity arising from intrauterine malposition, which is flexible and may have slight forefoot varus but does not have hindfoot equinus and varus. Proximal femoral focal deficiency, arthrogryposis, amniotic band syndrome, myelodysplasia, diastrophic dwarfism, Pierre Robin syndrome, Larsen syndrome, Möbius syndrome, Freeman–Sheldon syndrome and Charcot–Marie–Tooth disease and fibula hemimelia are associated with CTEV, so the whole child must be examined carefully. There is no standardized grading system, but those by Pirani et al. [1995] and Dimeglio et al. [1995] have recently become popular.

A lateral radiograph of the ankle with maximum dorsiflexion and an anteroposterior view of the foot provide the most complete radiographic picture. A talocalcaneal angle of less than 20° of an anteroposterior view indicates hindfoot varus, whereas a value of less than 35° of a lateral view indicates a hindfoot equinus. A talus–first metatarsal angle on the anteroposterior view of more than 0° indicates medial deviation of the foot at either the distal or the proximal tarsal row. Inability of the long axes of talus and calcaneus to converge on forced lateral dorsiflexion indicates an equinus contracture, as does a tibiocalcaneal angle of more than 90°. However, radiography in CTEV can be inaccurate, as the bones are small and ossification centers lie eccentrically. Therefore, many clinicians treat clinical rather than radiographic parameters.

Treatment

Treatment of CTEV should be based on reducing the congenital subluxation of the talocalcaneonavicular complex. The talar head is similar to that of the femur, with the medially displaced navicular,

distal end of the calcaneus, cuboid, the spring and Y-bifurcated ligaments acting as the acetabulum, so that in CTEV the socket is medially displaced on the 'ball'. The structures of the acetabulum pedis move in unison and need to be rotated laterally on the talar head. Its similarity to the hip gives it the name 'coxa pedis'.

Non-surgical treatment is the initial choice and should be started at birth. It includes manipulative correction, restoration of movement and maintenance of correction. Three methods are available to achieve these goals. Taping and strapping is restricted to premature infants who are in neonatal intensive care units and whose feet are required for venous access, but this is ineffective in correcting a stiff forefoot deformity, although Ghali et al. [1983] had 94% success, provided the treatment started at birth. Functional treatment by Bensahel et al. [1995] is to align the foot while retaining active mobility and suppleness, and provide gentle manipulation, active physiotherapy and splinting. Correction of the deformity is attempted sequentially: first, the talonavicular joint and forefoot adduction by stabilization of the global adduction of the calcaneus–forefoot block; and finally by progressive reduction of the heel varus and equinus. Each session lasts 30 min per foot and is followed by active physiotherapy and splintage. Below-knee splints are made of elastic tape, holding the foot in a slightly undercorrected position. This is performed daily from birth to 4–12 weeks. If there has been improvement, the manipulations are decreased to three sessions per week, continuing during infancy. In a 10-year follow-up of 350 feet using his technique, there was a significant difference between the results achieved by well-trained versus less trained therapists. Multiplanar continuous passive motion during sleeping periods in addition to the functional treatment resulted in 74% not requiring surgery and 46% of severe and 30% of moderate CTEV cases requiring less extensive surgical correction.

Manipulation and casting was developed by Ponseti [1992] and is based on sequential manipulative correction followed by retentive casts. Controversy still exists as to whether to correct all components of the deformity at the same time except equinus, as advocated by Ponseti, or to correct them sequentially starting from the forefoot adductus followed by hindfoot varus and finally the equinus, as advocated by Kite [1972]. The manipulation is started with the correction of cavus by supinating the forefoot and dorsiflexing the first metatarsal, to align the forefoot and midfoot in one plane, creating an effective lever arm to correct hindfoot varus by adducting the forefoot with counter-pressure of the thumb on the talar head. This method provides a fulcrum for abduction to the talonavicular joint, whereas others use the calcaneocuboid joint as the fulcrum. As the calcaneus abducts and everts by rotating and sliding under the talus, heel varus is corrected. No attempt at equinus correction is made until the foot can be fully abducted on the talus past neutral. An above-knee cast gives control of eversion and is less likely to slide off. Once the cavus and varus have been corrected, a percutaneous heel cord release is performed in the office. The postoperative care requires casting for 6–12 weeks followed by reverse-last shoes or a Denis Browne bar for several years. Some patients (30–40%) may ultimately require anterior tibialis tendon transfer.

The senior author's primary treatment protocol involves casts changed at weekly intervals for the first month and the foot manipulated at each cast change. We follow a simple rule of 70, 20, 10, i.e. manipulating forefoot adductus 70 times, hindfoot varus 20 times and stretching the heel 10 times at each visit. Casts are changed at biweekly intervals for the next month and then monthly until the third month. At this time the foot is reassessed clinically and radiographically and a decision taken for future management. A lateral maximum dorsiflexion view accesses correction of equinus. If equinus is corrected, the child is placed in corrective reverse-last shoes, whereas if it still persists, a percutaneous heel cord release is performed followed by casting and corrective shoes until the child begins walking.

At this stage the response to non-surgical treatment is assessed. A clinical assessment can score a foot on either the Dimeglio or the Pirani scale to add objectivity regarding the response to treatment. Weightbearing anteroposterior, lateral and a stress dorsiflexion lateral radiograph still remain the gold standard for evaluation of the residual deformity. The stress dorsiflexion view will show three signs of a fixed equinovarus deformity, i.e. no dorsiflexion of the calcaneus (tibiocalcaneal angle more than 90°), failure of the long axes of talus and calcaneus to converge, and no overlap of the distal end of the calcaneus and talus, i.e. the sinus tarsi remains open.

If this evaluation shows that the deformity is yielding to non-surgical treatment and the radiographic parameters are within the normal limits, it is advisable to continue with a further cast change for a month followed by straight or reverse-last shoes and a Denis Browne bar. Full-time corrective shoes are gradually weaned to night-time use only, at which time the shoes are stabilized with a bar to keep the feet externally rotated. Other forms of passive management include bivalved cast and knee–ankle–foot orthoses worn at night. The duration for the use of corrective shoes in an attempt to rebalance the musculotendinous units varies from 1 year to 6 years, with no objective data supporting either approach. If the deformity still persists, confirmed by radiographic parameters, the options are either limited surgical correction or immediate or delayed definitive surgical correction.

Limited surgical correction

Outpatient heel cord tenotomy can be carried out under local anesthersia for persistent equinus despite improvement in the cavus and adduction deformities. The foot is then placed in a cast for 3 weeks, when a lateral radiograph is taken to confirm the convergence of talocalcaneal axes. The foot is placed in a full-time corrective shoe for 3 months, and is gradually weaned to night-time use for a variable period of time. Cooper and Dietz [1995] reviewed the long-term results of Ponseti's protocol and reported that, of the 71 feet initially treated by serial casting, 27 required a heel cord tenotomy and 38 required a subsequent anterior tibial tendon transfer. They reported a 78% excellent function outcome in their patients, whereas Tibrewal et al. [1992] reported six of 25 feet requiring a further surgical procedure. Dal Monte et al. [1983] performed a limited posterior release by a sagittal plane Z lengthening of the Achilles tendon, posterior tibiotalar and talocalcaneal capsulotomy in 100 feet, with 71% good results in mild deformities and 34% in severe deformities. They concluded that this approach should be limited to mild deformities. The authors also compared 100 patients who underwent posterior release to 100 cases who underwent a posterior and medial release and concluded that, for grades II and III feet, both posterior and medial release were required. Porter [1987] treated 125 feet with a limited posterolateral release by Z lengthening of the invertors and reefing of the peroneus brevis as a one-stage procedure around 6 weeks of age, but 66 of these feet required a second-stage operation for forefoot correction. The treatment algorithm is shown in Figure 1 as designed by Dr Crawford.

Definitive surgical procedure

The timing of surgery does not reflect failure for the treating physician but mere recognition that the deformity will take more than manipulation to yield.

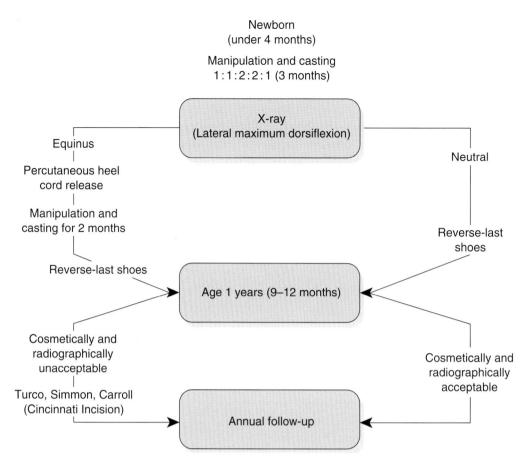

Figure 1

Treatment algorithm

Early surgical intervention will allow remodeling but predisposes the foot to iatrogenic cartilage and physeal damage. A comparison of the results of surgical correction performed at birth [Pous and Dimeglio 1978, Ryoppy and Sairanen 1983] and at approximately 1 year [Ghali et al. 1983] suggests no advantage for earlier intervention. Harrold and Walker [1983] reported on the results of surgical correction under 3 months of age; half of the feet required further surgery. Tibrewal et al. [1992] operated on 11 of 28 patients who had undergone a subtalar realignment at 6 weeks of age. Most surgeons recommend surgical correction between 9 and 12 months.

Controversy exists about the type and extent of the surgical correction. Turco [1979] described his technique of posteromedial release with pin fixation. Controversy still surrounds release of the talocalcaneal interosseous ligament as proposed by Simons [1995] and the deltoid ligament as proposed by Goldner [1990]. Surgeons must recognize that all CTEV are not the same, so a single recipe does not serve all (i.e. surgery is tailored to the need of the foot).

Turco [1979] used a single posteromedial incision, which makes release of the posterolateral structures difficult. The Cincinnati incision [Crawford et al. 1982] or the two-incision approach of Carroll [1997] overcomes this. The former allows excellent circumferential access to all parts of the deformity, which is beneficial for visualization of the pathology and for training residents. Skin necrosis is a potential concern, but Ferlic et al. [1997] reported their series of 31 feet where they left the medial part of the Cincinnati incision open by 10 mm and all but one wound healed within 6 weeks. Mountney et al. [1998] found no difference in the quality of the scar in those that had healed primarily or by secondary intention. The twin incision avoids potential skin necrosis but limits the approach.

Most surgeons advocate one, two or three pins to hold the correction. A single smooth pin is used to hold the reduced talonavicular articulation. Others use a smooth pin to hold the talocalcaneal and the calcaneocuboid articulation. Postoperative casting is mandatory for about 3 months, with removal of wires at 6 weeks.

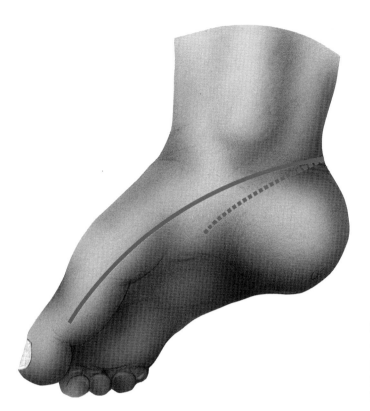

Figure 2

The skin incision begins just proximal to the medial aspect of the first metatarsophalangeal joint, crosses the medial malleolus and continues to a point directly posterior on the calf

Our approach is a posterior medial lateral release through the Cincinnati incision with the child supine and the leg prepared to allow sight of the patella to determine the angle of foot progression. The incision is outlined with a skin marker. The first step is a percutaneous release of the plantar fascia. With the foot held in maximum forced dorsiflexion a small tenotome is placed just anterior to the attachment of the plantar muscles and fascia to the base of the calcaneus at a point located one finger's breadth posterior to the medial malleolus, which avoids the neurovascular bundle and an iatrogenic arteriovenous fistula. A tenotome is inserted percutaneously and, with a swivelling mediolateral motion, all structures between the skin and the calcaneus are incised. The medial limb of the incision (Figure 2) is made, the neurovascular bundle isolated and protected (Figure 3). This illustration shows release of the abductor muscle from the laceniate ligament. An alternative to continuing the medial dissection is to perform a lateral subtalar release (Figure 4). By performing the lateral subtalar release first, the Y-bifurcate ligament is resected to give a direct approach to the lateral talonavicular joint and the calcaneocuboid joint. This prevents osteotomy of the talar neck while the talonavicular joint is being exposed. A small periosteal elevator is used to confirm the adequacy of release. The Achilles tendon is exposed at its insertion on the calcaneus and 'Z' lengthened. There is minimal

scarring from a previous percutaneous release, and the tendon is intact. The flexor hallucis longus lies in its small groove in the posterior talus. The oblique, lateral, talofibular and calcaneofibular ligaments are then released.

This direct posterior view after all the releases exemplifies the power of the Cincinnati incision. The flexor digitorum longus and posterior tibialis tendons are now lengthened, preserving the retinaculum. The distal posterior tibialis tendon stump is retracted and scissors are used to incise the capsule of the talonavicular joint (Figure 5). This is the most dangerous part of the medial release because the talar head is directed laterally and the navicular is articulating on the medial talar neck. Strong traction applied to the posterior tibial tendon opens the joint, preventing a talar neck osteotomy. An elevator can be passed through the joint to assist medial dissection.

With medial, anterior, posterior and lateral subtalar joint release, the talocalcaneal interosseous ligament is left intact. The foot is rotated into its normal progression angle and an antegrade pin is driven through the talus into the navicular (Figure 6). Thumb pressure keeps the navicular in line with the talus and prevents its dorsal subluxation. A radiograph taken in maximum forced dorsiflexion identifies the pin position and convergence of the talus and calcaneus. We now approach the medial spin. Small Steinman pins are placed in the midaxial

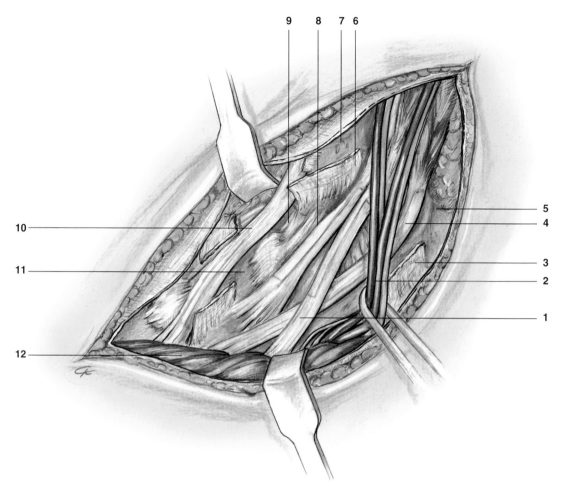

Figure 3

The tibialis posterior, flexor hallucis longus and flexor digitorum longus tendons are lengthened by Z-plasty as far distally as possible. The length of the Z is approximately one-quarter of the length of the foot

1 Flexor digitorum longus tendon
2 Neurovascular bundle
3 Flexor retinaculum and laceniate ligament (incised)
4 Flexor hallucis longus tendon
5 Calcaneus
6 Flexor retinaculum and laceniate ligament (incised)
7 Tibia
8 Tibialis posterior tendon
9 Talar neck
10 Tibialis anterior tendon
11 Navicular
12 Abductor hallucis muscle

position of the talus and the calcaneus. The calcaneal pin is usually directly posterior and adjacent to the fibula. Following correction of medial spin by bringing the calcaneus medially, its pin goes from just posterior and adjacent to the fibula to medial to the talar pin. We feel that this rotational correction of medial spin is important; it can be achieved only following release of the calcaneofibular and talofibular ligaments. We add a second talocalcaneal pin to prevent recurrence of the medial spin through the subtalar joint.

The retinaculum, digitorum longus and tibialis posterior tendons are repaired and a tenotomy of the flexor hallucis longus is performed. There is often an accessory joint on the medial malleolus, where the navicular had articulated. There is a finger-breadth width of talar articular cartilage exposed. The incision is closed with a subcuticular

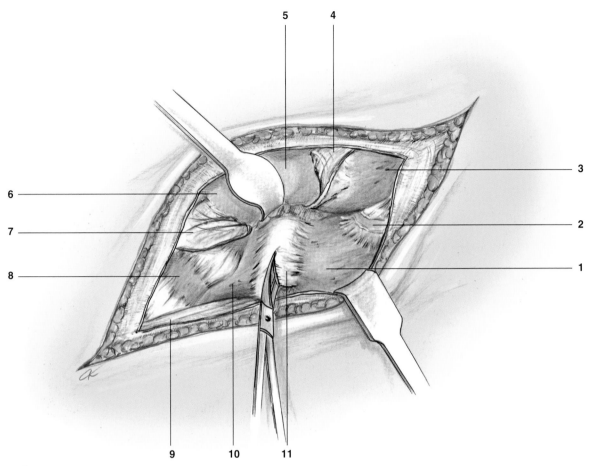

Figure 4

After identification and release from its fibrous sheath the peroneus longus tendon is protected, and then the calcaneocuboid joint capsule is identified and divided

1 Calcaneus
2 Capsule of subtalar joint (incised)
3 Talus
4 Capsule of talonavicular joint (incised)
5 Talar head
6 Navicular
7 Capsule of talonavicular joint (incised)
8 Medial cuneiform
9 Peroneus longus tendon
10 Cuboid
11 Capsule of calcaneocuboid joint

suture. Following skin closure, Steri-strips are placed over the wound with a layer of non-adhesive dressing. We then apply a sponge dressing above and below the foot. A skintight snug cast is unnecessary, as there is rigid internal fixation. An above-knee cast is applied with the knee bent to 90° and the foot in approximately 30° of external rotation. This cast is maintained for 6 weeks, at which time the pins are removed. The foot is then recast for 1 month. The child is placed in reverse-last shoes for daily wear. The shoes are attached to a Denis Browne bar at night for not less than 1 year.

In conclusion, a percutaneous tenotomy is useful as a primary limited procedure between 6 and 12 weeks. Extensive release before 9–12 months is avoided. Retention is maintained of the talocalcaneal interosseous ligament with a circumferential release, pre-fixation of subtalar and talonavicular joints after achieving correct alignment, and intraoperative radiography. The posterior tibialis tendon is lengthened, not released. Extreme valgus and abduction in the cast should be avoided.

Residual deformities do occur, and these require secondary procedures. Turco and Spinella [1982]

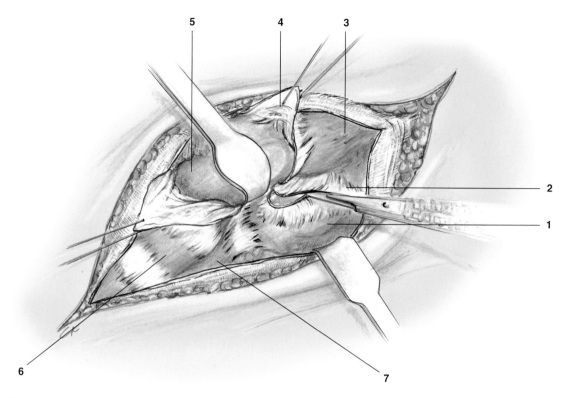

Figure 5

A curved blunt dissector is passed around the talar head and the subtalar joint is identified. The medial capsule of the subtalar joint, which takes an S-shaped curve, is divided

1 Calcaneus
2 Capsule of subtalar joint
3 Talus
4 Capsule of talonavicular joint (incised)
5 Navicular
6 Medial cuneiform
7 Cuboid

believe that residual deformities result from primary undercorrection and insufficient splinting for tarsal bones to remodel. Bensahel et al. [1995] agreed that no recurrence occurs after a foot is completely corrected and maintained, and if a relapse does occur after an initial successful operation a neurological cause should be considered. Tarraf and Carroll [1992] evaluated 159 feet which required a reoperation and reported an 8% incidence of adduction, 49% supination, 38% heel varus, 29% cavus and 24% equinus. Forefoot supination and adduction leading to an internal foot progression angle are reportedly the most common residual deformities in an operated CTEV. Otremski et al. [1987] reported that, in 21 of 28 clinically adducted feet, the main cause of the deformity was a metatarsus adductus. Tarraf and Carroll [1992] believed that failure to release the calcaneocuboid joint

was significant in producing a residual forefoot adduction. An imbalance between a strong tibialis posterior and a weak peronei results in a supination deformity. Asprheim et al. [1995], evaluating the residual deformities in operated CTEV utilizing gait analysis, showed that all except one patient in their series with intoeing had increased activity of the tibialis anterior during stance phase. Karol et al. [1997], in their gait analysis of patients with internal foot progression angle following release, showed that the most common cause was persistent internal tibial torsion, with only a minority of their patients showing an increase in the activity of the tibialis anterior during stance phase. Various procedures have been described to correct this deformity. Lateral transfer of the tibialis anterior to the third cuneiform is the most commonly utilized procedure. Cooper and Dietz [1995] reported 38 of

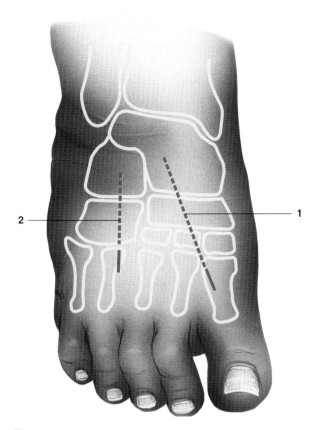

Figure 6

Placement of one pin from posterolateral through the talar body into the navicular (1). A second pin is driven from the dorsum of the foot through the cuboid into the calcaneus (2)

71 feet requiring a transfer of the anterior tibial tendon, with six of these patients requiring a further re-operation. Others have advocated a split transfer of the anterior tibial muscle. Hui et al. [1998], in an elegant biomechanical study, showed the axis of the fourth metatarsal for split transfer and that of the third metatarsal for the whole tendon transfer as being the ideal sites for insertion of the tendon. They found no difference in the maximum dorsiflexion achieved by split versus whole tibialis anterior tendon transfer. Open wedge osteotomy of the first cuneiform has been utlized to correct the residual adduction of the forefoot. This approach has been justified by later studies by Ostermski et al. [1987] who showed that most of the forefoot adduction was attributed to metatarsus adductus. Hofman et al. [1984] evaluated their results of talar opening wedge osteotomy along with radical plantar release and reported a 72% correction of adduction. Evans wedge resection and fusion of the calcaneocuboid joint has been greatly utilized to correct relapsed CTEV with the intention of reducing the navicular on the head of the talus by

shortening the lateral column. Graham and Dent [1992] evaluated the results of this procedure in 60 feet at a mean patient age of 29 years. They reported that function was satisfactory in 68% of the feet, and that 90% of the patients were able to perform all desired activities. Addison et al. [1983] evaluated their results of a modified Evans procedure in 45 feet. They reported satisfactory results in 30 feet, with the majority of the patients being able to participate in recreational activities. An opening wedge medial cuneiform osteotomy and a closing wedge cuboid osteotomy have been proposed to correct a bean-shaped foot, i.e. forefoot adduction with supination. McHale and Lenhart [1991], in an elegant cadaveric experiment, showed that forefoot adduction changed in direct proportion to the width of the talar wedge used, and that cuboid wedge resection allowed correction of the midfoot. They reported short-term results of this procedure in seven feet, with six of them showing correction of forefoot adductus and bean shape of the foot.

Treatment, results and analysis

The goal of surgery for CTEV is to render a near anatomically normal, pain-free plantigrade foot with reasonable mobility that fits into a normal shoe and maintains lasting correction. It is often difficult to compare the results of various surgical techniques, owing to the fact that no two CTEVs are alike and to the non-existence of a universal grading and evaluation system. Manzone [1999] compared the results of posteromedial release to that of a complete circumferential release performed by the same surgeon. Both groups were similar, according to radiographic evaluation. They found no difference in the radiographic and clinical results between these groups at a follow-up of 2 years. Haasbeek and Wright [1997] compared the long-term results of posterior release to those of Carroll's [1997] comprehensive release performed at the same institution and found that, although the two groups did not differ on the function-weighted Ponseti scale, the patients in the comprehensive group had fewer complications, more complete correction of heel varus and improved subtalar motion. Manzone et al. [1999] compared the results of the Carroll [1997] procedure, the McKay [1983] procedure and the Turco [1979] procedure and found similar excellent results. Blakeslee and DeValentine [1995] carried out a meta-analysis of the results of various surgical techniques in the literature and found 42% excellent results with posterior release only, 56%

excellent results with posterior and partial medial release, 65% excellent results with the Turco procedure and 64% excellent results with posteromediolateral release (McKay or Carroll procedures). Aronson and Puskarich [1990] reported on the deformity and disability from treated clubfoot in 29 patients with unilateral deformity and compared them to the contralateral normal foot. The most significant limitations in these treated clubfeet averaged a 65% decrease in normal dorsiflexion, a 24% decrease in plantarflexion strength, which correlated directly with the number of heel cord lengthenings, and a 10% decrease in calf girth unrelated to the total time spent in the cast. Miller and Bernstein [1986] reviewed the radiographic appearance of 24 feet undergoing a Turco procedure at a mean of 7 years' follow-up. They noted wedging of the navicular with dorsal displacement in 16 feet, flattening of the trochlear surface of the talus in 13 feet, and relative shortening of the talar neck and head in nine patients. Kuo et al. [1998] reported a 7.1% incidence of dorsal subluxation of the tarsal navicular. They created an anatomic model to explain that this radiographic appearance was due to a rotatory subluxation of the navicular in the coronal plane. They stressed the need to check the rotation of the navicular at the time of internal fixation. It is our contention that dorsal navicular subluxation may in some cases be iatrogenic. Special attention should be directed towards assessing anatomic positioning and pinning of the navicular, with radiographic confirmation.

Overcorrected severe, unacceptable flat-foot deformity is being increasingly recognized as a complication of aggressive surgical treatment of clubfoot. Initially attributed to release of the talocalcaneal interosseous ligament and early age at surgery, an increasing incidence of this complication has been reported in series without these variables. Turco [1979], in the long-term follow-up study of his posteromedial release, attributed 75% of his unsatisfactory outcomes to overcorrection. Clinically this deformity is characterized by a contracted anterior tibial tendon, limited plantarflexion, severe flatfoot with heel valgus, concavity of the sinus tarsi and hallux flexus with a dorsiflexed first ray. These patients may have a clinical dorsal bunion. These feet are functionally and cosmetically worse than undercorrected feet. Hypotonia, joint laxity, a fine transverse skin crease around the heel, lateral insertion of the heel cord and a higher incidence of gestational diabetes may be predisposing factors. Once these features are recognized, extreme caution should be exercised to avoid extensive

release and dorsal subluxation of the navicular on the talus.

References

Addison A, Fixsen JA, Lloyd-Roberts GC (1983) A review of the Dillwyn Evans type collateral operation in severe club feet. J. Bone Joint Surg 65B: 12–14

Aronson J, Puskarich CL (1990) Deformity and disability from treated clubfoot. J Pediatr Orthop 10: 109–119

Asprheim MS, Moore C, Carroll NC, Dias L (1995) Evaluation of residual clubfoot deformities using gait analysis. J Pediatr Orthop B 4: 49–54

Bensahel H, Dimeglio A, Souchet P (1995) Final evaluation of clubfoot. J Pediatr Orthop B 4: 137–141

Blackeslee TJ, DeValentine SJ (1995) Management of the resistent idiopathic clubfoot: the Kaiser experience from 1980–1990. J Foot Ankle Surg 34: 167–176

Cahuzac JP, Baunin C, Luu S et al. (1999) Assessment of hindfoot deformity by three-dimensional MRI in infant club-foot. J Bone Joint Surg 81B: 97–101

Carroll NC (1997) Clubfoot: what have we learned in the last quarter century? J Pediatr Orthop 17: 1–2

Ching GH, Chung CS, Nemechek RW (1969) Genetic and epidemiological studies in clubfoot in Hawaii: ascertainment and incidence. Am J Hum Genet 81: 97–101

Cooper DM, Dietz FR (1995) Treatment of idiopathic clubfoot. A thirty year follow-up note. J Bone Joint Surg 77A: 1477–1489

Crawford AH, Durrani AA (0000) Clubfoot. Orthopaedic Knowledge Update, POSNA Pediatrics no. 2 203–213

Crawford AH, Marxen JL, Osterfeld DL (1982) The Cincinnati incision: a comprehensive approach for surgical procedures of the foot and ankle in childhood. J Bone Joint Surg 64A: 1355–1358

Cuevas de Alba C, Guille JT, Bowen JR et al. (1998) Computed tomography for femoral and tibial torsion in children with clubfoot. Clin Orthop 353: 203–209

Dal Monte A, Manes E, Araoz S, Zajia A (1983) Congenital clubfoot: results and therapeutic guidelines. Ital J Orthop Traumatol 9: 25–38

Dimeglio A, Bensahel H, Souchet P et al. (1995) Classification of clubfoot. J Pediatr Orthop B 4: 129–136

Dimeglio A, Bonnet F, Mazeau P, DeRosa V (1996) Orthopaedic treatment and passive motion machine: consequences for the surgical treatment of clubfoot. J Pediatr Orthop B 5: 173–180

Evans D (1986) Treatment of the unreduced or 'relapsed' clubfoot in older children. Proc R Soc Med 61: 782–783

Ferlic RJ, Breed AL, Mann DC et al. (1997) Partial wound closure after surgical correction of equinovarus foot deformity. J Pediatr Orthop 17: 486–489

Ghali NN, Smith RB, Clayden AD, Silk FF (1983) The results of pantalar reduction in the management of congenital talipes equinovarus. J Bone Joint Surg 65B: 1–7

Goldner JL (1990) Operative treatment of congenital idiopathic clubfoot. J Bone Joint Surg 72A: 307–309

Graham GP, Dent CM (1992) Dillwyn Evans operation for relapsed clubfoot. Long-term results. J Bone Joint Surg 74B: 445–448

Haasbeek JF, Wright JG (1997) A comparison of the long term results of posterior and comprehensive release in the treatment of clubfoot. J Pediatr Orthop 17: 29–35

Harrold AJ, Walker CJ (1983) Treatment and prognosis in congenital clubfoot. J Bone Joint Surg 65B: 8–11

Hofmann AA, Constine RM, McBride GG, Coleman SS (1984) Osteotomy of the 1st cuneiform as treatment of residual adduction of the fore part of the foot in clubfoot. J Bone Joint Surg 66: 985–990

Hui JH, Goh JC, Lee EH (1998) Biomechanical study of tibialis anterior tendon transfer. Clin Orthop 349: 249–255

Johnson CE 2nd, Hobatho MC, Baker KJ, Baunin C (1995) Three dimensional analysis of clubfoot deformity by computed tomography. J Pediatr Orthop B 4: 39–48

Karol LA, Concha MC, Johnson CE 2nd (1997) Gait analysis and muscle strength in children with surgically treated clubfoot. J Pediatr Orthop 17: 790–795

Kite JH (1972) Nonoperative treatment of congenital clubfoot. Clin Orthop Relat Res 84: 29–38

Kuo KN, Jansen LD (1998) Rotatory dorsal sublaxation of the navicular: a complication of clubfoot surgery. J Pediatr Orthop 18: 770–774

Lochmiller C, Johnston D, Scott A et al. (1998) Genetic epidemiology study of idiopathic talipes equinovarus. Am J Med Genet 79: 90–96

McHale KA, Lenhart MK (1991) Treatment of residual clubfoot deformity – the 'bean-shaped' foot – by opening wedge medial cuneiform osteotomy and closing wedge cuboid osteotomy. Clinical review and cadaver correlations. J Pediatr Orthop 11: 374–381

McKay DW New concept of an approach to clubfoot treatment: section 1. J Pediatr Orthop 1982; 2: 347–356, section 2 J Pediatr Orthop 1983; 3: 10–21, section 3 J Pediatr Orthop 1983; 3: 141–148

Manzone PJ (1999) Clubfoot surgical treatment: preliminary results of a prospective comparative study of two techniques. J Pediatr Orthop B 8: 246–250

Miller JH, Bernstein SM (1986) The roentgenographic appearance of the corrected clubfoot. Foot Ankle 6: 177–183

Mountney J, Khan T, Davies AG, Smith TW (1998) Scar quality from partial or complete wound closure using the Cincinnati incision for clubfoot surgery. J Pediatr Orthop B 7: 223–225

Otremski I, Salama R, Khermosh O, Wientroub S (1987) An analysis of the results of a modified one stage posteromedial release (Turco operation) for the treatment of clubfoot. J Pediatr Orthop 7: 149–151

Palmer RM, Conneally PM, Yu PL (1974) Studies of the inheritance of idiopathic talipes equinovarus. Orthop Clin North Am 5: 99–108

Pirani S, Outerbridge H, Moran M, Sawatski B (1995) A method evaluating the virgin clubfoot with substantial inter-observer reliability. POSNA Miami Florida

Ponseti IV (1992) Treatment of congenital clubfoot. J Bone Joint Surg 74A: 448–454

Ponseti IV (1997) Common errors in the treatment of congenital clubfoot. Int Orthop 21: 137–141

Porter RW (1987) Congenital talipes equinovarus: a staged method of surgical management. J Bone Joint Surg 69B: 826–831

Pous JG, Dimeglio A (1978) Neonatal surgery in clubfoot. Orthop Clin North Am 9: 233–240

Ryoppy S, Sairanen H (1983) Neonatal operative treatment of clubfoot. A preliminary report. J Bone Joint Surg 65B: 320–325

Seringe R (1999) Congenital equinovarus clubfoot. Acta Orthop Belg 65: 127–153

Simons GW (1995) Calcaneocuboid joint deformity in talipes equinovarus: an overview and update. J Pediatr Orthop B 4: 25–35

Tarraf YN, Carroll NC (1992) Analysis of the components of residual deformity in clubfeet presenting for reoperation. J Pediatr Orthop 12: 207–216

Tibrewal SB, Benson MK, Howard C, Fuller DJ (1992) The Oxford Clubfoot Programme. J Bone Joint Surg 74B: 528–533

Turco VJ (1979) Resistant congenital clubfoot: one stage posteriomedial release with internal fixation. A follow-up report of a 15 year experience. J Bone Joint Surg 61A: 805–814

Turco VJ, Spinella AJ (1982) Current management of clubfoot. Instr Course Lect 31: 218–234

44

Surgical management of acute infections and of acute compartment syndrome of the foot

Thomas Mittlmeier

Introduction

Anatomy

The typical arrangement of the fascial spaces of the foot (Figures 1 and 2) has been the subject of recent studies, owing to recognition of the clinical importance of the spread of deep infections and the generation of acute compartment syndromes [Loeffler and Ballard 1980, Manoli 1990, Manoli and Weber 1990, Mittlmeier et al. 1991]. The anatomy of the plantar side of the foot provides biomechanical stability. This is supplied, in part, by the plantar aponeurosis, which only separates in the distal forefoot as its terminal fibers insert into the toes. The anatomy of the nine compartments of the foot with their strong and rigid septa also add to this stable construct. However, little space is available for any acute volume changes [Sarrafian 1983, Manoli and Weber 1990, Pisan and Klaue 1994].

Pathogenesis and clinical appearance

Acute infection

Local superficial infection of the foot is common in the forefoot and toes. It often results from mechanical irritation, from ingrown toenails, blisters or minor injuries of soft tissues with secondary overgrowth by skin organisms, such as *Staphylococcus aureus* or β-hemolytic streptococci. Deep acute infection may also result as a complication after penetrating trauma, such as puncture wounds, or after blunt trauma [Frierson and Pfeffinger 1993]. Infection is rarely caused by micro-organisms carried by vascular or lymph channels [Frierson and Pfeffinger 1993]. Predisposing factors for infection may be abnormal flow in the vascular system, gangrene, hematoma formation, penetrating wounds or blunt trauma, foreign bodies or chemical irritation. The clinical appearance of an acute infection may be clearly seen in a normal patient; this includes swelling, redness, temperature increase, tenderness, lymphangitis, pain and dysfunction. Infecting organisms are numerous: aerobic and anaerobic bacteria, mycobacteria, fungi, parasites and viruses. Concomitant infections may also occur, as in fungal infections which may lead to a skin lesion serving as a portal for bacterial infections. The early diagnosis of the underlying type and extent of the infection and the proper selection of treatment are crucial to avoid complications, such as penetration of the infection to deeper tissue levels or the development of an acute or chronic

a

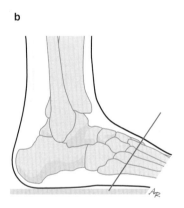

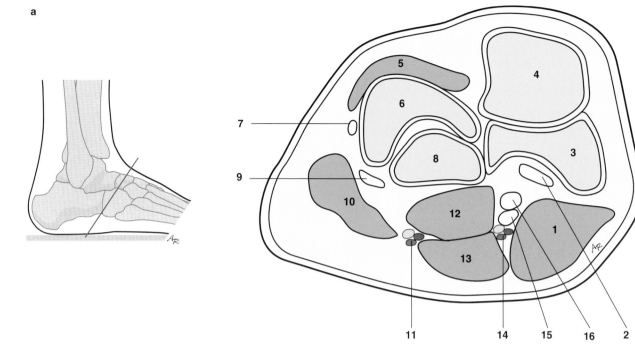

b

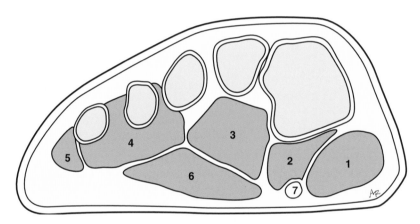

Figure 1

a
Cross-section of a right foot at the Chopart joint level
  1 Medial compartment (abductor hallucis muscle)
  2 Tibialis posterior tendon
  3 Navicular bone
  4 Talar head
  5 Extensor digitorum brevis muscle
  6 Anterior calcaneal process
  7 Peroneus brevis tendon
  8 Cuboid
  9 Peroneus longus tendon
 10 Lateral compartment (abductor digiti minimi muscle)
 11 Lateral plantar neurovascular bundle
 12 Deep central compartment (quadratus plantae muscle)
 13 Superficial central compartment (flexor digitorum brevis muscle)
 14 Medial plantar neurovascular bundle
 15 Flexor digitorum longus tendon
 16 Flexor hallucis longus tendon

b
Cross-section of a right foot at the proximal metatarsal level
  1 Abductor hallucis muscle
  2 Flexor hallucis brevis muscle
  3 Adductor hallucis muscle (oblique head)
  4 Interossei dorsales muscles 3 and 4 and interossei plantares muscles 3–5
  5 Lateral compartment (abductor digiti minimi muscle and flexor digiti minimi brevis muscle)
  6 Superficial central compartment (flexor digitorum longus et brevis tendons 2–5 and lumbrical muscles 2–5)
  7 Flexor hallucis longus tendon

osteomyelitis [Jahss 1982, Frierson and Pfeffinger 1993]. Owing to the limited elasticity of the plantar aponeurosis, even plantar infections may become apparent as dorsal swelling alone. In patients at risk, e.g. diabetic or immunosuppressed patients, superficial infection after local skin breakdown may rapidly

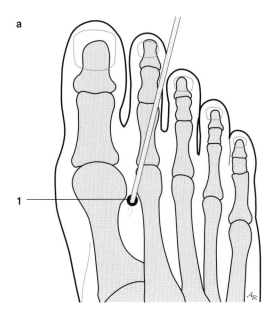

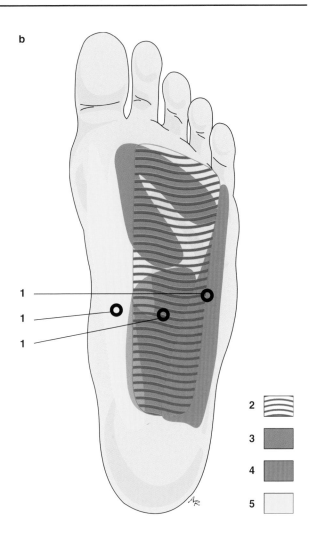

Figure 2

Standard measuring sites for compartment pressures.
a. dorsal aspect; b. plantar aspect

a
1 Measuring site

b
1 Measuring sites
2 Superficial central compartment
3 Deep central compartment
4 Lateral compartment
5 Medial compartment

progress to deep infection, which may culminate in local necrosis, osteitis, septic arthritis or propagation of the infection to the proximal foot or the lower leg. This may occur in particular if pain sensation is missing or attenuated owing to neuropathy, or if the typical appearance of an infected foot with redness, tenderness, swelling, fluctuation and increased skin temperature is altered by chronic pre-existing foot deformity. In this case, additional diagnostic tools such as a 99m-technetium-labeled patient-specific leukocyte scan or gadolinium-enhanced magnetic resonance imaging may be necessary to differentiate chronic non-inflammatory changes (such as in Charcot feet) from infection, and to evaluate the extent of the infection [Frierson and Pfeffinger 1993, Crim et al. 1996].

Acute compartment syndrome

In the acute compartment syndrome, an increased pressure within a limited fascial space compromises the circulation and function of the tissues contained within that space [Whitesides et al. 1975, Matsen 1980]. This generally accepted definition of

a compartment syndrome also applies to the foot. If untreated, this clinical entity may lead to the formation of claw toes (contractures of the short foot muscles), possibly resulting in the development of a cavus deformity with stiffness and paresthesia in the plantar nerve distribution or permanent pain [Manoli 1990, 1994, Mittlmeier et al. 1991, Myerson 1991, Pisan and Klaue 1994, Zwipp 1994].

Clinically, a foot with a compartment syndrome is usually held in slight plantarflexion and adduction [Pisan and Klaue 1994]. The metatarsophalangeal joints are often swollen. Pain usually increases with passive extension of the toes and the ankle joint [Pisan and Klaue 1994]. Dysesthesia or hypoesthesia can be found if the patient is conscious. Capillary filling is generally intact and the peripheral pulses remain palpable in the acute phase. Simultaneous manifestation of a compartment syndrome of the foot and the lower leg may occur [Zwipp 1994].

If compartment syndrome of the foot is suspected clinically, pressure measurements should always be performed, since palpation is an unreliable diagnostic tool. Owing to the specific anatomical arrangement of the nine fascial spaces of the foot, four standard measuring sites should be used [Manoli and Weber 1990, Manoli 1994] (Figure 2).

Treatment

Indications for surgery

Infection

Local infection of the foot may be treated by oral or intravenous antibiotics and other conservative measures, if it appears that only a cellulitis is present. However, abscess formation in the foot must be treated surgically.

Acute compartment syndrome

The pressure limit at which fasciotomy should be performed is controversial. Some authors recommend fasciotomy at pressures greater than 30 mmHg [Matsen 1980, Mittlmeier et al. 1991, Pisan and Klaue 1994]. Others perform fasciotomy if the compartment pressure is less than 10–30 mmHg below the diastolic blood pressure. This is particularly helpful in a hypotensive patient with multiple injuries [Whitesides et al. 1975, Manoli 1994].

Fasciotomy has been found necessary after 41% of crush injuries to the foot [Myerson 1991], 4–17% of calcaneal fractures [Mittlmeier et al. 1991, Myerson 1991] and up to 40% of Lisfranc and Chopart joint fracture–dislocations [Zwipp 1994]. A rare indication is a foot compartment syndrome developing after long-standing ischemia and following vascular reconstruction in the leg.

Surgical technique

Fasciotomy or incision for deep infection should generally be performed under regional or general anesthesia. The patient is usually positioned on the operating table in a supine or slightly oblique position, tilted towards the affected side, with free access to the entire lower leg. A tourniquet must not be used in decompression of the foot compartments or in infection, since its use could cause additional post-ischemic swelling.

If all compartments of the foot are to be released, three incisions will be necessary: a medial hindfoot incision (Figure 3) and two parallel incisions on the dorsum of the foot (see Figure 5) [Manoli 1994]. This approach may also be necessary after crush trauma of the foot, but has to be modified according to the individual situation and the specific tissue pressure

recordings. Therefore, a three-incision approach for decompression of all foot compartments should not be practiced routinely in any case of a foot compartment syndrome. The extent of the procedure should include the compartments with significantly increased pressure levels or those compartments where a pressure increase could be expected, e.g. after crush trauma. In Lisfranc fracture–dislocation, the standard single-incision technique for open reduction and internal fixation on the dorsum of the foot will usually suffice to decompress the foot compartments involved. However, this does not give access to the superficial central and the medial compartments. If a simultaneous compartment syndrome of the foot and the lower leg is present, the unilateral incision of the lower leg can be extended to the dorsum of the foot [Zwipp 1994].

For adequate drainage of all the plantar fascial spaces an incision has been described which combines both mediodorsal and plantar approaches [Loeffler and Ballard 1980]. In general, a less extensive approach will be sufficient for adequate debridement and drainage or decompression of the contents of the plantar compartments, and the midsole of the foot does not need to be exposed.

In an acute local plantar infection, a straight longitudinal incision directly over the involved area may be chosen, either medially, laterally or dorsally. A linear incision is generally preferable to a curved or S-shaped one because it minimizes the risk of injury to the sensory branches of the medial and lateral plantar nerves [Jahss 1982]. Plantar incisions should avoid the metatarsal heads or the calcaneus, since weightbearing occurs at the fat pads of these areas [Jahss 1982]. In general, plantar approaches do not cause local healing problems [Jahss 1982].

Using the medial approach (Figure 3) all five plantar compartments can be decompressed [Manoli 1990, 1994, Pisan and Klaue 1994]. The incision follows the edge of the abductor hallucis muscle. It begins about 4 cm from the posterior aspect of the heel, 3 cm from the plantar surface, and is about 6–8 cm long. The fascia of the abductor hallucis muscle is opened along the line of the skin incision. When the muscle is pulled plantarwards with a blunt retractor, the thick fascia of the deep calcaneal compartment can be identified (see Figure 4) [Pisan and Klaue 1994]. Alternatively, the abductor hallucis muscle is lifted dorsally to expose the deep central intermuscular septum [Manoli 1994]. The intermuscular septum should be opened with caution, starting with a small opening which is widened by careful dissection, to avoid injury to the medial plantar neurovascular bundle.

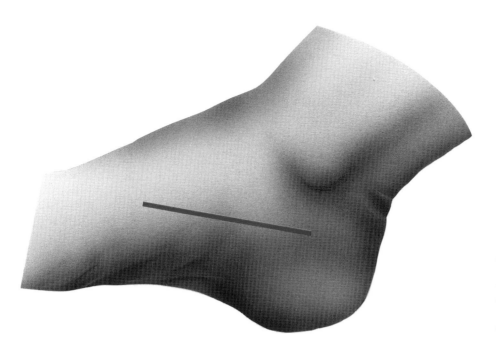

Figure 3

Skin incision of the medial approach for a decompression of all four plantar compartments

The neurovascular bundle usually runs in intimate contact with the medial border of the calcaneal compartment or in the septum between the calcaneal and the central superficial compartments (see Figure 4b). The lateral neurovascular bundle contains vessels which are 80% higher than the corresponding diameters of the vessels of the medial bundle. The lateral bundle crosses the deep central compartment from medial to lateral. Usually, the medial plantar nerve follows the vessels laterally. The lateral plantar nerve, however, is usually located medial to its accompanying vessels (see Figure 4b). An adequate release of the calcaneal compartment may become obvious by considerable bulging of the quadratus plantae muscle around the lateral neurovascular bundle [Manoli 1994].

The next step is the release of the superficial central compartment containing the flexor digitorum brevis muscle, approaching the corresponding fascia from the plantar side and retracting the fat from the medial side plantarwards [Manoli 1994]. The flexor digitorum brevis muscle should be mobilized and retracted plantarwards to identify the medial border of the lateral compartment. This is opened with the help of dissecting scissors, to decompress the abductor digiti minimi muscle and more anteriorly the flexor digiti minimi muscle [Manoli 1994].

A release of the compartments of the forefoot is usually performed by two separate 6–8-cm longitudinal incisions on the dorsum of the forefoot (Figure 5): the first is situated medial to the second metatarsal, and the second lateral to the fourth metatarsal, to avoid a narrow skin bridge which may result in skin problems. Through these incisions the corresponding four dorsal and plantar interossei compartments can be released. Dissecting from the first interspace along the second metatarsal with a sharp elevator, and keeping the interosseous muscle to the medial side, the fascia of the adductor muscle can be approached and opened (see Figure 5). From the lateral incision, the lateral plantar compartment of the forefoot can be decompressed.

Postoperative care

The incisions should be kept open and covered with skin substitute, which should be changed every 2–3 days until delayed skin closure or split-thickness skin grafting become possible; the timing of these procedures depends on the residual swelling and soft-tissue conditions [Manoli 1994, Zwipp 1994]. In deep infection, regular surgical revisions with debridement and lavage are superior to the closed suction–irrigation technique [Frierson and Pfeffinger 1993]. With the use of these techniques, the postoperative cosmetic appearance of the scars will be acceptable.

Fractures of the forefoot should be stabilized at the time of the fasciotomy [Manoli 1994, Zwipp 1994]. Comminuted fractures of the calcaneus should not be repaired at the primary intervention, because this would require an additional skin incision. They should be stabilized later, after healing of the fasciotomy wounds [Manoli 1994, Zwipp 1994]. If considerable instability is present after fasciotomy in complex and comminuted fractures or

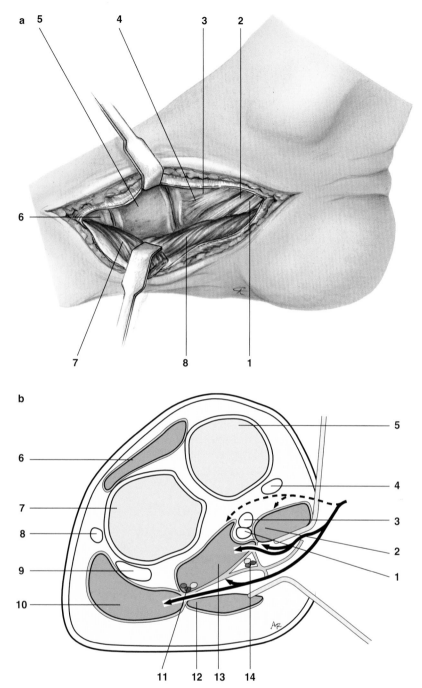

Figure 4

a. Medial approach for the decompression of all four plantar compartments.
b. the abductor hallucis muscle may either be retracted plantarwards (dotted arrow), where a lesion of the neurovascular bundle is hardly probable, or be lifted dorsally (solid arrow) to expose the deep central intermuscular septum

a
1   Flexor hallucis longus tendon
2   Flexor digitorum longus tendon
3   Navicular bone
4   Tibialis posterior tendon
5   Medial cuneiform
6   First metatarsal
7   Flexor hallucis brevis muscle
8   Abductor hallucis muscle

b
1   Flexor digitorum longus tendon
2   Medial compartment
3   Flexor hallucis longus tendon
4   Tibialis posterior tendon
5   Talar head
6   Extensor digitorum brevis muscle
7   Anterior calcaneal process
8   Peroneus brevis tendon
9   Peroneus longus tendon
10   Lateral compartment
11   Lateral plantar neurovascular bundle
12   Superficial central compartment
13   Deep central compartment
14   Medial plantar neurovascular bundle

fracture–dislocations of the foot, which cannot immediately be stabilized, tibiometatarsal transfixation can provide stability as a precondition for soft-tissue healing [Zwipp 1994]. The transfixation may be combined with minimal internal fixation or may be replaced by internal fixation at a second-stage intervention.

Complications

The major risk in acute deep infection or compartment syndrome of the foot is an incomplete release of the fascial structures, or starting the procedure too late to stop the disease progression [Manoli 1990, 1994, Myerson 1991, Pisan and Klaue 1994]. Skin scarification, an obsolete and insufficient method of decompression using only multiple dermal or transdermal short incisions, does not relieve compartment pressures and should not be used.

Fasciotomy itself is not a risky procedure: care should be taken to place the medial incision not too dorsally, to protect the medial calcaneal branches of the tibial nerve [Manoli 1994]. Damage to the two deep neurovascular structures of the sole of the foot can be avoided if the deep central compartment is

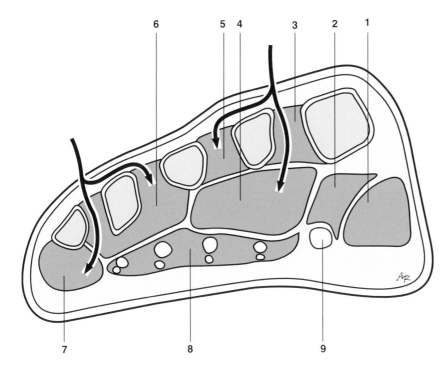

Figure 5

Two-incision technique of the forefoot for decompression of the interossei compartments, the adductor compartment and the lateral compartment

1 Abductor hallucis muscle
2 Flexor hallucis brevis muscle
3 First dorsal interosseous compartment
4 Adductor hallucis muscle (oblique head)
5 Second dorsal interosseous compartment
6 Interossei dorsales muscles 3 and 4 and interossei plantares 3–5 muscles
7 Lateral compartment
8 Superficial central compartment
9 Flexor hallucis longus tendon

carefully released, starting dissection with a small opening supported by digital palpation [Manoli 1994]. If the two dorsal incisions are placed at maximum distance from each other, skin slough or necrosis can be avoided.

References

Crim JR, Cracchiolo A, Hall RL (1996) Imaging of the Foot and Ankle. London, Martin Dunitz

Frierson JG, Pfeffinger LL (1993) Infections of the foot. In: Mann RA, McCoughlin MJ (eds) Surgery of the Foot and Ankle, 6th edn. St Louis, Mosby, pp 859–876

Jahss MH (1982) Surgical principles and the plantigrade foot. In: Jahss MH (ed) Disorders of the Foot. Philadelphia, Saunders, pp 144–194

Loeffler RD, Ballard A (1980) Plantar fascial spaces of the foot and a proposed surgical approach. Foot Ankle 1: 11–14

Manoli A (1990) Compartment syndromes of the foot. Current concepts. Foot Ankle 10: 340–344

Manoli A (1994) Compartment releases of the foot. In: Johnson KA (ed) Master Techniques in Orthopaedic Surgery: The Foot and Ankle. New York, Raven Press, pp 257–267

Manoli A, Weber TG (1990) Fasciotomy of the foot: an anatomical study with special reference to release of the calcaneal compartment. Foot Ankle 10: 267–275

Matsen FA (1980) Compartmental Syndromes. New York, Grune & Stratton

Mittlmeier T, Mächler G, Lob G et al. (1991) compartment syndrome of the foot after intraarticular calcaneal fracture. Clin Orthop 269: 241–248

Myerson M (1991) Management of compartment syndromes of the foot. Clin Orthop 271: 239–248

Pisan M, Klaue K (1994) Compartment syndrome of the foot. Eur J Foot Ankle Surg 1: 29–36

Sarrafian SK (1983) Anatomy of the Foot and Ankle. Philadelphia, Lippincott

Whitesides TE, Henry TC, Morimoto R et al. (1975) Tissue pressure measurements as a determinant for the need of fasciotomy. Clin Orthop 113: 43–51

Zwipp H (1994) Chirurgie des Fusses. Berlin, Springer

45

Surgical considerations in the diabetic foot

Patrick Laing
Nilesh Makwana

Introduction

Recent advances in our understanding of the pathogenesis of diabetes provide indisputable evidence that near-normal blood glucose control can reduce the development of complications in diabetic patients [Diabetes Control and Complications Trial Research Group 1993]. However, with increasing longevity the incidence of diabetes mellitus is rising, leading to more foot problems and a greater need for surgery. Foot problems occur in diabetic patients because of neuropathy, vascular disease, infection, or a combination of these. Surgical treatment of the diabetic foot is aimed at preserving as much of the foot as possible. The more proximal the level of amputation the greater the metabolic cost of walking [Waters et al. 1976]. Every procedure must be carefully planned, bearing in mind considerations for the future and taking the opposite limb into account. Regrettably, 'creeping amputation' is too frequently seen. It must be remembered that each part of the foot lost imposes greater forces on the remainder.

The neuropathic foot is often cavus with clawed toes, warm, dry skin, dilated veins and palpable pulses, and lacks protective sensation. High pressures develop under the metatarsal heads and heel, and the dorsa of the toes rub inside footwear. Without protective sensation, ulceration may occur at these areas of high pressure and infection can then supervene. Neuropathic ulcers are commonly surrounded by hyperkeratosis, are painless to touch or debride and have a pink, punched-out base which bleeds readily (Figure 1). Within the diabetic foot,

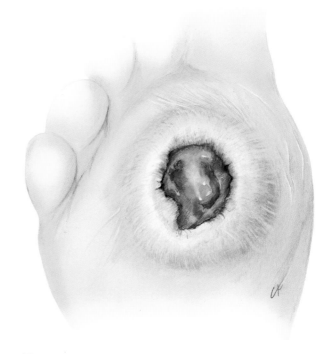

Figure 1

Plantar neuropathic ulcer in a diabetic patient

infection may spread rapidly along tissue planes, leading to abscess formation and osteomyelitis.

An important clinical point is the presence of pain in a normally painless foot; this is indicative of deep infection. It is possible to quantitate the sensory deficit by testing vibration sense with a biothesiometer and light touch with Semmes–Weinstein hairs; the latter has recently been shown to be a more reproducible method [Klenerman et al. 1996]. Semmes–Weinstein hairs are nylon monofilaments of different diameters which buckle at a defined force. They are numbered, each number referring to the logarithm of 10 times the force in milligrams required to buckle the hair [Bell-Krotoski and Tomancik 1987]. The 5.07 hair delivers a force of approximately 10 g, and from work on diabetic and leprosy patients [Birke and Sims 1986] this has been identified as the level of protective sensation. In contrast, a normal foot can perceive a force of as little as 1 g on the plantar surface. A small number of patients may develop neuropathic ulceration despite being able to feel a 5.07 hair.

Atherosclerosis occurs in the diabetic patient at a younger age, shows less male bias, is more often bilateral and progresses more quickly than in non-diabetics. The pattern of disease tends to involve the infrageniculate vessels, anterior tibial, posterior tibial and peroneal arteries. The distal dorsalis pedis or distal posterior tibial arteries may be preserved, making distal bypass reconstruction a possibility. Peripheral vascular disease may lead to ischemic ulceration and gangrene; this may be wet or dry and further complicated by osteomyelitis. The typical ischemic ulcer occurs in a foot with absent pulses, loss of hair, and shiny, atrophic and cold skin. The ulcer is not surrounded by hyperkeratosis, has a dull fibrotic base which does not bleed easily and is usually painful to debride. The peripheral circulation can be assessed by Doppler measurement of the dorsalis pedis and posterior tibial pulse pressures. This can be compared with the brachial pressure to give the ankle–brachial index (ABI). In a normal person this is usually greater than 1. However, the index may be falsely high because of calcification of the arterial tunica media, known as Mönckeberg's sclerosis. This appears to be a complication of neuropathy and can occur in non-diabetic patients following lumbar sympathectomy. It is classically seen with a calcified 'pipe-stem' appearance on radiographs and makes the vessel relatively incompressible; it is not uncommon to record ABIs of 2 or more in neuropathic patients. The ABI therefore is not an absolute guide to whether healing of an ulcer, or a surgical wound, will occur. An ABI of 0.45 or more has been cited as the lowest level at which healing will occur, but this cannot be relied upon. Pulse volume recording and continuous-wave Doppler waveform can be used, but are limited, as they are qualitative measures. In both cases the transition from triphasic to monophasic is indicative of large-vessel occlusion. Toe pressures may be helpful; a pressure of more than 45 mmHg is associated

with an 85% healing rate [Apelquist et al. 1989]. Transcutaneous oxygen tension measurements may be used to determine a viable level in the foot, but again these are only an adjunct to a clinical decision. A level of below 10 mmHg is indicative of severe skin ischemia.

Instead of neuropathic or ischemic ulceration, the diabetic foot may present with cellulitis. This may occur secondary to minor trauma, through fissuring in the dry skin or through the toe webs. Because there is little soft-tissue cover on the dorsum of the foot, osteomyelitis may develop secondary to cellulitis. A particularly severe form of cellulitis is necrotizing fasciitis (Figure 2), which is an acute infection of the subcutaneous fascia, resulting in necrosis along with gangrene of the overlying skin. The pathognomonic signs are dusky, purple patches developing over a cellulitic area. Although usually due to *Streptococcus pyogenes*, it may be caused by *Staphylococcus aureus*. In the past it has been associated with a high mortality rate in diabetic patients, and early diagnosis is important. It should also be noted that infections in the diabetic foot are usually polymicrobial, involving both aerobic and anaerobic bacteria. Gas in the soft tissues is not uncommon and does not imply clostridial infection; in diabetic patients it is usually caused by aerobic organisms such as coliforms and streptococci.

The diagnosis of osteomyelitis in diabetic patients is not straightforward because of the bony changes of diabetic osteopathy. These include periosteal reaction, osteoporosis, juxta-articular cortical defects and osteolysis. Osteolysis of the distal ends of the metatarsals and bases of the proximal phalanges leads to a 'pencil in cup' deformity. Therefore, bony changes in the presence of infection do not necessarily imply osteomyelitis. Technetium bone scans have high sensitivity for osteomyelitis, but low specificity with many false positives due to soft-tissue inflammation and periosteitis. Indium-labeled white-cell scans will rule out infection if negative, but if positive a simultaneous technetium bone scan may help differentiate osteomyelitis from infection limited to soft tissue [Jeffrey et al. 1996]. A combination of technetium- and indium-labeled white-cell scans can give a diagnostic accuracy of approximately 90% [Crerand et al. 1996]. An alternative is magnetic resonance imaging (MRI), which can now give similar accuracy but may not differentiate between infection, a neuropathic joint and fracture. Invasive techniques such as bone biopsy through an area not contiguous with the ulcer may provide both culture and histology for definitive diagnosis. It may yield the organism to guide antibiotic therapy.

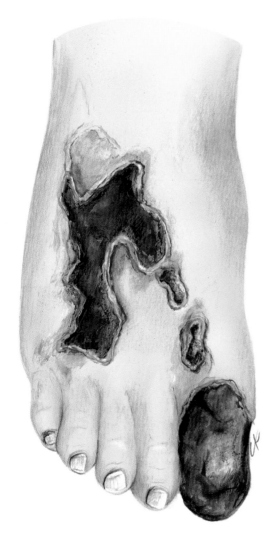

Figure 2

Necrotizing fasciitis on the dorsum of the foot

Indications for surgery

When faced with ulceration or infection in the diabetic foot, the first priority is to establish whether the etiology is neuropathic or ischemic. If it is ischemic, then consideration should be given to revascularization prior to debridement or any partial amputations. The rationale is that revascularization, if possible, will limit the extent of any subsequent amputation. However, this is not always possible, as the most important consideration is to control any acute infection and drain any abscesses. Sometimes a guillotine amputation will allow control of infection prior to revascularization and definitive amputation. The oxygen requirements of infected tissue are much higher than those of normal tissue; by controlling infection first, necrosis of flaps may be avoided. One of the advances in the management of the diabetic foot has been the development of distal revascularization techniques with anastomosis

to vessels at the level of the foot and ankle. Results with 56 vein grafts to the dorsalis pedis demonstrate a graft patency of 92% and limb salvage of 98% at 3 years [Tannenbaum et al. 1992].

Callosities on the plantar aspect of the foot are commonly found at sites of high plantar pressures. Preulcerative and ulcerated lesions are frequently seen underneath these areas, and removing the callosity may lead to a significant reduction in plantar pressure [Young et al. 1992]. These callosities can often be pared down in outpatients.

Uncomplicated neuropathic ulceration without evidence of deep infection, i.e. abscess formation or osteomyelitis, does not require surgery, as the ulceration will heal if high pressures are relieved, e.g. in a total contact cast. In the authors' experience uncomplicated ulceration does not require antibiotics, although wound swabs will reveal a polymicrobial culture [Laing et al. 1992].

Abscesses require prompt drainage, and osteomyelitis usually requires removal of the infected bone to achieve healing. Broad-spectrum antibiotics such as co-amoxiclav (amoxicillin–potassium clavulanate, Augmentin®) are needed with aerobic and anaerobic cover. If a toe is involved in osteomyelitis then amputation of the whole toe is generally necessary. There may be some advantage in preserving a stump of proximal phalanx to discourage drift to the other toes. If a metatarsal head is infected then resection of the head will be necessary. If the adjacent proximal phalanx is also involved then a partial ray amputation may be preferable to avoid leaving a short, floppy toe. Extensive infection or gangrene may necessitate more proximal amputation (see Chapter 44). The level will depend on the amount of foot involved and the vascularity. The possible levels are transmetatarsal, Lisfranc, Chopart, Syme, below-knee and above-knee. Osteomyelitis of the heel is a difficult problem, but a partial calcanectomy may be possible through a Gaenslen's midline incision [Gaenslen 1931]. As the alternative is a below-knee amputation it should be considered if possible, as good results have been reported. Preoperative criteria for partial calcanectomy may be an ABI of over 0.45, a transcutaneous Po_2 over 28 mmHg, an albumin level over 30 g/l and a total lymphocyte count of over 1500/ml. Using these criteria, ten out of 12 patients healed and nine patients maintained their preoperative mobility [Smith et al. 1992].

In chronic foot problems the indication for surgery is recurrent ulceration in the presence of a fixed deformity which cannot be controlled by footwear and insoles. Surgery will usually be in the nature of an exostectomy, but sometimes a resection type of forefoot arthroplasty may be necessary. A chronic heel ulcer may also be dealt with by partial or complete calcanectomy.

Treatment

Surgical technique

The patient is positioned supine, except in the case of osteomyelitis of the calcaneus, when a prone position is used. It is often unnecessary to use general anesthesia as most procedures can be carried out either under regional anesthetic blockade or spinal anesthesia. The neuropathic patient may need little or no anesthesia if the neuropathy is dense.

Amputation of toe or ray

A 'racket' incision is used, with extension of the racket dorsally if a ray amputation is being performed (Figure 3). This will ensure that the plantar skin is preserved for weightbearing without scarring. Frequently a partial ray amputation is adequate, with resection of the metatarsal at midshaft level. If this is done, then it is important to bevel the metatarsal on the plantar surface (Figure 3). One or two loose, deep sutures may be placed to shape the wound, but these wounds should not be closed primarily as this usually invites infection. The wound may be packed with an alginate dressing, such as Kaltostat. Postoperatively the patient can be managed in a total contact cast, if there is any plantar wound, or in a postoperative shoe until the wound is healed. It is then imperative that the patient wear a bespoke shoe with a custom-made insole to protect the foot from further ulceration.

Debridement for necrotizing fasciitis

Debridement is standard surgery but it must be aggressive and thorough. Inadequate resection of devitalized tissue in an effort to retain function is a mistake. Once this is done there may be exposed tendons on the dorsum of the foot. It is important to keep these moist and obtain early soft-tissue cover as the tendons will otherwise necrose. Split skin grafts may be used on the dorsum of the foot, but on the weightbearing plantar areas these will tend to break down. Subatmospheric pressure techniques (vacuum-assisted wound closure) may provide a solution in helping to close these difficult wounds. In a randomized study, satisfactory healing of postoperative foot wounds was achieved quicker with

this technique than with standard saline-moistened gauze [McCallon et al. 2000] (Figure 4).

Partial or complete calcanectomy

The objective in osteomyelitis and chronic ulceration of the calcaneus is to remove the infected bone as demarcated on plain radiographs, bone scan or MRI. The operation is best performed with the patient positioned prone under general anesthesia. A midline heel-splitting incision is used to expose the whole of the undersurface of the calcaneus and provides excellent, wide exposure of the calcaneus (Figure 5) [Gaenslen 1931]. If an ulcer is present the margins are excised. All the infected bone is removed until bleeding healthy bone is revealed (Figure 5). Originally, only the cancellous bone was removed, but it is usually necessary to remove axial slices of the calcaneus roughly parallel to the posterior subtalar joint. In so doing it may be necessary to sacrifice the attachment of the Achilles tendon and allow it to retract proximally. This area may be necrotic. Once the infected dead bone has been resected or, in the case of chronic ulceration, sufficient bone has been removed to allow the soft tissues to come together, then, if there is no osteomyelitis, the wound may be closed, or left partially open. A plaster of Paris backslab is applied to keep the foot in some equinus to relieve tension, and the patient is kept from weightbearing until the wound is soundly healed. A custom-made, solid ankle–foot orthosis is necessary once the patient starts walking again. Despite Achilles tendon release, most patients are able to perform a heel raise, presumably using the tibialis posterior. Occasionally, complete excision of the calcaneus may be necessary and the patient will require an ankle–foot orthosis permanently after this has been done.

Amputations

Both Lisfranc's and Chopart's amputations have fallen into disuse because of the tendency of the foot to fall into an equinovarus position (see Chapter 44). This occurs because of the pull of the more powerful tibialis posterior and Achilles tendons. The equinovarus deformity can be avoided if the foot is 'balanced' at the time of surgery by suturing the long extensors and peroneus brevis laterally. An advantage of a Lisfranc's amputation is that the patient can wear a normal boot or slightly oversized shoe. A Syme's amputation requires a prosthesis virtually as large as for a below-knee amputation, but does give an end-bearing stump and requires less energy consumption.

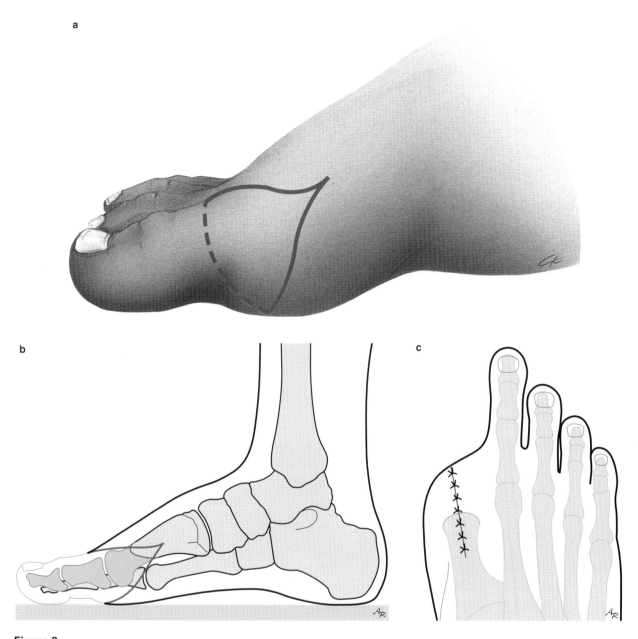

Figure 3

Ray amputation. a. skin incision; b. the plantar aspect of the resection surface is beveled (medial aspect); c. following skin closure (superior aspect)

Charcot foot

Neuroarthropathy or Charcot foot is a non-infective, destructive lesion of a bone or joint occurring in patients with peripheral neuropathy, most commonly due to diabetes. It affects fewer than 1% of patients and occurs most commonly in the fifth and sixth decades. It is a chronic, painless degenerative process that progresses through three stages [Eichenholtz 1966]. Stage I is characterized by acute inflammation, hyperemia and swelling. During this stage spontaneous fractures and dislocations with bone fragmentation are common. In stage II the swelling and erythema start to settle and radiological evidence of new bone formation is seen. In stage III bony consolidation and healing occur. By this stage the Charcot's foot may have become markedly misshapen, with either a rocker-bottom or a banana-shaped deformity. The acute stage I Charcot's foot may be mistaken for osteomyelitis or septic arthritis, which can lead to inappropriate surgery or amputation. The etiology is unknown, although both neurovascular and neurotraumatic theories have been advanced. Neuropathy is always

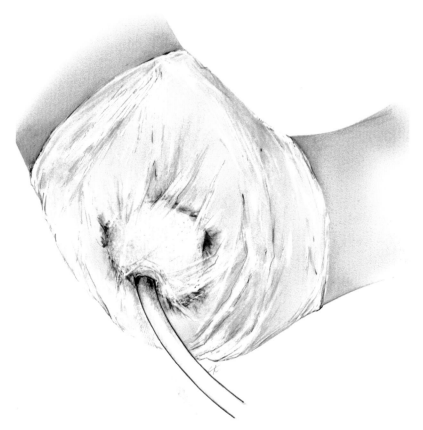

Figure 4

Vacuum-assisted wound closure device in place

a

b

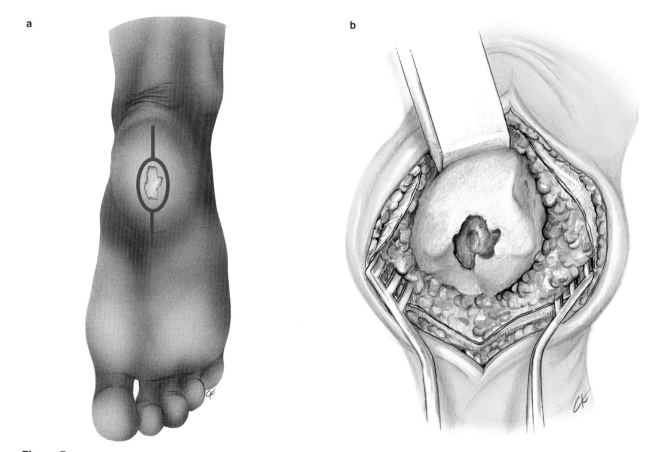

Figure 5

Partial or complete calcanectomy. a. midline heel incision; b. intraoperative aspect

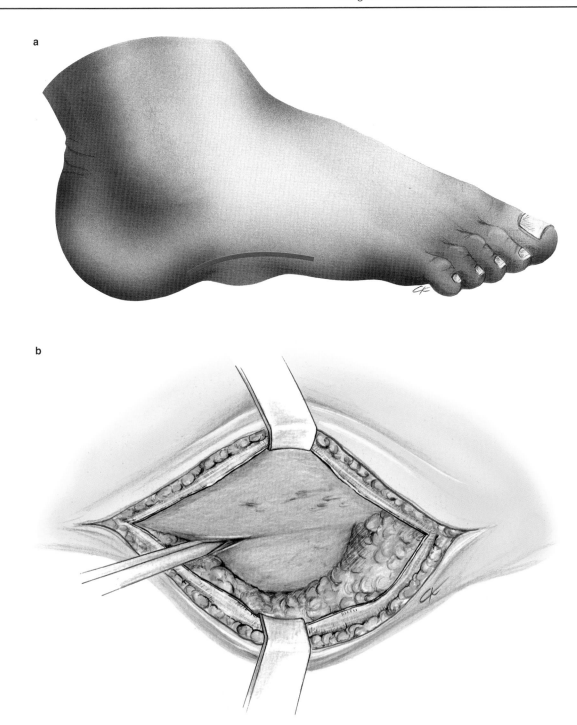

Figure 6

Exostectomy in Charcot's foot deformity. a. skin incision; b. intraoperative aspect

present, and although there may be some pain in stage I this is not in proportion to the changes seen on radiographs. The midtarsal joints are most commonly affected, in approximately 60% of cases. A good blood supply is essential as Charcot's foot is not seen with ischemia but has been reported in revascularized feet. The three stages run their course over a period of 2–3 years and the patient is then left with a painless, deformed foot that is prone to ulceration because of pressure over bony prominences. It is important to try to maintain the shape of the foot during stage I while the bone is soft, as the final aim is a plantigrade foot. A total-contact cast is effective for this but may need to be worn for 6–9 months, and it is important that the patient understands the need for this. Despite a plaster cast the deformity may progress. Surgical intervention should normally be avoided during stages I and II, as attempted bony fusions or reductions are likely to fall apart with bony fragmentation. The only possible exception to this may be the acute, unstable but manually reducible fracture–dislocation, if diagnosed before bony fragmentation or periosteal new bone formation is apparent on radiographs. In these circumstances it is possible to obtain an adequate purchase in bone and achieve stabilization [Myerson et al. 1994]. This is not recommended surgery for those inexperienced in the management of the diabetic foot. In stage III Charcot's foot most patients can be treated with bespoke shoes and insoles. Plantar deformities causing recurrent ulceration may be treated by simple exostectomy (Figure 6). An unstable hindfoot which it is not possible to brace may require stabilization by arthrodesis. Although it is possible to achieve arthrodesis with screw fixation, an intramedullary nail introduced through the calcaneus, subtalar and ankle joints is an effective means of stabilization. Surgical reconstruction of the midfoot to achieve a plantigrade braceable foot can be achieved with joint decompression and arthrodesis, but meticulous care and attention to detail is required. Surgical reconstruction may avoid the need for a below-knee amputation [Sammarco and Conti 1998].

Exostectomy of rocker-bottom foot

If localized skin pressure beneath a bony prominence with a sharp point cannot be relieved by orthoses and suitable shoes it may be necessary to remove the point. In the neuropathic foot anesthesia may not be necessary. After elevation to allow exsanguination, an ankle tourniquet is applied. An incision is made parallel to either the medial or the lateral border of the foot (see Figure 6). A full-thickness skin flap is raised. The bony projection is cleared of all soft tissue. As much as possible of the projection is excised using an osteotome and the bone is reduced to a concavity with a bone nibbler (see Figure 6). A coexisting contracture of the Achilles tendon may be lengthened percutaneously to reduce the forefoot pressure if equinus is present. The wound is closed with loose, widely spaced skin sutures. For the first 2 weeks the patient is mobilized without weightbearing on crutches. The foot is then protected in bespoke shoes and insoles.

Ankle fractures

Diabetic patients with peripheral neuropathy require special consideration if they sustain an ankle fracture. The same orthopedic principles are applied as for non-diabetic patients, except that a higher complication rate is expected and a prolonged period in a non-weightbearing cast is used. Usually this is double the time for a non-diabetic patient, which may be up to 3 months. A weightbearing cast is then used for up to 4–5 months to prevent the late development of a Charcot joint. If features of a Charcot foot in Eichenholtz stage 1 exist acutely with the fracture, then treatment with a total contact cast is indicated.

References

Apelquist J, Castenfors J, Larsson J (1989) Prognostic value of systolic ankle and toe blood pressure levels in outcome of diabetic foot ulcer. Diabetes Care 12: 373–378

Bell-Krotoski J, Tomancik E (1987) The repeatability of testing with Semmes–Weinstein monofilaments. J Hand Surg 12A: 155–161

Birke JA, Sims DS (1986) Plantar sensory threshold in the ulcerative foot. Lepr Rev 57: 61–67

Crerand S, Dolan M, Laing P et al. (1996) Diagnosis of osteomyelitis in neuropathic foot ulcers. J Bone Joint Surg 78B: 51–55

Diabetes Control and Complications Trial Research Group (1993) The effect of intensive treatment of diabetes on the development and progression of long-term complication in insulin-dependent diabetes mellitus. N Engl J Med 329: 977–986

Eichenholtz SN (1966) Charcot Joints. Springfield, Thomas

Gaenslen FJ (1931) Split-heel approach in osteomyelitis of the os calcis. J Bone Joint Surg 13: 759–772

Jeffrey J, Kennedy EJ, Shereff M et al. (1996) Prospective study of bone, indium-111-labelled white blood cell, and gallium-67 scanning for the evaluation of osteomyelitis in the diabetic foot. Foot Ankle Int 17: 10–16

Klenerman L, McCabe C, Cogley D et al. (1996) Screening for patients at risk of diabetic foot ulceration in a general diabetic outpatient clinic. Diabetic Med 13: 561–563

Laing P, Cogley D, Klenerman L (1992) Neuropathic foot ulceration treated by total contact casts. J Bone Joint Surg 74B: 133–136

McCallon SK, Knight CA, Valiulus JP et al. (2000) Osteotomy Wound Manage 46: 28–34

Myerson MS, Henderson MR, Saxby T, Short KW (1994) Management of midfoot diabetic neuroarthropathy. Foot Ankle Int 15: 233–241

Sammarco GJ, Conti SF (1998) Surgical treatment of neuroarthropathic foot deformity. Foot Ankle Int 19: 102–109

Smith DG, Stuck RM, Ketner L et al. (1992) Partial calcanectomy for the treatment of large ulcerations of the heel and calcaneal osteomyelitis. J Bone Joint Surg 74A: 571–576

Tannenbaum G, Pompposelli GB, Maraccio EJ (1992) Safety of vein bypass grafting to the dorsal pedal artery in diabetic patients with foot infection. J Vasc Surg 15: 982–990

Waters R, Perry J, Antonelli D, Hislop H (1976) Energy cost of walking on amputees. The influence of the level of amputation. J Bone Joint Surg Am 56A: 42–46

Young MJ, Cavanagh PR, Thomas G et al. (1992) The effect of callus removal on dynamic plantar foot pressure in diabetic patients. Diabetic Med 9: 55–57

46

Amputations John Angel

Introduction

The most common conditions leading to amputation in the foot or at the ankle are trauma and diabetes mellitus. In the early stages after a severe injury an amputation may be needed as a means of wound closure, or at a later stage it may be used to remove gangrenous tissue once it is demarcated, as may occur following a crush injury or cold damage. In diabetes the involvement of the distal vascular tree hastens the appearance of localized gangrene but makes digital and transmetatarsal amputations possible; this is rarely the case in arteriosclerosis uncomplicated by diabetes. Infections induced by diabetic neuropathy in the absence of ischemia can usually be controlled, at least initially, by means other than amputation. Occasionally amputations are required for congenital problems and tumors.

Compared with the results of amputation in the rest of the lower limb, those in the foot are often disappointing because of either delayed healing or difficulties in rehabilitation. It is important to select a level of amputation that produces not only *viable skin flaps* but a foot that is *plantigrade* and free from areas of high plantar *pressure* and, more importantly, excessive *shear*. The weight of the body must be carried on plantar skin with adequate sensibility. The only amputation level where load-bearing is tolerated by anesthetic skin is the Syme amputation (see Figure 6) or its variants, where shear forces can be eliminated by good prosthetic fitting.

Assessment and preparation

The amputation level is largely dependent on the extent of the pathological process. However, there are other factors to be borne in mind. Syme's amputation produces a stump that is unacceptable to most women because of the bulky shape of the prosthesis, the transtibial level being preferable. A fixed joint deformity or unbalanced paralysis may also force a higher amputation level than would otherwise be the case. Often it is necessary to opt for amputations at indeterminate levels or using alternative flaps; this should not be a problem as long as the principles emphasized above are adhered to. Ray resections come into this category, as each one is tailor-made to suit the situation.

All amputations should be covered by prophylactic antibiotic therapy. This should guard against *Clostridium perfringens* infection as well as controlling any organisms isolated in the distal part of the limb. A combination of penicillin with a broader spectrum antibiotic is often suitable [Friis 1987]. Before embarking on an amputation some thought should be given to the disposal of the amputated part so that the relevant preparations can be made in good time. The side and digits are clearly marked with an indelible pen.

Foot amputations can be performed under local anesthetic block at the ankle or under general anesthesia. Amputation of the terminal segment of a lesser toe is best performed under ring block at the base of the toe. In all but the most ischemic cases a pneumatic tourniquet is helpful.

Treatment

Principles

With regard to the handling of the various tissues in the course of foot amputations there are a number of points common to all levels. The skin flaps should always be marked with a pen before the knife is applied to the skin. The soft tissues are generally cut in a raked fashion so that the scalpel meets the bone at the level of section or a little proximal to it. This

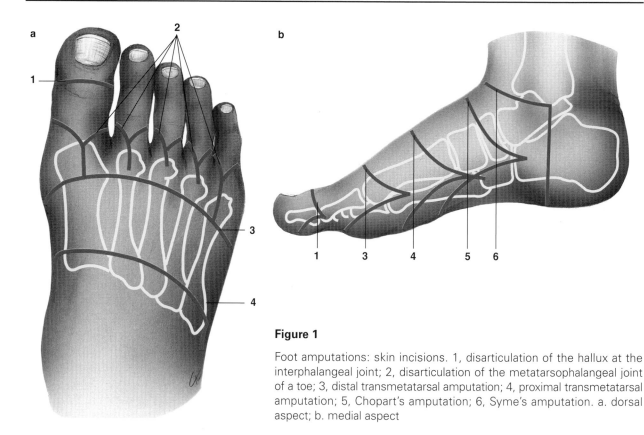

Figure 1

Foot amputations: skin incisions. 1, disarticulation of the hallux at the interphalangeal joint; 2, disarticulation of the metatarsophalangeal joint of a toe; 3, distal transmetatarsal amputation; 4, proximal transmetatarsal amputation; 5, Chopart's amputation; 6, Syme's amputation. a. dorsal aspect; b. medial aspect

allows the skin flaps to fall comfortably together. The fat loculi of the plantar skin should not be disrupted. Tendons not required for tenodesis are best pulled down and cut as high as possible. This applies particularly in diabetic patients, in whom connective tissue is particularly prone to slough in the presence of infection. Hemostasis can, on the whole, be secured by diathermy, but in the case of the dorsalis pedis and medial and lateral plantar vessels and the saphenous vein, absorbable transfixion ligatures are required. Nerves should be pulled down and cut high with scissors so that the retracting end forms a terminal neuroma within its fatty tunnel. Bones are best cut with an oscillating saw with the blade well cooled with saline. The deep fascia is closed with a 2–0 or 3–0 absorbable suture and either staples or interrupted nylon sutures are used for the skin. Where there has been heavy contamination the wound is either left unsutured or partially closed over a pack to allow delayed primary closure. The wound of the Syme amputation inevitably contains dead space, and suction drainage helps to minimize this. Drainage of amputations more distal to this level is generally not necessary.

Disarticulation of the hallux at the interphalangeal joint

Following the incision (Figure 1), the short dorsal flap is retracted and the extensor tendon divided to allow a knife to enter the interphalangeal joint and release the capsule circumferentially (Figure 2). The flexor tendon is divided and the plantar flap fashioned. At this point it may be desirable to reduce the bulk of the condyles of the proximal phalanx. The wound is closed with skin sutures alone. The stump of the toe is dressed with paraffin gauze, wool and crêpe. Restricted heel-walking is allowed later the same day. The sutures are removed at 10–15 days.

Partial lesser toe amputations

The lesser toes are particularly prone to deformity due to tendon imbalance, so that it is not recommended to amputate a toe between the levels of the distal interphalangeal and the metatarsophalangeal joints, at least not without specific measures to counteract the threatened deformity [Baumgartner 1988]. It is also easy to produce a troublesome bulbous end to a distal toe amputation. This is avoided by fashioning the plantar flap of good length but the width no greater than one-third of the circumference of the digit at that level and ruthlessly trimming redundant soft tissue and skin.

Disarticulation at the distal interphalangeal joint of a lesser toe is a simple and effective procedure for dealing with resistant, painful callus formation due to fixed mallet toe in the elderly. Ring block local anesthesia at the base of the toe and a rubber catheter tourniquet work well. The dorsal skin

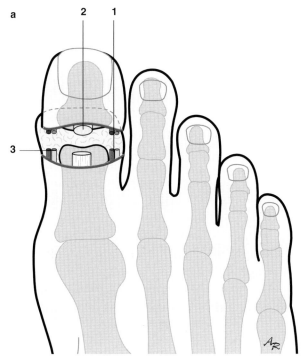

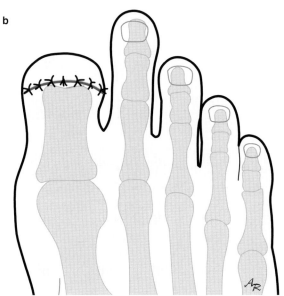

Figure 2

Disarticulation through the interphalangeal joint of the great toe. a. creation of a plantar skin flap; b. following closure

a
1   Lateral neurovascular bundle
2   Long extensor tendon
3   Medial neurovascular bundle

incision goes straight into the distal interphalangeal joint. The base of the long plantar flap takes up hardly more than one-third of the circumference of the digit. The flexor tendon is cut and the distal phalanx filleted from the plantar flap. The vascular bundle is cauterized and the digital nerve on its plantar aspect is pulled down and cut high. The wound is closed with four or five interrupted sutures.

Postoperatively heel-walking is allowed within a few hours, followed by a gradual return to normal activities over 1–2 weeks. The sutures are removed at 10–15 days.

Disarticulation of the metatarsophalangeal joint of a toe

The operation is most commonly performed to deal with gangrene but it is contraindicated if the process has spread to involve the root of the toe. In the case of the hallux there may be an advantage in preserving the base of the proximal phalanx in order to retain the attachment of the sesamoids [Ademoglu et al. 2000]. It is conducted in the supine position under infiltration local anesthesia with the foot end of the table elevated.

A racket incision that encircles the toe is used (Figure 1). At the sides, the incision passes 3 or 4 mm distal to the base of the toe to form flaps that fall together. The handle of the 'racket' is used to gain access to the metatarsophalangeal joint, which is disarticulated after the extensor tendon is sectioned (Figure 3). The remaining soft tissues are divided and the vessels cauterized. If conditions allow, the skin is closed with three or four interrupted monofilament sutures. Where the wound has to be left open because of the degree of contamination, it often heals just as rapidly and with a linear scar. Postoperatively the wound is dressed with gauze or non-adherent dressing and a pressure bandage. Heel-walking is allowed later the same day. The sutures are removed at 10–14 days.

Ray amputation

This may be required in circumstances where there is insufficient skin to close a digital amputation. It is most commonly undertaken on the first and fifth rays but can be performed successfully on one or possibly two of the central three rays. The results of this type of surgery have on the whole been disappointing [Gianfortune et al. 1985], although once healing has been achieved they are as favorable as other foot amputations [Santi et al. 1993]. It is particularly worth considering when used in conjunction with successful reconstructive vascular surgery [Chang et al. 1995].

The digit is removed using a circumferential, wedge-shaped skin incision (Figure 4) which is extended through the deeper tissues to include the metatarsal head. Circumstances often dictate a rather ad hoc arrangement of the skin flaps. In diabetic patients it is recommended that the entire

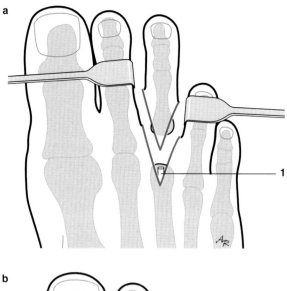

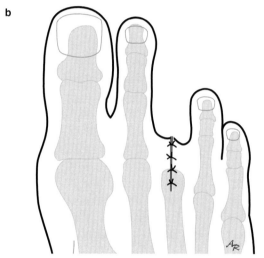

Figure 3

Amputation of lesser toe at metatarsophalangeal joint.
a. exposure of the metatarsophalangeal joint through a
racket incision; b. following closure

a

1 Extensor tendon

head should be removed using a powered instrument in order to reduce the risk of hypertrophic
bone formation [Armstrong et al. 1999a]. It is often
necessary to suture the wound loosely over a pack
with a view to delayed closure.

Transmetatarsal amputation

Transmetatarsal amputation has been used to treat
frostbite and the complications of diabetes mellitus
[McKittrick et al. 1949]. The line along which the
metatarsals are to be resected is marked on the
dorsum of the foot (see Figure 1). It is gently curv-
ing and oblique, sloping proximally towards the
head of the fifth metatarsal. It passes through the

proximal parts of the heads of the first and fifth
metatarsals and the necks of the middle three.
Amputation through the relatively avascular
metatarsal shafts should be avoided, especially in
the presence of infection, and if the more distal
level is not practicable then it is better to move
higher to the proximal ends of the metatarsals
[Baumgartner 1988]. The flaps are marked to allow
sufficient skin and soft tissue to cover the ends of the
bones, which usually means making the flaps longer
over the medial aspect where the bones are thicker.
The plantar flap will extend virtually to the root of the
toes. The short dorsal flap is fashioned (Figure 5),
with the extensor tendons pulled down and cut high.
The base of the plantar flap is closer to the sole of
the foot than the dorsum. The flap contains the fatty
loculi of the sole together with the plantar fascia and
the septa connecting it to the flexor tunnels. The tendons themselves and the muscles of the sole are cut
level with bone section. The metatarsals are cut with
a powered saw. They are trimmed at the plantar
aspect (Figure 5) and then smoothed with a rasp.
The tourniquet is released, hemostasis is secured
and the wound is closed.

Postoperatively the wound is covered with a single layer of gauze and a thick layer of plaster wool,
and the limb is immobilized in a below-knee cast.
This counteracts the tendency for chronic debility
and pain to lead to an equinus deformity of the
ankle. If this deformity is already present, Achilles
tenotomy, serial plasters or even an external fixator
may be required to correct it. The healed stump
is fitted with a toe filler attached to a sole plate
designed to cause the shoe to 'break' at the usual
place just behind the toe cap.

Chopart's amputation

Chopart's amputation is used mainly in trauma.
It is contraindicated in the presence of fixed deformity, tendon imbalance or peripheral neuropathy.
Lengthening of the Achilles tendon, subtalar arthrodesis and tenodesis should be used liberally in the
prevention of postoperative contractures [Christie
et al. 1980, Armstrong et al. 1999b].

The skin flaps are fashioned from two points
2 cm below and 2 cm in front of each malleolus
(see Figure 1). They must be long enough to cover
the posterior components of the midtarsal joint
together with the rather stiff, thick subcutaneous
tissue of the sole. The tibialis anterior tendon is
traced distally and cut close to its insertion. Raking
incisions are made down to the midtarsal joint,

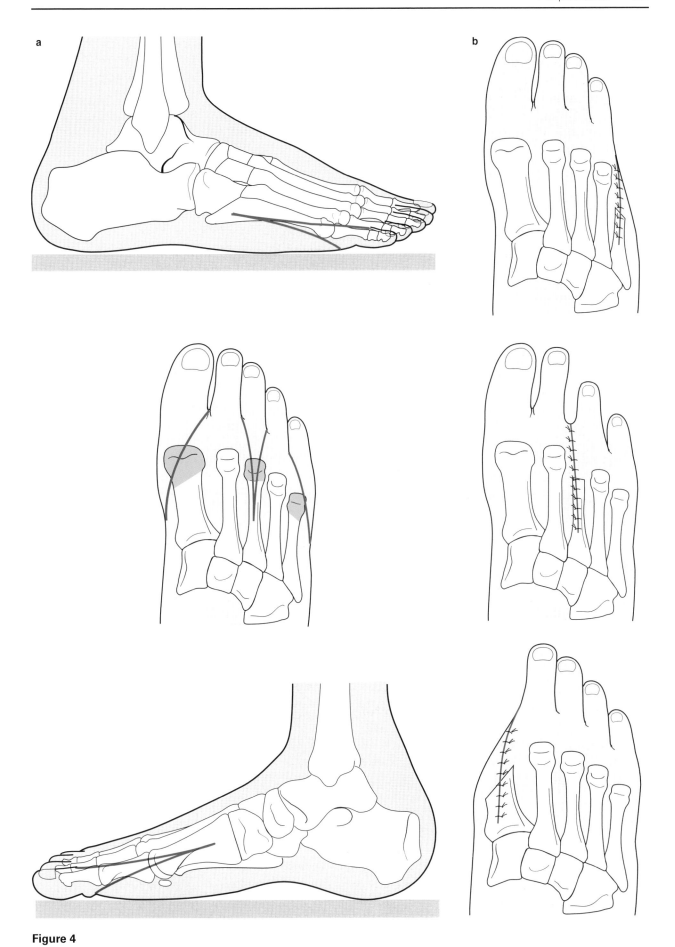

Figure 4

a. Examples of incisions used in ray resection; b. examples of ray resections

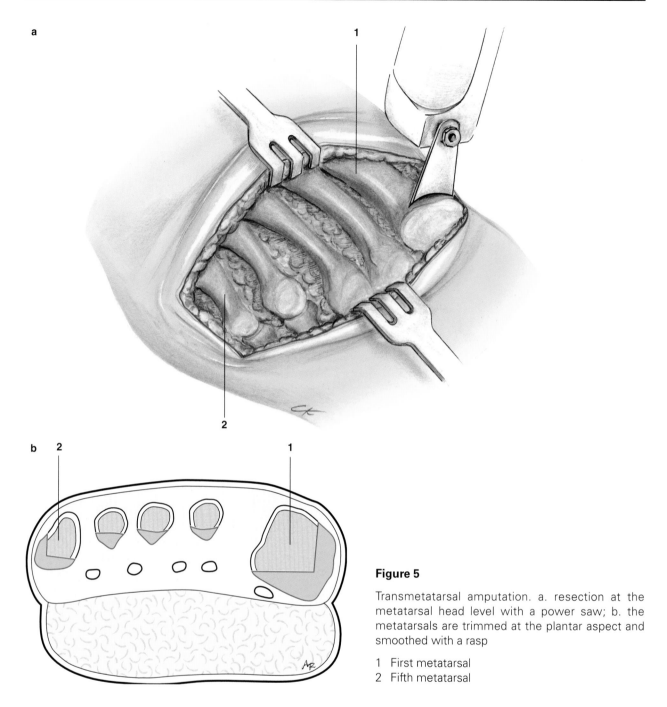

Figure 5

Transmetatarsal amputation. a. resection at the metatarsal head level with a power saw; b. the metatarsals are trimmed at the plantar aspect and smoothed with a rasp

1   First metatarsal
2   Fifth metatarsal

cutting through all the soft tissues. The joint is disarticulated (Figure 6). The tourniquet is released, hemostasis is secured and the named nerves are sought, pulled down and cut high. The tibialis anterior tendon is then attached to the head of the talus under slight tension using either a staple or a drill hole. Where there is contamination it is better to stitch the tendon to the plantar fascia while closing the wound. If the tibialis anterior tendon is not viable, percutaneous Achilles tenotomy should be performed. The plantar fascia is stitched to the extensor retinaculum using 2–0 absorbable sutures and the skin is closed with staples. A rigid plaster

dressing is applied to protect the tenodesis and maintain slight dorsiflexion of the ankle.

Postoperatively, ambulation with full weight-bearing is allowed once the wound has healed. The tenodesis needs to be protected with a cast for 5 weeks. This level of amputation requires an artificial foot and hence the attention of a prosthetist rather than an orthotist. There are a variety of prostheses available. Those that encroach only up to the level of the ankle have good cosmesis but produce an awkward gait with no 'push-off'. For a normal gait it is necessary to fit a rigid limb extending up to the tibial tubercle.

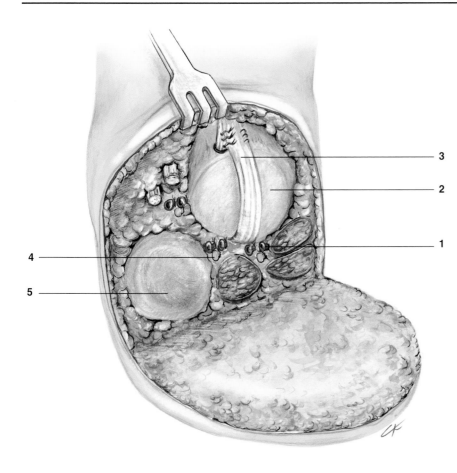

Figure 6

Chopart's amputation. The tibialis anterior tendon is attached to the head of the talus under slight tension

1   Medial plantar vessels
2   Talus
3   Tibialis anterior tendon
4   Lateral plantar vessels
5   Calcaneus

Syme's amputation

The Syme amputation, essentially an ankle disarticulation utilizing the heel pad to cover the distal end of the tibia, produces a particularly robust stump [Harris 1956, Gaine and McCreath 1996]. If the heel is ulcerated an anterior flap can be used [Robinson 1999, Atesalp et al. 2000]. With adequate prosthetic care it can provide good function, even if completely anesthetic, and so it is used in peripheral neuropathy and trauma. Its value in the management of congenital deformity has also been confirmed [Naudie et al. 1997, Birch et al. 1999, McCarthy et al. 2000].

The flaps are marked from the tips of the malleoli (see Figure 1 and Figure 7). The anterior incision takes the shortest route across the front of the ankle. The plantar incision drops on each side perpendicularly to the sole of the foot with a slightly oblique interconnecting section beneath the heel pad. The plantar incision is deepened in a raking cut to meet the bone, dividing on the way all the vessels and tendons. In the course of making the dorsal incision the extensor tendons are pulled down and cut high, and then severed distally to prevent their distal ends from obstructing the view of

the wound. The ligaments of the ankle are divided and the talus is drawn forward with the aid of a sharp hook inserted into its dome. The periosteum is stripped from the back of the talus and then from the os calcis. Once the back of the os calcis is reached it is possible to transfer the hook into that bone. In order to free the rest of the back of the os calcis it is necessary to free the sides of the bone and also its inferior surface. By working round and round the bone the final posteroinferior angle will be cleared and the foot can be discarded, leaving an empty heel pad. The distal end of the tibia is supported on a receiver, allowing the heel pad to hang free. Clamps are applied to the remaining tendons which are used to retract the soft tissues from the distal end of the tibia. The malleoli are removed with a saw. The plane of the cut must be at right angles to the long axis of the tibia and the level such as barely to clear the subchondral bone of the tibial plafond. Any higher and the cross-sectional area of the tibia is likely to be reduced, with an adverse effect on eventual load-bearing. The tendons are trimmed. The medial and lateral plantar vascular bundles are ligated and the related nerves are pulled down and cut high. The anterior tibial neurovascular bundle is

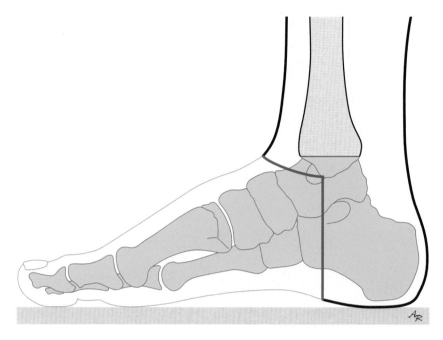

Figure 7

Syme's amputation

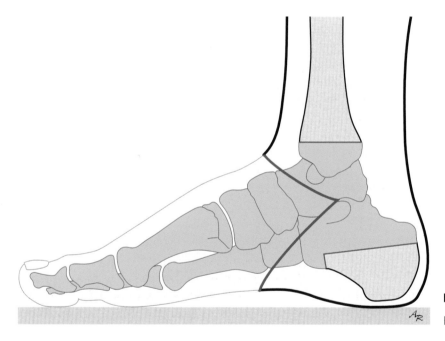

Figure 8

Boyd's amputation

similarly treated. The wound is cleared of poorly vascularized soft-tissue tags. The extensor digitorum brevis is preserved in order to fill some of the dead space of the heel pad. The tourniquet is released and hemostasis secured. A suction drain is inserted up behind the inferior tibiofibular ligament and passed laterally and proximally out through the skin. The plantar fascia is sutured to the extensor retinaculum and the skin is closed with staples. A plaster cast is applied and moulded to centralize the heel pad which at this stage is vulnerable to displacement.

Postoperatively, the drain is removed at 2 days and the plaster is changed at 5 days to allow the wound to be inspected. At 3 weeks the sutures are removed and a fiberglass cast is applied and fitted with a rocker to allow weightbearing. Postoperative swelling and calf atrophy usually delay the definitive prosthetic fitting for some 3 months.

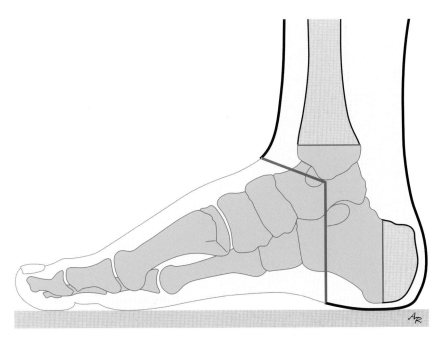

Figure 9

Pirogoff's amputation

Boyd and Pirogoff amputations

These alternatives to Syme's amputation have a role in certain situations. For example, the Boyd amputation (Figure 8) is marginally more durable than the Syme procedure and might be preferred when the heel pad has less than optimal sensibility. It should also be used where the distal end of the tibia is atrophic or has been badly damaged. It has been shown to be superior to the Syme amputation for longitudinal deficiency of the fibula [Felp et al. 1996]. Its main disadvantages are the extra length, which may compromise the height and function of the artificial foot, and its unsuitability for infected cases.

Although it is necessary to fashion skin flaps significantly longer than for the Syme level, the first part of the dissection proceeds similarly, with a disarticulation of the ankle and a dissection of the soft tissues off the upper part of the calcaneus. The calcaneocuboid and subtalar joints are then disarticulated, allowing the main part of the foot to be removed. Using a sagittal saw the tibia is trimmed at the same level as for the Syme procedure, immediately proximal to the subchondral bone, and the upper half of the calcaneus is removed. The calcaneus is fixed to the tibia by means of a wire mattress suture, a screw or a Charnley clamp.

The Pirogoff amputation (Figure 9) is generally less satisfactory than the Boyd procedure because of the thinner heel pad. In practice a compromise is often necessary, producing a stump that is somewhere between the two. The technique is similar to that used in Boyd's amputation, except that greater stripping of the calcaneum is required and the bone is cut vertically. An interesting modification of the Boyd amputation which does not require a prosthesis has been described [Kornah 1996].

References

Ademoglu Y, Ada S, Kaplan I (2000) Should the amputations of the great toe be replanted? Foot Ankle Int 21: 673–679

Armstrong DG, Hadi S, Nguyen HC, Harkles LB (1999a) Factors related to bone regrowth following diabetes-related partial amputation of the foot. J Bone Joint Surg 81A: 1561–1565

Armstrong DG, Stachpoole-Shea SB, Nguyen H, Harkles LB (1999b) Lengthening of the Achilles tendon in diabetic patients who are at high risk for ulceration of the foot. J Bone Joint Surg 81A: 535–538

Atesalp S, Yildiz C, Robinson KP (2000) Disarticulation at the ankle using an anterior flap. J Bone Joint Surg 82B: 462

Baumgartner RF (1988) Partial foot amputations: aetiology, principles, operative techniques. In: Murdoch G (ed) Amputation Surgery and Lower Limb Prosthetics. Oxford, Blackwell, pp 97–104

Birch JG, Walsh SJ, Small JM et al. (1999) Syme amputation for the treatment of fibular deficiency. An evaluation of long-term physical and psychological functional status. J Bone Joint Surg 81A: 1511–1518

Chang BB, Jacobs RL, Darling RC 3rd et al. (1995) Foot amputations. Surg Clin North Am 75: 773–782

Christie J, Cloughs CB, Lamb DW (1980) Amputations through the middle part of the foot. J Bone Joint Surg 62B: 473–474

Felp T, Davids JR, Leslie CM, Blackhurst DW (1996) Longitudinal deficiency of the fibula. J Bone Joint Surg 78A: 674–682

Friis H (1987) Penicillin G versus cefuroxime for prophylaxis in lower limb amputations. Acta Orthop Scand 58: 666–668

Gaine WJ, McCreath SW (1996) Syme's amputation revisited: a review of 46 cases. J Bone Joint Surg 78B: 461–467

Gianfortune P, Pulla RJ, Sage R et al. (1985) Ray resections in the insensitive or dysvascular foot: a critical review. J Foot Surg 24: 103–107

Harris RI (1956) Syme's amputation: the technical details essential for success. J Bone Joint Surg 38B: 614–632

Kornah B (1996) Modified Boyd amputation. J Bone Joint Surg 78B: 149–150

McCarthy JJ, Glancy GL, Chang FM, Eilert RE (2000) Fibular hemimelia: comparison of outcome measurements after amputation and lengthening. J Bone Joint Surg 82A: 1732–1735

McKittrick LS, McKittrick JB, Risley TS (1949) Transmetatarsal amputation for infection or gangrene in patients with diabetes mellitus. Ann Surg 130: 826–842

Naudie D, Hamdy RC, Fassier F et al. (1997) Management of fibular hemimelia. J Bone Joint Surg 79B: 1040–1041

Robinson KP (1999) Disarticulation to the ankle using an anterior flap. J Bone Joint Surg 81B: 617–620

Santi MD, Thoma BJ, Chambers RB (1993) Survivorship of healed partial foot amputations in dysvascular patients. Clin Orthop 292: 245–249

47

Surgical considerations for tumors

Stephen Parsons

Introduction

Patients complaining of localized prominences, swellings or tumors present frequently to specialists dealing with foot and ankle complaints. Most of these swellings are benign, but primary and secondary malignancies do occur. An accurate diagnosis is obtained through recording a careful history, performing a thorough examination and undertaking the appropriate investigations. The management, whether conservative or surgical, depends on that diagnosis, the size, the site and the effect of the lesion on foot function.

There is a wide variation in the characteristics of tumors or tumor-like swellings in the foot and ankle (Table 1). Congenital abnormalities include duplications, hemangiomas, hematomas and arteriovenous fistulae; trauma gives rise to neuromas, inclusion dermoids, deep-seated foreign bodies, displaced fractures, callus formation and Charcot's disease. Ganglia, mucous cysts and osteophytes are found in degenerative processes. Other miscellaneous lesions include epidermal cysts, granuloma annulare, fibromatosis, skeletal chondromas, simple and aneurysmal bone cysts and fibrodysplasia.

Benign neoplasic lesions can be staged surgically into three groups [Enneking et al. 1980, Wolfe and Enneking 1996] (Table 2). Latent tumors are intracapsular or surrounded by mature bone, do not change in size, may be asymptomatic and may spontaneously resolve. Active lesions are intracapsular, or bony lesions which expand and are surrounded by reactive bone, but barriers are not breached. Fractures can occur but spontaneous resolution is

Table 1 Tumor characteristics

Type
Congenital
Traumatic
Degenerative
Miscellaneous
Neoplastic

Tissue of origin
Skin
Fat
Fibrous tissue
Muscle
Blood vessels
Nerve
Synovium
Cartilage
Bone
Uncertain

Behavior
Benign
Low-grade malignancy
High-grade malignancy

Site
Superficial soft tissues
Weightbearing areas
Deep soft tissues
Forefoot skeletal
Hindfoot skeletal

uncommon. Aggressive tumors, although benign, cross compartmental barriers.

Primary malignancies are rare [Murari et al. 1989] and are staged by histological features (i.e. low or high grade), the presence or absence of metastases,

Table 2   Surgical staging [Enneking et al. 1980]

Benign
I   Latent
II   Active
III Aggressive

Malignant
I   Low-grade, no metastasis
    A   Intracompartmental
    B   Extracompartmental
II   High-grade, no metastasis
    A   Intracompartmental
    B   Extracompartmental
III Low- and high-grade, with metastasis
    A   Intracompartmental
    B   Extracompartmental

and by intra- or extracompartmental location [Enneking et al. 1980, Enneking 1986, Wolfe and Enneking 1996] (Table 2). As an example, stage I sarcomas are histologically low-grade with a pseudocapsule, are slowly invasive, are restricted by anatomical barriers and rarely metastasize. Radiological features are active but not aggressive.

Stage II sarcomas are histologically high-grade with little or no pseudocapsule, are destructive, are rapidly growing, are invasive and are not restrained by natural barriers or compartments. Skip lesions and metastases are common and early. Stage III sarcomas are either low- or high-grade with metastases.

A tumor or tumor-like lesion can arise from any tissue, and this tissue, e.g. skin or bone, determines the type, site and subsequent behavior of the tumor. The granular cell tumor, malignant fibrous histiocytoma and epithelioid sarcoma are of uncertain origin.

The surgical treatment will depend on staging and symptoms. If a lesion is benign but increasing in size and giving functional problems, excision is indicated with a warning of potential recurrence. Malignancies, depending on grade, will need wide or radical excision. The site also influences the surgical technique. Smaller lesions on the dorsum of the foot may be removed by marginal excision and primary closure. Larger lesions on the sole of the foot may require rotation or free vascularized flaps. Bony lesions in the forefoot requiring wide excision are simply treated, but in the hindfoot complex fusions may be required.

Preoperative assessment

A careful history records the start of swelling, alteration in appearance or size, symptoms, disability,

associated lesions and medical history. Examination includes the position, mobility, shape, consistency and surface of the lesion and its effect on the local anatomy and foot function. Weightbearing dorsoplantar, lateral and oblique radiographs show expansion, cavitation, destruction, erosion, calcification and size. Real-time ultrasonography is useful to evaluate soft-tissue swelling. Technetium bone scanning demonstrates local bone activity [Williams et al. 1991] and metastatic disease. Spiral computed tomography (CT) scanning provides multiplanar imaging of the shape, size and constitution of lesions in bone and soft tissue. Linear tomography is useful if CT is not available. Magnetic resonance imaging (MRI) is highly effective for soft-tissue lesions [Crim et al. 1992], complementing CT for bony or soft-tissue lesions and marrow spread, so that knowledge of size, position, extent and relationship to normal tissues allows accurate surgical planning.

High-resolution Doppler ultrasound scanning is useful for hemangiomas, arteriovenous fistulae and vascular tumors, while angiography gives greater detail and permits embolization. General investigations are needed for preoperative assessment of malignant disease, e.g. serological analysis of bone and liver activity, a chest radiograph and CT, liver ultrasound and technetium bone scans.

Treatment

General surgical considerations

Surgery is undertaken under general or regional anesthesia. A tourniquet assists dissection but exsanguination should not be used for aggressive lesions. Draping must give access to all parts of the foot and ankle and the iliac crest if grafting is required. The surgical approach is determined by the position and size of the lesion and the proposed technique. Preoperative planning and incisions must minimize the risk to neurovascular bundles and cutaneous nerves. After removal of the tumor, the tourniquet is released to allow for hemostasis. Closed suction drainage reduces hematoma, and non-constricting dressings must be supportive, absorbent and applied to give soft tissue support. Elevation prevents postoperative swelling and hematoma.

After major resections and amputations, plaster slabs, casts or splints prevent deformity. Function can be enhanced by the use of insoles, shoe modifications, prostheses and physiotherapy.

Diagnostic surgical techniques

Large lesions should be biopsied prior to definitive surgery for diagnosis and grading [Simon 1982, Heare et al. 1989, Simon and Biermann 1993]. Percutaneous or needle biopsies can be performed under local anesthesia by palpation or guided by CT imaging, but only if an appropriate sample can be obtained. With this technique, minimal anatomical structures are compromised and the biopsy tract can be included in the definitive surgery. The alternative is an open incisional biopsy under general or local anesthesia. Incisions must not compromise the definitive surgery, and should reflect local anatomy and avoid weightbearing areas. The biopsy is removed through an adequate longitudinal incision with a minimum of soft-tissue dissection and undermining of the skin flaps. Closure is by subcuticular suture to avoid a wide suture track. Suction drainage is best avoided, but if there is a significant cavity the position of the drain must be in the line of the subsequent definitive surgery.

Therapeutic surgical techniques

Surgical excisions can be classified into four groups based on the margin of excision [Enneking et al. 1980].

Intralesional excision

Intralesional excision removes the tumor from within its pseudocapsule; this involves curettage, incisional biopsy or debulking. Tumor will inevitably be retained, so the technique is for lesions that do not recur or those that require adjuvant therapy. For example, in curettage and bone grafting the bony wall over the lesion is identified. Using drill holes linked by an osteotome a cortical window is reflected on a periosteal hinge (Figure 1). The contents are curetted and saved for histological examination. A burr is used to abrade the wall to a bleeding surface, cleaning all crevices. For more aggressive lesions, various forms of adjuvant therapy, e.g. acrylic cement [Persson and Wouters 1976], liquid nitrogen [Marcove et al. 1978] or phenol [McDonald et al. 1986] have been used. Autogenous bone can be harvested using a separate trolley of instruments. For larger volumes human allograft can be used. After morcellization the bone graft is packed into the cavity and the cortical window replaced or a corticocancellous graft fashioned to fit the defect. The soft tissues are closed in layers over a drain.

Marginal excision

The tumor is removed at the level of the pseudocapsule, but microscopic extensions of aggressive tumors may be retained. This technique is useful for stage I and II foot and ankle soft-tissue lesions (Figure 2). The resection is performed under general or regional anesthesia with a tourniquet. The incision depends upon the position of the neoplasm, and dissection is undertaken in a meticulous fashion, preserving, if possible, vital structures while ensuring complete removal. Closure is without tension, in layers with closed suction drainage. The wound is dressed, supported by wool and crêpe bandage or casting for extensive lesions.

Wide excision

Benign aggressive tumors and stage I low-grade malignancies require wide excision [Rydholm and Rööser 1987], i.e. the removal of all the tumor with a cuff of normal tissue, but skip lesions may be retained if the technique is used for a higher-grade tumor. In the forefoot, wide excision requires a ray amputation. In the midfoot and hindfoot the resection may result in loss of bone and joint. Arthrodesis is required to restore functional stability. The loss of skin may require plastic surgical reconstruction. When choosing wide excision or partial amputations, it is important to consider the best functional outcome. Resected low-grade tumors in the distal tibia can be replaced by arthrodesis [Tadross and Checketts 2000], block allograft arthrodeses [Mankin et al. 1996] or custom prostheses.

Radical excision

Radical excision is used for stage II high-grade malignancies and involves the en bloc removal of involved tumor, which in the foot means amputation, because the wide resection would result in considerable functional loss. The site, size and local condition of the tumor and the patient's general medical state dictate the level. For digits it is ray amputation, in the midfoot a Syme's amputation and in the hindfoot or ankle a below-knee amputation.

Surgery for specific tumors and tumor-like lesions

Skin tumors

Benign tumors constitute a heterogeneous group presenting to the surgeon or dermatologist (Table 3). Although the commonest malignant skin neoplasm

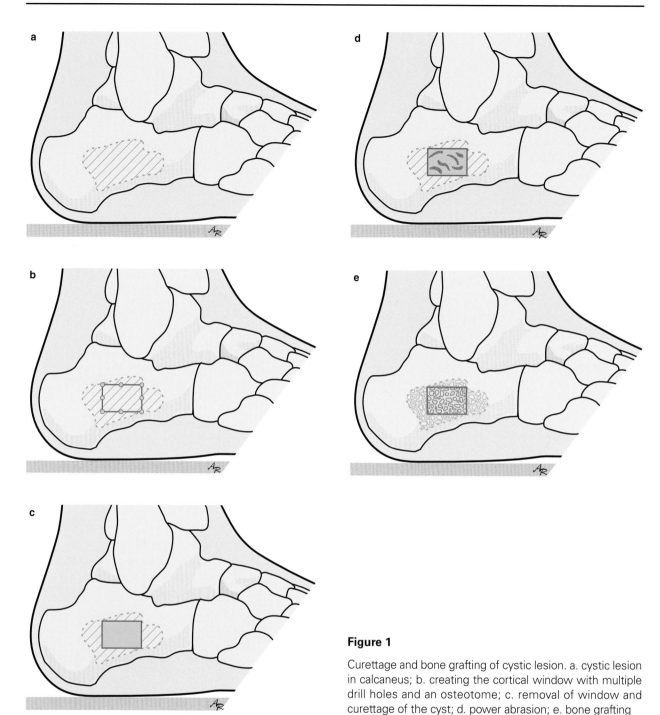

Figure 1

Curettage and bone grafting of cystic lesion. a. cystic lesion in calcaneus; b. creating the cortical window with multiple drill holes and an osteotome; c. removal of window and curettage of the cyst; d. power abrasion; e. bone grafting

is the basal cell carcinoma, only 2% occur on the legs [Kurzer and Patel 1979]. Those in the foot usually occur on the dorsum [Roenigk et al. 1986]. However, basal cell carcinoma of the sole has been reported [Robinson 1979]. Treatment is wide excision with split skin grafting. Squamous cell carcinoma arises in skin damaged by sun, hydro-carbon or radiation exposure, from scars, e.g. from burns, lupus vulgaris or in sinuses for osteomyelitis, or in the immunosuppressed patient; it can take the form of keratotic or fungating nodules or as ulcers. In situ squamous cell carcinoma, i.e. Bowen's disease,

appears as a red, scaly patch with slow growth before becoming a true squamous cell carcinoma. The diagnosis of subungual squamous cell carcinoma is often delayed; treatment is by toe amputation. On the sole, epithelioma cuniculatum or verrucous carcinoma can invade deep tissue, but rarely metastasizes. The treatment is by wide excision with split skin grafting.

The prevalence of melanoma is increasing. The median age at presentation is the early 40s [Smith 1979], and the 5-year survival is between 10 and 99% according to the histology and clinical stage [Vollmer 1989]. Early detection, diagnosis and

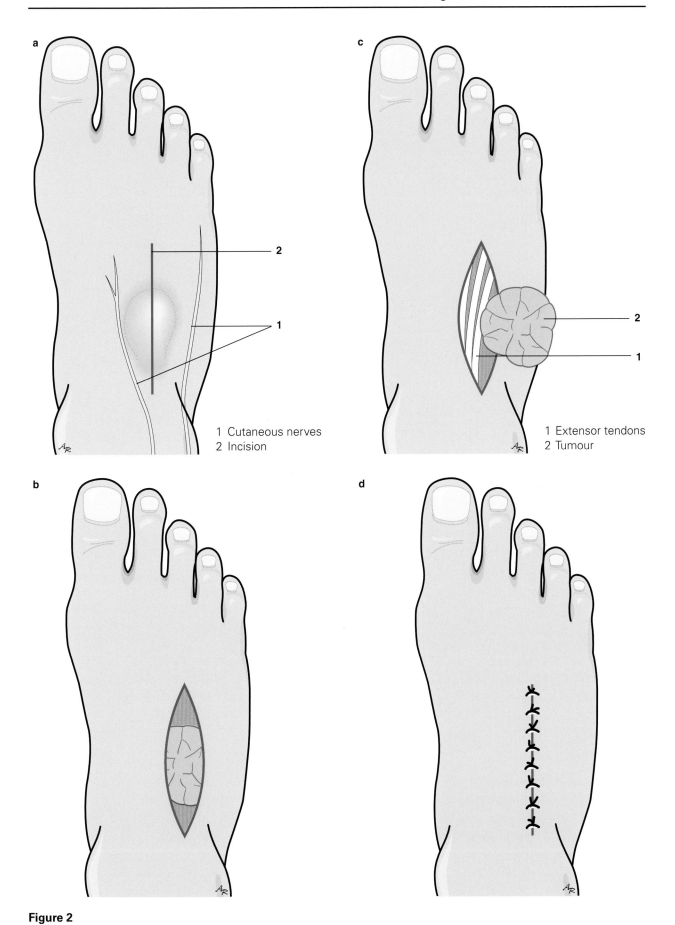

1 Cutaneous nerves
2 Incision

1 Extensor tendons
2 Tumour

Figure 2

Marginal excision of a soft-tissue tumor. a. incision; b. demonstration of the lesion; c. dissection and removal of the complete lesion; d. wound closure

Table 3   Skin tumors

Congenital
Hemangioma
Lymphangioma
Neurofibroma
Hamartoma

Traumatic
Inclusion dermoid cysts

Miscellaneous
Epidermal cysts
Granuloma annulare

Neoplastic
Benign

    Basal cell papilloma
    Benign fibrous histiocytoma
    Acquired digital fibrokeratoma
    Dermatofibroma
    Eccrine poroma
    Melanocytic nevi
    Pyogenic granuloma

Malignant

    Basal cell carcinoma
    Squamous carcinoma
    Malignant melanoma
    Kaposi's sarcoma
    Dermatofibrosarcoma protuberans
    Malignant eccrine poroma
    Neurofibrosarcoma

treatment [Friedman et al. 1991] have improved the overall 5-year survival rate to 80%. In the foot a melanoma is the most common malignant lesion; 1–9% of malignant melanomas occur on the sole, a quarter from a pre-existing nevus [Dwyer et al. 1993], but they also occur on the dorsum of the foot. There are three histological types. The superficial spreading melanoma has a 'buckshot' spread over the invasive component and is flat or pigmented black to blue or red. The acral lentiginous melanoma is plantar or subungual, spreading along the basal layer (i.e. lentiginous spread), starting as a flat, irregular brown or black lesion which becomes raised. The nodular melanoma invades into the dermis and is found as a brown, black or amelanotic nodule. Melanomas on the foot are detected late because they are mistaken for benign nevi, subungual or traumatic hematomas, blisters, dermatofibromas, cysts, verrucas or pyogenic granulomas [Hughes et al. 1985]. Prevention by self-examination has been emphasized [Friedman et al. 1991]. To differentiate benign from malignant moles the ABCD criteria are useful: A, asymmetry; B, irregular border; C, variegate color; D, increasing diameter [Smith 1994].

Oozing, crusting, bleeding and altered sensation are significant [Healsmith et al. 1994].

Staging may be based on recommendations of the American Joint Commission on Cancer [Beahrs et al. 1992]. Histopathological stages are classified according to depth or level of invasion [Breslow 1970]. The thickness of the lesion is measured in millimeters from the granular layer in the epidermis to its deepest part: thin, less than 1 mm; intermediate, 1–4 mm; thick, more than 4 mm. This is the most important prognostic factor [Vollmer 1989, Dywer 1993]. The level of invasion [Clark et al. 1969] is more subjective but correlates with the depth:

- Level I, in situ melanoma confined to the epidermis
- Level II, invasion in the papillary dermis
- Level III, invasion of the junction of the papillary and reticular dermis
- Level IV, invasions of the reticular dermis
- Level V, invasion of the subcutaneous fat.

After biopsy, the histological assessment of the thickness dictates the margin of surgical excision [Veronesi et al. 1988; Balch et al. 1993]: for thickness under 1 mm, the surgical margin is 1 cm; for thickness of 1–2 mm, the surgical margin is 1–2 cm; for thickness of 2–4 mm, the surgical margin is 2 cm; and for thickness over 4 mm, the surgical margin is 3 cm.

Lesions on toes are amputated. More radical amputations, e.g. at the Lisfranc level, are required for level IV or V lesions in the forefoot. Prophylactic groin node dissection in stage I or stage II disease is less popular now [Beahrs et al. 1992] and has many complications [Fortin et al. 1995]. The 5-year and 10-year survival rates of patients with foot and ankle melanomas are lower than the rates for all sites [Dwyer et al. 1993, Saxby et al. 1993, Barnes et al. 1994, Fortin et al. 1995] because of the delay in diagnosis [Saxby et al. 1993, Barnes et al. 1994, Fortin et al. 1995]. Skin defects require grafting and those on the sole will result in loss of weight-bearing skin. Split skin grafts have been successful [Woltering et al. 1979] but tend to be protected by alteration of the patient's gait [Sommerlad and McGrouther 1978]. In the more active patient, local transposition flaps, island pedicle flaps or free flaps may be required.

Soft-tissue tumors

The modification of the World Health Organization classification recognized 82 distinct benign and

Table 4   Benign soft-tissue tumors

Congenital
Hamartomas
Arteriovenous malformations

Traumatic
Traumatic neuroma
Traumatic aneurysm
Deep foreign bodies

Miscellaneous
Ganglion
Plantar fibromatosis
Local pigmented villonodular synovitis
Diffuse pigmented villonodular synovitis
Synovial chondromatosis
Digital mucous cyst
Infantile digital fibroma
Fibromatoses
Extraskeletal chondroma

Neoplastic (benign)
Lipoma
Fibroma
Neurofibroma
Neurilemmoma
Leiomyoma
Angioleiomyoma
Hemangioma
Glomus tumor

malignant soft-tissue lesions arising in the distal leg (Table 4) [Enzinger and Weiss 1985]. The majority are benign [Jahss 1982, Kirby et al. 1989, Craigen et al. 1991]. Malignant lesions have been found to have an incidence of 2.4% [Craigen et al. 1991], 4.2% [Jahss 1982] and 13% [Kirby et al. 1989]. Sites can be described as occurring in prescribed zones of the foot [Kirby et al. 1989] (Figure 3).

Benign soft-tissue lesions

Ganglia are degenerative multilocular cysts arising commonly in zones 1 and 3, where synovial joints and tendon sheaths are superficial, and at 49% are the commonest soft-tissue swellings [Craigen et al. 1991]. They can resolve spontaneously and are removed for pain and difficulties with shoe wear. They can arise as subperiosteal or interosseous lesions [Avison et al. 1994]. Under local regional anesthesia with a tourniquet to visualize extensions to tendon sheath or joint capsule, a longitudinal incision allows extension for larger lesions and avoids undue traction. Finding the correct plane allows complete excision with the underlying degenerate tissue, which lowers the recurrence rate. Routine skin closure is performed with a compression bandage.

Local pigmented villonodular synovitis, i.e. giant cell tumor of the tendon sheath, is slow-growing, is commoner in women, and arises from joint or tendon sheaths [Byers et al. 1968]. Radiographs may show a soft-tissue swelling or erosion of bone. Surgical removal is indicated for pain and increasing size. A generous incision is necessary to trace its full length, but recurrence rates can be as high as 30% [Enzinger and Weiss 1985]. Diffuse pigmented villonodular synovitis affects larger joints, giving pain, tenderness, limitation of movement and joint swelling. Radiographs reveal a soft-tissue mass with bone erosions. Synovectomy with curettage of bone is either open or, in the ankle, arthroscopic. Regardless of the technique, complete removal is required, but a recurrence rate up to 50% can be expected [Enzinger and Weiss 1985].

Open synovectomy of the ankle is through a standard anterior approach. The ankle capsule is opened and the abnormal synovium removed piecemeal using rongeurs. The posterior recess is difficult to see without distraction, so a posterior exposure is therefore required. Arthroscopic synovectomy is performed through anterolateral and anteromedial portals with power suction shavers. Extensive joint damage requires arthrodesis.

Synovial chondromatosis is of two types. Primary chondromatosis has benign nodules of metaplastic chondroid tissue in synovial soft tissues, is mono-articular, affecting larger joints including the ankle and toes [Murphy et al. 1962, Jeffreys 1967], and may present at any age as a painful swelling and restriction of movement. Radiographs may show only a soft-tissue swelling with some erosion of the related bone. Treatment is by marginal excision. Recurrence can occur. In secondary chondromatosis or synovial osteochondromatosis loose bodies of bone and cartilage are present in the joint and synovia of larger joints including the foot and ankle [Nihal et al. 1999]. Treatment is excision of symptomatic lesions.

The lipoma is a benign neoplasm arising from fat, containing fibrous and vascular stroma presenting as a subcutaneous soft swelling or within the tendon sheaths or bone. Surgery is under local anesthesia for small lesions but under regional or general anesthesia with a tourniquet for larger ones. An incision over the swelling allows enucleation.

Fibromas are benign localized lesions in soft tissue and bone and are commonly slow-growing, forming subcutaneous, immobile hard nodules. Resection is by a direct incision over the lesion, and removal is easy, owing to a well-defined plane between normal and abnormal tissue.

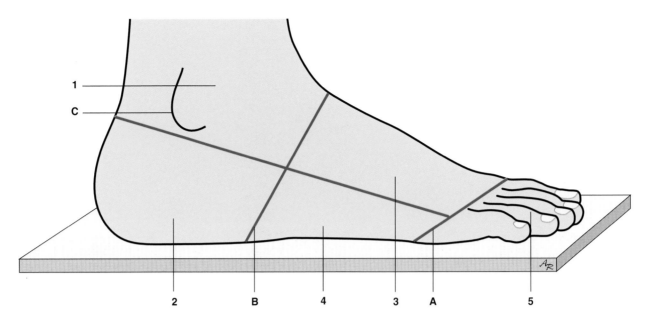

Figure 3

Zones of the foot. 1, ankle; 2, heel; 3, dorsum; 4, sole; 5, toes; A, transverse line across metatarsophalangeal joints; B, oblique line from the dorsal aspect of the midtarsal joint to the posterior limit of the posterior longitudinal plantar arch; C, longitudinal line from the metatarsal heads to the insertion of the Achilles tendon

Plantar fibromatosis is a benign condition that usually occurs in the fourth and fifth decades of life, as either solitary or multiple nodules in the sole of the foot, most commonly towards the medial side or the apex of the medial arch. It may involve the dermis of the plantar skin or extend deeply via the fascial bands to the metatarsals. Treatment is conservative, by footwear modification. Surgery is indicated for larger, painful lesions. It must include complete excision of the medial band of the plantar fascia or recurrence is likely [Allen et al. 1955, Lee et al. 1993, Durr et al. 1999, Sammarco and Mangone 2000]. Surgery is performed with the patient supine or prone (Figure 4), under general or spinal anesthesia with exsanguination. The traditional medial incision described by Henry [1963] requires an extensive subcutaneous dissection with the risk of skin breakdown [Curtin 1965]. A longitudinal incision on the sole of the foot medial to the midline is curved distally and proximally [Curtin 1965, Cracchiolo 1995, Sammarco and Mangone 2000], and skin flaps are raised to expose the plantar fascia proximal to distal, carefully preserving the medial and lateral plantar nerves. The plantar fascia is elevated from the flexor digitorum brevis and distally to the metatarsal heads, protecting the common digital nerves. With dermal involvement, skin is included. The tourniquet is deflated for meticulous hemostasis with bipolar diathermy. A narrow suction drain is inserted, the skin flap closed with interrupted nylon sutures and a firm compression

bandage or a below-knee plaster cast applied. The limb is elevated for 7 days. Sutures should be retained for a minimum of 14 days and weightbearing permitted when healed.

A traumatic neuroma presents on the dorsum of the foot as a result of previous crush or laceration injury. It appears as a painful or tender nodule with a positive Tinel's sign and distal dysesthesia. Surgery is indicated if the nodule is sufficiently symptomatic and unresponsive to conservative treatment. The operation is performed under general or regional anesthesia with a tourniquet and magnification loupes. The nerve is identified proximally, dissected along its length, pulled distally and sectioned as proximally as possible to allow retraction away from the incision.

The neurilemmoma or schwannoma is a rare encapsulated lesion arising from the nerve sheath; it is slow growing in patients 20–50 years old. It may give pain or neurological symptoms. After exposure under general or regional anesthesia with a tourniquet, the tumor is dissected carefully from the nerve under loupe magnification.

Neurofibromas are solitary or multiple lesions and present in childhood or in young adults. The solitary neurofibroma is the commonest nerve tumor in the foot [Berlin et al. 1975]; multiple lesions occur as part of von Recklinghausen's disease, i.e. neurofibromatosis, and can be plexiform or diffuse, lax and variable in their size. The plexiform

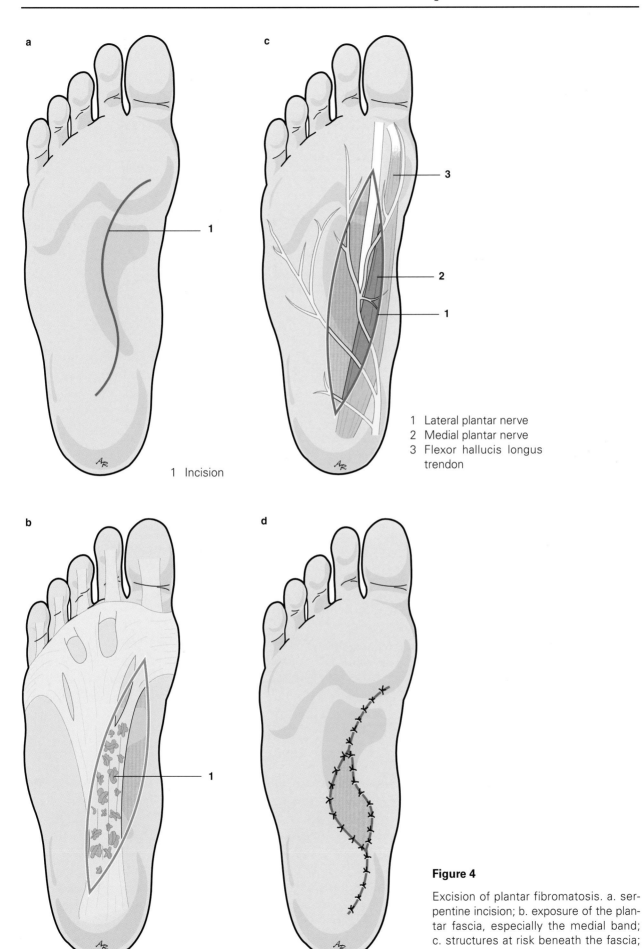

a

1 Incision

c

1 Lateral plantar nerve
2 Medial plantar nerve
3 Flexor hallucis longus trendon

b

1 Plantar fascia

d

Figure 4

Excision of plantar fibromatosis. a. serpentine incision; b. exposure of the plantar fascia, especially the medial band; c. structures at risk beneath the fascia; d. wound closure with grafting if required

type causes nerve distortion and may extend into skin and have skeletal deformities, such as giantism or bony dysplasia. Solitary neurofibromas are excised by sacrificing the nerve as for a traumatic neuroma. A plexiform neurofibroma is difficult to excise completely because it is diffuse and involves the skin. A larger lesion may require reduction in size, and anatomical structures do not need to be sacrificed. The residual cavity requires closed suction drainage and a compression bandage.

Smooth muscle tumors, i.e. leiomyomas or angioleiomyomas, have a predilection for females in their fourth to sixth decades and for the lower limb, more commonly in the foot and ankle [Spinosa 1985, Kirby et al. 1989, Craigen and Anderson 1991]. Pain or tenderness is often disproportionate to the size of the lesion. Calcification can occur in the deeper, larger tumors. With the patient under general or regional anesthesia and using a tourniquet, the lesion is excised with an ellipse of skin if there is dermal involvement.

Hemangiomas and vascular tumors are the most common tumors of infancy and childhood but are rare in the foot, occurring in skin, subcutaneous tissue, muscle and bone. They are poorly defined, palpable masses, initially increasing in size, but they may resolve spontaneously. Initially no treatment is indicated. Deeper subcutaneous or paraosseous capillary hemangiomas present as a more localized tender swelling identified by MRI. Preoperative embolization is useful for larger vascular tumors. Surgical excision is performed under regional or general anesthesia and with the aid of a thigh tourniquet through a direct incision. Careful dissection of soft tissues exposes the tumor, and feeding vessels are ligated. After excision the wounds are closed in layers over a suction drainage. A compression bandage is applied.

A glomus tumor, a hamartoma of the glomus body, is a collection of arteriovenous anastomoses surrounded by a nerve plexus. In the foot these are found in the dermis of the sole or under toenails, and cause severe pain localized by direct pressure at a specific point or provoked by cold. They are spherical and small (less than 0.5 cm in diameter) and are localized by technetium bone scanning. Surgery is for relief of pain, and the nail is removed under digital block and tourniquet (Figure 5). A longitudinal incision is made in the nail bed, which is reflected medially and laterally. The tumor is identified by its usually blue or violet color, and is removed and its bed curetted. The nail bed is repaired with absorbable sutures and covered with a non-adherent dressing, which should be changed after 48 h.

Malignant soft-tissue tumors

Malignant soft-tissue tumors (Table 5) of the foot and ankle are rare [Seale et al. 1988] but aggressive. Treatment is by wide or radical excision. Synovial sarcoma affects young adults. Twenty per cent occur in the foot and ankle [Wright et al. 1982, Enzinger and Weiss 1985, Davis and Henderson 1992, Vila et al. 1999], making it the most common primary malignant soft tissue tumor in the foot [Kirby et al. 1989]. As a painless swelling it may have been present for some time [Enzinger and Weiss 1985, Davis and Henderson 1992]. Treatment is by radical excision. Tumors in the digits are removed by ray amputation and those in the midfoot or hindfoot require removal by proximal amputation, usually below the knee. The 5-year survival rate is between 36 and 55% [Buck et al. 1981, Wright et al. 1982, Enzinger and Weiss 1985].

Clear cell sarcoma occurs in young women, with 50% of tumors arising in the foot. A painless mass is often present for several months or years, arising from tendons and aponeurosis, usually on the plantar aspect of the foot. Melanin is found in approximately 50% of the tumors, which gives the unusual appearance on MRI scanning with high intensity on T_1 and low intensity on T_2. Treatment is by radical excision, depending on site. The tumor frequently metastasizes.

Two per cent of malignant fibrous histiocytomas occur in the foot, where they constitute approximately 11% of malignant tumors. Presenting most commonly in men in their seventh decade, they arise from skeletal muscle or rarely subcutaneous tissue as a painful, rapidly increasing swelling. Treatment is by radical resection or amputation.

Two per cent of fibrosarcomas occur in the foot, comprising between 5 and 10% of sarcomas arising from fascia, aponeurosis or fibrous tissue in patients in their fifth decade. The tumor presents as a slowly growing painless mass. Treatment is by radical resection.

Tumor and tumor-like lesions arising in bone

Bony lesions in the foot and ankle are uncommon [Dahlin and Unni 1986, Murari et al. 1989, Helm and Newman 1991] and present with pain, bony swelling and pathological fracture, or are a chance radiological finding as a cyst or a solid intraosseous or extraosseous lesion. Solid lesions arise from bone or cartilage, but the cystic lesions are a heterogeneous group (Table 6).

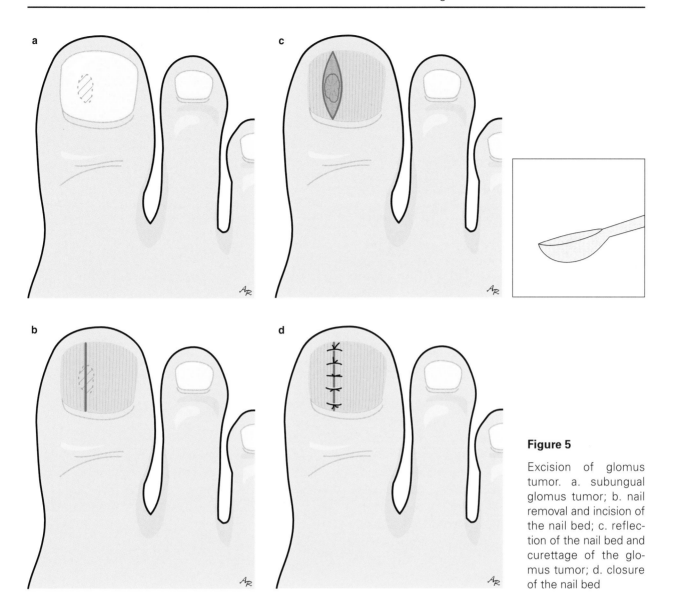

Figure 5

Excision of glomus tumor. a. subungual glomus tumor; b. nail removal and incision of the nail bed; c. reflection of the nail bed and curettage of the glomus tumor; d. closure of the nail bed

Table 5   Malignant soft-tissue tumors

Synovial sarcoma
Clear cell sarcoma
Malignant fibrous histiocytoma
Fibrosarcoma
Liposarcoma
Rhabdomyosarcoma
Leiomyosarcoma
Malignant schwannoma
Granular cell tumor
Epithelioid sarcoma

Cysts in the calcaneus can arise from any of its constituent tissues [Smith and Smith 1974, Malawer and Vance 1981, Campanacci et al. 1986, Avison et al. 1994, Sochart 1995, Davis et al. 1996, Stukenborg-Colsman et al. 1999]. Surgical treatment is indicated for symptomatic larger or expansile lesions. Surgical management is curettage and bone grafting. The extended lateral approach permits a wide exposure of the lateral wall. The incision is along the posterior ankle and foot, anterior to the Achilles tendon, to the level of the plantar skin of the heel, turning abruptly distally along the infralateral aspect of the foot to the base of the fifth metatarsal. The abductor digiti minimi is split and a full-thickness flap is elevated from the calcaneus, protecting the peroneal tendons and the sural nerve.

Cysts of the talus have similar pathology, presentation and treatment but the surgical approaches are more difficult, owing to the extensive articular surface. Lesions in the medial head and neck are approached through a dorsomedial incision, retracting the tibialis anterior. Lesions in the lateral head and neck are approached through a dorsolateral approach, protecting lateral branches of the

Table 6   Benign cystic lesions in bone

Solitary bone cyst
Fibrous dysplasia
Non-ossifying fibroma
Intraosseous ganglion
Intraosseous lipoma
Intraosseous schwannoma
Intraosseous neurofibroma
Hemangioma
Lymphangioma
Hemangioendothelioma
Hemangiopericytoma
Eosinophilic granuloma
Solitary enchondroma
Ollier's disease
Maffucci's syndrome

superficial peroneal nerve and reflecting the belly of the extensor digitorum brevis inferiorly. Approaches to the body depend on the site of the lesion. Expansile lesions permit a direct approach, while anterior lesions are approached through the extra-articular proximal talar neck via a dorsomedial incision. Posterior lesions are approached through a posterolateral incision, protecting the sural nerve and passing through the interval between the peroneus brevis and the flexor hallucis longus. Medial talar lesions can be grafted through a medial approach after a medial malleolar osteotomy. An incision is made on the medial side of the ankle joint, centered at the tip of the medial malleolus. A small arthrotomy is made anteriorly in the ankle joint and the tibialis posterior is identified posteriorly and reflected. The medial malleolus is prepared with two 2.5-mm drill holes for subsequent internal fixation. An osteotomy is performed using a low-speed saw and completed with an osteotome at the level of the dome of the talus. The medial malleolus is reflected inferiorly with the deltoid ligament. A limited dissection of the soft tissue can be made more inferiorly to expose the non-articular segment and it can be extended distally with exposure at the medial side of the head and neck of the talus. After removal of the cortical window the lesion is curetted and grafted as previously described. The medial malleolus is replaced and compressed using two partially threaded cancellous screws. The osteotomy is protected with a below-knee cast until satisfactory consolidation of the lesion and union of the malleolus have been achieved.

Enchondromas, benign tumors of mature cartilage, can occur singly, or as multiple lesions in Ollier's disease and in association with hemangiomas in Maffucci's syndrome. Larger, solitary or symptomatic lesions can be treated by curettage and grafting. Metatarsal lesions (Figure 6) are exposed by a dorsal incision, retracting the extensor tendons, protecting cutaneous nerves and incising the periosteum. Through a cortical window the lesion is curetted and grafted. Digital lesions are excised via a dorsal serpentine incision to gain greater exposure laterally and medially. Proximal phalangeal lesions in lesser rays are excised, with interposition of the extensor tendon into the gap beneath the metatarsal head and passed plantar to dorsal through a small drill hole. Distal lesions are treated by amputation.

Benign solid lesions (Table 7), for example osteochondromas (cartilage-capped exostoses), are found proximal to the ankle joint, or in the metatarsals or proximal phalanges [Fuselier et al. 1984]. Surgery is required for painful lesions that cause functional disability (Figure 7). Incision is made directly over the lesion and the soft tissues are retracted to expose its base; an osteotome is used to obtain complete removal.

The subungual exostosis is found adjacent to or beneath the toenail, usually in the hallux [Paul et al. 1991, de Palma et al. 1996] as a painful, enlarging mass, elevating the nail and bed, as confirmed on a lateral radiograph. Under local anesthesia and with a digital tourniquet, the nail is avulsed. A longitudinal incision is made in the nail bed remnant (Figure 8), which is carefully peeled using a sharp periosteal elevator. The subungual exostosis is identified to its base, and removed using a small, sharp osteotome. The nail bed is then repaired using fine interrupted, absorbable sutures.

An osteoid osteoma presents in children or young adults and can be found in the foot [Shereff et al. 1983], mainly in the tarsal bones [Capanna et al. 1986, Amendola et al. 1994], but rarely in the forefoot, e.g. the great toe [Khan et al. 1983, Spinosa et al. 1985]. Pain is present both on activity and at night, and is eased by anti-inflammatory medication. Diagnosis can be difficult [Kenzore and Abrams 1981], but isotope bone scanning and computerized axial tomography can localize the area of sclerotic bone surrounding a cystic area, with a calcified nidus. Treatment can be conservative with anti-inflammatory agents (Kneisl and Simon 1992). Lesions in the great toe and the tubular bones of the forefoot are treated in a similar manner to the cystic lesions described above. Superficial osteoid osteomas in the tarsus can be localized by CT and the nidus marked using a 2-mm bone biopsy needle inserted under local or general anesthesia

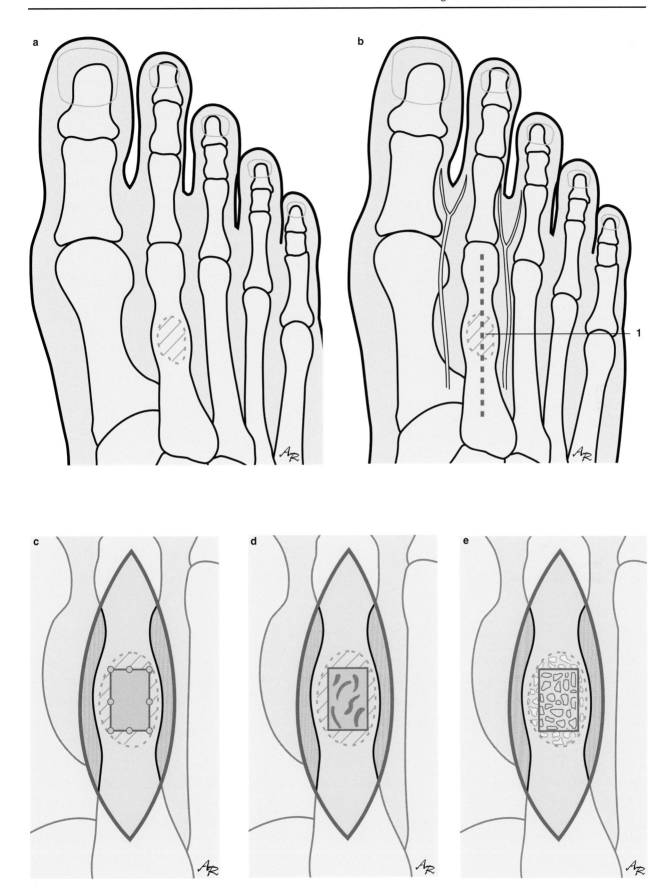

Figure 6

Grafting of cystic lesion in a metatarsal. a. lesion in the metatarsal; b. incision over the metatarsal avoiding the cutaneous nerves; c. cortical window removed and bone curetted; d. power abrasion; e. bone grafting

1 Incision

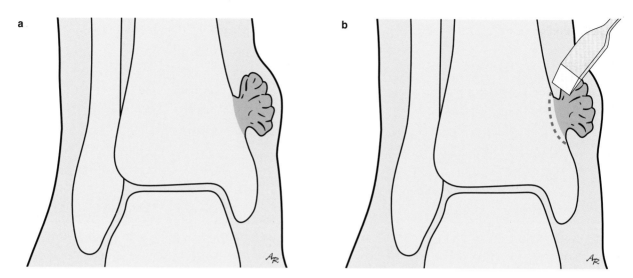

Figure 7

Excision of osteochondroma. a. osteochondroma of the distal tibia; b. excision of the osteochondroma at its base

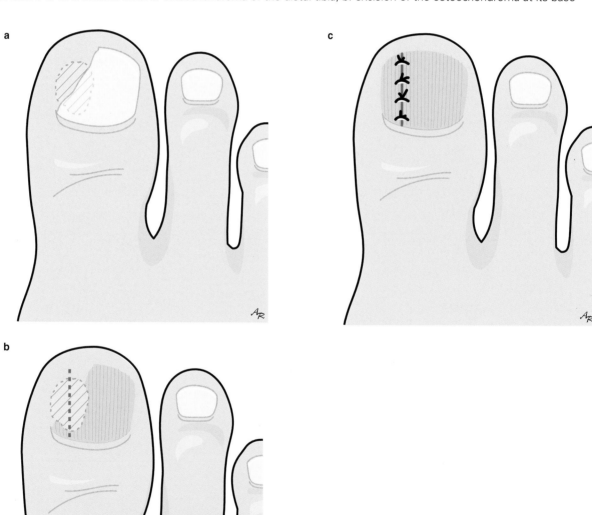

Figure 8

Excision of subungual exostosis. a. exostosis with partial loss of the nail; b. nail removed, incision in the nail bed; c. repair of the nail bed remnant

Table 7   Benign solid tumors in bone

Non-neoplastic
Duplications
Accessory bones, e.g. navicular
Osteophytes
Fracture callus
Bony spurs
Induced skeletal abnormalities
    Traumatic
    Neurogenic
Hamartomas
Neurofibromatosis

Neoplastic
Osteochondroma
Subungual exostosis

Table 8   Benign aggressive tumors in bone

Giant cell tumors
Aneurysmal bone cysts
Chondromyxoid fibroma
Chondroblastoma
Osteoblastoma
Desmoplastic fibroma

[Amendola et al. 1994, Chakrabarti et al. 1995, Turan et al. 1995, Donley et al. 2000]. Percutaneous radiofrequency ablation [Rosenthal et al. 1998, Barei et al. 2000, Lidner et al. 2001] and laser photocoagulation [Witt et al. 2000] have been reported as effective procedures. Traditionally the lesion was excised en bloc or by curettage of the nidus after imaging.

Benign aggressive bone tumors

Benign aggressive bone tumors are listed in Table 8. The giant cell tumor or osteoclastoma occurs in young to early middle-aged adults mainly in the epiphyseal region of long bones, but may occur anywhere in the tarsal or metatarsal bones [Goldenberg et al. 1970, McGraith 1972, Sung et al. 1982, Mechlin et al. 1984, O'Keefe et al. 1995, Casadei et al. 1996]. The patient presents with a painful swelling and a lytic lesion on radiographs. The recurrence rate after curettage is 36–48% [Goldenberg et al. 1970, McGraith 1972, Sung et al. 1982, Dahlin and Unni 1986] and metastatic lesions can occur. The chondroblastoma can be confused with unicameral bone cysts, but the majority of the latter occur in the anterior calcaneum. A chondroblastoma occurs close to articular or apophyseal surfaces where they can be seen as lytic expansile symptomatic lesions [Fink et al. 1997].

Most osteoblastomas occur in the tarsal bones, especially the talar neck. They are larger than osteoid osteomas, less sclerotic, and expansile if near to the cortex. Optimal treatment is en bloc excision and bone grafting, but recurrence can occur over long periods [Temple et al. 1998].

For benign aggressive tumors, wide excision with the surrounding shell of cortical bone is the optimal treatment, but problems arise if the tumor involves the hindfoot. In the midfoot and forefoot, wide excision is performed through a dorsal incision over the appropriate tarsal bone [Arenson and Cohen 1998]. The soft tissues are dissected, and the adjacent anatomical structures preserved. The entire midfoot tarsal bone is excised by division of its soft-tissue attachments. In proximal tarsal bones two incisions may be necessary, and reconstruction with a cortical autograft will be required for arthrodesis between the proximal and distal adjacent bones (Figure 9), restoring the length and stability of the medial or lateral columns [Fraipont and Thordarson 1966]. Compression plates on the plantar surface give added stability until revascularization and fusion occur. In the talus, the site and size of the lesion dictate the treatment program. Tumors localized to the head and neck can be treated by partial resection with talonavicular fusion [Malawer and Vance 1981]. A dorsomedial approach exposes the neck of the talus and the talonavicular joint. Larger lesions should be replaced by a combination of morcellized and tricortical graft with internal fixation. The foot may require protection for a minimum of 3 months in a below-knee cast, with partial weightbearing after 6 weeks. An ankle–foot orthosis may be needed until consolidation. Extensive lesions in the body of the talus require partial or complete talectomy through lateral and medial incisions to permit a complete en bloc removal. The position of the incisions will depend on the expansion and distortion of the bone. After the astragalectomy, the articular surfaces of the calcaneus and the tibial plafond are removed to bleeding cancellous bone. Good internal fixation can be achieved using partially threaded cancellous screws (Figure 10) or an external fixator [Casadei et al. 1994]. In the calcaneus, smaller lesions are treated by wide excision. The anterior calcaneus can be widely excised with a good surrounding cuff of bone through a lateral approach (Figure 11). To provide adequate stability a fusion of the posterior subtalar

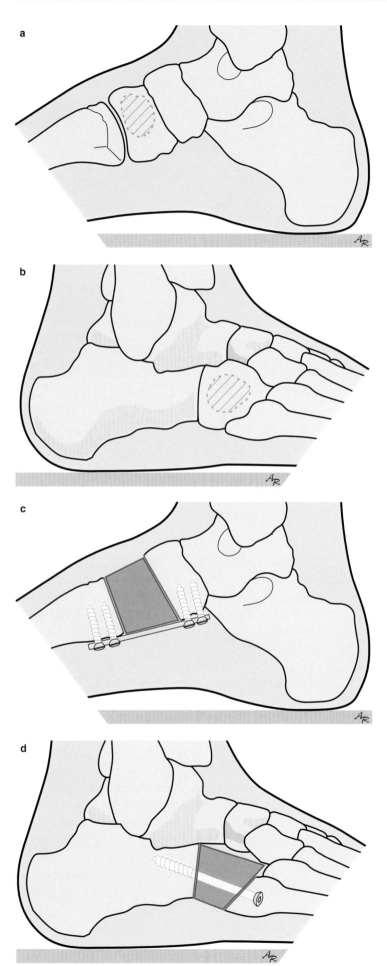

Figure 9

Excision and grafting of midfoot lesion. a. site of the medial midtarsal lesion; b. site of the lateral midtarsal lesion; c. following insertion of a bone graft and internal fixation, medial lesion; d. lateral lesion

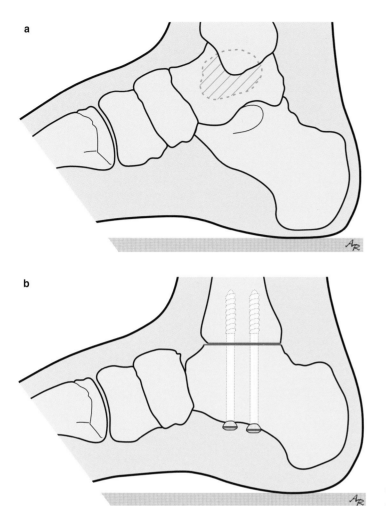

Figure 10

Excision of talus with tibiocalcaneal fusion. a. extensive lesion in the talus; b. tibiocalcaneal arthrodesis with screw fixation

joint with autogenous grafting of the residual calcaneus to the cuboid is optimal. In the body of the calcaneus, excision has been advocated with satisfactory function, using a shoe with an inbuilt heel raise [Seth and Shah 1972]. An alternative is curettage with an adjunct such as acrylic cement [Persson and Wouters 1976], liquid nitrogen [Marcove et al. 1978] or phenol [McDonald et al. 1986]. Amputation should be considered only for recurrent lesions.

Chondromyxoid fibroma is a potentially locally recurrent lesion occurring in the second and third decades of life and involving the long bones, particularly of the lower limbs and in the foot [Crisafulli et al. 1990]. The patient presents with pain and local tenderness. Radiographs show a circumscribed area, occasionally expansile. Surgery is by local excision as recurrences are possible after curettage.

Primary malignant tumors of bone and cartilage

Malignant bone tumors are not common (Table 9) [Dahlin and Unni 1986, Murari et al. 1989].

Ewing's sarcoma is rare in the foot and ankle [Leeson and Smith 1989]. The patient, usually under the age of 20 years, has symptoms of pain and swelling. Pyrexia may accompany a palpable tender swelling, so it can be confused with osteomyelitis. Radiologically the lesion is lytic, on occasions giving rise to the typical 'onion skin' appearance of subperiosteal reactive new bone. It is treated by a combination of amputation and aggressive chemotherapy [Leeson and Smith 1989]. Tumors in the metatarsals can be amputated at the Syme's level; if more proximal, a below-knee amputation is required.

Osteosarcomas commonly arise between the ages of 10 and 20 years, more often in boys, with 1–2% in the ankle or foot [Revell 1981]. Clinical presentation is usually with pain and local swelling. Plain radiographs and MRI scanning demonstrate bone destruction and a soft-tissue mass. Careful preoperative staging and assessment for metastatic disease should be performed. Treatment is based on a combination of wide resection of the lesion, adjuvant chemotherapy and radiotherapy. Lesions arising in the hindfoot and ankle usually require

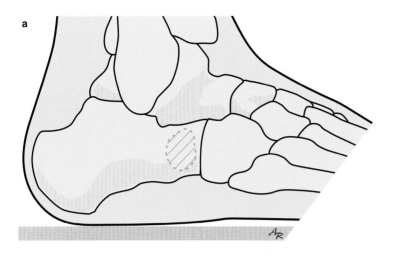

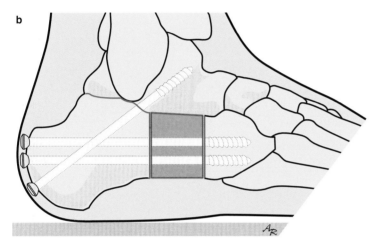

Figure 11

Excision of anterior calcaneus with subtalar fusion. a. smaller lesion in the anterior calcaneus; b. bone grafting with subtalar and calcaneocuboid fusion

Table 9   Malignant tumors in bone
Ewing's sarcoma
Osteosarcoma
Chondrosarcoma
Neuroectodermal tumors of bone
Paget's sarcoma
'Soft tissue' sarcomas within bone
Lymphoma
Myeloma
Metastatic tumors

a below-knee amputation. Only if a lesion is diagnosed particularly early, with little soft-tissue involvement and less aggressive histological features, can limb preservation be undertaken, because of the limited soft-tissue envelope.

Chondrosarcoma occurs most frequently in the third to fifth decades, but is extremely rare in the foot and ankle [Patcher and Alpert 1964, Dahlin and Salvadore, 1974]. Presentation is with local pain and swelling. Radiographic examination demonstrates an expansile destructive mass, with mottled calcification or ossification within the lesion. Treatment is by radical excision. For lesions in the forefoot, a Syme's amputation may be appropriate [Dhillon et al. 1992].

Secondary malignant bone tumors

The foot and ankle are an infrequent site for metastatic disease, but any part may be involved. Presentation is by pain and swelling, or a pathological fracture. Tumors may be difficult to distinguish from infection or inflammatory processes. Treatment is usually non-surgical and allied to the management of the overall condition, the aim being to maintain maximum mobility with pain relief. The foot and ankle may also be involved in lymphomas and myelomatous processes. The treatment in these cases is usually non-surgical, with management of the underlying condition through chemotherapy and radiotherapy as the mainstay of treatment.

References

Allen RA, Woolner LB, Ghormley RK (1955) Soft tissue tumors of the sole. J Bone Joint Surg 37A: 14–26

Amendola A, Vellett D, Willits K (1994) Osteoid osteoma of neck of talus: percutaneous computed tomography; guided technique for complete excision. Foot Ankle 15: 429–432

American Joint Committee on Cancer. (1992) Malignant melanoma of the skin (excluding eyelid). In: Beahrs OH, Henson DE, Hutter RVP, Kennedy BJ eds. American Joint Committee on Cancer, Manual for Staging of Cancer, 4th edn. Philadelphia, Lippincott, pp 143–148

Arenson DJ, Cohen MD (1998) Structural and functional reconstuction after resection of aneurysmal bone cyst of the fifth metatarsal: a case study. Foot Ankle Int 19: 405–410

Avison G, Irwin A, Howie CR (1994) Intraosseous ganglion of calcaneum. Foot 4: 163–165

Balch CM, Urist MM, Karakaisis CP et al. (1993) Efficacy of 2 cm surgical margins for intermediate thickness melanomas (1–4 mm): results of a multi-institutional randomised surgical trial. Ann Surg 218: 262–267

Barei DP, Moreau G, Scarborough MT, Neel MD (2000) Percutaneous radiofrequency ablation of osteoid osteoma. Clin Orthop 373: 115–124

Barnes BC, Seiguler HF, Saxby TS et al. (1994) Melanoma of the foot. J Bone Joint Surg 76A: 892–898

Berlin SJ, Donick II, Block LD, Costa AJ (1975) Nerve tumours of the foot: diagnosis and treatment. J Am Podiatr Assoc 65: 157–166

Breslow A (1970) Thickness, cross sectional areas and depth of invasion in the prognosis of cutaneous melanoma. Ann Surg 172: 902–908

Buck P, Mickelson MR, Bonfiglio M (1981) Synovial sarcoma: a review of 33 cases. Clin Orthop 156: 211–215

Byers PD, Cotton RE, Deacon OD et al. (1968) The diagnosis and treatment of pigmented villonodular synovitis. J Bone Joint Surg 50B: 290–305

Campanacci M, Capanna R, Picci P (1986) Unicameral and aneurysmal bone cysts. Clin Orthop 204: 25–36

Capanna R, Van Horn J, Ayala A et al. (1986) Osteoid osteoma and osteoblastoma of talus: a report of 40 cases. Skel Radiol 15: 360–364

Casadei R, Ruggieri P, Giuseppe T et al. (1994) Ankle resection arthrodesis in patients with bone tumor. Foot Ankle Int 15: 242–249

Casadei R, Ruggieri P, Moscato M et al. Aneurysmal bone cyst and giant cell tumor of the foot. (1996) Foot Ankle Int 17: 487–495

Chakrabarti I, Greiss ME, Jennings P (1995) Osteoid osteoma of os calcis: computed tomography; guided diagnosis and excision. Foot 5: 153–154

Clark WH, Fron L, Bernardino EA, Mihm MC (1969) The histogenesis and biological behaviour of primary human melanomas of the skin. Cancer Res 29: 705–727

Cracchiolo A (1995) Plantar fibromatosis. In: Helal B, Myerson M, Rowley D, Cracchiolo A (eds) Surgery of Disorders of the Foot and Ankle, 2nd edn. London, Martin Dunitz

Craigen MAC, Anderson EG (1991) Smooth muscle tumours in the foot. Foot 1: 33–34

Craigen MAC, El Gawad MA, Anderson EG (1991) Soft tissue swelling of the foot. Foot 1: 113–116

Crim JR, Seeger LL, Yao L et al. (1992) Diagnosis of soft tissue masses with MR imaging: can benign masses be differentiated from malignant ones? Radiology 185: 581–586

Crisafulli JA, Adams D, Sakhurja R (1990) Chondromyxoid fibroma of a metatarsal. J Foot Surg 29: 164–168

Curtin JW (1965) Fibromatosis of the plantar fascia: surgical technique and design of skin incision. J Bone Joint Surg 47A: 1605

Dahlin DC, Salvadore AH (1974) Chondrosarcoma of bones of hand and feet: a study of 30 cases. Cancer 34: 755–760

Dahlin DC, Unni KK (1986) Bone Tumours: General Aspects and Data on 8542 Cases, 4th edn. Springfield, CC Thomas

Davis RI, Henderson SA (1992) Synovial sarcoma: an under diagnosed swelling of the foot. Foot 1: 169–173

Davis RI, Swain D, Barr RJ et al. (1996) Tumours of the os calcis: a report of 2 rare tumours. Foot 6: 43–46

De Palma L, Gigante A, Specchia N (1996) Subungual exostosis of the foot. Foot Ankle Int 17: 758–763

Dhillon MS, Singh DP, Mittal RL et al. (1992) Primary malignant and potentially malignant tumours of the foot. Foot 2: 19–26

Donley BG, Philbin T, Rosenberg GA et al. (2000) Percutaneous CT guided resection of osteoid osteoma of the tibial plafond. Foot Ankle Int 21: 596–598

Durr HR, Krodel A, Trouillier H et al. (1999) Fibromatosis of the plantar fascia: diagnosis and indications for surgical treatment. Foot Ankle Int 20: 13–17

Dwyer PK, Mackie RM, Watt DC, Aitchison TC (1993) Plantar malignant melanoma in a white Caucasian population. Br J Dermatol 128: 115–120

Enneking WF, Spanier SS, Goodman MA (1980) A system for the surgical staging of musculoskeletal sarcoma. Clin Orthop 153: 106–120

Enneking WF (1986) A system of staging musculo-skeletal neoplasms. Clin Orthop 204: 9–24

Enzinger FM, Weiss SW (1985) Soft Tissue Tumours, 2nd edn. St Louis, Mosby

Fink BR, Temple HT, Chiricosta FM et al. (1997) Chondroblastoma of the foot. Foot Ankle Int 18: 236–242

Fortin PT, Freiberg A, Rees R et al. (1995) Malignant melanoma of foot and ankle. J Bone Joint Surg 77A: 1396–1403

Fraipont MJ, Thordarson DB (1996) Aneurysmal bone cyst of the navicular; a case report and review of the literature. Foot Ankle Int 17: 709–711

Friedman RJ, Reigel DS, Silverman MK et al. (1991) Malignant melanoma in the 1990s: the continued importance of early detection and the role of the physician examination and self examination of the skin. Cancer J Clin 41: 201–226

Fuselier CO, Billing T, Kushner T, Kirchwehm W (1984) Solitary osteochondroma of foot: an in-depth study with case reports. J Foot Surg 23: 3–24

Goldenberg RR, Campbell CJ, Bonfiglio M (1970) Giant cell tumour of bone: analysis of 218 cases. J Bone Joint Surg 52A: 692

Hayes AG, Nadkarni JB (1996) Extensile posterior approach to the ankle. J Bone Joint Surg 78B: 468–470

Healsmith MF, Bourke JF, Osbourne JE, Graham-Brown RAC (1994) An evaluation of the revised 7 point check list for the early diagnosis of cutaneous and malignant melanoma. Br J Dermatol 130: 48–50

Heare TC, Enneking WF, Heare MH (1989) Staging techniques and biopsy of bone tumours. Orthop Clin North Am 20: 273

Helm RH, Newman RJ (1991) Primary bone tumors of the foot: experience of the Leeds Bone Tumour Registry. Foot 1: 135–138

Henry AK (1963) Extensile Exposure. Baltimore, Williams & Wilkins

Hughes LE, Horgan K, Taylor BA, Laidler P (1985) Malignant melanoma of the hand and foot: diagnosis and management. Br J Surg 72: 811–815

Iossifidis A, Sutaria PD, Pinto T (1995) Synovial chondromatosis of ankle. Foot 5: 44–46

Jahss MH (1982) Disorders of the Foot. Philadelphia, WB Saunders

Jeffreys TE (1967) Synovial chondromatosis. J Bone Joint Surg 49B: 530–534

Kenzore JE, Abrams RC (1981) Problems encountered in the diagnosis and treatment of osteoid osteotomy of the talus. Foot Ankle 2: 172–178

Khan MD, Tiano FJ, Lillie RC (1983) Osteoid osteoma of the great toe. J Foot Surg 22: 325–328

Kirby EJ, Shereff MJ, Lewis MM (1989) Soft tissue tumors and tumor like lesions of the foot. J Bone Joint Surg 71A: 621–626

Kneisl JS, Simon MA (1992) Medical management compared with operative treatment for osteoid osteoma. J Bone Joint Surg 74A: 179–185

Kurzer A, Patel M (1979) Basal cell carcinoma of the foot. Br J Plast Surg 32: 300–301

Lee TH, Wapner KL, Hecht PJ (1993) Current concepts review: plantar fibromatosis. J Bone Joint Surg 75A: 1080–1084

Leeson MC, Smith MJ (1989) Ewing's sarcoma of the foot. Foot Ankle 10: 147–151

Lidner NJ, Ozaki T, Roedi R et al. (2001) Percutaneous radiofrequency ablation in osteoid osteoma. J Bone Joint Surg 83B: 391–396

Malawer MM, Vance R (1981) Giant cell tumour and aneurysmal bone cyst of talus: clinico-pathological review and 2 case reports. Foot Ankle 4: 235–244

Mankin HJ, Gebhardt MD, Jennings CL et al. (1996) Long-term results of allograft replacement in the management of bone tumors. Clin Orthop 324: 86–97

Marcove RC, Veiss ID, Vhehairvalla MR et al. (1978) Cryosurgery: the treatment of giant cell tumors of bone: report of 52 consecutive cases. Cancer 41: 957–969

McDonald DJ, Sim FH, McLeod RA, Dahlin DC (1986) Giant cell tumor of bone. J Bone Joint Surg 68A: 235–242

McGraith PJ (1972) Giant cell tumour of bone: an analysis of 52 cases. J Bone Joint Surg 54B: 216–227

Mechlin MB, Kricun M, Stead J, Schwann H (1984) Giant cell tumours of the tarsal bones. Skel Radiol 11: 266–270

Murari TM, Callaghan JJ, Berrey BH, Sweet DE (1989) Primary benign and malignant osseous neoplasms of the foot. Foot Ankle 10: 68–80

Murphy FP, Dahlin DC, Sullivan CR (1962) Articular synovial chondromatosis. J Bone Joint Surg 44A: 77–86

Nihal A, Read CJ, Henderson DC, Malcolm AJ (1999) Extra-articular giant solitary synovial chondromatosis of the foot; a case report and literature review. Foot Ankle Surg 5: 29–32

O'Keefe RJ, O'Donnell RJ, Temple HT et al. (1995) Giant cell tumour of bone in the foot and ankle. Foot Ankle Int 15: 242–249

Patcher MR, Alpert M (1964) Chondrosarcoma of the foot skeleton. J Bone Joint Surg 46A: 601–607

Paul AS, Ohiorenaya B, Meadows TH (1991) Subungual exostosis presenting as an ingrowing toe nail. Foot 1: 125–126

Persson BM, Wouters HW (1976) Curettage and acrylic cementation in surgery of giant cell tumours of bone. Clin Orthop 120: 125–133

Revell P (1981) Diseases of bone and joints. In: Berry CL (ed) Paediatric Pathology. Berlin, Springer

Robinson JK (1979) Gigantic basal cell carcinoma on the plantar arch of the foot: report of a case. J Dermatol Surg Oncol 5: 958–960

Roenigk RK, Ratz JL, Bailin PL, Wheeland RG (1986) Trends in the presentation and treatment of basal cell carcinomas. J Dermatol Surg Oncol 12: 860–865

Rosenthal DI, Hornicek FJ, Wolfe MW et al. (1998) Percutaneous radiofrequency coagulation of osteoid osteoma compared with operative treatment. J Bone Joint Surg 80A: 815–821

Rydholm A, Rööser B (1987) Surgical margins for soft tissue sarcoma. J Bone Joint Surg 69A: 1074–1078

Sammarco GJ, Mangone PG (2000) Classification and treatment of plantar fibromatosis. Foot Ankle Int 21: 596–598

Saxby TS, Barnes B, Harrelson JM, Seigler HF (1993) Melanoma of the foot and ankle. Orthop Trans 16: 786

Seale KS, Lange TA, Munson D, Hackbarth DA (1988) Soft tissue tumours of the foot and ankle. Foot Ankle 9: 19–27

Seth RD, Shah SN (1972) Osteoclastoma of os calcis. Int Surg 57: 748–749

Shereff MJ, Cullivan W, Johnson K (1983) Osteoid osteoma of the foot. J Bone Joint Surg 65A: 638–641

Simon MA (1982) Current concepts review: biopsy of musculoskeletal tumors. J Bone Joint Surg 64A: 1253–1257

Simon MA, Biermann JS (1993) Biopsy of bone and soft tissue lesions. J Bone Joint Surg 75A: 616

Smith AG (1994) Skin tumours of the foot. Foot 4: 175–179

Smith RW, Smith CF (1974) Solitary unicameral bone cyst of calcaneum. J Bone Joint Surg 56A: 45–56

Smith T (1979) The Queensland Melanoma Project. An exercise in health education. Br Med J 1: 253–294

Sochart DH (1995) Intraosseous schwannoma of calcaneum. Foot 5: 32–40

Sommerlad BC, McGrouther DA (1978) Resurfacing the sole. Br J Plast Surg 31: 107–116

Spinosa AF (1985) Leiomyoma of the foot. J Foot Surg 24: 68–70

Spinosa AF, Freundlich WA, Roy PP (1985) Osteoid osteoma of the hallux. J Foot Surg 24: 370–372

Stukenborg-Colsman C, Wulker N, Wirth CJ (1999) Cystic bone lesions of the calcaneus and the talus: report of five cases. Foot Ankle Surg 5: 33–38

Sung HW, Kuo DP, Shu WP et al. (1982) Giant cell tumor of bone: 210 cases in Chinese patients. J Bone Joint Surg 64A: 755–761

Tadross TS, Checketts RG (2000) Retrograde intramedullary nail for metastatic lesion of the lower tibia. Foot Ankle Int 21: 683–685

Temple HT, Mizel MS, Murphey MD, Sweet DE (1998) Osteoblastoma of the foot and ankle. Foot Ankle Int 19: 698–704

Turan RA, Gunter P, Hardstedt C, Fellander LT (1995) Osteoid osteoma of the talus: percutaneous radical excision followed by computed tomographic-guided indication of the lesion under local anaesthesia. Foot 5: 149–151

Veronesi W, Casanelli N, Adamus J et al. (1988) Thin stage I primary cutaneous malignant melanoma: comparison of excision width margin of 1 or 3 cm. N Engl J Med 318: 1159–1162

Vollmer RT (1989) Malignant melanoma: a multivariate analysis of prognostic factors. Pathol Ann 24: 383–407

Vila J, Larrainzar R, Llanos LF, Martinez-Tello FJ (1999) Synovial sarcoma of the foot: a review of five cases. Foot Ankle Surg 5: 191–196

Williams PH, Monagham D, Barrington NA (1991) Undiagnosed foot pain: the role of the isotope bone scan. Foot 1: 145–149

Witt JD, Hall-Craggs MA, Ripley P et al. (2000) Intersitial laser photocoagulation for the treatment of osteoid osteoma. J Bone Joint Surg 82B: 1125–1128

Wolfe RE, Enneking WF (1996) The staging and surgery of musculoskeletal neoplasms. Orthop Clin North Am 27: 473–481

Woltering EA, Thorpe WP, Reed JK, Rosenberg SA (1979) Split thickness skin grafting of the plantar surface of the foot after wide excision of neoplasms of the skin. Surg Gynaecol Obstet 149: 229–232

Wright PH, Sim FH, Soule EH et al. (1982) Synovial sarcoma. J Bone Joint Surg 64A: 112–122

48

Techniques of soft tissue coverage of the foot and ankle

Alain C. Masquelet

Introduction

Soft tissue coverage of the foot and ankle is always a difficult problem, for several reasons:

1. Defects are of a great variety and may involve soft tissues, bones and tendons. For example, compound avulsion of the heel remains an unsolved problem.
2. The tissue qualities at the foot and ankle vary considerably, which requires specific procedures of repair for each area. Before choosing a surgical technique it is necessary to take into account the original qualities of the avulsed tissues. The repair should provide a comparable tissue, as far as possible.

   - At the dorsal aspect of the foot and of the perimalleolar region, the skin is very thin and pliable. Extensor tendons, bones and joint structures are often exposed or even avulsed.
   - The plantar aspect of the foot comprises the weightbearing area of the forefoot, the plantar vault and the weightbearing zone of the heel. Surgical procedures cannot restore the weightbearing capacity of the soft tissues. It remains controversial whether sensation in patients without neurological deficits can be restored. The main complications of coverage of weightbearing areas are related to the thickness of the graft or to lack of adherence of the flap to the underlying tissues.

   - The hindfoot includes very distinct zones, i.e. the lower part of the Achilles tendon, the small area of insertion of the tendon at the calcaneal tuberosity and the rubbing area of the heel.

3. Soft-tissue repair may be complicated by medical disorders, such as arteritis, diabetes, venous dystrophy and neurological disorders. A thorough assessment of the extremity prior to surgery is required to avoid failure.
4. The non-specialized surgeon may find it difficult to choose the best technique out of the huge armamentarium of surgical procedures now available. This choice must take into account the size of the defect, the features of the tissues to be restored, the exposed structures, the local conditions with respect to all involved pathological problems and the requirements of the patient.

General principles of soft-tissue repair

The principles of soft-tissue repair have been reviewed elsewhere by the author [Masquelet 1994].

Simple flaps are preferable to more complicated ones, if possible. For instance, a local or regional procedure such as raising a pedicled flap should be preferred to a more sophisticated operation such as a free flap.

If granulation tissue is present, it should be covered with a split-thickness skin graft. Over weightbearing areas, which require optimum coverage, this is generally only a temporary solution.

There is no ideal technique to restore a large defect of the weightbearing aspect of the heel. Myocutaneous flaps should be avoided because they do not adhere to the underlying tissues. Fasciocutaneous flaps are preferable. A muscle flap covered with a skin graft may also be used.

The optimum treatment of compound injuries involving bone and soft tissues is open to debate. Composite flaps are not easy to construct. Matching the flap to the recipient site is difficult and the morbidity at the donor site is frequently unacceptable. A two-stage reconstruction is usually possible with good results. A sensitive flap is always preferable, when possible [Harrison and Morgan 1981, Morrison et al. 1983, Duncan et al. 1985, Chang et al. 1986], but it is not mandatory at the weightbearing area of the foot in healthy patients. A sensitive flap does not avoid ulceration and hyperkeratosis, which are usually the consequence of lack of adherence of the flap.

The postoperative regimens are similar, irrespective of the flap employed. It is advocated that patients remain in bed for 4–5 days with the foot slightly elevated to just above the level of the heart. If the flap is used to restore a weightbearing area, walking with crutches is allowed after 5–6 days. Partial ground contact should be avoided for 3 weeks; full contact is not allowed for 6 weeks. Compressive garments are used to improve the appearance of the flap and to enhance lymphatic and venous drainage.

Vascular anatomy should be revised in order to understand the basis of the flaps at the ankle and foot (Figure 1).

The following flaps and their indications, advantages and disadvantages are described in this chapter (Figure 2):

- Pedicle flaps: dorsalis pedis flap, lateral supramalleolar flap, medial plantar flap, medialis pedis flap, distally based sural flap, abductor hallucis muscle flap, extensor digitorum brevis muscle flap, peroneus brevis flap, medial saphenous cross-leg flap
- Free flaps: scapular, latissimus and serratus muscle flaps.

Dorsalis pedis flap

Indications

The dorsalis pedis flap [Man and Acland 1980, Zuker and Manktelow 1986] is used for coverage of a defect that requires thin and pliable skin. The indications for this flap have diminished. It is not indicated for coverage of the weightbearing area of the foot. The dorsalis pedis flap can be used as a free flap or as a pedicled island flap.

Advantages

Advantages of the dorsalis pedis flap are:

- Wide arc of rotation
- Reliable
- Can be used as a sensory flap.

Disadvantages

Disadvantages are:

- Difficult dissection
- Functional deficit at the donor site
- Sacrifice of a main vascular axis of the foot.

Anatomy

The vascular axis of the flap is the dorsalis pedis artery. The vascular supply is provided by small arterioles which issue from the short segment lying between the extensor hallucis longus tendon and the tendon of the first head of the extensor digitorum brevis muscle.

Surgical technique

The medial border of the flap overlaps the tendon of the extensor hallucis longus (Figure 3a). The distal end is at the level of the midpoint of the metatarsal bones. The vessels of the pedicle and the superficial peroneal nerve are isolated through a longitudinal incision proximal to the flap. The flap is elevated from medial to lateral. The medial vein is included. The deep branch of the dorsalis pedis artery is ligated and divided after transecting the tendon of the extensor hallucis brevis (Figure 3b). The tendon of the extensor hallucis longus is retracted medially to include the artery into the flap.

Laterally, the extensor digitorum longus tendons are retracted. The plane of dissection should leave areolar tissue over the tendons to provide a well-vascularized bed for subsequent skin graft coverage (Figure 3c). Following elevation of the flap, the tendons of the extensor digitorum brevis and extensor hallucis longus are joined together by sutures and a split-thickness skin graft is applied to cover the donor site (Figure 3d).

a

1
2
3
4

5
6
7

18
17
16
15
14

13
12
11
10
9
8

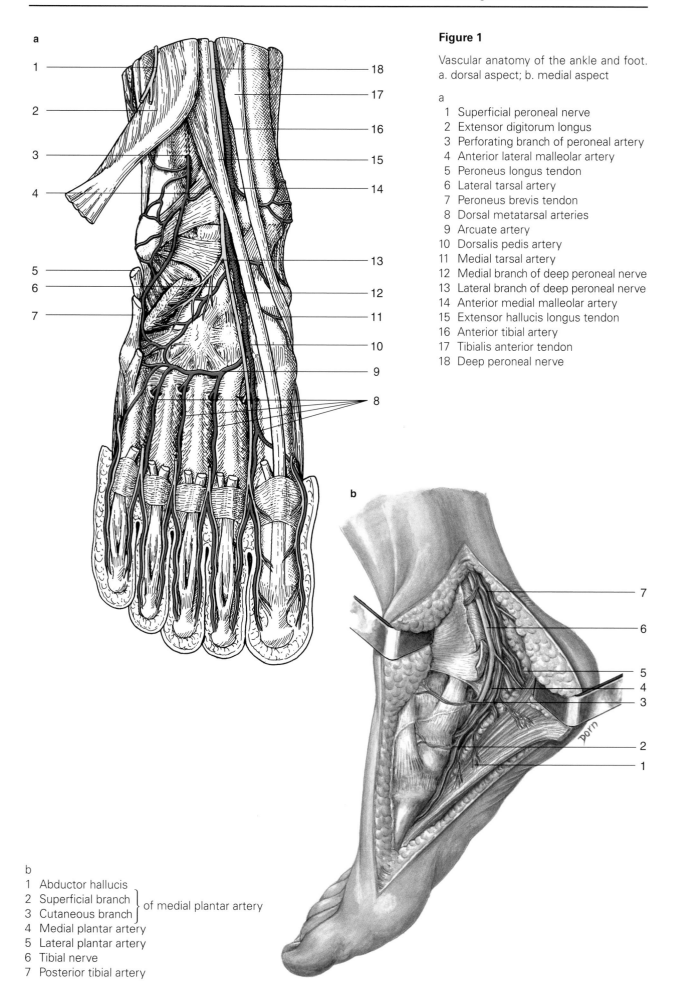

Figure 1

Vascular anatomy of the ankle and foot.
a. dorsal aspect; b. medial aspect

a
1 Superficial peroneal nerve
2 Extensor digitorum longus
3 Perforating branch of peroneal artery
4 Anterior lateral malleolar artery
5 Peroneus longus tendon
6 Lateral tarsal artery
7 Peroneus brevis tendon
8 Dorsal metatarsal arteries
9 Arcuate artery
10 Dorsalis pedis artery
11 Medial tarsal artery
12 Medial branch of deep peroneal nerve
13 Lateral branch of deep peroneal nerve
14 Anterior medial malleolar artery
15 Extensor hallucis longus tendon
16 Anterior tibial artery
17 Tibialis anterior tendon
18 Deep peroneal nerve

b

7
6
5
4
3
2
1

b
1 Abductor hallucis
2 Superficial branch ⎫ of medial plantar artery
3 Cutaneous branch ⎭
4 Medial plantar artery
5 Lateral plantar artery
6 Tibial nerve
7 Posterior tibial artery

Lateral supramalleolar flap

Indications

The indications for the lateral supramalleolar flap [Masquelet et al. 1988] depend on the type of flap. The distally based peninsular flap is used for coverage of the distal quarter of the leg. The distally based island pedicle flap is used for coverage of the dorsum of the foot, of the lateral and medial arches and of the posterior aspect of the heel. The lateral supramalleolar flap is not suitable for the medial aspect of the heel because of the impaired venous return. The weight-bearing area of the heel is not an indication for the flap, as the skin quality is not suitable for weightbearing.

Advantages

Advantages of the lateral supramalleolar flap are:

- No sacrifice of a main artery
- Wide arc of rotation
- Easy and reliable dissection.

Disadvantages

Disadvantages are:

- Sacrifice of the superficial peroneal nerve, which is included in the flap
- Cosmetic disfigurement at the donor site, which may be unacceptable to women.

Anatomy

The flap is raised on the lateral aspect of the lower leg. It is supplied by a recurrent cutaneous artery issued from the ramus perforans of the peroneal artery. The latter anastomoses with the lateral tarsal artery.

Surgical technique

The patient is positioned supine with a sandbag under the ipsilateral buttock.

The proximal end of the incision should not extend beyond the middle of the lower leg (Figure 4a). The anterior border of the flap is along the course of the tibialis anterior tendon. The posterior extension of the flap is limited by the fibula. The distal end must include the emergence of the ramus perforans of the peroneal artery, which is located at the distal tibia and the fibula. The skin is incised distally in continuity with the anterior margin of the flap and anterior to the lateral malleolus.

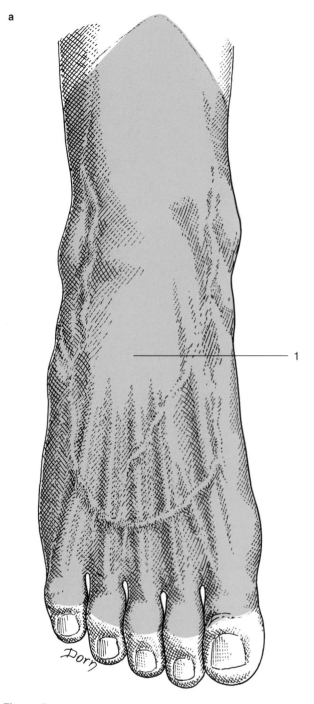

a

1

Figure 2

Indications and total area which can be covered by each local flap. In some locations, e.g. the posterior heel, several solutions are possible. The final choice depends on the local tissue conditions of the lower limb (the skin, pre-existing scars and the vascular pattern) and on the general condition and the demands of the patient

a. anterior aspect

1 Lateral supramalleolar flap, distally based sural flap

(Continued)

The distal pedicle with the ramus perforans is first identified deep to the extensor retinaculum. Branches of the superficial peroneal nerve are cut

b. medial aspect

1 Medialis pedis flap
2 Abductor hallucis muscle flap
3 Medial plantar flap, distally based sural flap

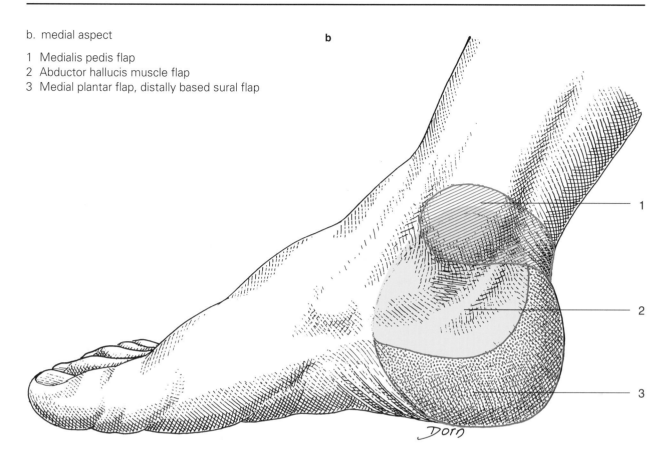

c. lateral aspect

1 Extensor digitorum brevis muscle flap
2 Lateral supramalleolar flap, distally based sural flap

(Continued)

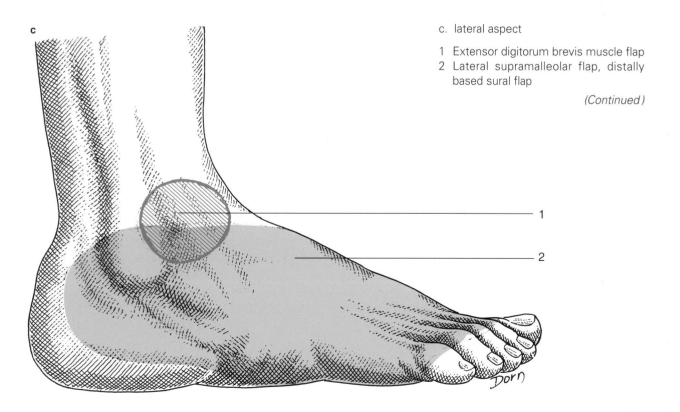

d

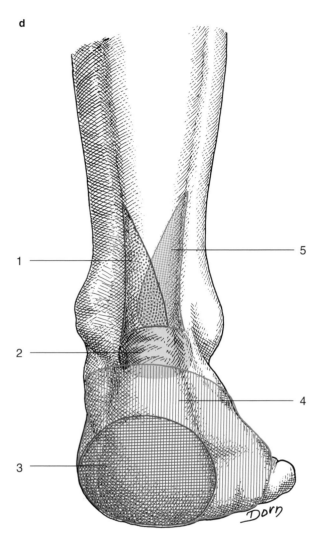

Figure 2   (Continued)

d. posterior aspect

1 Flexor hallucis longus flap
2 Medialis pedis flap, distally based sural flap
3 Medial plantar flap, distally based sural flap
4 Lateral supramalleolar flap, distally based sural flap
5 Peroneus brevis flap

distally (Figure 4b). The common trunk of the nerve is severed proximally.

The posterior skin hinge of the flap is maintained and the vascular pattern is identified. The anterior lateral malleolar artery is severed. The ramus perforans of the peroneal artery is also severed proximal to the cutaneous branch, which supplies the flap. A small incision of the interosseous membrane may facilitate the ligature. The pedicle is released down to the sinus tarsi, which is the pivot point of the pedicle (Figure 4c). The posterior margin of the flap is then released subperiosteally from the fibula to protect the cutaneous branch.

The arc of rotation of the lateral supramalleolar flap allows coverage of the medial aspect of the

lower leg, the posterior aspect of the heel and the dorsum and the borders of the foot (Figure 4d). Its design with a subcutaneous fascial pedicle (Figure 4e) allows an increase in the arc of rotation of a limited-size skin paddle. When the ramus perforans is destroyed at the ankle, the emergence of the ramus perforans of the peroneal artery is used as the pivot point of the pedicle.

Medial plantar flap

Indications

The medial plantar flap [Harrison and Morgan 1981, Morrison et al. 1983] is indicated for the repair of confined defects of the weightbearing area of the heel.

Advantages

Advantages of the medial plantar flap are:

- Excellent quality of the skin for the above-mentioned indication
- It is a sensory flap.

Disadvantages

Disadvantages are:

- Difficult dissection
- Functional impairment at the donor site when the flap is very large.

Anatomy

The flap is raised from the plantar vault, i.e. the non-weightbearing area of the foot. It is supplied by the medial plantar artery. Sensation is supplied by a branch from the medial plantar nerve.

Surgical technique

The design of the flap is limited by the surface of the non-weightbearing area of the foot (Figure 5a). The origin of the medial plantar artery is identified. The fascia of the abductor hallucis muscle and the plantar aponeurosis are included in the flap. The abductor hallucis muscle is divided to release the pedicle (Figure 5b). The key to the dissection is to identify and to preserve the medial digital nerve of the great toe. Proximally, the medial plantar nerve is separated from the vascular pedicle. The small branch supplying the flap must be identified and released by an intraneural

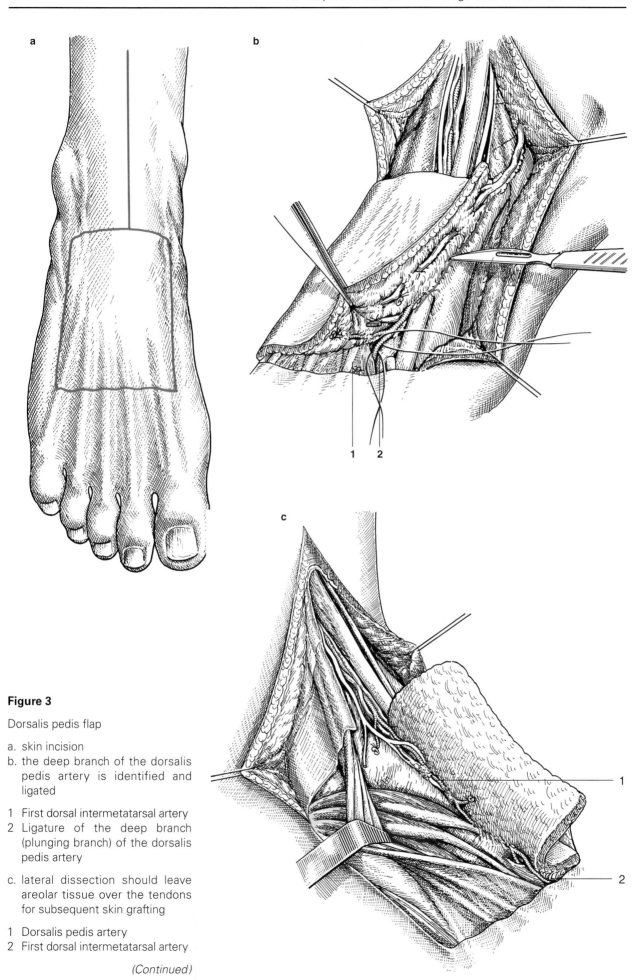

Figure 3

Dorsalis pedis flap

a. skin incision
b. the deep branch of the dorsalis pedis artery is identified and ligated

1 First dorsal intermetatarsal artery
2 Ligature of the deep branch (plunging branch) of the dorsalis pedis artery

c. lateral dissection should leave areolar tissue over the tendons for subsequent skin grafting

1 Dorsalis pedis artery
2 First dorsal intermetatarsal artery

(Continued)

d

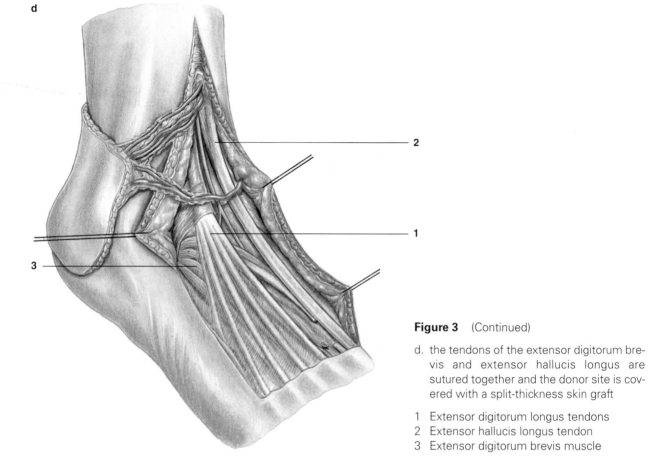

Figure 3   (Continued)

d. the tendons of the extensor digitorum brevis and extensor hallucis longus are
   sutured together and the donor site is covered with a split-thickness skin graft

1 Extensor digitorum longus tendons
2 Extensor hallucis longus tendon
3 Extensor digitorum brevis muscle

a

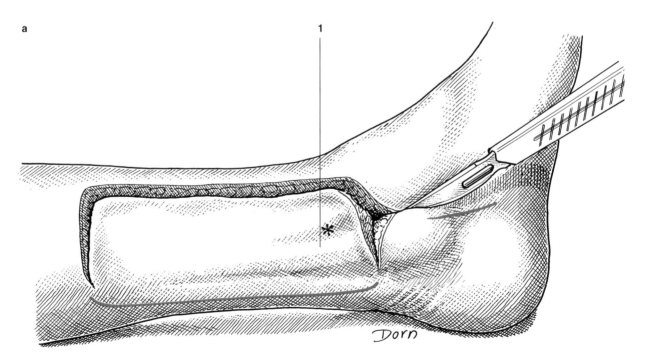

Figure 4

Lateral supramalleolar flap.

a. skin incision

1 Location of the ramus perforanus of the peroneal artery

b

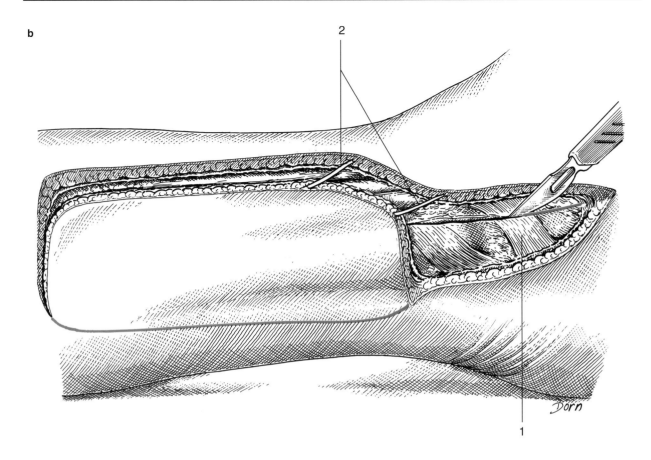

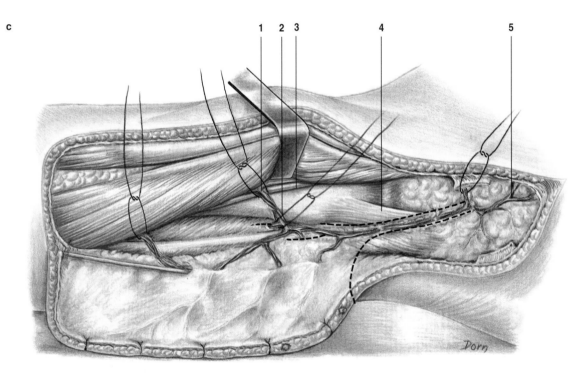

b. the pedicle lies on the tibiofibular ligament and is isolated with its surrounding loose areolar tissue

1 Extensor retinaculum
2 Branches of the superficial peroneal nerve

c. vascular structures and nerves at the tibiofibular space

1 Ligature of the anterior lateral malleolar artery
2 Ligature of the emergence of the perforating branch of the peroneal artery
3 Deep peroneal nerve
4 Inferior tibiofibular syndesmosis
5 Anastomosis with the lateral tarsal artery

(Continued)

d

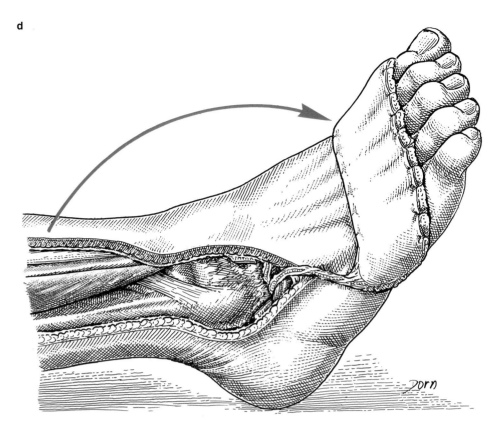

e

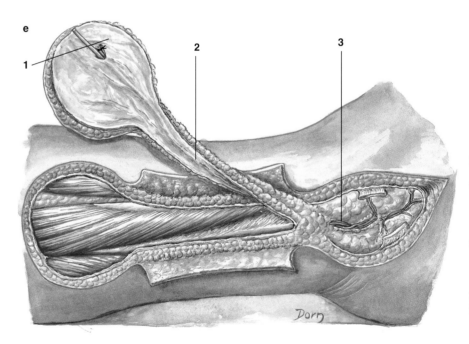

Figure 4 (Continued)

d. the arc of rotation of the lateral supramalleolar flap allows coverage of all dorsal, medial and lateral zones of the foot

e. lateral supramalleolar flap with a subcutaneous fascial pedicle

1 Fasciocutaneous island
2 Subcutaneous fascial pedicle
3 Ramus perforans of peroneal artery

dissection as far as needed, in order to provide a long neurovascular pedicle (Figure 5c). The deep branch of the medial plantar artery and pedicles supplying the flexor digitorum brevis should be ligated and divided.

The arc of rotation of the pedicle is limited by the bifurcation of the posterior tibial artery (Figure 5d). The donor site is closed by suturing the abductor hallucis and the flexor digitorum brevis and applying a split-skin graft.

a

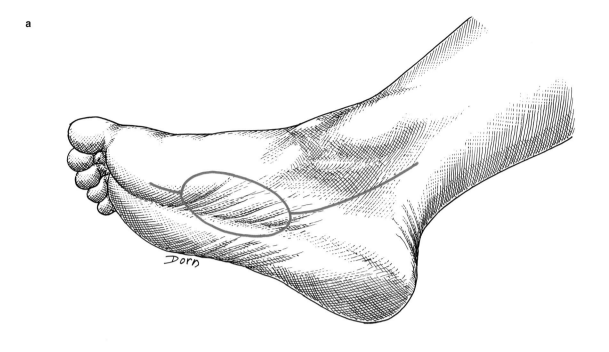

b

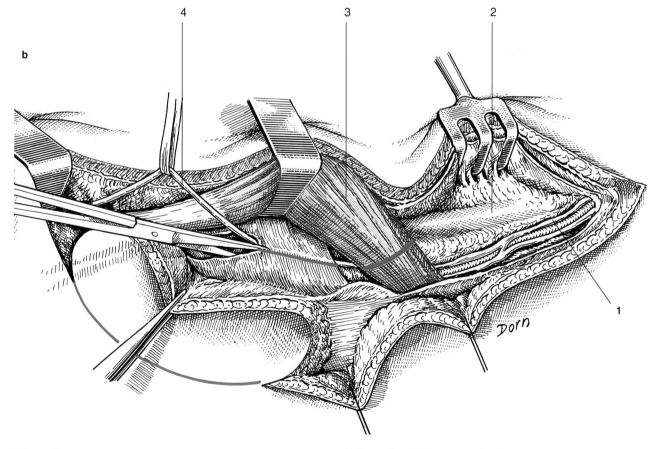

Figure 5

Medial plantar flap.

a. skin incision
b. the abductor hallucis muscle is cautiously divided,
    exposing the medial plantar artery

1 Posterior tibial artery and veins
2 Flexor hallucis longus tendon
3 Abductor hallucis
4 Medial digital nerve to the great toe

(Continued)

c

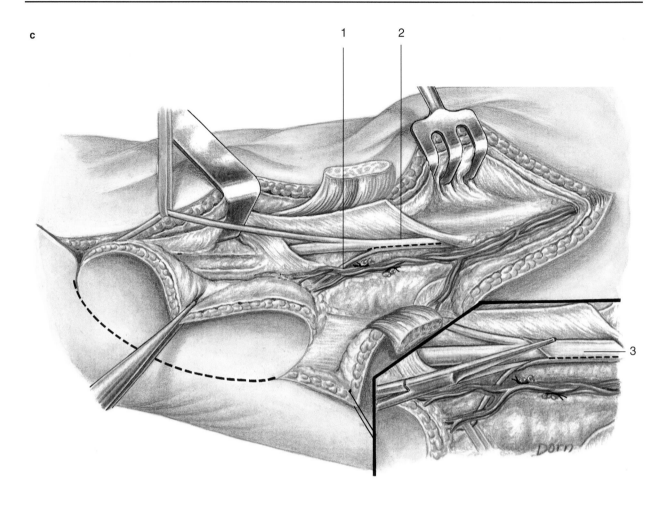

d

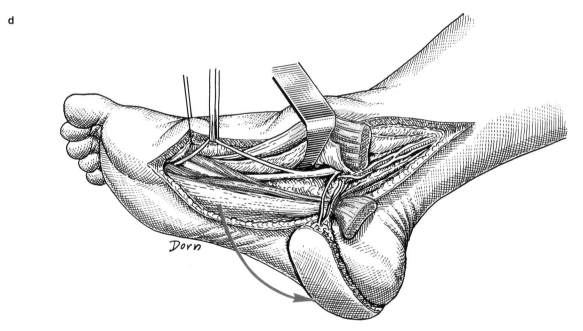

Figure 5   (Continued)

c. the neurovascular bundle is released up to the bifurcation of the posterior tibial vessels
1 Sensory branch to the flap
2 Medial plantar nerve
3 Intraneural dissection of the branch

d. the arc of rotation provided by the pedicle allows the weightbearing area and the posterior aspect of the heel to be covered

Medialis pedis flap

Indications

Indications for the medialis pedis flap [Masquelet and Romaña 1990] include confined defects of the medial side of the calcaneus, the tip of the medial malleolus, which is not well covered by the abductor hallucis muscle flap, and of the insertion of the Achilles tendon.

Advantages

Advantages of the medialis pedis flap are:

- Supple and pliable skin
- Fast and easy surgical technique.

Disadvantages

The disadvantage of this flap is the limited arc of rotation provided by the medial plantar artery.

Anatomy

The flap is supplied by a constant cutaneous branch which is issued either from the medial plantar artery or from its deep branch. This cutaneous branch runs upward on the distal end of the tibialis posterior tendon, back to the tuberosity of the navicular and then obliquely parallel to the medial border of the foot. The pedicle of the flap consists of the medial plantar artery which is released to its bifurcation.

Surgical technique

The design of the flap includes the prominence of the tuberosity of the navicular bone and the slight skin depression at the distal part of the tibialis posterior tendon (Figure 6a). The flap can be extended distally along the medial border of the foot to the middle of the first metatarsal.

The flap is raised from anterior to posterior (Figure 6b). The deep dissection is performed close to the navicular and to the posterior tibial tendon to include the cutaneous branch of the medial plantar artery within the flap. The posterior hinge of the flap is maintained to allow safe exposure of the blood supply. The fascia is then incised, the origin of the medial plantar artery is identified and the anterior border of the abductor hallucis muscle is released and retracted plantarwards.

The vascular pattern is exposed (Figure 6c). Several arterial branches must be ligated and severed: the deep branch of the medial plantar artery, the superficial branch distal to the flap and

a

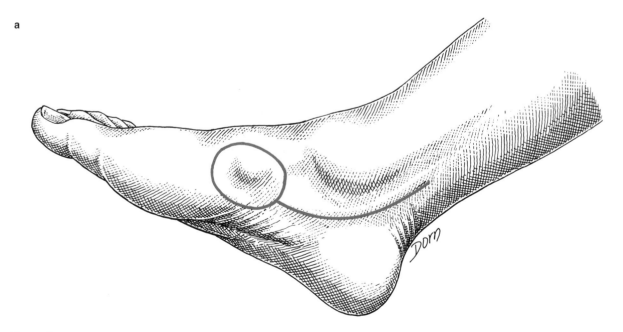

Figure 6

Medialis pedis flap

a. skin incision

(Continued)

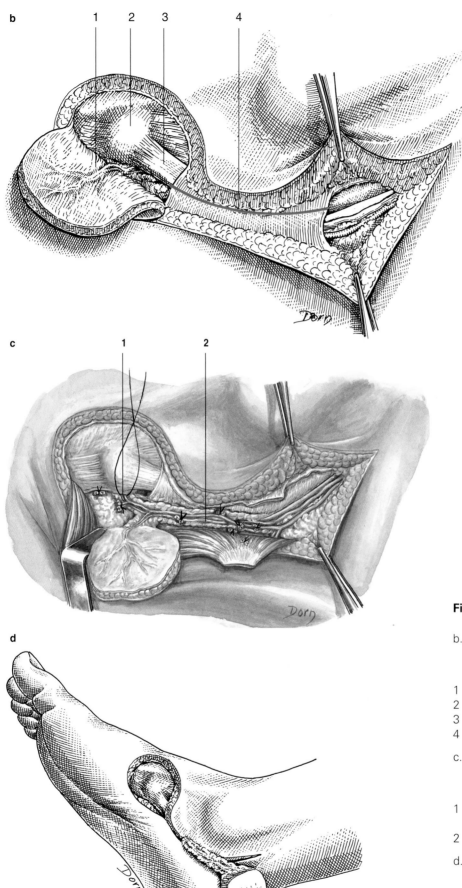

b

1 2 3   4

c

1   2

d

Figure 6 (Continued)

b. the flap is progressively raised and retracted from anterior to posterior

1 Supplying branch to flap
2 Tuberosity of navicular bone
3 Tibialis posterior tendon
4 Incision of fascia

c. the pedicle is released as far as the division of the posterior tibial artery

1 Deep branch of the medial plantar artery (to be ligated)
2 Medial plantar vessels

d. the donor site is covered with a split skin graft. The arc of rotation provided by the pedicle allows the distal insertion of the Achilles tendon to be covered

numerous branches supplying the abductor hallucis muscle. The medial plantar artery is released as far as the bifurcation.

The donor site (Figure 6d) is covered with a split-skin graft.

Distally based neurocutaneous sural flap

Indications

Like the lateral supramalleolar flap, the neurocutaneous sural flap is raised from the lower leg [Masquelet et al. 1992]. Its wide arc of rotation allows coverage of the anterior, lateral and posterior aspects of the instep. Large defects of the weight-bearing area are a good indication for this flap, in particular defects of the heel. Coverage of the medial aspect of the instep, i.e. the medial malleolus and the medial aspect of the hindfoot, is not advocated because of the risk of torsion of the pedicle.

Advantages

Advantages of the neurocutaneous sural flap are:

- Fast, easy and reliable procedure
- Good matching of the flap tissue with the recipient site.

Disadvantages

Disadvantages are:

- Sacrifice of the sural nerve
- Owing to its bulk the pedicle may have to be thinned in a second procedure.

Anatomy

The flap is supplied by the vascular axis that accompanies the sural nerve. If a small flap is used it should not be obtained proximal to the middle of the calf because the sural nerve runs deep to the fascia at this level.

The vascular axis is perfused by anastomoses from the peroneal artery. The most important and distal anastomosis is located three fingerbreadths proximal to the tip of the lateral malleolus. It constitutes the pivot point of the pedicle of the flap,

which is composed of subcutaneous and fascial tissue, including the sural nerve, its vascular network and the sural vein.

Surgical technique

The flap is outlined at the junction of the relief of the two heads of the gastrocnemius muscle (Figure 7a). The pivot point is identified as described. Two skin flaps are retracted in order to isolate a subcutaneous fascial pedicle 1.5 cm wide (Figure 7b). The fascia is also included in the flap. The dissection is very rapid. Small arteries arising

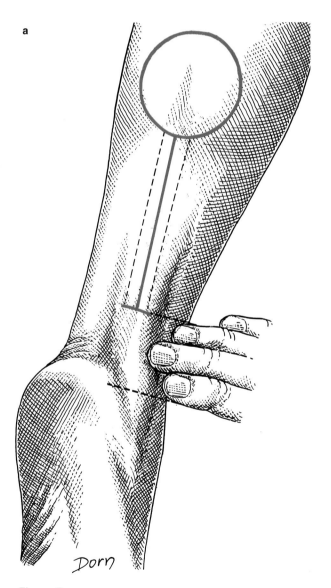

Figure 7

Distally based neurocutaneous sural flap

a. outline of the flap.

(Continued)

b   c

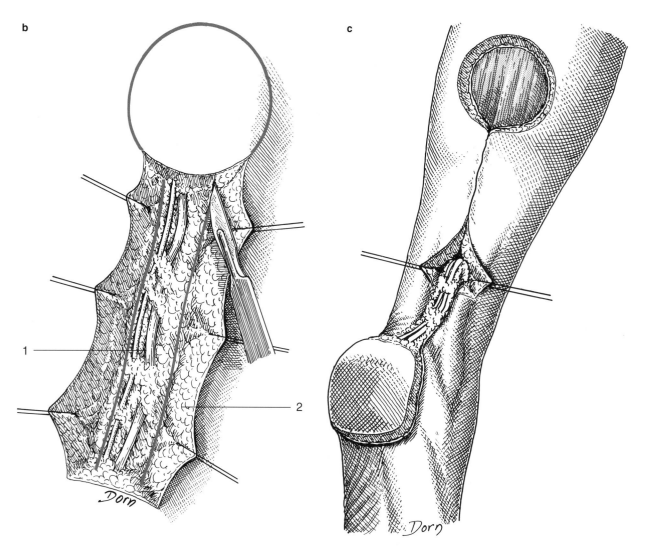

Figure 7   (Continued)

b. the subcutaneous fascial pedicle is isolated

1 Sural vein and nerve
2 Subdermal dissection

c. the arc of rotation provided by the pedicle allows the heel to be covered

from the peroneal artery should be ligated and divided.

The skin is closed to bury the pedicle (Figure 7c). The donor site and the pedicle are covered with a split-thickness skin graft.

Abductor hallucis muscle flap

Indications

The abductor hallucis muscle flap [McCraw 1979] is especially indicated in osteomyelitis with fistula formation at the medial aspect of the hindfoot.

Advantages

The advantage of the abductor hallucis muscle flap is that there is no functional defect at the donor site.

Disadvantages

Disadvantages are:

• The arc of rotation is limited
• The muscle belly does not cover the medial malleolus if it is attached at its proximal pedicle.

Anatomy

The muscle is supplied by one main proximal pedicle and several small pedicles issued from the medial plantar artery. The muscle can be rotated on its proximal pedicle or pedicled on the medial plantar artery, which increases the arc of rotation. Ligature of the lateral plantar artery to increase the arc of coverage is not advocated.

Surgical technique

A long, slightly curved incision is made on the medial side of the foot (Figure 8a). Incision of the fascia allows exposure of the muscle belly.

According to the coverage needed, the muscle is pedicled on the medial plantar artery, in which case distal pedicles should be spared, or the muscle is rotated on the proximal supply pedicle (Figure 8b).

Extensor digitorum brevis muscle flap

Indications

The extensor digitorum brevis muscle flap [Landi et al. 1985] is not commonly used. It is applied to cover limited defects of the perimalleolar area.

Advantages

The advantages of the extensor digitorum brevis muscle flap are:

- Minimal functional impairment
- Suitable for small defects.

Disadvantages

The disadvantage is that most of the time, the dorsalis pedis artery must be ligated to provide a sufficient arc of rotation.

a

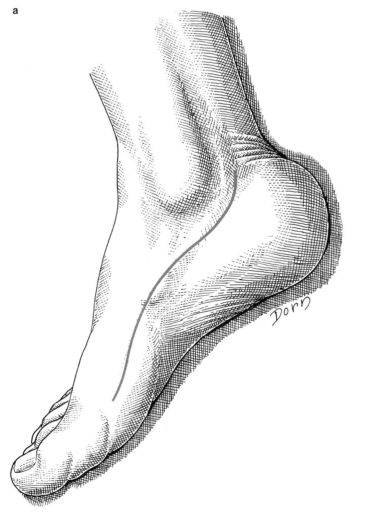

Figure 8

Abductor hallucis muscle flap

a. skin incision

(Continued)

b

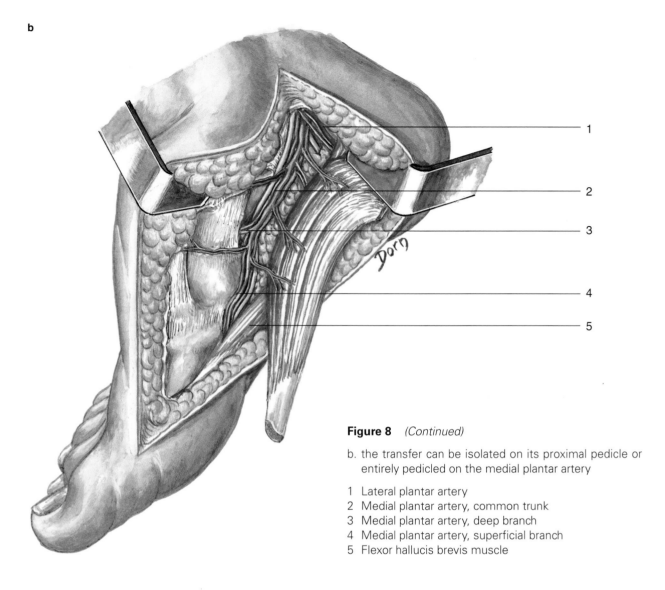

1

2

3

4

5

Figure 8 *(Continued)*

b. the transfer can be isolated on its proximal pedicle or entirely pedicled on the medial plantar artery

1 Lateral plantar artery
2 Medial plantar artery, common trunk
3 Medial plantar artery, deep branch
4 Medial plantar artery, superficial branch
5 Flexor hallucis brevis muscle

Anatomy

The extensor digitorum brevis flap is supplied by the lateral tarsal artery, which issues from the dorsalis pedis artery. The muscle flap can be pedicled on the lateral tarsal artery, but the arc of rotation is short. The muscle flap is usually based proximally or distally on the dorsalis pedis artery.

The lateral digitation of the muscle to the fourth toe is not well vascularized by the supply system from the dorsalis pedis artery. Therefore, it should usually be excised.

Surgical technique

A curved incision is made on the dorsum of the foot to expose the anterior tibial artery and the extensor digitorum brevis muscle (Figure 9a). Care must be

taken to minimize the size of the skin flaps to avoid postoperative necrosis.

The inferior extensor retinaculum and the fascia are incised along two lines in order to mobilize the extensor tendons laterally and medially (Figure 9b). The lateral branch of the superficial peroneal nerve must be identified and preserved.

The muscle is released from the calcaneus by retracting the extensor tendons medially (Figure 9c). The tendons of the muscle are cut distally. The medial tarsal artery is ligated and divided. The lateral tarsal artery is identified on the lateral aspect of the muscle. It is also ligated and severed.

The extensor tendons are then retracted laterally to raise the muscle in continuity with the pedicle (Figure 9d). The dorsalis pedis artery is ligated and severed distal to the muscle. The vascular pedicle is separated from the deep peroneal nerve. The motor branch to the muscle is cut. The skin is closed over a suction drain.

Peroneus brevis muscle flap

Indications

The distal portion of the muscle belly provides good coverage for the Achilles tendon. However, the distal insertion of the tendon cannot be covered with the muscle. The peroneus brevis muscle can be used in association with the distal portion of the flexor hallucis longus muscle to cover a large defect exposing the Achilles tendon [Masquelet and Gilbert 1995].

Advantages

Advantages of the peroneus brevis muscle flap are:

- Fast and easy procedure
- The distal tendon of the peroneus brevis is preserved.

Disadvantages

The disadvantage is the risk of adhesions between the muscle and the Achilles tendon.

Anatomy

The muscle is supplied by small branches from the peroneal artery. Only the distal half of the muscle can be elevated without risk of necrosis.

Surgical technique

A sandbag is placed under the patient's ipsilateral buttock to provide slight internal rotation of the limb. The incision is made behind the fibula (Figure 10a).

The peroneus brevis muscle is identified and released from the tendon of the peroneus longus (Figure 10b). The distal half of the muscle is separated from the tendon and rotated backwards to cover the Achilles tendon. The muscle is covered with a split-thickness skin graft.

Medial saphenous cross-leg flap

Indications

The cross-leg flap procedure using the medial saphenous fasciocutaneous flap has attracted new interest. Its main indication is the repair of defects involving the posterior and the plantar aspect of the heel [Barclay et al. 1983, Roggero et al. 1993].

If no local procedure is suitable, the cross-leg flap is an excellent alternative to a free flap. Free flaps are mostly used following acute injuries; the cross-leg flap is used mostly for late sequelae. In avulsion of the heel with a poor arterial pattern at the recipient site, the cross-leg flap is the procedure of first choice.

Advantages

After separation of the cross-leg flap, the matching of the flap is excellent. It is not too bulky. Its thickness is

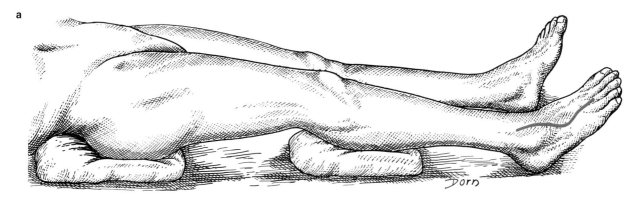

a

Figure 9

Extensor digitorum brevis muscle flap

a. skin incision

(Continued)

b

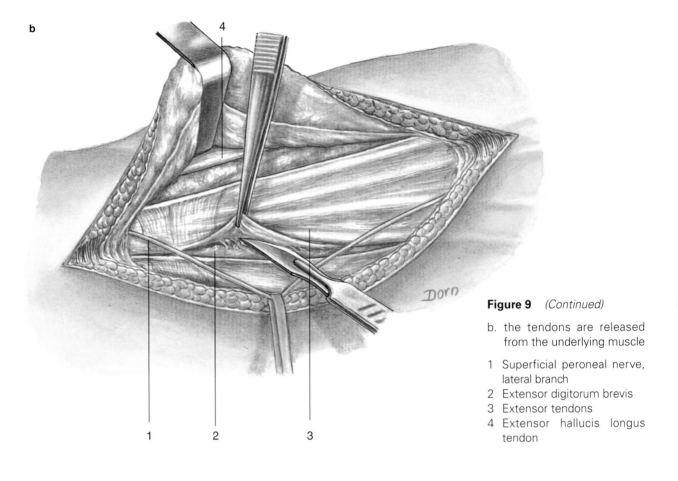

Figure 9 *(Continued)*

b. the tendons are released from the underlying muscle

1 Superficial peroneal nerve, lateral branch
2 Extensor digitorum brevis
3 Extensor tendons
4 Extensor hallucis longus tendon

c

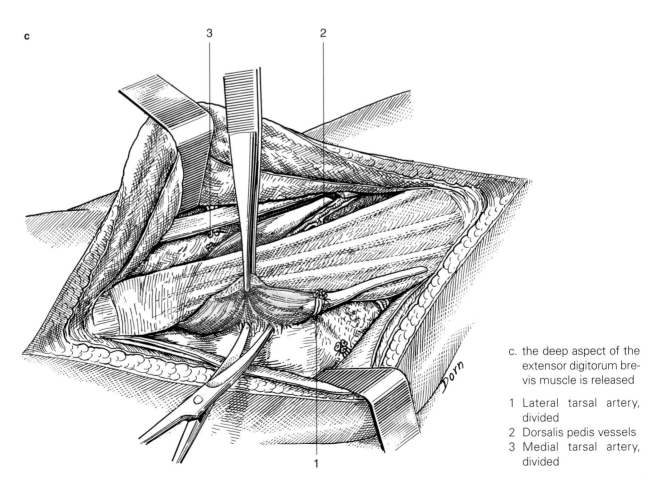

c. the deep aspect of the extensor digitorum brevis muscle is released

1 Lateral tarsal artery, divided
2 Dorsalis pedis vessels
3 Medial tarsal artery, divided

d

4 3

2

1

Dorn

1   2

d. the muscle is passed beneath the extensor tendons to be isolated on the lateral tarsal artery

1 Deep peroneal nerve
2 Dorsalis pedis vessels
3 Arcuate vessels
4 Dorsalis pedis vessels

sufficient and the skin is supple and resistant. In addition, the flap can be resensitized by suturing the saphenous nerve to a recipient nerve.

Disadvantages

Disadvantages of the cross-leg flap are:

• Immobilization of the patient
• The duration of hospitalization
• The main risk is infection.

Surgical technique

The flap is created on the medial aspect of the opposite leg. The distal portion of the flap covers

the posterior aspect of the heel, and the proximal portion is tubulated or covered with a skin graft. Immobilization of both lower limbs with an external fixator is strongly advocated. After 3 weeks the flap is cut at its origin. It is detubulated or the skin graft is removed and the proximal portion of the flap is used to repair the plantar aspect of the heel.

Free flaps

Indications

Free flaps [Serafin et al. 1977, May et al. 1985, Gidumal et al. 1986, Hentz and Pearl 1987] are indicated in large defects that cannot be treated by local procedures. Two main techniques are routinely

a

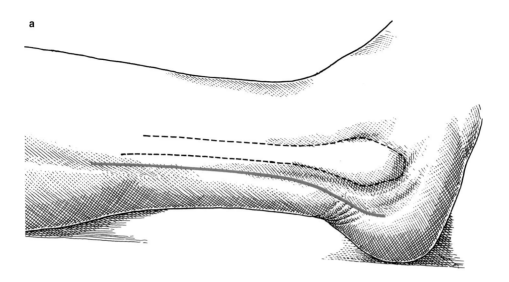

b

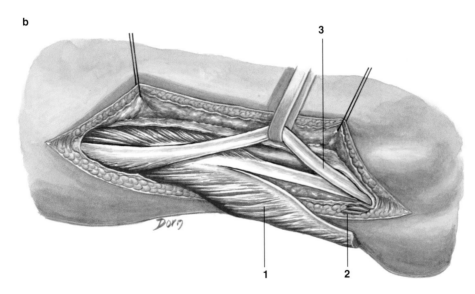

Figure 10

Peroneus brevis muscle flap

a. skin incision
b. the distal half of the muscle is separated from the tendon and rotated backwards to cover the Achilles tendon

1 Peroneus brevis, split
2 Sural vein and nerve
3 Peroneus longus tendon

used. The latissimus dorsi is employed for large defects of the ankle and dorsum of the foot. The scapular or parascapular flaps are used to repair large defects involving the plantar vault and the heel. Repair of the heel can also be performed with a latissimus dorsi muscle flap covered with a split-thickness skin graft.

Advantages

Free flaps often allow salvage of the foot. Little impairment occurs at the donor site.

Disadvantages

The risk of vascular failure is inherent in free flap surgery; it occurs in about 10% of cases. Functional deficits may result from salvage of the foot, i.e. lack of sensitivity of the flap and chronic ulceration. Free flaps are often too bulky and require several secondary procedures to match the flap to the recipient site.

Anatomy

The vascular pedicle is the subscapular artery and its divisions. Scapular and parascapular flaps are based on the circumflex scapular artery. The latissimus dorsi flap is supplied by the dorsal branch of the dorsal thoracic artery. Smaller defects can be covered with a free serratus anterior muscle flap, which is an alternative to a partial latissimus dorsi muscle flap.

References

Barclay TL, Sharpe DT, Chisholm E (1983) Cross leg fascio cutaneous flap. Plast Reconstr Surg 72: 843–847

Chang KN, DeArmond SJ, Buncke J (1986) Sensory reinnervation in microsurgical reconstruction of the heel. Plast Reconstr Surg 78: 652–664

Duncan MJ, Zuker RM, Manktelow RT (1985) Resurfacing weight-bearing areas of the heel. The role of the dorsalis pedis innervated free tissue transfer. J Reconstr Microsurg 1: 201–208

Gidumal R, Carl A, Evanski P et al. (1986) Functional evaluation of nonsensate free flaps to the sole of the foot. Foot Ankle 7: 118–123

Harrison DH, Morgan BG (1981) The instep island flap to resurface plantar defects. Br Plast Surg 34: 315

Hentz VR, Pearl RM (1987) Application of free tissue transfers to the foot. J Reconstr Microsurg 3: 309–320

Landi A, Soragni O, Monteleone M (1985) The extensor digitorum brevis muscle island flap for soft tissue loss around the ankle. Plast Reconstr Surg 75: 892–897

Man D, Acland RD (1980) The micro arterial anatomy of the dorsalis pedis flaps and its clinical applications. Plast Reconstr Surg 65: 419–423

Masquelet AC (1994) Principles of soft tissue repair at the foot and ankle. Eur J Foot Ankle Surg 1: 55–66

Masquelet AC, Gilbert A (1995) An Atlas of Flaps in Limb Reconstruction. London, Martin Dunitz

Masquelet AC, Romaña MC (1990) The medialis pedis flap: a new fascio cutaneous flap. Plast Reconstr Surg 5: 769–772

Masquelet AC, Beveridge J, Romaña MC, Gerber C (1988) The lateral supramalleolar flap. Plast Reconstr Surg 82: 74–81

Masquelet AC, Romaña MC, Wolf G (1992) Skin island flap supplied by the vascular axis of the sensitive superficial nerves: anatomic study and clinical experience in the leg. Plast Reconstr Surg 89: 1115–1121

May JW, Halls MJ, Simon SR (1985) Free microvascular muscle flaps with skin graft reconstruction of extensive defects of the foot: a clinical and gait analysis study. Plast Reconstr Surg 75: 627–641

McCraw JB (1979) Selection of alternative local flaps in the leg and the foot. Clin Plast Surg 6: 228

Morrison WA, Crabb DM, O'Brien BM, Jenkins A (1983) The instep of the foot as a fascio-cutaneous island and as a free flap for heel defects. Plast Reconstr Surg 72: 56–65

Roggero P, Blanc Y, Krupp S (1983) Foot reconstruction in weightbearing areas – long-term result and gait analysis. Eur J Plast Surg 16: 186

Serafin D, Georgiade NG, Smith DH (1977) Comparison of free flaps with pedicled flaps for coverage of defects of the leg or foot. Plast Reconstr Surg 59: 492

Zuker RM, Manktelow RT (1986) The dorsalis pedis free flap. Technique of elevation, foot closure and flap application. Plast Reconstr Surg 77: 93–104

Index

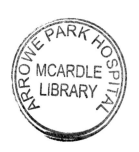